LITHIUM RESEARCH
AND THERAPY

LITHIUM RESEARCH AND THERAPY

Edited by

F. N. JOHNSON

Lecturer in Psychology, University of Lancaster, England

1975

ACADEMIC PRESS
LONDON   NEW YORK   SAN FRANCISCO

A Subsidiary of Harcourt Brace Jovanovich, Publishers

ACADEMIC PRESS INC. (LONDON) LTD.
24/28 Oval Road,
London NW1

United States Edition published by
ACADEMIC PRESS INC.
111 Fifth Avenue
New York, New York 10003

Library of Congress Catalog Card Number: 74-17997
ISBN: 0-12-386550-6

PRINTED IN GREAT BRITAIN BY
Page Bros (Norwich) Ltd, Norwich

CONTRIBUTORS

A. AMDISEN, *Director of Research, Psychopharmacology Research Unit, Statshospitalet v. Aarhus, DK-8240 Risskov, Denmark*

D. K. ANDERSON, *Research Service, Veterans Administration Hospital, 13000 North 30th Street, Tampa, Florida 33612, U.S.A.*
and *Assistant Professor, Department of Physiology, College of Medicine, University of South Florida, Tampa, Florida 33620. U.S.A.*

S. C. BERENS, *Assistant Professor of Medicine, University of California, Los Angeles, California 90024, U.S.A.*

S. BERL, *Research Professor of Neurology, Department of Neurology, Mt. Sinai School of Medicine, Fifth Avenue and 100th Street, New York, New York 10029, U.S.A.*

P. A. BOND, *Medical Research Council Unit for Metabolic Studies in Psychiatry, University Department of Psychiatry, Middlewood Hospital, P.O. Box 134, Sheffield S6 1TP, England*

J. F. J. CADE, *Psychiatric Superintendent, Psychiatric Hospital, Royal Park, Private Bag 3, Parkville 3052, Victoria, Australia*

D. D. CLARKE, *Professor of Biochemistry, Chemistry Department, Fordham University, Bronx, New York 10458, U.S.A.*

THE LATE H. I. COOMBS, *One time Honorary Consulting Pathologist, St. Bernard's Hospital, Southall, Middlesex, England*

R. R. H. COOMBS, *14 Museum Mansion, 63A Great Russell Street, London W.C.1, England*

M. DIMITRAKOUDI, *Research Assistant in Psychiatry, Medical Research Council Unit for Metabolic Studies in Psychiatry, Middlewood Hospital, P.O. Box 134, Sheffield S6 1TP, England*

J. FORN, *Departamento de Farmacologia, Facultad de Medicina, Universidad de Barcelona, Barcelona, Spain*

B. FYRÖ, *Assistant Professor, Karolinska Institute, Department of Psychiatry, St. Görans Hospital, Box 125 00, S-11281 Stockholm, Sweden*

M. D. GOLDFIELD, *The Langley Porter Neuropsychiatric Institute, 401 Parnassus Avenue, San Francisco, California 94122, U.S.A.*

K. GREENSPAN, *Columbia-Presbyterian Medical Center, 161 Fort Washington Avenue, New York, New York 10032, U.S.A.*

R. P. HULLIN, *Director Regional Metabolic Research Unit, High Royds Hospital, Menston, Ilkley, Yorkshire LS29 6AQ, England*
and *Reader in Biochemistry, University of Leeds, Yorkshire, England*

F. A. JENNER, *Professor of Psychiatry, Medical Research Council Unit for Metabolic Studies in Psychiatry, University Department of Psychiatry, Middlewood Hospital, P.O. Box 134, Sheffield S6 1TP, England*

F. N. JOHNSON, *Department of Psychology, University of Lancaster, Bailrigg, Lancaster, Lancashire, England*

S. JOHNSON, *Department of Psychology, University of Lancaster, Bailrigg, Lancaster, Lancashire, England*

O. S. JØRGENSEN, *Psychochemistry Institute, Rigshospitalet, Blegdamsvej 9, DK-2100 Copenhagen Ø, Denmark*

R. J. KERRY, *Consultant Psychiatrist, Middlewood Hospital, Sheffield S6 1TP, England*

N. S. KLINE, *Director, Research Center, Rockland State Hospital, Orangeburg, New York 10962, U.S.A.*

S. MACNEIL, *Medical Research Council Unit for Metabolic Studies in Psychiatry, University Department of Psychiatry, Middlewood Hospital, P.O. Box 134, Sheffield S6 1TP, Yorkshire, England*

U. G. MEE, *The Pathology Laboratory, St. Bernard's Hospital, Southall, Middlesex, England*

E. T. MELLERUP, *Psychochemistry Institute, Rigshospitalet, Blegdamsvej 9, DK-2100 Copenhagen Ø, Denmark*

J. MENDELS, *Professor of Psychiatry, University of Pennsylvania,* and *Chief, Affective Diseases Research Unit, Veterans Administration Hospital, University and Woodland Avenues, Philadelphia, Pennsylvania 19104, U.S.A.*

E. S. PAYKEL, *Consultant Psychiatrist, Department of Psychiatry, St. George's Hospital, Blackshaw Road, London, S.W.17, England*

M. PEET, *Senior Registrar, Royal Dundee Liff Hospital, By Dundee DD2 5NF. Scotland* and *Honorary Lecturer in Psychiatry, University of Dundee, Dundee, Scotland*

R. F. PRIEN, *Assistant Chief, Central Neuropsychiatric Research Laboratory, Veterans Administration Hospital, Perry Point, Maryland 21902, U.S.A.*

L. D. PROCKOP, *Professor of Medicine, Chief, Neurology Section, College of Medicine, University of South Florida, Tampa, Florida 33620, U.S.A.* and *Neurology Consultant, Veterans Administration Hospital, 13000 North 30th Street, Tampa, Florida 33612, U.S.A.*

O. J. RAFAELSEN, *Professor of Biological Psychiatry, Psychochemistry Institute, Rigshospitalet, Blegdamsvej 9, DK-2100 Copenhagen Ø, Denmark*

M. SCHOU, *Professor of Biological Psychiatry and Director of Research, Psychopharmacology Research Unit, Aarhus University, Institute of Psychiatry, DK-8240, Risskov, Denmark*

G. SEDVALL, *Associate Professor of Neuropsychopharmacology, Department of Pharmacology, Karolinska Institute, S-104 01 Stockholm 60, Sweden*

D. M. SHAW, *External MRC Staff, Department of Psychological Medicine, Whitchurch Hospital, Cardiff, Glamorgan, Wales*

G. SIMPSON, *Principal Research Psychiatrist, Research Center, Rockland State Hospital, Orangeburg, New York 10962, U.S.A.*

K. THOMSEN, *Research Associate, Psychopharmacology Research Unit, Aarhus University, Institute of Psychiatry, Psychiatric Hospital, DK-8240 Risskov, Denmark*

L. VACAFLOR, *Director, In-patient Service, The Montreal General Hospital, Montreal 109, Canada*

E. S. VIZI, *Associate Professor of Pharmacology, Department of Pharmacology, Semmelweis University of Medicine, 1085 Budapest, Hungary*

M. R. WEINSTEIN, *Associate Professor of Psychiatry in Residence, University of California at San Francisco, San Francisco, California 94143, U.S.A.* and *Senior Psychiatrist, The Langley Porter Neuropsychiatric Institute, 401 Parnassus Avenue, San Francisco, California 94143, U.S.A.*

J. WOLFF, *Associate Chief, Clinical Endocrinology Branch, National Institute of Arthritis, Metabolism and Digestive Diseases, National Institutes of Health, Bethesda, Maryland 20014, U.S.A.*

PREFACE

The discovery, in 1949, that the salts of the metallic element lithium had therapeutic properties in certain types of psychiatric illness, did not make an immediate impact on clinical practice: now, some 25 years later, that discovery is considered by many of those working in the field of psychiatric research to have been one of the most significant in the history of pharmacotherapy. It has opened up whole new areas of investigation and has been responsible for promoting research into diverse matters which had not previously been seen as closely linked.

In editing this survey of the therapeutic uses of lithium salts and the research which has been, and is being, conducted into the biochemical, physiological and behavioural aspects of these substances, I have been conscious of the multiple roles which the completed text would have to fulfill. The form in which the text now appears represents what I hope will be the most useful, bearing in mind the different categories of readership which will be attracted to it.

Whilst I have had to make some decisions as to which areas should be covered by individual chapters and which merged into single chapters I have usually been inclined to expand coverage rather than to contract it, on the grounds that, at this stage, it is not possible to prejudge what aspects of lithium research may become important at some future time—indeed, if our experiences with lithium tell us anything it is that even the most casual and apparently isolated finding may eventually prove to have an importance out of all proportion to that attached to its initial discovery. The survey is, I hope, as comprehensive as it can reasonably be made and though I do not doubt that there are certain studies published before the book went to press which do not find coverage in this work they will be few in number.

The primary function of the text is as a reference work, a statement of the position in lithium research and therapy at the time of going to press. It will, for those who choose to use it in this way, provide a background against which to place, and to assess, future trends in this rapidly developing area.

Whilst holding to the primary aim of comprehensiveness I have also tried to keep in mind the special requirements of particular groups of readers: accordingly, the text has been organized into two major parts. In the first of these the practicing psychiatrist will find the information needed to make an assessment of the efficacy of lithium therapy in the various conditions for which it has been indicated, as well as a guide to the practicalities of lithium treatment procedures. In the second part the results of laboratory investigations of lithium effects are brought together.

The role of an editor of a text such as this goes beyond the mere commissioning and collating of chapters: he has to undertake the unification of the disparate manuscripts into a meaningful whole. I have tried to see some overall structure in present research endeavours involving lithium and to reflect this structure in the disposition of the chapters. There are, of course, dangers inherent in an attempt to crystallize prematurely any area of research in which the very lack of obvious structure is an indication of the vigour with which the subject is being pursued on many different fronts. On the other hand, the provision of at least a minimal framework may be of value in drawing attention to those issues which require more intensive investigation than others at any particular time. Some brief explanation of the rationale behind the organization of the text is, therefore, called for.

As far as the coverage of the clinical applications of lithium was concerned the structure was, from the start, fairly obvious. After a short introductory section in which the nature of lithium and the historical trends in lithium research are outlined, the therapeutic profile of lithium is indicated in six chapters. Major indications, such as the affective disorders, are naturally dealt with first and then some consideration is given to the various other possible uses to which lithium therapy might be put in conditions not primarily associated with affective dysfunctioning. One of the questions which quite properly occurs to the clinician faced with a decision about using lithium, relates to the relative advantages or disadvantages which lithium therapy has compared with other drugs which might also, *prima facie*, be indicated: is lithium better, or worse, than the alternatives? I asked Dr. Robert Prien to handle this question and his balanced account provides a different perspective on the matters contained in the preceding four chapters.

The demand for a proper evaluation of the therapeutic effectiveness of lithium has provided a unique stimulus to the development of rigorous clinical trial methodology, and this too is an issue dealt with at some length in this part of the text.

Having come to the conclusion that lithium medication may be appropriately prescribed for a particular patient, the clinician then has to face the practical problems which such a course of treatment necessarily entails. Dr. Kerry outlines the general principles of patient management and his chapter provides an introduction to more specific issues such as the techniques involved in monitoring lithium levels in the body, and the characteristics of sustained release preparations.

The questions of the likely toxic and side reactions to be expected from any pharmaceutical product, together with considerations of special contra-indications, are clearly of vital importance, and all the more so in the case of lithium since the margin between the therapeutic and toxic dose levels for this drug is so narrow. These matters have, therefore, been covered in some detail. The special case of lithium usage during pregnancy is given priority, and techniques for alleviating or combating lithium poisoning are reviewed.

The second part of the text was more difficult to organize. One of the reasons for this may lie in the state of development of laboratory-based experimental work on lithium. There are, I suspect, several readily discernible stages in the evolution of research on any psychoactive compound. The initial discovery is inevitably followed by replications aimed at supporting the original findings or disconfirming them, and by toxicity tests to determine how safe the medication is likely to be. The drug is then typically applied to other conditions in an attempt to delineate the degree of specificity of its therapeutic actions. When biochemical and physiological studies are undertaken (and this may be early or late in the sequence of clinical studies—relatively later in the case of lithium) they tend at first to be concerned with a few of the more obvious characteristics, such as effects on neurotransmitter metabolism, but the investigations then rapidly spread over a wide front according to the particular interests of individual investigators, and depending upon whether the emphasis is upon changes produced in the bodies of patients undergoing active treatment or in specially set up *in vitro* or *in vivo* laboratory situations. If lithium research were in this latter stage, life might have been much easier from an editor's point of view, for the disparate, discrete, disorganized state of the field could merely have been reflected in a more or less random organization of the chapters. As it is, however, lithium research has moved into the next phase, in which advances in individual areas of study have revealed links with other areas: this has not, however, proceeded to the point of identifying with any certainty the relative importance of each of these points of connection. We are therefore at a transition point in the fortunes of lithium: each line of attack has some points of contact with most other lines, but the full pattern has yet to emerge. This leads to two effects as far as this text is concerned. First, the sequence of chapters as presented here may be subject to considerable modification within a fairly brief space of time as the interrelationships between the areas are clarified; and secondly, there is, inevitably, some degree of overlap between some of the chapters.

As a matter of editorial policy I have tried to keep overlap to a minimum, particularly where this was a matter of straightforward duplication of material, but it rapidly became apparent that to eliminate overlap entirely was seriously to misrepresent the flavour of lithium research. In arranging the chapters I therefore paid particular attention to material held in common between the various investigatory approaches.

The second half of the text commences with a review of the fate of lithium in the body—how it is taken up, what happens to its distribution amongst the tissues, and the factors governing its elimination. These are important matters, not only in their implications for the physiological effects which lithium produces, but also from the point of view of the clinician, and the first three chapters of part two of the text form an appropriate bridge with part one.

Before dealing with the various physiological and biochemical characteristics of lithium effects, I have exercised an editor's privilege to be slightly self-indulgent, and have included a coverage of behavioural studies of lithium, an area which, though undoubtedly still in its infancy, promises much to the eventual understanding of the subjective changes noted by patients during successful lithium therapy.

An outline of the place which lithium occupies amongst the Group I elements (the alkali metals) and the implications, in broad terms, which this may have for the biological properties of the lithium ion, precedes quite naturally a discussion of electrolyte balance effects. Carbohydrate metabolism is considered next in view of the possibility that lithium actions on this system are intimately associated with effects on electrolytes. Neurotransmitters, in the form of acetylcholine, catechol- and indole-amines, and various amino acids, are obvious targets for lithium action, and a chapter is devoted to each class of transmitter. The links between amine and amino acid are emphasized in the chapter by Professor Berl and Dr. Clark. In their discussion of the endocrine changes produced by lithium, Drs. Berens and Wolff note effects on antidiuretic hormone action: this potentially important area is given more intensive scrutiny in the following chapter on lithium and polyuria. The discussion of lithium effects on cyclic AMP which then follows has clear implications for both thyroidal and renal hormonal systems. Side effects and toxic reactions are again brought up by the chapters on endocrine effects and polyuria, and the survey of EEG changes associated with lithium therapy may also be important in this respect. A few of the pathological changes which have been reported as accompanying lithium administration are collected together in a speculative chapter concerning some possible mechanisms underlying side effects. The second part of the text is wound up by returning to a consideration of what is probably the fundamental question in biochemical and physiological studies of lithium, namely the relationship between lithium and other cations.

In order to make the text maximally valuable to medical students and to those lacking specialist knowledge in some of the areas, I have encouraged authors to provide brief accounts of the biochemical or physiological concepts which they employ.

Those readers who have either been personally engaged in, or who have had some association with, lithium research, will find in this text contributions from many investigators whose names are familiar. The contributions are, however, all entirely new, and authors have endeavoured (and very successfully, I feel) to provide fresh viewpoints, up to date coverage, and reintegrations of their particular areas. Whilst it may be invidious to single out particular authors for special attention, I am sure that none of the other contributors will feel slighted if I express especial pleasure at securing the services of both Dr. John Cade and Professor Mogens Schou. Dr. Cade, as is now well known, was the original discoverer of the therapeutic actions of lithium in states of excitement, whilst it was Professor Schou who, more than anyone, put lithium on the psychiatric map and his name is inseparable from any discussion of almost any aspect of lithium research and therapy.

Whilst the book was still in the early stages of preparation I learned of the sudden death of Dr. H. I. Coombs who had agreed to undertake the preparation of the chapter on serum lithium estimation. I had never met Dr. Coombs, but from my correspondence with him I know that he viewed the task of writing his chapter with considerable eagerness and enthusiasm. At the time of his death he had already prepared the basic groundwork for his chapter and it was, therefore, with great pleasure that I accepted the offer of his son, Dr. R. R. H. Coombs to complete the preparation of the chapter in association with Miss U. G. Mee who had worked with Dr. H. I. Coombs on his serum analysis technique. The final version of the chapter, which I am sure Dr H. I. Coombs would have approved, carries his name as senior author and is dedicated to his memory.

It has been a great privilege to be associated with so many excellent investigators in the preparation of this text, and I owe to all of them a debt of thanks for the great amount of work which they have put into the project. They have suffered, uncomplainingly, my often stridulent urgings to get synopses, first drafts and final scripts in to my office by the various deadline dates: I am only too aware of the pressures of other, unexpected committments which make compliance with such requests exceedingly difficult, and it is to their credit that all contributors kept so closely to the dates I imposed upon them.

I must acknowledge with especial gratitude the generous financial assistance of Delandale Laboratories Ltd., of Canterbury, England, pioneers in the use of controlled release lithium carbonate (Priadel) in lithium therapy; through their help it was possible to provide essential secretarial services to expedite the editorial process. In particular, I wish to express my appreciation of the technical assistance, in the form of the provision of lithium bibliographies and copies of papers relating to lithium, which was extended to myself and all contributors by Dr. Anne Wickham, Director of the Medical Services Department of Delandale Laboratories Ltd. Many of the contributors who benefited from this invaluable service have expressed their thanks to me, and it is fitting that I should convey these sentiments in this preface.

The Lithium Corporation of America also provided technical information, and for this too I am grateful.

Various publishers have kindly agreed to allow the reproduction in this text of material previously published elsewhere: specific acknowledgements are given with the appropriate table or figure, in the body of the text.

To those colleagues, both my own and of other contributors, who have been involved in reading and commenting upon earlier drafts of chapters, and who are too numerous to be listed here by name, I would record my thanks. Any errors which remain in the text are, of course, not theirs.

Mrs Lynda Teale proved to be a most efficient and helpful secretarial assistant; without her efforts the final manuscript would have been much delayed. Mrs. Carol Goss undertook at short notice the task of typing the index, which she completed both expeditiously and with total accuracy.

Finally I must record my indebtedness to my wife, Susan, who not only contributed the final chapter to the text, but who also bore with great fortitude the frequent expressions of editorial anguish. My daughter, Jenny, and son, Reuben, also played their part, though they are too young to realize how.

Neil Johnson
Lancaster, 1974.

CONTENTS

PART I: CLINICAL STUDIES AND PRACTICAL ISSUES
SECTION A: INTRODUCTION

Chapter 1. Lithium

F. N. Johnson

Chapter 2. The Historical Background to Lithium Research and Therapy

F. N. Johnson and J. F. J. Cade

SECTION B: THE THERAPEUTIC PROFILE OF LITHIUM

Chapter 3. Lithium in the Acute Treatment of Mania

M. Peet

Chapter 4. Lithium in the Acute Treatment of Depressive States

J. Mendels

Chapter 5. Lithium Prophylaxis of Recurrent Endogenous Affective Disorders

M. Schou and K. Thomsen

Chapter 6. Lithium in the Treatment of Conditions Other Than the Affective Disorders
N. S. Kline and G. Simpson

Chapter 7. The Clinical Effectiveness of Lithium: Comparisons with Other Drugs
R. F. Prien

Chapter 8. Methodological Issues in Research on Lithium Therapy
E. S. Paykel

SECTION C: PATIENT MANAGEMENT: PRACTICE AND PROBLEMS

Chapter 9. The Management of Patients Receiving Lithium Treatment
R. J. Kerry

Chapter 10. Methods of Serum Lithium Estimation
The Late H. I. Coombs, R. R. H. Coombs and U. G. Mee

Chapter 15. Administration of Lithium During Pregnancy
M. R. Weinstein and M. D. Goldfield

PART II: PHYSIOLOGICAL, BIOCHEMICAL AND BEHAVIOURAL STUDIES

SECTION A: UPTAKE, DISTRIBUTION AND EXCRETION

Chapter 16. Lithium Absorption and Distribution in Body Tissues
D. K. Anderson and L. D. Prockop

SECTION B: BEHAVIOURAL EFFECTS

Chapter 24. Lithium and Acetylcholine Metabolism
E. S. Vizi

Chapter 25. Lithium and Amine Metabolism
D. M. Shaw

Chapter 26. Lithium and Amino Acid Metabolism
S. Berl and D. D. Clarke

PART I

CLINICAL STUDIES AND PRACTICAL ISSUES

SECTION A.

INTRODUCTION

1

LITHIUM

F. N. Johnson

I. Discovery of the Element

Petalite, a milky white or clear aluminium silicate mineral resembling quartz and often found in close association with quartz deposits, was discovered in the early 19th Century by Jose Bonifacio de Andrade Silva, a Brazilian. In 1817 Johann Auguste Arfwedson, a Swedish chemist, analyzed samples of petalite found on Utö, an island off the Swedish coast. Arfwedson was working under the direction of J. J. Berzelius and had been given the task of providing a full analytic description of petalite: he found, however, that he was unable to account for some 4% of the sample. Assuming that the loss had occurred as a result of a technical error during the analytic procedure, he adopted a different approach and obtained a salt which he at first thought might be the sulphate of either potassium or sodium but which, after observing the low solubility of the carbonate, he eventually decided contained a hitherto unknown alkali metal.

Berzelius proposed the name *lithion* for this new element, based on the Greek word meaning a stone, or mineral. Arfwedson subsequently demonstrated the presence of lithion in two further mineral ores, lepidolite and spodumene. In the following year, 1818, Sir Humphry Davy isolated small quantities of lithium metal by electrically decomposing its oxide, but there followed a gap of 37 years before Bunsen and Mattheisen, using an electrolytic process, were able to prepare the metal in any quantity from molten lithium chloride.

II. Abundance

Lithium is of widespread occurrence, being found in most rocks of igneous origin. In the region of 0·006% of the earth's crust consists of lithium (Fleischer, 1953), an abundance greater than that of such metals as tin, lead, silver or gold. Despite its almost ubiquitous presence, however, lithium only rarely appears in concentrations sufficient to make mining an economic proposition.

In 1961, Schreck reported that the annual lithium production (in the form of the carbonate) had increased from a pre-World War II level of a few hundred thousand pounds weight to several million pounds, but precise production figures are difficult to obtain, particularly for recent years.

III. Sources

A. Major sources

1. *Minerals*

At least 145 minerals have been reported to contain lithium (Schreck, 1961) but only four of these, occurring mainly in pegmatites, provide commercially viable sources.

(a) *Spodumene:* Containing up to 8% lithium oxide in the richer deposits, spodumene provides the major source of lithium in North America. It also occurs as gem varieties such as the lilac-coloured kunzite (after Dr. G. F. Kunz) and the emerald-coloured hiddenite (after W. E. Hidden).

(b) *Amblygonite:* This mineral, a complex phosphate which may contain as high as a 10% fraction of lithium, does not occur in large deposits and, as a consequence, its early status, along with lepidolite, as the most important of the commercial sources of lithium, has been lost to spodumene.

(c) *Lepidolite:* Sometimes referred to as lithium mica, lepidolite has a variable composition but usually contains some 3–4% of lithium. It also bears rubidium and caesium salts.

(d) *Petalite:* This is the least important of the commercial lithium ores, containing a maximum of 4–5% of lithium.

2. Brines

Sea water contains little lithium—only about 0·1 part per million (Bach *et al.*, 1967)—but certain brines have been located in which the lithium content may be as much as several thousand times greater than this, and these brines occasionally provide useful commercial sources of lithium. The Searle's Lake in California is extensively exploited, whilst the Great Salt Lake in Utah contains an estimated four million tons of lithium chloride.

B. Minor sources

1. Minerals and mineral waters

There are many minerals which contain small and generally unworkable. deposits of lithium salts. In California certain clays have been found in which the lithium content is as high as 1·2% (Schreck, 1961), but generally the levels are much lower than this.

Mineral springs may also contain measurable amounts of lithium salts (0·039 g of the chloride, for example, in each litre of mineral water from Durkheim in Germany).

2. Biological materials

(a) *Animal tissues:* Schou (1957) has listed the animal tissue sources of lithium. These include most human organ tissues—brain, bones, teeth, kidney, lung, spleen, liver, muscles, gut and skin. Human blood, bile, lymph and urine also apparently contain traces of lithium. In other animals, lithium has been found in hair, nails, blood, muscles and milk. Both vertebrates and invertebrates seem to harbour small quantities of lithium salts, but whether, and to what extent, lithium operates as a physiologically important trace element remains an unanswered question (Cade, 1949).

(b) *Plant tissues:* The ash of many plants shows, on analysis, small traces of lithium, but again the metabolic significance, if any, of the metal is obscure.

IV. Geographical Distribution

Unlike sodium and potassium—chemically related elements—lithium does not occur in feldspars, but it is generally to be found, along with quartz and mica, wherever there are pegmatite deposits. Large deposits of lithium-bearing minerals occur in the United States, Canada and Western Australia, and some Central African countries are also major producers. Smaller, though still commercially quite important, deposits occur in South America (Argentina and Brazil particularly), in Europe (Czechoslovakia, France, East Germany, Portugal, Spain, Sweden and the U.S.S.R.) and in certain Asian countries (India and Korea).

V. Extraction

Spodumene, a lithium aluminium silicate obtained in the form of raw ore, is crushed and heated to between 1075 and 1110°C. The chemical reactivity of the lithium aluminium silicate is thereby enhanced and, when mixed with sulphuric acid and roasted to 250°C, it becomes converted to lithium sulphate which may then be leached out of the ore residue with water. The lithium sulphate solution is first purified by processes which precipitate out magnesium and calcium salts, and then concentrated. Aluminium impurities are next moved. The lithium is next precipitated as the relatively insoluble carbonate, extracted and dried.

Lithium metal, in liquid form, may be obtained from a molten lithium chloride-potassium chloride mix by electrolysis at 460°C, and it can then be cast into ingots, or produced as rod, wire or shot.

Other variants of this extraction procedure are also available.

VI. Properties of the Element

A. Physical properties

The physical characteristics of lithium are summarized in Table I. Lithium, the lightest of all solid elements, has a silver-white appearance indicative of its metallic nature. Its atomic structure is relatively simple, the nucleus comprizing three or four neutrons and three protons. Two of the three electrons occur in an inner shell whilst the remaining electron occupies a distant outer shell from which it is readily lost.

Lithium ions pack in body-centred cubic lattices which permit a high degree of electron mobility and thus provide a low electrical resistance.

One curious physical property of lithium is its ability to dissolve in liquid ammonia to produce a saturated solution possessing the lowest known density of any liquid.

B. Chemical properties

The ready loss of the second shell electron from the lithium atom is a major determinant of the element's chemical properties, resulting, in particular, in powerful reducing properties. The metal even reacts with the relatively inert element nitrogen at room temperature to form lithium nitride. With more readily reactive oxidants the reactions are naturally even more easily achieved, and often with some vigour.

Lithium burns in air or oxygen when heated, it reacts with water to release hydrogen (which does not, however, burn—unlike similar reactions involving sodium or potassium), it gives a stable hydride on reaction with hydrogen, and it combines readily with all the halogen elements, and violently with mineral acids.

TABLE I. Physical Properties of Lithium (reproduced by permission of the Lithium Corporation of America).

Property	Value
Symbol	Li
Atomic number	3
Ionic radius Å (Li^+)	0·60
Stable isotopes	*Natural abundance (atomic %)*
6	7·4
7	92·6
Atomic Weight (natural isotopic composition)	6·939
Melting point, °C	180·5
Boiling point, °C	1336
Density, g/cm³ at 20°C	0·531
Specific heat at 25°C, cal/gram	0·849
Specific heat of liquid at mp, cal/gram	1·05
Heat of fusion, cal/gram	103·2
Heat of vaporization, cal/gram	5100
Electric resistivity, at 20°C, ohm-cm	$9·446 \times 10^{-6}$
Characteristic spectrum lines, Å	
red	6708
orange	6103

Vapor pressures			
°C	mm Hg	°C	mm Hg
702	0·49	1002	41·0
802	2·82	1052	70·5
902	12·1	1077	91·0

VII Non-Medical Uses of the Element and Its Compounds

The full diversity of the uses to which lithium is now put is remarkable, and all the more so since commercial exploitation of the metal and its products has only been undertaken to any degree during the past thirty years or so.

In 1918 an alloy of lead and lithium was developed and used quite widely in Germany, but its production was virtually discontinued less than fifteen years later, following the development of superior alloys.

In the early nineteen-forties lithium hydride, a light and compact substance, was used to produce hydrogen: when the hydride contacted water, large volumes of hydrogen were produced and this was used to inflate balloons used for a variety of military purposes. Later during the war period various lithium alloys were tested in the United States, including the very light magnesium–lithium combinations which, at the present time, are finding an important role in the aerospace industry. In addition to the lithium–magnesium alloys, with their economically valuable characteristics of great strength and extreme light-ness, there are several other binary alloys which either are, or are likely to become, useful in industry: these include lithium-lead, lithium-copper, lithium-silver and lithium-aluminium.

Lithium (in the form of the stearate) is used as a constituent of lubricating greases which are characterized by their ability to maintain their action over wide temperature ranges and also in the presence of water. Certain lithium compounds are highly hygroscopic, taking up large quantities of moisture from the air, and are thus ideally suited for use in air-conditioning and dehumidifying systems.

Lithium catalysts are extensively employed in the rubber industry, polymerization processes being facilitated by the metal in a dispersed form. High energy batteries capitalize upon the high electrochemical equivalent and oxidation potential of lithium. Other uses include metal cleaning in welding processes (the chloride and fluoride), carbon dioxide absorption (the anhydrous hydroxide), the modulation of laser beams (the tantalate), water sanitization (the hypochlorite), and as catalysts (the organo-lithium compounds).

The lithium minerals, particularly spodumene and lepidolite, also find commercial uses in their own right. The ceramics and glass industries employ the minerals for fluxing and for producing resistance to cracking, warping and sagging. Glazes are improved by the addition of spodumene.

This brief survey cannot, of course, hope to do justice to the versatility of lithium and its compounds, and it is certain that the full range of applications to which this element may eventually be put has hardly begun to be apparent.

References

Bach, R. O., Kamienski, C. W. and Ellestad, R. B. (1967). *Encycl. Chem. Technol.* **12,** 529–556.

Cade, J. F. J. (1949). *Med. J. Aust.* **36,** 349–352.

Fleischer, M. (1953). *Geom. Survey Circ.* No. 285.

Schou, M. (1957). *Pharmac. Rev.* **9,** 17–58.

Schreck, A. E. (1961). "Lithium: A Materials Survey". U.S. Department of the Interior, Bureau of Mines, Washington.

2

THE HISTORICAL BACKGROUND TO LITHIUM RESEARCH AND THERAPY

F. N. JOHNSON and J. F. J. CADE

I. Introduction

The past decade has seen an enormous proliferation in the number of publications dealing (many of them exclusively) with the biology and pharmacology of the lithium ion. An analysis of the bibliographies prepared by Schou (1969, 1972) shows that the present yearly output of lithium papers averages around 250, or in the region of five a week (Table I), and this rate of output betrays no immediate signs of slackening off. It is clear that the recognition of lithium as a substance of biological importance can be traced to 1949, the first year in which the number of publications on the topic reached double figures.

Not all of the published material deals, even indirectly, with the use of lithium in psychiatric treatment, but it is nevertheless certain that this use of lithium is the major factor behind the explosion of interest in the element and its compounds.

In addition to their psychiatric applications, lithium and its salts are also employed in other branches of medicine, particularly in the manufacture of a variety of pharmaceutical products: vitamin A, certain antihistaminic compounds and oral contraceptives, for example, are synthesized by processes which at some stage involve the use of lithium. Lithium oxalate is a useful anticoagulant in analytic work involving blood, the citrate has been used in antirheumatic and diuretic preparations, and lithium fluoride finds a place in radiation therapy.

There is no doubt, however, that by far the most important medical application of lithium compounds lies in the treatment of the affective disorders, and it is with this aspect of their use that this book is mainly concerned.

The history of lithium usage in psychiatry is already well-documented. The discovery of the specific anti-manic actions of lithium compounds has been described in detail in three papers (Cade, 1949, 1967, 1970). Schou (1959) and Gershon (1970b) reviewed the position at intervals of ten and twenty years respectively since the initial discovery. Other reviews, dealing in greater or lesser detail with historical trends in lithium research, have been presented by many different authors including Kline (1969a), Fieve (1970–71), Gattozzi (1970), Gershon (1970a, 1972), Leung (1970), Tupin (1970), Maletzky and Blachly (1971), Prien et al. (1971), Malitz (1972), and Saran and Gaind (1973). Schou and his colleagues have, in many excellent papers too numerous to detail here, dealt with the historical development of many aspects of lithium therapy. More recently, Kline (1973) has produced a highly entertaining narrative account covering the history of lithium therapy to date.

These diverse accounts, taken in conjunction with several thorough pharmacological reviews dealing specifically with lithium (e.g., Schou, 1957; Davis and Fann, 1971) and the two extensive bibliographies provided by Schou (1959, 1972) provide detailed coverage of the literature relating to the history of lithium in psychiatry. The purpose of the present chapter will be to present an

TABLE I. Numbers of papers published during the period 1800 to 1972 in which details have been given relating to the biology and pharmacology of the lithium ion (data derived from bibliographies prepared by Schou, 1969, 1972).

Decade	Total number of papers	Year	Number of papers
1800–1809	0		
1810–1819	2		
1820–1829	0		
1830–1839	1		
1840–1849	0		
1850–1859	0		
1860–1869	5		
1870–1879	3		
1880–1889	5		
1890–1899	12		
1900–1909	29		
1910–1919	4		
1920–1929	40		
1930–1939	36		
1940–1949	44	1940	2
		1941	5
		1942	3
		1943	4
		1944	4
		1945	2
		1946	1
		1947	8
		1948	1
		1949	14
1950–1959	206	1950	20
		1951	22
		1952	21
		1953	18
		1954	11
		1955	28
		1956	12
		1957	27
		1958	23
		1959	24
1960-1969	890	1960	21
		1961	29
		1962	39
		1963	36
		1964	49
		1965	79
		1966	104
		1967	122
		1968	213
		1969	198
1970–1979	—	1970	257
		1971	241

historical framework against which the contents of subsequent chapters may be seen, and in so doing several issues will be touched upon lightly which will be dealt with in more detail later in the book.

II. Early Uses in Medicine (Pre-1949)

A. Non-psychiatric uses

In the nineteenth century a variety of putative medicinal properties were ascribed to lithium, including a possible effectiveness in the treatment of certain conditions in which uric acid and the insoluble urates had been implicated. It was known that in the presence of uric acid lithium salts became converted into lithium urate, and since this was the most soluble of all urates it was argued that uric acid excretion would be enhanced and the conditions supposedly caused by it would thereby be alleviated (Garrod, 1859). The laboratory-based prediction failed to be confirmed in practice, however, and the use of lithium in treating gout, rheumatism and similar conditions has never gained general acceptance amongst medical practitioners, despite occasional resurgences of interest even in the last decade.

Weiss (1924) claimed a beneficial effect for lithium in a number of diabetic patients, but other workers (e.g., Depisch, 1924; Isaac, 1924) rejected the claim and the matter has received little further investigation.

In the latter part of the nineteen-forties, patients suffering from various forms of cardiovascular disease or hypertension were given lithium chloride as a taste substitute for sodium chloride, the latter being contraindicated in such conditions. This use was discontinued in 1950 following several reports of fatalities or serious side-effects linked to lithium chloride ingestion, and the elucidation of the toxic effects of lithium salts.

B. Psychiatric uses

Kline (1973) has noted that the first indication of the anti-manic properties of lithium salts may be found in the writings of Soranus of Ephesus as recorded by Caelius Aurelianus in the fifth century A.D. Soranus advocated the use of alkaline waters from various mineral springs to treat manic excitement. As has often been pointed out, the alleged medicinal properties of spa waters is interesting in view of their relatively high lithium content. Even in recent years the level of naturally-occurring lithium in drinking water has been linked to the incidence of mental illness of various kinds (Dawson *et al.*, 1970, 1972) though others have raised objections to the interpretation placed on the available data (Pokorny *et al.*, 1972).

Schou (1957) has drawn attention to four papers by Lange, published in 1897, in which the use of lithium salts in the treatment of "uric acid diathesis" was described: this condition apparently involved both gout and mental depression and some improvement was noted in the latter.

In the late nineteen-twenties lithium made a brief appearance in psychiatric usage, the bromide being variously employed as a tonic, hypnotic, or anti-epileptic agent, but attention centred mainly on the bromide component and interest in the drug was not sustained: no great use was made of lithium bromide in any of these three capacities.

III. Early Experimental Studies of Physiological Effects (Pre-1949)

Schou (1957) has given a detailed account of those physiological studies involving lithium which were carried out prior to 1949. He points out that as early as the eighteen-nineties work was in progress which demonstrated the influence of lithium upon developmental processes in various embryonic life forms, and upon tissue regenerative processes (e.g. in planarian worms). Associated lithium-induced protoplasmic and metabolic changes were also described, but little information was forthcoming which provided any really satisfactory or comprehensive explanation of the effects on morphogenesis.

At the turn of the present century studies of the effects of lithium ions on various bioelectric phenomena were commenced with the general aim of comparing lithium with the other more commonly occurring alkali metal ions, sodium and potassium, in such systems.

Lithium salts were subsequently observed in a wide range of situations—on the movements of cilia and amoebae, on the motility and metabolism of spermatozoa, on bacteria and fungi, on excretory processes in unicellular organisms, and in many other model systems. Few of these studies have any clear relevance to the present medical usage of lithium salts.

More interest, from the clinical point of view, attaches to studies of lithium toxicity. When used, briefly, as an anti-gout medication, lithium was associated with toxic symptoms—muscle tremors and gastrointestinal effects being among the more evident of these. Good (1903) produced a fairly detailed study of the effects of large doses of lithium salts on cats, and demonstrated many of the toxic symptoms and side-effects with which later physicians have become all too familiar.

The toxicological investigations of the late nineteen-forties confirmed the findings of Good and the early experimenters and, as will be noted later, were in many ways instrumental in impairing the ready acceptance of lithium therapy.

IV. Discovery of the Anti-Manic Action of Lithium

A. The experimental work

The studies which led to the eventual establishment of the anti-manic properties of lithium were carried out in 1948 and 1949 in Australia by J. F. J. Cade, working single-handed in a laboratory attached to a chronic mental hospital.

The guiding hypothesis, or rationale, was simply that mania might be a state of intoxication produced by a circulating excess of some metabolite, whilst depression, where it was associated with mania, might be due to the corresponding absence or relative lack of such a substance. The manic patient, it was argued, would be expected to excrete either the offending chemical itself, or at least one of its catabolic products, to an extent greater than that shown by other categories of patient or by normal individuals, and accordingly tests were made on urine samples from manic, depressive, schizophrenic and normal control subjects.

These tests were relatively crude, but nonetheless effective. The concentrated urine samples were injected intraperitoneally into guinea pigs. Whilst all the urine samples generally proved fatal to the animals, the urine from some of the manic patients was soon found to be by far the most toxic.

It was clear that the toxicity was due to the presence of urea in the urine, but since this did not appear in greater quantities in the urine excreted by manics than in samples from any of the other categories of subjects, it was proposed that the urea toxicity might itself be enhanced by the presence of uric acid, and that this enhancement might occur to the greatest degree in manic patients.

On the basis of this hypothesis, tests were next carried out using mixtures of urea and a soluble uric acid salt—which happened to be lithium urate, chosen because of its high degree of water solubility. Far from potentiating the effect of urea as had been expected, the lithium urate appeared to exert some kind of protection and to reduce urea toxicity. Moreover, and what was equally surprising, the guinea pigs given the lithium urate lost their natural timidity and their usual frantic righting reflex, and became instead placid, tranquillized, and generally lacking in responsiveness to stimulation.

Further experiments involving injections of lithium carbonate solution confirmed that this calming action was due to the lithium ion alone and not to the urate component.

B. The clinical studies

After repeated self-administration of lithium carbonate and lithium citrate failed to reveal any untoward effects of either, Cade took the decision to employ lithium salts in the treatment of patients having illnesses characterized in large part by excitement or mania, arguing that if the lithium ion did indeed produce a calming effect in animals, possibly by protecting against the actions of some metabolite like urea, then the same should also be true in humans in whom the matabolite might be expected to be present in excess.

In all, ten manic patients, six schizophrenics, and three chronically depressed patients, were treated. The results were gratifying and little short of dramatic. Whilst there was little effect in either the schizophrenics or the depressed patients (although the hyper-excitability component of their syndrome tended to show some lessening), all ten manic patients showed rapid and marked improvement.

Lithium, it seemed, possessed a powerful and specific anti-manic action.

C. Retrospective comments on the discovery

"Serendipity" is a term which is frequently applied to the discovery of lithium's specific anti-manic potential. For example, Gershon (1970b) commented that "... serendipity played a significant role in the discovery...." (p. 333), and again in another paper (Gershon, 1970a) "... serendipity seems to have been the midwife for lithium...." (p. 169), whilst more recently Blackwell (1972) has referred to "this serendipitous observation" (p. 140).

It is, of course, true that the decision to use lithium in the experiments rested solely upon the known solubility of its urate; nevertheless, it is clear that the progression from the hypothesis of a metabolic basis for mania right through to the clinical trial of lithium salts in the treatment of mania, was inevitable and that the final conclusion could not have been otherwise. That the therapeutic efficacy of lithium was unsuspected when the experimental work was commenced, in no way makes the final outcome entirely the product of chance.

V. Early Clinical Studies on the Psychiatric Use of Lithium (1949–1954)

The report of Cade's successful use of lithium salts, which appeared in the September 1949 issue of the *Medical Journal of Australia* (Cade, 1949), stimulated a number of other clinical investigations of a similar nature.

Between 1949 and 1953 four papers arose from Australia, four from France and one from Italy (Kline, 1969a). By the end of 1954 nine papers had been published in which lithium was used as the sole physical treatment for mania (Schou, 1959). Out of a total number of 75 patients involved in the studies reported, only 11 failed to show any improvement. Only one of the reports (and this involved only two patients) failed to discern any therapeutic effect of lithium.

VI. Obstacles to the General Acceptance of Lithium Therapy

Despite the excellent results obtained by Cade, and the support given by such other studies as were carried out in the following five-year period, lithium therapy failed to gain any degree of general acceptance among psychiatrists. In retrospect, it is possible to point to three major reasons why this should have been so.

A. Toxicity

The use, during the late nineteen-forties, of lithium chloride as a salt substitute has already been mentioned. Several patients who had been placed on such a diet subsequently showed either severe toxic reactions or actually died. By 1950 lithium had been labelled as a dangerously poisonous substance, despite a valiant rearguard action by Talbott (1950) who vigorously defended its use as a salt substitute.

Understandably, clinicians were reluctant to use a new and potentially hazardous drug until much more became known about the nature and frequency of the associated dangers, particularly since at least one fatality was reported following the use of lithium therapy in a case of mania (Roberts, 1950).

B. Other psychoactive drugs

1953 marked the beginning of the era of psychoactive drugs. It is perhaps unfortunate that lithium should have been recognized as a therapeutic agent at the same time as chlorpromazine was being tested in Europe for almost precisely the same psychiatric indications. The very wide safety margins of chlorpromazine, as well as its astonishing effectiveness in controlling the more overt manifestations of schizophrenia (two attributes notably absent in lithium) gave it, and the other subsequently developed phenothiazine drugs, distinctly the edge over lithium.

The next few years saw the introduction into clinical usage of several new classes of drugs—the butyrophenones, the benzodiazepines, the thioxanthenes, and the Rauwolfia alkaloids—and all of them appeared to have enormous advantages, both in terms of their wide range of possible indications and their relatively low toxcities, over a substance so notoriously toxic as lithium.

C. Economic issues

Several writers have hinted that other than purely medical consisderations may have been involved in the difficulties experienced in getting lithium accepted as a viable therapeutic tool.

Amongst the vast array of pharmaceutical products, lithium is remarkably cheap, the price per pound of the carbonate having fallen from $1.50 in 1926 to $0.67 in 1959 (Schreck, 1961): its use, moreover, is not, and cannot be, patented. The suggestion that drug manufacturers saw little prospect of making anything like a substantial profit out of lithium preparations and made a definite economic decision not to pursue the investigation of such substances or to undertake their marketing, may well carry some force (Cole, 1968). It was indeed not until 1970 that lithium appeared on the American market and, as Kline (1973) remarks, the companies involved "have probably proceeded to lose money consistently on the product."

VII. The Reintroduction of Lithium Therapy

The turning point in the fortunes of lithium therapy undoubtedly came in 1954 when, according to Maletzky and Blachly (1971), the director of Aarhus State Psychiatric Hospital at Risskov in Denmark suggested to a research associate, Dr. (now Professor) Mogens Schou, that the reports about lithium looked interesting and possibly worth following up. Schou and his associates took up the matter and commenced by examining the claim that lithium possessed a specific anti-manic action.

A. The acute treatment of mania

Schou *et al.* (1954), in their first published report, came down strongly in favour of the view that lithium did indeed show a significant anti-manic potential, though they added a cautionary note about the associated dangers of toxic reactions. To Schou and his colleagues, the importance of lithium treatment extended beyond the therapeutic context, offering as it did "... new possibilities for a study of the pathophysiology of the manic-depressive psychoses...." (p. 256).

The interest of clinicians in lithium therapy was stimulated afresh by this report and by the many different lines of investigation which it opened up. By 1972 it was possible to point to more than 70 reports on the treatment of mania with lithium (Gershon, 1972) and to estimates of between 60 and 100% improvement rates.

B. The prophylactic treatment of manic-depressive psychosis

In his clinical trials, Cade had demonstrated only that lithium was effective against an existing, ongoing manic condition. It was found not to be beneficial against an established depressive mood, nor did the trial enable anything to be said about the ability of lithium to·*prevent* the recurrence of either a manic or depressive episode. As early as 1951, however, a report appeared which did mention that, following lithium treatment, there seemed to be some degree of protection established against a recurrence of the manic phase (Noack and Trautner, 1951), and this was later also briefly noted by Schou *et al.* (1954).

It was not until 1959 that a report came from England that this prophylactic effect might extend also to recurrent depressions (Hartigan, 1959), a suggestion based on casual observations in the first instance but later confirmed formally (Hartigan, 1963).

In fact, as Schou (personal communication) has pointed out, Baastrup in Denmark saw the prophylactic effect of lithium against depressive recurrences at the same time as, and quite independently of, Hartigan. Both investigators wrote to Schou in 1960, informing him of their observations and asking whether he had noted similar effects. Schou subsequently visited Hartigan and saw the patients on lithium maintenance treatment; although the patients were few in number they were, by Schou's report, very striking, and included patients who had suffered from recurrent depressions for many years but who, during their two years on lithium therapy, had been free from depressive episodes. Baastrup's observations were of an almost identical nature and Schou urged both investigators to publish their findings: this they did (Hartigan, 1963; Baastrup, 1964).

Subsequent work, mainly by Baastrup and Schou and their colleagues in Denmark, and followed by a wide range of studies in the United States and elsewhere, leaves little doubt that lithium does indeed exert a prophylactic effect against both mania and depression.

C. The acute treatment of depression

All the early indications were that lithium possessed little, if anything, in the way of effectiveness as an antidepressant when administered acutely during a depressive episode. Neither Cade (1949) nor Noack and Trautner (1951) had been able to demonstrate an antidepressant potential of lithium salts, and this opinion prevailed amongst reviewers of lithium research around the late nineteen-sixties (Gershon, 1968; Platman and Fieve, 1968; Schou, 1968).

At about this same time however, a few reports began to appear suggesting that the dismissal of an acute antidepressant action of lithium might have been premature. Zall et al. (1968) found, for example, that in some patients who had hitherto failed to respond to a variety of antidepressant medications some improvement might be obtained by adding lithium to the existing treatment regime. Dyson and Mendels (1968) argued that if manic-depression were indeed a unitary medical condition then lithium ought to show an antidepressant as well as an anti-manic action, and they presented evidence which they felt supported their contention.

These early reports have led to further examination of this issue, but at the present time the status of lithium as an effective acute medication for depression is still undergoing clarification.

D. Establishment of safe dosage regimes

One of the most influential factors in the resurgence of interest amongst practising physicians in the use of lithium therapy, lay in the development of adequate serum lithium monitoring techniques, and in the demonstration that a definite relationship existed between serum lithium levels and the nature of the clinical response—particularly the onset of side-effects and toxic reactions.

These advances enabled safe limits to be established for lithium dose levels, and provided a rational basis for patient management in lithium therapy.

VIII. The Lithium Controversy

The issues associated with clinical trial methodology are nowhere more clearly, or indeed dramatically, illustrated than in the controversy which has surrounded lithium therapy.

Fascinating insights are provided into the involvement of human personalities in research endeavours and their evaluation, by an examination of the heated and occasionally vituperous exchanges which have enlivened the pages of otherwise austere scientific journals wherever lithium has been the subject under discussion.

A. The acute treatment of mania

In 1969 a flurry of correspondence in the pages of *The Lancet* occurred in response to an editorial charge that no strong or convincing evidence had been presented to show that lithium was an effective anti-manic agent or that it possessed any therapeutic superiority over alternative, and possibly safer, medications for manic conditions. In the following year Shull and Sapira (1970) reviewed the efforts made up to that time to demonstrate an anti-manic potential of lithium, and they reached the same gloomy conclusion that little hard evidence, free from serious methodological deficiencies, had been provided on the matter.

B. The prophylactic treatment of manic-depressive psychosis

The anti-lithium arguments reached their most extreme expression on the matter of the prophylactic treatment of recurrent endogenous affective disorders of a bipolar nature. In an extraordinary and forceful paper, Blackwell and Shepherd (1968) labelled the claims for this aspect of lithium's therapeutic effectiveness as a "therapeutic myth", drawing a fierce rebuttal from Baastrup and Schou (1968). When Kline (1968) also made enthusiastic claims for lithium as a prophylactic agent, Blackwell (1969) again leapt to the attack, adopting the language of comic opera, with Kline replying in kind (Kline, 1969b).

The clashes still continue with unabated vigour. A report by Baastrup *et al.* (1970) of a double-blind discontinuation trial of lithium led to further methodological criticisms and equally spirited defences.

IX. The Recent History of Lithium Research

In April 1970 the Food and Drug Administration (FDA) of the United States Department of Health, Education and Welfare issued a statement to the effect that it had approved three new drug applications from commercial companies for the production of lithium carbonate for clinical uses. Kline (1973) reports that there had for some considerable time prior to this been a clamour from psychiatrists in the United States for such approval to be given. Even when it came, however, approval was only partial: the FDA announcement stated that "... the sole indication for the use of lithium carbonate at this time is for control of manic episodes of manic depressive psychosis. ..." The prophylactic properties of lithium were not acknowledged or even mentioned.

Since the FDA announcement things have moved quickly. Clinical trial methodology has been refined in many successive attempts to establish the therapeutic value of lithium: indeed, this has extended beyond the use of lithium in treating the affective disorders and lithium salts have been incorporated into clinical trials involving a wide range of other conditions. As Kline comments wryly "... it seems if we only wait long enough everyone in the world will try lithium for everything. ..." (Kline, personal communication).

There has been a dramatic increase in the number of physiological studies which have concentrated upon lithium as distinct from considering it as only one among many variables; these studies have been pursued vigorously and have utilized an extensive battery of *in vivo* and *in vitro* techniques. Many of the effects which lithium produces on electro-physiological, endocrine, and metabolic processes are rapidly being elucidated. Whilst the very complexity of the picture which is emerging has effectively destroyed earlier hopes that anything approaching a simple physiological model of lithium action (and hence of the affective disorders themselves) might be discerned, it is nevertheless an exhilarating experience to observe the intense activity which currently attends lithium research.

There are already exciting indications that out of the mass of data some overall patterns are beginning to emerge, and we may surely look forward to the structuring of this wealth of information into a viable unified hypothesis of lithium action in the affective disorders within the next decade.

Acknowledgements

The authors are grateful to Professor Mogens Schou and Dr. Nathan Kline for reading the manuscript in draft form and for contributing many helpful comments.

References

Baastrup, P. C. (1964). *Compreh. Psychiat.* 5, 396–408.
Baastrup, P. C., Poulsen, J. C., Schou, M., Thomsen, K. and Amdisen, A. (1970). *Lancet* 2, 326–330.
Baastrup, P. C. and Schou, M. (1968). *Lancet* 1, 1419–1422.
Blackwell, B. (1969). *J. Amer. med. Ass.* 125, 1131.
Blackwell, B. (1972). *Amer. Heart J.* 83, 139–141.
Blackwell, B. and Shepherd, M. (1968). *Lancet* 1, 968–971.
Cade, J. F. J. (1949). *Med. J. Aust.* 36, 349–352.

Cade, J. F. J. (1967). *Aust. N.Z. J. Psychiat.* **1**, 61–62.
Cade, J. F. J. (1970). *In* "Discoveries in Biological Psychiatry" (F. J. Ayd and B. Blackwell, eds.) pp. 218–229. Lippincott, Philadelphia.
Cole, J. O. (1968). *Am. J. Psychiat.* **125**, 556–557.
Davies, J. M. and Fann, W. E. (1971). *A. Rev. Pharmac.* **11**, 285–302.
Dawson, E. B., Moore, T. D. and McGanity, W. J. (1970). *Dis. nerv. Syst.* **31**, 811–820.
Dawson, E. B., Moore, T. D. and McGanity, W. J. (1972). *Dis. nerv. Syst.* **33**, 546–556.
Depisch, F. (1924). *Wien. Klin. Wochenschr.* **37**, 1216.
Dyson, W. L. and Mendels, J. (1968). *Curr. ther. Res.* **10**, 601–608.
Fieve, R. R. (1970-71). *Int. J. Psychiat.* **9**, 375–412.
Garrod, A. B. (1859). "Gout and Rheumatic Gout". Walton and Maberly, London.
Gattozzi, A. A. (1970). "Lithium in the Treatment of Mood Disorders". National Clearinghouse for Mental Health Information; NIMH Publication No. 5033.
Gershon, S. (1968). *Am. J. Psychiat.* **124**, 1452–1456.
Gershon, S. (1970a). *Clin. Pharmac. Ther.* **11**, 168–187.
Gershon, S. (1970b). *Dis. nerv. Syst.* **31**, 333–335.
Gershon, S. (1972). *A Rev. Med.* **23**, 439–452.
Good, C. A. (1903). *Am. J. med. Sci.* **125**, 273–284.
Hartigan, G. P. (1959). Paper read to the Southern Branch of the Royal Medico-Psychological Society. Reported by Gattozzi, A. (1970). "Lithium in the Treatment of Mood Disorders". National Clearinghouse for Mental Health Information: NIMH Publication No. 5033.
Hartigan, G. P. (1963). *Br. J. Psychiat.* **109**, 810–814.
Isaac, S. (1924). *Wien. Klin. Wochenschr.* **37**, 1263.
Kline, N. S. (1968). *Am. J. Psychiat.* **125**, 558–560.
Kline, N. S. (1969a). *In* "Modern Problems of Pharmacopsychiatry" (F. A. Freyhan, N. Petrilowitsch and P. Pichot, eds.) Vol. **3**, pp. 1–90. Karger, Basel.
Kline, N. S. (1969b). *J. Am. med. Ass.* **125**, 1131–1132.
Kline, N. S. (1973). *In* "Lithium: Its Role in Psychiatric Research and Treatment" (S. Gershon and B. Shopsin, eds.), pp. 5–13. Plenum Press, New York.
Leung, A. S. (1970). *Can. psychiat. Ass. J.* **15**, 189–199.
Maletzky, B. and Blachly, P. H. (1971). "The Use of Lithium in Psychiatry". CRC Press, Cleveland.
Malitz, S. (1972). *Bull. N.Y. Acad. Med.* **48**, 767–778.
Noack, C. and Trautner, E. (1951). *Med. J. Aust.* **38**, 219–222.
Platman, S. R. and Fieve, R. R. (1968). *Archs gen. Psychiat.* **19**, 659–663.
Pokorny, A. D., Sheehan, D. and Atkinson, J. (1972). *Dis. nerv. Syst.* **33**, 649–652.
Prien, R. F., Caffey, E. M. and Klett, C. J. (1971). *Dis. nerv. Syst.* **32**, 521–531.
Roberts, E. L. (1950). *Med. J. Aust.* **37**, 261–262.
Saran, B. M. and Gaind, R. (1973). *Clin. Toxicol.* **6**, 257–269.
Schou, M. (1957). *Pharmac. Rev.* **9**, 17–58.
Schou, M. (1959). *Psychopharmacologia* **1**, 65–78.
Schou, M. (1968). *In* "Psychopharmacology: A Review of Progress 1957–67". (D. H. Efron, J. O. Cole, J. Levine and J. R. Wittenborn, eds.), pp. 701–718. United States Government Printing Office, Public Health Service Publication No. 1836, Washington D.C.
Schou, M. (1969). *Psychopharmac. Bull.* **5**, 33–62.
Schou, M. (1972). *Psychopharmac. Bull.* **8**, 36–62.

Schou, M., Juel-Nielsen, N., Strömgren, E. and Voldby, H. (1954). *J. Neurol. Neurosurg. Psychiat.* **17**, 250–260.

Schreck, A. E. (1961). "Lithium: A Materials Survey". United States Department of the Interior: Bureau of Mines, Washington D.C.

Shull, W. K. and Sapira, J. D. (1970). *Am. J. Psychiat.* **127**, 218–222.

Talbott, J. H. (1950). *Archs intern. Med.* **85**, 1–10.

Tupin, J. P. (1970). *Hosp. Commun. Psychiat.* **21**, 73–80.

Weiss, H. (1924). *Wien. Klin. Wochenschr.* **37**, 1142.

Zall, H., Therman, P. O. G. and Myers, J. M. (1968). *Amer. J. Psychiat.* **125**, 549–555.

PART I

SECTION B

THE THERAPEUTIC PROFILE OF LITHIUM

3

LITHIUM IN THE ACUTE TREATMENT OF MANIA

M. PEET

I. Introduction

The first report on the use of lithium in the treatment of manic illness was that of Cade (1949). He was led to try lithium in the treatment of psychotic excitement by his earlier observation that guinea-pigs became lethargic when injected with lithium salts. A marked reduction in symptoms occurred in all ten manic patients treated. Six patients with dementia praecox, and three melancholics were also treated, and showed no notable improvement. Soon afterwards, Noack and Trautner (1951) reported a similarly encouraging response to lithium treatment in 29 out of 30 manic patients. The introduction of the phenothiazine drugs, and the deaths which occurred due to the uncontrolled use of lithium as a salt substitute, initially led to a relative neglect of lithium as a treatment for mania. However, lithium therapy, both in acute mania and, more controversially, as a prophylactic measure in recurrent affective illness, has gained increasing acceptance. This chapter will begin with a review of the

25

evidence relating to the therapeutic activity of lithium in mania; associated clinical aspects will then be discussed.

II. Clinical Trials

A. Open trials

A general survey of the literature indicates that about 80% of manic patients improve when treated with lithium salts. Schou (1968) was able to find 42 published reports in the world literature on the use of lithium for mania, and all but one were favourable. Many more reports have been published since then. However, the great majority of these studies have serious methodological deficiencies. In particular, most of the data come from studies in which no attempt is made to use a double-blind technique, and no control group is included. The deficiencies of uncontrolled trials are now well known. It is therefore important to examine the controlled trials in more detail.

B. Controlled trials

There are several more specific problems involved when a trial of treatment for manic patients is attempted. Diagnostic problems are considerable. The self-limiting and recurrent nature of mania emphasises the need for control data, and may raise problems when cross-over trials are attempted. There is a lack of adequate rating devices for mania; a psychiatrist's rating must generally be used, since disturbed manic patients are unable to complete self-rating scales reliably. The use of placebo medication in severely disturbed patients presents ethical as well as management problems, and the use of concomitant medication may be unavoidable at times. The nature of the illness may lead to a high dropout rate, and to the exclusion of more severely ill patients. Lithium has well-recognized side-effects which are discussed in Chapter 13, and these may affect the "blindness" of the rater. Since blood samples must be taken during lithium treatment for serum lithium estimation, it is also necessary to take samples from the control group in order to preserve blindness.

Bearing these problems in mind, the double-blind trials will now be considered individually.

1. *Schou et al.* (*1954*)

The first controlled trial of lithium salts in the treatment of manic illness was carried out in Denmark by Schou and his colleagues. The 38 patients for whom data are presented were divided into a group of 30 typical cases, in whom there was no doubt as to the diagnosis at any stage in the disease, and a group of 8 atypical cases. Details of diagnostic and selection criteria are not given. There was usually a short period without medication, following which an unspecified number of patients were treated with lithium on an open basis, and the remainder received lithium or placebo medication on a double-blind basis. In these cases, treatment was randomly varied, usually at two-week intervals. The changes used were lithium–placebo, placebo–lithium, lithium–lithium, or placebo–placebo. Supplementary medication was avoided as far as possible. Lithium was given as carbonate, citrate, or chloride in a variable dosage, but the criteria by which the dosage was determined are not given. Blood was taken during treatment with both lithium and placebo, and the plasma lithium level was usually between 0·5 mEq/l and 2·0 mEq/l. The number of patients who developed side-effects is not given. Lumbar puncture was carried out in order to measure cerebro-spinal fluid lithium levels in six patients. The degree of mania was rated on a 0,+,++,+++ scale each day. After the trial period, a global rating of response to lithium treatment was made on a 3-point scale as + effect, possible effect, and − effect. The data from selected individual patients were presented in graphical form, and from these it could be seen that the length of the periods during which the effects of varying medication were observed varied from a few weeks in some patients to eight months or more in others. The allocation of some patients to the "+ effect" category appears to have been based, at least in part, on evidence of the prophylactic activity of lithium rather than on its therapeutic effect against an established acute episode of mania. Thus, one of the criteria for a + effect is: "In a patient with manic attacks occurring at regular intervals, lithium was able to prevent these attacks". The results are shown in Table I. In the 30 typical cases, a + effect was observed in

TABLE I. The Efficacy of Lithium Treatment During Mania: The Study of Schou *et al.* (1954). (Reproduced with permission from Schou *et al.*, 1954.

| | No. of cases | | | |
	+ Effect	Possible effect	− Effect	Total
Typical cases	12	15	3	30
Atypical cases	2	3	3	8
Total	14	18	6	38

12 and a possible effect in 15. In the eight atypical cases, a + effect was observed in two and a possible effect in a further two. The presented data are insufficient to allow the effects of lithium and placebo treatment to be compared by statistical analysis.

Whilst this work suggests that lithium administration is associated with a reduction of manic symptoms in many patients, it does not provide conclusive evidence that lithium is superior to placebo in the treatment of manic states. This is largely due to the inclusion of data from an open trial, and the lack of any statistical analysis of the results.

2. Maggs (1963)

In 1963, Maggs treated 28 patients with lithium and placebo medication in a double-blind cross-over trial. The selection criteria included the ability of the patient to co-operate during the trial. This involved the exclusion of more severely ill patients. The patients, who had received no previous anti-manic treatment during the current attack, were treated in three phases, each of two weeks duration. The subjects were randomly assigned to either Group A (lithium–rest period–placebo) or Group B (Placebo–rest period–lithium). Lithium carbonate was given in a fixed dose of 0·5 g three times daily. This resulted in toxicity necessitating withdrawal from the trial in two patients, and may have resulted in inadequate plasma lithium levels in other patients. Details of the plasma lithium levels achieved are not given. Blood samples were taken from both the lithium-treated and the placebo groups. The clinical state of the patients was assessed using the psychiatric rating scale devised by Wittenborn et al. (1953). Cluster V (schizophrenic excitement), which reflects many manic symptoms, was considered individually together with cluster III (manic states).

Only 18 of the initial 28 patients completed the trial. The drop-outs included five patients who became severely disturbed, and exclusion of such patients could have biased the results of the trial in a direction depending on which phase of treatment these patients were undertaking when they were excluded. Apart from two patients excluded due to lithium toxicity, side-effects were noted in two patients only, one on lithium and the other on placebo treatment. Statistical analysis showed that the patients on lithium treatment fared significantly better than those on placebo medication after two weeks of treatment, as assessed using Wittenborn clusters III or V. The treatment effect was less marked after one week of medication.

This work provides evidence that lithium is superior to placebo in the treatment of acute manic illness, within the limitations imposed by the high drop-out rate. However, patients with a severe degree of mania were not studied.

3. Bunney et al. (1968); Goodwin et al. (1969a, b)

In 1968, Bunney et al. reported a pilot study carried out on two manic patients, for whom detailed case histories are given. A period of lithium therapy was interrupted at intervals by placebo substitution for a few days, on a double-blind basis. Lithium carbonate was administered in a variable dose, and daily plasma lithium levels were obtained during the trial period. The patient's clinical state was rated each day by nursing staff on a 15-point scale (Bunney et al., 1963), and a global rating was made by a psychiatrist. The psychiatrist's rating, which correlated highly with the nurse's rating, was used alone in the assessment of the results. It was found that there was a clear increase of manic symptoms following withdrawal of lithium, usually occurring within 24 hours. The association between a fall in plasma lithium level and an increase in manic symptoms reached statistical significance in one patient. The reduction of manic symptoms following reinstatement of lithium was less immediate, and was not included in the statistical calculations.

This work was criticized (*Lancet*, 1969a,b) on the grounds that the assignment of treatment periods was not random. This comment was accepted by the authors (Goodwin *et al.*, 1969b), who in their reply stressed that the purpose of this pilot study was to evaluate the temporal relationships on a day-to-day basis between changes in medication, lithium blood-levels, and clinical change, rather than to prove the efficacy of lithium in mania.

Using the same experimental design, this group of workers (Goodwin *et al.*, 1969b) extended their trial to include 12 patients (including the original two) with manic illness. Treatment was started with lithium carbonate in doses calculated from the age and body weight of the patient to give blood levels between $0 \cdot 8$ and $1 \cdot 3$ mEq/l. The actual lithium levels achieved during the trial are not given, and there is no mention of the plasma lithium levels being monitored.

At predetermined times during the course of the lithium treatment, placebo medication was substituted, on a double-blind basis, for varying periods of time. Occasional doses of chloral hydrate were given in some cases. The clinical state was rated by two independent nurse raters on a 15-point scale. After the trial period, a global rating of the overall response of the patient was made. A

TABLE II. The Efficacy of Lithium Treatment During Mania: The Study of Goodwin *et al.* (1969b). (Reproduced with permission from Goodwin *et al.*, 1969b).

Response	Manic-Depressive		Noncyclic depressive
	Manic	Depressed	
Complete response	3	5	0
Unequivocal	4	3	
Probable	4	2	
Partial response	1	5	2
Unequivocal	1	4	1
Probable	0	1	1
No response	0	1	3
Worse	3	2	0
Total	12	13	5

complete and unequivocal response was defined as a cessation of all manic symptoms within two weeks of starting lithium, together with a return of symptoms during the placebo period. A partial and unequivocal response was defined as a decrease of ratings of at least 3 points within two weeks of starting lithium, with an increasing score during placebo periods. The significance of any unusual fluctuations in ratings was established statistically. Probable improvement was defined as initial remission or decrease of symptoms within two weeks of starting lithium with no consistent return of symptoms during placebo periods. In these cases, it appears impossible to determine whether remission was due to the effects of treatment or to spontaneous improvement. The results are shown in Table II. Complete or partial unequivocal response was observed in 5 (42%) of the patients, 4 had a probable response, and 3 became worse.

The design of this trial is such that the statistical comparison of periods of lithium and placebo treatment is not possible. However, the finding that 75% of patients improved with lithium treatment and that 42% subsequently relapsed on placebo substitution supports the idea that lithium has a therapeutic effect in mania.

4. *Johnson et al.* (*1968, 1971*)

In 1968, Johnson *et al.* produced an interim report on a double-blind evaluation of lithium and chlorpromazine in the treatment of manic states. A total of 27 manic patients and 14 patients with schizoaffective illness were included in the trial. Many patients were unable or unwilling to co-operate in the study, and thus some of the more severely ill patients were probably excluded.

Following a baseline period of placebo treatment, which averaged 5 days, the patients were randomly allocated to treatment with either lithium carbonate or chlorpromazine. Five patients received more than one trial of treatment, due to either readmission to the trial or crossover to the alternative medication following treatment failure. The duration of treatment was not constant, but was stated to average 3–4 weeks. The drug dosage was increased until either a therapeutic response or toxic symptoms occurred. Chlorpromazine dosage varied between 200 and 1800 mg. daily, and lithium levels reached 1·0 mEq/l or above in all patients. Blood samples were taken twice weekly during the study. It is stated that "owing to the differential effects of these two drugs, on occasions it was impossible not to have guessed with a reasonable degree of certainty which medication was being used" (p. 564).

The patients' clinical state was rated by nursing and medical staff and by a psychologist, using several different rating scales. The response to treatment was then globally rated as marked, moderate, or minimal improvement, no change or worse. The outcome in the manic group only will be considered here (Table III). Of the 18 periods of lithium treatment, 14 resulted in marked improvement, and two in moderate improvement. Of the 11-periods of treatment with chlorpromazine, four resulted in marked improvement and four in moderate improvement.

The authors argue that "the results of this study show unequivocally the superior therapeutic efficacy of lithium in manic states" (p. 568), since marked improvement occurred in 78% of the lithium-treated patients as compared with 36% of the chlorpromazine-treated patients. However, analysis of the

TABLE III. The Efficacy of Lithium Treatment During Mania: The Study of Johnson *et al.* (1968). (Reproduced with permission from Johnson *et al.*, 1969).

Global change	Manic-depressive		Schizo-affective		Chronic mania	
	Lithium	Chlorpro-mazine	Lithium	Chlorpro-mazine	Lithium	Chlorpro-mazine
Marked Improvement	14	4	0	3	—	—
Moderate Improvement	2	4	1	5	—	—
Minimal Improvement	1	3	0	2	—	—
No Change	1	0	0	0	1	1
Worse	—	—	6	—	—	—
Total	18	11	7	10	1	1

published figures by a chi-square test with Yates' correction reveals that the difference between the effects of the two treatments fails to reach the 5% level of statistical significance.

In a later paper (Johnson *et al.*, 1971), further data are presented on a group of 21 manic patients treated with lithium carbonate or chlorpromazine in a double-blind trial. Some of these findings were included in the earlier report. The methodology of this study was essentially the same as that of the earlier trial. The patients were allocated to treatment with either lithium or chlorpromazine for a three-week period. Again, the drug dose was increased until either a therapeutic response or toxic effects occurred. The plasma lithium levels attained ranged from $1 \cdot 0 – 2 \cdot 5$ mEq/l. The number of patients who developed side-effects is not given. The table of results gives data for 5 chlorpromazine-treated patients and 6 lithium-treated patients. Reasons for drop-out included leaving hospital against medical advice, and refusal of medication. The patients' clinical state was rated at intervals during the study using a variety of rating scales. Using the baseline and terminal scores only, both lithium and chlorpromazine treatment were shown to be associated with a statistically significant reduction in severity of symptoms as assessed by the Brief Psychiatric Rating Scale and a "Clinical Global Impression" rating. Assessment by the Nurses' Observation Scale for In-patient Evaluation failed to demonstrate any significant improvement in either group, and analysis of the scores obtained by the Treatment Response Assessment Method indicated that only the lithium-treated patients improved significantly. The authors were unable to demonstrate any significant difference between the overall therapeutic effects of lithium and chlorpromazine in the treatment of mania, although there was a trend in favour of lithium.

5. *Spring et al. (1970)*

From 40 patients considered for entry to this trial, 14 were selected according to stated clinical criteria. Treatment was given on a double-blind basis with either lithium carbonate or chlorpromazine for a three-week period. In nine patients, lithium carbonate was given in a fixed dose of 1800 mg daily for one week, following which the dosage was increased to a maximum of 3 g daily depending on clinical response. In five patients, chlorpromazine was given in doses of up to 1600 mg daily. Amylobarbitone was given for sleeping and occasionally to control agitation on a temporary basis. Clinical ratings were made twice weekly by two psychiatrists on a 0–3 + scale, for each of eight target symptoms.

Two patients did not complete the trial for reasons unconnected with their psychiatric state. The incidence of side-effects was not specified, although it was stated that the common side-effects of lithium were also frequent with chlorpromazine, and the authors did not consider that this problem biased their results.

Six out of seven patients on lithium and three out of five patients on chlorpromazine were considered to have responded to treatment. The two chlorpromazine failures were crossed over onto lithium, and remitted. The lithium failure was crossed over to chlorpromazine, and failed to respond. The lithium responders all had plasma lithium levels not exceeding 1·3 mEq/l, but the range of levels is not given. It is not clear whether blood was taken from both groups of patients.

With these small groups of patients, the authors were unable to demonstrate any significant difference in efficacy between the two treatments.

6. *Platman (1970)*

Thirty patients were selected for this trial. The diagnostic and selection criteria are not stated. Seven of the more severely ill patients were unable to complete a baseline two-week placebo period and were therefore dropped from the study. Patients were randomly assigned to treatment with either lithium carbonate or chlorpromazine in starting doses of 1,200 mg daily and 400 mg daily respectively. The dosage was subsequently varied. Morning plasma lithium levels were above 0·8 mEq/l in all patients, but there is no mention of whether blood samples were taken from both groups. The authors considered that side-effects reduced the "blindness" of the trial.

The patients' clinical state was rated weekly by ward staff on six scales from the Psychiatric Evaluation Form. No statistically significant difference between the two treatments was demonstrated, although there was a trend in favour of lithium.

7. *Stokes et al.* (*1971*)

Stokes *et al.* (1971) selected 38 patients who had been diagnosed by three psychiatrists as suffering from typical manic-depressive illness. Alternate patients were given lithium or placebo medication at the start of the trial. Thereafter, four 7–10 day periods of alternating lithium or placebo medication were used in each case. Nursing staff reported the behaviour of the patients on a daily basis, and the reports were quantified by a psychologist on two 7-point scales for depression and mania. Global ratings on similar scales, made by psychiatrists on the basis of a clinical interview, were found to correlate highly with the psychologist's ratings.

Lithium chloride solution was given in a standard dose of 0·5 mg/kg body weight daily, unless the plasma lithium level rose above 1·5 mEq/l (which occurred in seven patients) or toxic symptoms occurred. The resulting reduction of lithium dosage was apparently known to the nursing staff, and this could have affected the blindness of the ratings in these patients. Chlorpromazine was given to eight patients and pentobarbitone at night to a few subjects. Blood samples were taken on six mornings per week during the study. The mean plasma lithium level was 0·93 mEq/l after 7 to 10 days of treatment.

There was a total of 98 manic treatment periods, prior to which mania ratings had been equal to, or greater than, 1 on the 7-point scale. Treatment periods beginning during a depressive episode were also included in the study, but will not be discussed here. Some of the results are illustrated in Table IV.

Improvement occurred in 75% of the lithium treatment periods, and worsening in 18%. In the placebo-treatment periods 40·5% of the patients improved and the same percentage worsened. During 56 lithium treatment periods there was a highly significant fall in mania ratings. During 42 placebo treatment periods there was no significant fall in these ratings. Median mania ratings during days 7 to 10 of lithium treatment were significantly lower than during days 7 to 10 of placebo treatment, even though the mania ratings at the beginning of the lithium treatment periods tended to be higher. In contrast to the report of Bunney *et al.* (1968), the authors were unable to demonstrate a significant change in behaviour during the first 24 hours of changeover to placebo treatment.

TABLE IV. The Efficacy of Lithium Treatment During Mania: The Study of Stokes *et al.* (1971). (Reproduced with permission from Stokes *et al.*, 1971).

Treatment	Periods			Total	No. of patients
	Improved	Worsened	No change		
Lithium	42 (75%)	10 (18%)	4 (7%)	56	28
Placebo	17 (40·5%)	17 (40·5%)	8 (19%)	42	28
Totals	59	27	12	98	34

8. *Prien et al.* (*1972a*)

In this multicentre trial, 255 manic patients were randomly assigned to treatment with lithium carbonate or chlorpromazine over a three-week period. The patients were classified into "highly active" and "mildly active" groups. Drug dosage was varied according to the patient's clinical state and the occurrence of side-effects. The median lithium level was 1·4 mEq/l for the highly active group and 1·2 mEq/l for the mildly active group. No other psychotropic drugs were given. The patient's clinical state was assessed using a number of different observer rating scales.

Amongst the highly active patients who completed the trial, no major difference in response was found between the lithium-treated and chlorpromazine-treated groups. However, there were significantly more early terminations on lithium than on chlorpromazine, and because of this the chlorpromazine-treated group as a whole fared significantly better than the lithium-treated group. Chlorpromazine controlled behaviour within a few days, whereas the therapeutic effect of lithium did not become evident until the tenth day of treatment.

In the mildly active group there was no significant difference in drop-out rate or in therapeutic response betwen the treatment groups.

A side-effects check-list was completed. The authors note that chlorpromazine produced more severe side-effects and left the patient feeling more fatigued and sluggish than did lithium.

C. Discussion

It is necessary to assess the evidence from two aspects. Firstly, is lithium therapeutically active against mania? Secondly, what is the relative efficacy of lithium as compared with other drugs?

Taken as a whole, the available evidence strongly supports the clinical impression that lithium salts have a therapeutic effect on mania which is greater than that of placebo. The comparison of the clinical effectiveness of lithium with that of other drugs is dealt with in detail in Chapter 7.

It appears that lithium is as effective as chlorpromazine in the treatment of mildly manic patients, but that more disturbed patients fare better on chlorpromazine. It is unfortunate that the antimanic effect of lithium has not been compared with that of other drugs such as haloperidol which many clinicians use in preference to chlorpromazine in the treatment of mania.

III. Factors Affecting Response to Lithium

The published data suggest that at least 20% of manic patients fail to respond to treatment with lithium. There is no clear evidence to suggest that the response to lithium treatment is influenced by the age or sex of the patient or by the number of previous episodes of affective illness. The major factors generally considered to be of importance in affecting the response to lithium are the symptomatology of the patient and the plasma lithium levels attained.

A. Symptomatology

Clinical experience indicates that lithium salts are effective not only against elated manic states, but also in the less common manic states in which irritability and hostility are predominant (Schou, 1963). There is evidence that patients with the classical symptoms of manic illness (Kraepelin, 1921) respond more favourably to lithium treatment than those with a less typical presentation. Thus, Schou et al. (1954) found that the presence of atypical symptoms, such as delusions without relation to mood, prolonged hallucinations, periods with reticence and contact difficulties, and gross hysterical symptoms, tended to be associated with a poor response to treatment.

The clinical criteria by which mania is diagnosed are variable and sometimes ill-defined. Marked differences in diagnostic usage have been found between psychiatrists in Britain and in the United States (Cooper et al., 1972). The borderline between schizophrenia and mania is a particularly difficult area, and the apparent co-existence of manic and schizophrenic symptoms in some patients had led to the use of the term "schizoaffective illness". It is of importance to assess the extent to which the response of manic patients is affected by the presence of an admixture of schizophrenic symptoms.

Although there are reports, based on uncontrolled observations, that lithium is of benefit to some patients diagnosed as schizophrenic (Carrere and Pochard, 1954; Glessinger, 1954; Margulies, 1955; Gershon and Yuwiller, 1960; Forssman and Wålinder, 1969; Meiers, 1970; Martorano, 1972), Shopsin et al. (1971) in a double-blind controlled trial were unable to demonstrate any therapeutic effect of lithium in these patients. There are several reports of improvement in patients with schizoaffective illness following lithium treatment (Rice, 1956; White *et al.*, 1966; Blinder, 1968; Gottfries, 1968; Zall *et al.*, 1968; Serry, 1969a,b; Sikes and Sikes, 1970). Most of these workers have stressed that although elevated mood and psychomotor excitement are reduced by lithium, the schizophrenic symptoms remain unchanged. In controlled trials, Johnson *et al.* (1968, 1971) could not demonstrate any beneficial effect from lithium treatment in a group of patients with schizoaffective illness. Prien *et al.* (1972b) found no clear differences in effect between chlorpromazine and lithium in the treatment of mildly active schizoaffective patients, but highly active patients clearly responded better to chlorpromazine.

The general impression is that although manic symptoms may decrease with lithium treatment, associated schizophrenic symptoms often worsen. This has led several authors (Zall *et al.*, 1968; Gattozzi, 1970) to suggest the use of lithium treatment as a differential diagnostic tool. However, the differences in response are probably not sufficiently clear-cut.

The evidence that the presence of schizophrenic or other atypical symptoms is associated with a less favourable response to lithium treatment emphasises the need for diagnostic criteria to be sharpened, standardized, and clearly defined, particularly in reports of clinical trials.

B. Dosage and plasma lithium levels

It is now standard practice to monitor plasma lithium levels during therapy. Clinical experience suggests that, 8–12 hours after the last dose of lithium, the plasma lithium level should be in the range $0 \cdot 8$–$1 \cdot 5$ mEq/l. However, the range recommended in the literature is variable (e.g. Warick, 1966; Gershon, 1970; Schou *et al.*, 1971; Brown, 1973). Until recently, no systematic work had been done on this topic. Prien *et al.* (1972c) examined the relationship between clinical response and plasma lithium levels in a group of manic patients given lithium or chlorpromazine in a double-blind trial. They found that levels exceeding $1 \cdot 4$ mEq/l, which are associated with an increased risk of toxic effects, produced no greater improvement in the clinical state of the patients. Patients with levels lower than $0 \cdot 9$ mEq/l responded poorly. An increased sodium intake is associated with a reduction in plasma lithium levels and an associated increase in manic symptoms (Platman and Fieve, 1969; Demers and Heninger, 1971).

A tendency for decreased lithium excretion during mania and increased excretion associated with recovery has been found by some workers (Trautner *et al.*, 1955; Greenspan *et al.*, 1968a, b; Serry, 1969a, b; Almy and Taylor, 1973), but not by all (Epstein *et al.*, 1965; Platman and Fieve, 1968; Platman *et al.*, 1968). Serry (1969a, b) developed a "lithium excretion test", based on measurement of urinary lithium excretion over a four-hour period following a loading dose of lithium carbonate. He found that the "lithium excreters" responded poorly to lithium therapy, whereas the "lithium retainers", who had lower plasma lithium levels, responded well. However, Stokes *et al.* (1972) found that the lithium excretion pattern did not predict the subsequent response to lithium therapy.

Trautner *et al.* (1955) reported that the doses of lithium required to treat manic patients were higher than normal subjects would tolerate, but that these high doses were no longer tolerated after recovery. Several authors (Gershon and Yuwiler, 1960; Schou, 1968; Prien *et al.*, 1971; Wren, 1972), have stated the need to reduce the dose of lithium after recovery from an acute manic attack. Conversely, an increase in lithium dosage is often of benefit in patients who have relapsed into mania whilst on prophylactic lithium therapy, particularly if the plasma lithium level is less than 0·8 mEq/l. Jacobson (1965) discusses the importance of recognizing the early signs of mania which he terms a "hypomanic alert", and it is at this stage that the dosage of lithium may often be increased with advantage.

In summary, the clinical response of manic patients to lithium therapy is reduced by the presence of atypical symptoms and by plasma lithium levels below 0·8 mEq/l. There remains, however, a proportion of typical manic patients who fail to improve despite adequate lithium levels. These non-responders cannot be clearly identified on clinical or biochemical grounds.

IV. Further Clinical Aspects

Lithium, when used as a therapeutic agent in an acute illness, is active primarily against manic states, although some success has been claimed in other disorders. Major tranquillizers, such as chlorpromazine, are active against a greater variety of states of agitation and overactivity. Several authors (Schou, 1968; Gershon, 1970; Wittrig and Coopwood, 1970; Shopsin and Gershon, 1971) have formed the clinical impression that lithium acts directly on the underlying manic process, whereas major tranquillizers merely suppress overactivity and restlessness, leaving the patient drugged and drowsy but still with the fundamental manic mood and ideation. Such an impression is very difficult to quantify. Johnson *et al.* (1968) considered that they had some evidence of such a differential effect. Prien *et al.* (1972a) were unable to demonstrate any clear differential action between chlorpromazine and lithium on manic mood or ideation, but chlorpromazine produced more drowsiness and sluggishness than lithium, and the rating scales used were not ideal for detecting these differences between the treatments. Further studies are necessary before the clinical impression can be confirmed or refuted.

It is generally agreed that the full therapeutic effects of lithium do not usually appear until the sixth to tenth day of lithium treatment. Because of this, lithium alone is unsuitable for treating highly active or disturbed patients in whom more rapid control is desirable. Several authors (e.g. Blinder, 1968; Schou, 1968; Baastrup, 1969; Tupin, 1970) recommend that treatment should be initiated with other drugs, either alone or in combination with lithium, in patients with severe manic illness. This suggestion was underlined by the finding of Prien *et al.* (1972a) that lithium was less effective than chlorpromazine in the treatment of a group of highly active manic patients.

Mildly manic patients, who may often be managed on an out-patient basis, can be treated with lithium alone, thus avoiding the drowsiness induced by tranquillizers. Lithium alone is also useful in the treatment of patients who are resistant or sensitive to tranquillizers (Wharton and Fieve, 1966).

The commonest drugs used in combination with lithium are the phenothiazines, such as chlorpromazine, or the butyrophenone haloperidol. The rationale behind such combinations is that the tranquillizer contains the behaviour of the patient until lithium cuts short the underlying manic process, at which stage the dose of tranquillizer can be reduced. It must be emphasized that the therapeutic superiority of such combinations over either treatment used alone has been observed clinically but not demonstrated by clinical trials.

Few other drugs have been used in combination with lithium in the treatment of mania, but there are some interesting possibilities. There are reports that imipramine may be of therapeutic benefit to some manic patients (Akimoto, *et al.*, 1960; Akimoto *et al.*, 1961). The use of a combination of amitriptyline and lithium in the treatment of mania is mentioned by Williamson (1966), and White *et al.* (1966) report success with a combination of imipramine and lithium in a manic patient who did not respond to lithium alone. The amino-acid tryptophan has been shown to be more effective than chlorpromazine in the treatment of mania (Wilson and Prange, 1972). A combination of lithium and tryptophan appears to be effective in some patients who fail to respond optimally to lithium alone, although again this impression requires confirmation by clinical trial. This observation may be of theoretical as well as practical importance, since there is evidence that lithium increases brain tryptophan levels and serotonin synthesis in rat brain (Tagliamonte *et al.*, 1971).

V. Summary and Conclusions

Most psychiatrists now accept that lithium has a useful part to play in the treatment of manic states. The evidence reviewed in this chapter supports this opinion. Patients must be carefully selected on clinical grounds, and adequate plasma lithium levels maintained. More severe cases of mania are probably best treated with a phenothiazine or haloperidol, either alone or in combination with lithium.

There is still room for further investigation. On the clinical side, further trials of lithium versus other antimanic agents, such as haloperidol or tryptophan, would be of great interest, as would trials attempting to examine the possible advantages of combination therapy. The impression that lithium acts primarily on the fundamental mood disturbance, whereas drugs like the phenothiazines have a much less specific tranquillizing effect, could be examined using sensitive rating scales designed for the purpose. It would be useful to have either a clinical or a biochemical method of identifying non-responders. It is necessary to investigate further the relationship between clinical response and plasma lithium levels. In the study by Prien *et al.* (1972c), the dose of lithium given was determined for each patient on clinical grounds. Ideally, dose-response studies should be carried out in which the patients are randomly allocated to various steady-state plasma levels of lithium.

The most fundamental problem is that of the mode of action of lithium, but consideration of this is outside the scope of the present chapter. If the mode of action can be established, then it may be possible to treat mania more specifically, rather than use lithium which appears to affect virtually every biochemical and physiological system which has been examined.

References

Akimoto, H., Nakakuki, M. and Machiyama, Y. (1960) *Dis. nerv. Syst.* **21**, 645–648.
Akimoto, H., Honda, Y., Takahashi, Y., Toyoda, J., Sasaki, K. and Machiyama, Y. (1961). *Proc. Third World Congr. Psychiat.* **2**, 958.
Almy, G. L. and Taylor, M. A. (1973). *Archs gen. Psychiat.* **29**, 232–234.
Baastrup, P. C. (1969). *Acta psychiat. scand. Suppl.* **207**, 12–18.
Blinder, M. (1968). *Int. J. Neuropsychiat.,* **4**, 26–27.
Brown, (1973). *Can. med. Ass. J.* **108**, 742–751.
Bunney, W. E., Jr. and Davis, J. M. (1963). *Archs gen. Psychiat.* **9**, 114–128.
Bunney, W. E., Goodwin, F. K., Davis, J. M. and Fawcett, J. A. (1968). *Am. J. Psychiat.* **125**, 499–511.
Cade, J. F. (1949). *Med. J. Aust.* **36**, 349–352.
Carrere, M. J. and Pochard, A. (1954). *Ann. med. psychol.* **112**, 566–572.
Cooper, J. E., Kendell, R. E., Gurland, B. J., Sharpe, L., Copeland, J. R. M. and Simon, R. (1972). "Psychiatric Diagnosis in New York and London" Maudsley Monograph No. 20, Oxford University Press, London.
Demers, R. G. and Heninger, G. R. (1971). *Amer. J. Psychiat.* **128**, 100–104.
Epstein, R., Grant, L., Herjanic, M. and Winokur, G. (1965). *J. Amer. med. Ass.* **192**, 149.
Forssman, H. and Wålinder, J. (1969). *Acta psychiat. scand. Suppl.* **207**, 34–39.
Gattozi, A. A. (1970). "Lithium in the treatment of mood disorders". National Clearing House for Mental Health Information: Washington D.C. Publication No. 5033.
Gershon, S. (1970). *Clin. Pharmacol. Ther.* **11**, 168–187.
Gershon, S. and Yuwiler, A. (1960). *J. Neuropsychiat.* **1**, 229–241.
Glessinger, B. (1954). *Med. J. Aust.* **41**, 277–283.
Goodwin, F., Murphy, D. and Bunney, W. (1969a). *Archs gen. Psychiat.* **21**, 486–496.
Goodwin, F. K., Murphy, D. L. and Bunney, W. E. (1969b). *Lancet* **2**, 212–213.
Gottfries, C. G. (1968). *Acta psychiat. scand. Suppl.* **203**, 157–167.
Greenspan, K., Green, R. and Durrell, J. (1968a). *Amer. J. Psychiat.* **125**, 512–519.
Greenspan, K., Goodwin, F. K., Bunney, W. E. and Durrell, J. (1968b). *Archs gen. Psychiat.* **19**, 664–673.
Jacobson, J. E. (1965). *Amer. J. Psychiat.* **122**, 295–299.

Johnson, G., Gershon, S. and Hekimian, L. J. (1968). *Compreh. Psychiat.* **9,** 563–573.

Johnson, G., Gershon, S., Burdock, A. F. and Hekimian, L. (1971). *Brit. J. Psychiat.* **119,** 267–276.

Kraepelin, E. (1921). "Manic Depressive Insanity and Paranoia", Livingstone, Edinburgh.

Lancet, (1969a), **1,** 709–710.

Lancet, (1969b), **1,** 83.

Maggs, R. (1963). *Brit. J. Psychiat.* **109,** 56–65.

Margulies, M. (1955). *Med. J. Aust.* **1,** 137–143.

Martorano, J. T. (1972). *Compreh. Psychiat.* **13,** 533–537.

Meiers, R. L. (1970). *Schizophrenia* **2,** 87–91.

Noack, C. H. and Trautner, E. M. (1951). *Med. J. Aust.* **38,** 219–222.

Platman, S. R. (1970). *Amer. J. Psychiat.* **127,** 351–352.

Platman, S. R. and Fieve, R. R. (1968). *Archs gen. Psychiat.* **19,** 659–663.

Platman, S. R. and Fieve, R. R. (1969). *Archs gen. Psychiat.* **20,** 133–137.

Platman, S. R., Rorlich, J. and Fieve, R. R. (1968). *Dis. nerv. Syst.* **29,** 733–738.

Prien, R. F., Caffey, E. M. and Klett, C. J. (1971). *Dis. nerv. Syst.* **32,** 521–531.

Prien, R. F., Caffey, E. M. and Klett, C. J. (1972a). *Archs gen. Psychiat.* **26,** 146–153.

Prien, R. F., Caffey, E. M. and Klett, C. J. (1972b). *Archs gen. Psychiat.* **27,** 182–189.

Prien, R. F., Caffey, E. M. and Klett, C. J. (1972c). *Br. J. Psychiat.* **120,** 409–414.

Rice, D. (1956). *J. ment. Sci.* **102,** 604–611.

Schou, M. (1963). *Brit. J. Psychiat.* **109,** 803–809.

Schou, M. (1968). *J. psychiat. Res.* **6,** 67–95.

Schou, M., Amdisen, A. and Baastrup, P. C. (1971). *Brit. J. hosp. Med.* **6,** 53–60.

Schou, M., Juel-Nielson, N., Strömgren, E. and Voldby, H. (1954). *J. Neurol. Neurosurg. Psychiat.* **17,** 250–260.

Serry, M. (1969a). *Lancet* **1,** 1267–1268.

Serry, M. (1969b). *Aust. N.Z. J. Psychiat.* **3,** 390–394.

Shopsin, B., Kim, S. S. and Gershon, S. (1971). *Brit. J. Psychiat.* **119,** 435–440.

Shopsin, B. and Gershon, S. (1971). *In* "Brain Chemistry and Mental Disease". (B. T. Ho and W. M. Isaac, eds.) pp. 319–377. Plenum Press, New York.

Sikes, J. C. and Sikes, S. C. (1970). *Dis. nerv. Syst.* **31,** 52–55.

Spring, G. K., Schweid, D., Gray, C., Steinberg, J. and Harwitz, M. (1970). *Amer. J. Psychiat.* **126,** 1306–1310.

Stokes, J. W., Shamoian, C. A., Stoll, P. M. and Patton, M. J. (1971). *Lancet* **1,** 1319–1325.

Stokes, J. W., Mendels, J., Secunda, S. K. and Dyson, W. L. (1972). *J. nerv. ment. Dis.* **154,** 43–48.

Tagliamonte, A., Tagliamonte, P., Perez-Cruet, J. and Gessa, G. L. (1971). *Nature New Biology* **229,** 125–126.

Trautner, E. M., Morris, R., Noack, C. H. and Gershon, S. (1955). *Med. J. Aust.* **2,** 280–291.

Tupin, J. P. (1970). *Hosp. Commun. Psychiat.* **21,** 73–80.

Warwick, L. H. (1966). *Dis. nerv. Syst.* **27,** 527–530.

Wharton, R. N. and Fieve, R. R. (1966). *Amer. J. Psychiat.* **123,** 706–712.

White, R. B., Schlagenhauf, G. and Tupin, J. P. (1966). *Curr. Psychiat. Ther.* **6,** 230–242.

Williamson, B. (1966). *Dis. nerv. Syst.* **27,** 775–782.

Wilson, I. C. and Prange, A. J. (1972). *Psychopharmacologia* **26,** (Suppl.), 76–78.

Wittenborn, J. R., Holzberg, J. D. and Simon, B. (1953). *Genet. Psychol. Monogr.* **47,** 301–306.

Wittrig, J. and Coopwood, W. E. (1970). *Dis. nerv. Syst.* **31,** 486–489.

Wren, J. C. (1972). *J. Maine med. Assoc.* **63,** 146–148.

Zall, H., Therman, P. O. G. and Myers, J. M. (1968). *Amer. J. Psychiat.* **125,** 549–555.

4

LITHIUM IN THE ACUTE TREATMENT OF DEPRESSIVE STATES

J. Mendels

I. Introduction

For more than a hundred years numerous claims have been made for the therapeutic efficacy of lithium salts in the treatment of a variety of specific medical disorders including gout, epilepsy and insomnia, as well as claims that it has more general functions as a "tonic" or "sedative" (Mendels and Secunda, 1972). It was 90 years after Garrod's (1859) original claims for a therapeutic role for lithium that Cade reported the successful treatment of ten manic patients with lithium salts (Cade, 1949). It took another 20 years for convincing proof to be gathered that lithium is an effective anti-manic agent and for a significant body of psychiatrists to be convinced of this.

    The more recent claims that lithium will reduce the frequency of relapses and recurrences in patients with manic-depressive (bipolar or biphasic) illness or recurrent unipolar or uniphasic depressive disorders has also been marked with controversy and uncertainty. It is only after some years of debate that a consensus is developing that lithium probably is effective in the prophylactic treatment of manic-depressive illness and perhaps (but less certainly) of recurrent depressive disorder.

Thus, it is not at all surprising that the suggestion that lithium carbonate may be effective in the treatment of yet another clinical condition, namely depression, should be regarded with reservation. This chapter will review the evidence for a possible role for lithium in the treatment of the clinical syndrome of depression. At the outset it should be said that controlled experience with lithium in the treatment of depression is very limited, and this review should therefore be viewed as a progress report rather than as a definitive statement.

Traditionally, psychobiology and psychopharmacology have tended to regard the clinical syndromes of mania and depression as polar opposite states. This is certainly supported by the more manifest symptomatology of these two syndromes. It is also clearly implied in the biogenic amine theories of affective illness which hold that there is a relative deficiency of one or other amine in depression and a relative excess of this amine in mania (Prange, 1964; Bunney and Davis, 1965; Schildkraut, 1965; Mendels and Stinnett, 1973; Mendels, 1974).

This has not always been the prevalent view. For example, Emil Kraepelin (1921) described a series of "mixed states" such as "depressive mania", "excited depression", "manic stupor", and "depression with flight of ideas". He noted that while these mixed states may occur during the transition from mania to or from depression, they also occurred as independent entities. Also, many psychoanalytic theorists have held that mania is not simply the opposite of depression but is a defense against an underlying depression.

My own interest in this area of investigation goes back about ten years when, in the course of a series of studies of the psycho-physiology of sleep with David R. Hawkins, we noted that the electroencephalographic sleep of a hypomanic patient (Mendels and Hawkins, 1971) was similar to that of a group of depressed patients who had been studied under the same conditions (Mendels and Hawkins, 1967)[1]. This led to a preliminary review of the literature in which we suggested that neurophysiological changes in depression and mania may have certain important characteristics in common (Whybrow and Mendels, 1969).

These observations led me to think that it was possible that lithium might exert an anti-depressant effect in selected depressed patients *because* it was an effective anti-manic agent (rather than *in spite* of the fact that it is an anti-manic agent as has been suggested). Subsequent investigations, to be reviewed later, provide some additional support for this view. Furthermore, a series of studies in our laboratory as well as by other investigators have provided additional data

---

[1] We have recently confirmed some of the main features of this finding (Chernik and Mendels, 1972).

pointing to the fact that mania and depression do share some important features and may not simply be polar opposite states.

The next section reviews reports from a number of investigators in which the anti-depressant effects of lithium were evaluated. For convenience, these reports are divided into two sections: uncontrolled and controlled studies.

II. Uncontrolled Studies

The anti-depressant effect of lithium was first evaluated by Cade (1949) who reported that lithium had no beneficial effect in a small group of depressed patients. Two years later another group of Australian investigators (Noack and Trautner, 1951) noted the absence of any therapeutic benefits in another small group of depressed patients given lithium carbonate. The absence of any details in their report makes it difficult to evaluate their finding.

Several years elapsed before other investigators pursued this line of investigation. There were then several reports from European investigators which suggested that there might be some therapeutic benefit from lithium. Vojtechovsky (1957) found that of 14 depressed patients who had failed to respond to treatment with electroconvulsive therapy, eight subsequently improved when given lithium. Andreani et al. (1958) reported that ten out of 24 very depressed patients appeared to benefit from lithium treatment. Hartigan (1963) reported that six out of eight manic-depressive patients (depressed type) who were treated with a combination of electroconvulsive therapy and lithium had a favourable response. While he implied that the lithium exerted some therapeutic effect, it is obviously difficult to separate this from the known anti-depressant benefits of electroconvulsive treatment.

There was an interval of several years before additional findings were published.

In 1968 William Dyson and I reported on the apparently successful treatment of 19 out of 31 depressed patients who were treated with lithium carbonate alone. The patients who showed a favorable response remained well for a mean follow-up period of 6·7 months[2]. It is important to note that we studied a heterogeneous group of inpatients and outpatients of varying degrees of severity of illness and almost certainly not all suffering from the same type of depression. While this was an uncontrolled study, several interesting trends emerged which we thought warranted further consideration. Of the 19 patients who improved, seven were diagnosed as suffering from manic-depressive illness, with a clear-cut history of both depressive and manic episodes, and ten gave a history suggestive of "cyclothymic personality". The other two responders had a history of recurrent depressive episodes. In contrast, nine of the patients who did not improve had a history of chronic depression which

---

[2] This does not mean that they then relapsed. The study was discontinued.

fluctuated in relationship to environmental events and three were diagnosed as suffering from an involutional depressive illness. Thus, bearing in mind the limitations of this uncontrolled study and the absence of predetermined criteria for making the diagnoses, our findings did suggest to us that there was a sub-group of depressed patients who responded to treatment with lithium and that these patients were more likely to have a history of recurrent (perhaps manic-depressive) illness. We also noted that the responders had a high incidence of family history of affective illness in contrast to the non-responders.

It is widely recognized that the clinical syndrome designated as depression almost certainly consists of a number of discrete subtypes with probable variations in symptomatology and pathophysiology, etiology and response to treatment (Mendels, 1968, 1970; Klerman, 1972; Robins et al., 1972). While a number of investigators have attempted to resolve this nosological problem, a simple solution continues to elude us. This obviously causes difficulties in evaluating reports of changes in groups of depressed patients. Some investi-gators do not provide any meaningful description of their patients at all. Others label them as unipolar or bipolar (or bipolar I and II); as endogenous or reactive; as neurotic or psychotic; as agitated or retarded; as primary or secondary; and so forth. While a detailed consideration of this problem is beyond the scope of this review, there is little doubt that there are important differences between groups of patients within the broad syndrome of depression and that continuing efforts must be made to define meaningful subtypes, be it in terms of response to a particular mode of treatment, a specific biochemical abnormality, the relationship to particular environmental events, etc.

With this in mind, we proceeded to a further examination of the clinical differences between the depressed patients who responded to treatment with lithium and those who did not respond. In addition to the fact that the responders seemed more likely to receive a diagnosis of manic-depressive illness or cyclothymic personality, and have a positive family history for affective illness, we found that they were characterized by symptoms usually associated with the syndrome of "endogenous" depression[3].

There are several other recent reports of uncontrolled observations of the anti-depressant effects of lithium. Zall et al. (1968) suggested that lithium alone was relatively ineffective in the treatment of acute depression. However, examination of their data shows that some of the patients who received lithium

---

[3] It should be noted that the use of the terms endogenous and reactive depression does not imply agreement with the etiological implications of these terms. They are simply used to designate descriptive clinical syndromes, the origins of which are undetermined at this time. This is discussed in greater detail elsewhere (Mendels and Cochrane, 1968). The findings in our review and the tentative conclusion that the clinical features associated with "endogeneous depression" may in fact represent the "core" of the syndrome of depression (Mendels, 1968, 1970) have recently been supported by Copeland et al. (1971). These conclusions are similar to those reached by Robins et al. (1972), in their concept of primary and secondary depressive illness.

did improve. They suggested that a combination of lithium with either a tricyclic anti-depressant or a monoamine oxidase inhibitor was a very effective form of treatment. They did not report any controlled evidence in support of this conclusion but did suggest that there may be a synergistic action between lithium on the one hand and tricyclics or monoamine oxidase inhibitors on the other.

Van der Velde (1970) reported no significant improvement in a small group of depressed patients who received lithium for 14 days and suggested that there may have been precipitation of a depression in association with lithium administration in a few patients. The absence of any controls makes it difficult to determine whether the depression in these patients was precipitated by the lithium or was a naturally occurring relapse (implying that the lithium was not exerting an effective prophylactic action).

Noyes et al. (1971) reported that four out of five depressed patients became symptom free when treated with lithium citrate. Furthermore, two of the four relapsed within 48 hours of placebo substitution. The fifth patient showed moderate improvement with lithium and also relapsed with placebo substitution.

Nahunek et al. (1970) reported that 54% of a group of 98 patients diagnosed as suffering from either "endogenous depression" or "involutional melancholia" improved when treated with lithium (300–2100 mg daily for an average of 26·4 days). Those who improved usually did so at the end of the first week or during the second week of treatment. This is a difficult study to evaluate. Not only was it uncontrolled but many of the patients received very low doses of lithium for short periods of time and thus may not have had an adequate exposure to the drug. In part, this appears to have been due to a high incidence of side effects. The authors concluded that lithium appeared to be as effective an anti-depressant as amitriptyline or imipramine. Furthermore, they suggested that lithium was not as effective as the demethylated tricyclic drugs (desimipramine, nortriptyline) in the treatment of retarded depressives but that it was more effective than those drugs in anxious and agitated depressives. These comparisons should be regarded with caution in that the drugs were not compared directly with each other nor was there randomization of patients between drug groups. They reflect the authors' clinical conclusions based on a series of consecutive studies. Further, the overall improvement rate of 54% noted in this study is probably not much better than the response to a placebo. However, in view of the fact that many of the patients probably did not receive an adequate trial of lithium, no conclusions can be reached.

Himmelhoch et al. (1972) recently reported the results of treating 21 depressed patients with a combination of lithium and tranylcypromine. Many of their patients showed a "modest but definite improvement" with lithium, and the addition of tranylcypromine seemed to "add the finishing touches". They note that all of the patients had previously had unsuccessful trials with tricyclic anti-depressants. The patients who responded were severely depressed, had hypersomnia and, while many had previous histories of mania, this did not appear to be a necessary prerequisite.

III Controlled Studies

Over the past few years there have been several controlled studies designed to evaluate the anti-depressant effectiveness of lithium.

A. Studies which report little or no anti-depressant action

The first study in this group was conducted by Hansen and his colleagues. Only a summary of this experiment has been reported (Schou, 1968) making interpretation of the findings difficult. They report no significant improvement in 12 patients with "severe endogenous depression" who were treated with lithium carbonate for two weeks. There was a cross-over between lithium and placebo and a criterion for improvement was that the patient relapsed when changed from lithium to placebo. Of the 12 patients studied only one demonstrated a clear-cut improvement with lithium followed by a relapse during the placebo period. Several other patients did improve with lithium administration but remained well when placebo was substituted, suggesting a spontaneous remission or a non-specific placebo response. It is not clear whether or not these patients had recurrent depressions and, if so, whether they were of the unipolar or bipolar type.

Fieve *et al.* (1968) compared the anti-depressant effects of lithium with imipramine in a group of 29 hospitalized depressed patients. They concluded that imipramine was clearly superior to lithium and that the latter had only a "mild anti-depressant effect".

Several points must be considered in evaluating their conclusions. They diagnosed their patients as suffering from manic-depressive illness but did not specifically report on a previous history of mania. Their diagnoses appear to have been based on a history of recurrent depressive episodes. Thus, while it is possible that these patients were indeed manic-depressives, it is equally likely (perhaps *more* likely in view of the relative frequency of the two states) that some of them may have suffered from recurrent uniphasic or unipolar depression. This may be an important point if there is a difference in the response to lithium between unipolar and bipolar depressive illness (see below).

Furthermore, their report does not include reference to the doses of lithium or imipramine or the plasma levels of lithium. Thus, we were not able to determine whether or not the differential response to the two drugs may have been related to dosage, or indeed whether the patients who were treated with lithium received an adequate dose and achieved a sufficient plasma level.

Clinical improvement was judged by changes in scores on several rating scales. Examination of the actual scores in their report does reveal a greater change in the patients who received imipramine than those who received lithium. However, no statistical tests are reported to show whether the response to imipramine was statistically superior to the response to lithium. This would have been useful before coming to any conclusion. Examination of the actual data presented in their report suggests that there was little apparent difference in the responses to lithium and imipramine after two weeks of treatment. At this time there was a definite change in both groups of patients (as reflected by the rating scale scores) with the response to imipramine proceeding at a faster rate than the response to lithium. However, there was continuing improvement with lithium treatment on three of the rating scales.

In the main, they determined clinical change by the use of two scales. One was the Zuckerman Multiple Affect Adjective Checklist (Zuckerman, 1960). We have reported elsewhere that there is some question as to whether this instrument provides a reliable and specific measure of changes in depression (Mendels et al., 1972c). They also used a single global depression item from the Psychiatric Evaluation Scale (Endicott and Spitzer, 1972). It is possible that the use of a global rating may not have been sufficiently sensitive adequately to reflect change in a complex clinical syndrome—as compared with a more broadly based rating scale.

Stokes et al. (1971) treated 18 patients with either lithium or placebo during 38 separate periods of depression (placebo during 21 and lithium during 17 periods). They found a statistically significant reduction in symptoms of depression during the period of lithium administration in comparison with depression ratings on the day prior to the institution of lithium treatment ($p < 0.005$), and also some impovement during the placebo periods. They suggest that there was no significant difference between the level of improvement achieved during the lithium and placebo periods.

They divided their patients into three categories: improved, worsened and no change. It would have been preferable if they had provided more specific details of the changes in the patients, as the therapeutic effect of lithium, if any, in depression is not absolute (as is the anti-depressant effect of the tricyclic drugs). Furthermore, they appear to have treated their patients with increasing doses of lithium for only ten days. This may not have been long enough. Thus, the trend towards improvement with lithium which is clearly suggested by their data may have been heightened by a longer treatment period or made more clear by a detailed description of the changes in their patients.

B. Studies which report significant anti-depressant activity

Goodwin et al. (1969, 1972) have reported two controlled studies during which patients received either a placebo or lithium on an alternating basis. There was a complete remission of symptoms in 15 patients and a partial remission in 21 patients out of 52 patients studied. One important criterion of improvement was that the patient should show significant improvement while receiving lithium and have a recurrence of symptoms with placebo substitution. A potential problem with this procedure is that the change in medication from lithium to placebo may be detected by the patient (for example, the disappearance of a fine lithium tremor or of the mild sedative effect which some patients experience with lithium). The published reports do not provide sufficient details of either the dose of lithium or plasma levels achieved and thus we cannot be certain that all of the patients had an adequate exposure to active treatment. It is thus conceivable that the remission rate may have been higher. They do confirm our original observation (Dyson and Mendels, 1968) that a significant therapeutic response is more likely to occur when there is a history of previous mania, as opposed to unipolar depressive illness.

Noyes *et al.* (1974) gave lithium to six bipolar and 16 unipolar patients in a placebo controlled study. All six of the bipolar and seven of the unipolar patients improved (Hamilton scores of 5 or less). Four of the seven unipolars who improved developed symptoms of lithium toxicity to "which their improvement appeared directly related". Of the 13 responders, nine had a "definite return of symptoms" with lithium withdrawal and placebo substitution. It is important to note that the unipolar patients who were studied had a relatively chronic history of depression and had often shown a poor response to previous therapies. The authors also suggest that an early age of onset of affective illness and a higher frequency of episodes may be factors associated with a positive response to lithium.

Johnson (1974) has reported on the successful treatment of ten hospitalized depressed patients of the "endogenous" type with lithium. The patients received placebo for an average of 9 days before lithium. Thereafter they were treated for a minimum of 21 days and attained serum lithium levels between 0·7–1·9 mEq/l. Striking improvement was noted in both Hamilton Depression Scale scores as well as in the Structured Clinical Interview. By global evaluation, five patients were judged to be "markedly" improved and five had a minimal improvement or no change. Johnson notes that the five patients who improved had been unresponsive to other drug treatments, hospitalization and placebo.

We have completed two controlled studies designed to evaluate the anti-depressant effects of lithium carbonate. In the first study (Mendels *et al.*, 1972b), we found that lithium was as effective as desmethylimipramine (DMI) in the treatment of selected depressed patients. This was a double-blind controlled study in which neither patients nor raters knew which drug was being administered. Twenty-four patients who scored at least 15 on the Hamilton Depression Rating Scale (Hamilton, 1960) and whose clinical profile was characterized by at least six of the following ten features were included in the study: at least two previous depressive episodes with a return to normal mood state in between; occurrence of mania or depression requiring hospitalization in a first-degree relative; lack of an apparent precipitating cause for the current episode; non-reactive (environmental events do not appear to exert a significant effect on the patient's mood or on the course of the illness); inevitability of clinical course (once begun the illness ran its course without the patient being able to influence significantly the presence or degree of symptomatology); self-blame rather than self-pity; poor concentration; loss of interest; sleep disturbance; suicidal thoughts or attempts.

The patients were randomly assigned to either desimipramine or lithium for an initial three-week treatment period. Desimipramine was given in doses of 100–200 mg daily and lithium carbonate in doses of 1000–2000 mg daily. All patients had blood drawn routinely for plasma lithium estimations and all bloods were processed whether or not the patient was receiving lithium. Dosage adjustments were allowed on study days 4, 7 and 14, depending on the patient's clinical response, emergence of signs of toxicity and, where appropriate, plasma lithium levels. These adjustments were made by a psychiatrist who had no direct contact with the patient and who was not involved in any of the evaluations or ratings.

In summary, nine of the 12 patients who received lithium improved by at least 50%[4], at the end of the three weeks of treatment. Six of the 12 patients who received desimipramine showed similar change (difference in improvement rates between the two drugs was not statistically significant). Further detailed analysis of the data indicated that the changes in the two groups were very similar (see Mendels *et al.,* 1972b for details). In this particular sample there was not a statistically significant difference in the rate of improvement between bipolar and unipolar patients. However, the numbers involved are small and no conclusions about this can be reached from this particular investigation. As noted in our earlier report (Dyson and Mendels, 1968), as well as in subsequent studies (Mendels and Frazer, 1973), there does appear to be a significant but not consistent association between clinical improvement and a diagnosis of manic-depressive illness.

One of the limitations of this study is the absence of a placebo group to control for the possibility of spontaneous remissions. However, the comparison with desimipramine is of interest in that it has been shown to be an effective anti-depressant agent. In their comprehensive review, Davis *et al.* (1968) noted

---

[4] Improvement was determined according to the percentage change on the Hamilton Depression Scale. We used the criterion of 50% as an index of improvement. It seemed to us that this answered the question of *how much* the patient changed during the study period. Thus, for example, a patient with an initial Hamilton score of 40 whose three-week score was 30 would be regarded as "less improved" (only 25% change) than a patient whose score went from an initial value of 25 to 15 (40%). Both patients had a 10 point change, while the second patient had a larger percentage improvement.

that, "in overall clinical efficacy, desimipramine is very much like its parent compound imipramine".

In a more recent study we have examined the effect of lithium carbonate on the clinical symptomatology of 21 severely depressed hospitalized patients with placebo control. It should be noted that this sample is not representative of the general syndrome of clinical depression in that all of the subjects were hospitalized males with a moderate or severe depression (mean Hamilton Depression score at time of entry into study was 28·1) and were studied on a research ward rather than in a general clinical setting.

The study involved the administration of increasing doses of lithium carbonate to either a point of clinical improvement, a dose of 2400 mg/daily, a plasma level of 1·5 mEq/l, or the development of significant toxicity. The period of lithium carbonate administration was preceded by 7–15 days of placebo administration and was followed by 7–22 days of placebo administration. Neither the patients nor staff were told when the changes in medication were made. Indeed, many of the staff were not even aware that a study was being conducted. The patients had signed a consent form in which they had been informed that, in addition to being treated with the active compound (i.e. lithium), they might receive an inactive placebo at some stage during the program. No further information was given which might have alerted them to the time of placebo administration. However, it is possible that they would have become aware of this as a result of some alteration in subjective or objective effects consequent on the lithium administration. Thus, while all efforts were made to keep the study double-blind, we cannot be certain that some patients might not have detected the changeover (see Chapter 8).

In this study, the primary criterion for improvement was that the patient had sufficient relief of symptomatology so as not to require any other form of active anti-depressant treatment. Using this criterion, 13 of the 21 patients showed

TABLE I. Clinical response to lithium

	n	Non-Responders	Responders	Responders Who Relapsed with Placebo substitution
Unipolar	8	4	4	1
Bipolar	13	4	9	6

unequivocal improvement. Of these 13 patients, seven relapsed with subsequent placebo administration (Table I).

The findings from this study, while not completely analyzed, together with the material reviewed here and elsewhere (Mendels, 1973), do support the view that at least some depressed patients do show a positive therapeutic response to treatment with lithium and that this is more likely to occur in patients with a diagnosis of manic-depressive illness. However, it is clear that not all patients with this diagnosis respond to treatment with lithium and that some patients with a diagnosis of recurrent unipolar depression appear to improve with lithium treatment. It is possible that at least some of the patients who were diagnosed as unipolar depressives will develop a manic episode in the future, necessitating a change in diagnosis. As we noted in our earlier study, improvement also was more likely to occur in the presence of a positive family history of affective illness. It is of interest to note that Mendlewicz et al. (1972) have reported that lithium appears more likely to exert a prophylactic effect in patients with a positive family history of affective illness.

Using a different approach, Lingjaerde et al. (1974) have reported that lithium enhances the anti-depressant action of tricyclic drugs, especially imipramine-N-oxide in "endogenous" depression. They conducted a double-blind study in which all of the patients received a tricyclic and either lithium or a placebo. The superiority of combination of the two drugs was evident after one and two weeks of treatment in the main sample in their study. (Forty-five patients were drawn from nine hospitals. Thirteen of the patients came from one unit, and it is in this group that positive findings emerged.) Age, sex or diagnosis (unipolar or bipolar) did not affect the outcome.

IV. Predicting Response to Lithium

A number of efforts have been made to develop an objective method of predicting which individual patients will respond to treatment with lithium. For example, Serry (1969) has suggested that improvement (in all groups of patients) is related to the amount of lithium excreted in the urine in a four-hour period after the ingestion of a single oral dose of 1200 mg of lithium. Unfortunately, we (Stokes et al., 1972) and others (Grof, personal communication; Gershon, personal communication) have not been able to confirm this claim. This lack of confirmation should be interpreted with caution in that we have also shown (Sugita et al., 1973) that there are significant differences in the rate of absorption of lithium depending on the particular commercial preparation being used. This could have contributed to our failure to replicate Serry's finding.

V. Intracellular Lithium Concentration

As part of our efforts to distinguish between responders and non-responders, we have recently examined the intra-erythrocyte (RBC) concentration of lithium under various conditions. We were interested in obtaining an intracellular measure of lithium as the plasma level of this cation is not always a good predictor of either clinical efficacy or pending toxicity. We assumed that the concentration of lithium in the brain is an important variable in determining the clinical response of individual patients and that an intracellular measure of lithium (e.g., RBC lithium) *might* provide a better correlation with brain lithium concentration than the extracellular or plasma measure does. We have now shown in rats that brain lithium concentration does have a significantly higher correlation with RBC lithium concentration than with plasma lithium under certain circumstances (Frazer *et al.*, 1973). This suggests that greater accuracy of predicting brain lithium concentration is achieved from knowing RBC lithium concentration than from knowing plasma lithium concentration. For example, the predictability of brain lithium concentration from RBC levels ranged between 64% and 88%. This contrasts with the predictability of brain lithium levels from a knowledge of plasma levels which ranged from a low of 17% to a maximum of 62%.

We hypothesized that depressed patients who respond to treatment with lithium would have higher RBC lithium concentration (for a given plasma lithium level) than patients who do not improve. In an early study (Mendels and Frazer, 1973) that we conducted to evaluate this hypothesis, we found that hospitalized male depressed patients who responded to treatment with lithium carbonate had a significantly higher RBC lithium concentration and RBC

TABLE II. Mean plasma and RBC Li and daily dose of lithium carbonate in patients who improved and who did not improve (from Mendels and Frazer (1973), with permission).

Patients	n	Daily dose of lithium carbonate (mg)	Plasma lithium (mEq/l)	RBC lithium (mEq/l RBC)	RBC lithium / Plasma lithium
Responders	8	$1572 \pm 92^*$	$1 \cdot 11 \pm 0 \cdot 07$	$0 \cdot 64 \pm 0 \cdot 07$	$0 \cdot 56 \pm 0 \cdot 03$
Non-responders	6	1836 ± 186	$1 \cdot 02 \pm 0 \cdot 06$	$0 \cdot 40 \pm 0 \cdot 03\dagger$	$0 \cdot 39 \pm 0 \cdot 02\ddagger$

$^*\overline{X} \pm$ S.E.M.
$\dagger$p $< 0 \cdot 02$ (Student's t test).
$\ddagger$p $< 0 \cdot 005$ (Mann Whitney U test).

lithium : plasma lithium ratio than depressed patients who did not respond to this treatment (see Table II). This difference was independent of the dose of lithium and the plasma lithium concentration, suggesting that the higher RBC lithium : plasma lithium ratio in the responders is a function of a proportionately higher red cell lithium concentration.

We have also found that male control subjects have a relatively low lithium ratio (0·3 mEq/l ± 0·02) as compared with our responders (mainly manic-depressives). Lyttkens et al. (1973) have reported that female manic-depressives have a significantly higher RBC lithium: plasma lithium ratio than control subjects but did not correlate the ratio with clinical change. These findings suggest that depressed patients who respond to treatment with lithium carbonate have some difference in cell membrane properties governing lithium entry into or out of the cell as compared with patients who do not respond to treatment with lithium. As we have noted, depressed patients who respond to treatment with lithium are more likely to have a previous history of mania than patients who do not. Thus, it is possible that people with manic-depressive illness may have some difference in cell membrane properties as compared with both control subjects and patients with other forms of depressive illness. We have elsewhere reviewed experiments that make it unlikely that the difference in red cell lithium: plasma lithium ratio between responders and non-responders is a function of differences in either dietary sodium intake or variations in plasma hormonal concentrations (Mendels and Frazer, 1974).

The RBC lithium: plasma lithium ratio appears to stabilize fairly early in treatment. Thus, there is little change in this ratio between day 7 and day 28 of lithium administration. Patients who have a relatively high ratio on day 7 do not usually change to a low ratio and, conversely, patients who have a low ratio at the end of one week of treatment do not usually develop a high ratio by day 28. We have noticed a tendency for the ratio to rise very slowly over months in a few patients and have wondered if this in any way correlates with Schou's (1968) suggestion that the long-term prophylactic effect of lithium may not be fully present in all patients for many months or even a year.

We have also examined changes in erythrocyte sodium concentration in depressed patients with particular reference to their relationship with RBC lithium concentration and clinical change. Erythrocyte sodium concentrations were measured by atomic absorption spectrophotometry, the value obtained being corrected for the amount of plasma trapped in the RBC column by the use of cobalt EDTA as an extracellular marker (Frazer et al., 1972).

At this time, information is available about changes in RBC sodium concentration in 12 depressed patients who were treated with lithium carbonate. A minimum of seven baseline (pretreatment) values were compared with values obtained during 21 days of lithium treatment during which the dose of lithium was either held constant or increased. During the baseline period there was no change in RBC sodium concentration, suggesting the stability of this measure, as noted by other investigators (Beilin et al., 1966a, b; Smith, 1972).

The effects of lithium on RBC sodium concentration are shown in Table III. The treatment period for each patient was divided into thirds, the mean for each period computed and a linear trend analysis done to determine the significance of changes in sodium concentration. There was a significant increase (F (linear)$= 5.60$; $p < 0.05$) in RBC sodium concentration with lithium administration, confirming our earlier finding in a single patient (Mendels et al., 1971). The increase in RBC sodium was most marked in patients who received the highest dose of lithium.

We also found an association between changes in RBC sodium concentration and alterations in the patients' clinical state. The depressed patients were

TABLE III. RBC Na change with Li

Li Dose	N	RBC Na (mEq/l)					P
		a	b	c	d	e	
>1500	7	7.8	7.9	7.9	8.4	9.1	$<.001$
<1500	8	8.1	8.2	8.3	8.6	8.6	NS

divided into two groups: (i) sodium increasers (the half of the sample that showed the largest increment in RBC sodium concentration during the period of lithium administration), and (ii) sodium non-increasers (the patients who showed little or no increase in RBC sodium concentration). Changes in depression rating scale scores for these two groups of patients are shown in Table IV. There was a significant decrease in the depression ratings for patients whose RBC sodium increased. In contrast, there was no significant change in ratings for the group of patients whose RBC sodium did not increase. This preliminary finding suggests that depressed patients who are treated with lithium carbonate and who show a subsequent increase in RBC sodium are more likely to improve than patients who are treated with lithium and who do not show an increase in RBC sodium concentration.

TABLE IV. Changes in depression ratings in groups classified by changes in RBC sodium[a]

	Nurses' depression score			Beck depression scores		
	a	b	c	a	b	c
Sodium Increase	8.4	8.2	5.8*	17.7	10.5	5.5**
No Sodium Increase	7.8	7.7	7.3†	19.8	13.4	14.4††
*F (lin)$= 8.8$ p<0.05				†F (lin) <1.0 NS		
**F (lin)$= 6.5$ p<0.05				††F (lin) $= 2.3$ NS		

[a]The treatment period was divided into equal thirds.

We have also shown that there is a statistically significant tendency for the RBC lithium : plasma lithium ratio to be higher in patients whose baseline sodium concentration is higher (Fig. 1). As noted above, there is a significant correlation between the higher RBC lithium : plasma lithium ratio and clinical improvement.

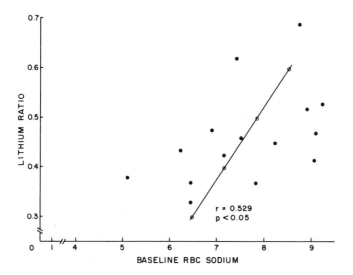

FIG. 1. Linear regression between baseline RBC Sodium and RBC Li: Plasma Li measured on day 14

We have done similar studies of changes in RBC potassium and magnesium and in plasma sodium, potassium and magnesium concentrations, and no significant changes have been found.

Our findings of associations between changes in RBC sodium, lithium administration and clinical improvement are compatible with the reports of Aronoff *et al.* (1971) and Baer *et al.* (1970) that patients who improved during lithium treatment had a significantly larger increment in the 24 hour exchangeable sodium than patients who did not improve.

Given these observations, it is obviously important to determine which systems are important in determining red cell lithium concentration. In a series of experiments (in collaboration with Alan Frazer, Ph.D., Arthur Schless, M.D. and Elizabeth Dorus, Ph.D), we have found that red cell lithum concentration is, at least in part, under genetic control and that the factors which regulate the distribution of lithium are similar to those which regulate sodium flux across the cell membrane. This suggests the possibility that there may be some genetically determined abnormality in sodium (and lithium) flux in these patients and that lithium may be useful in the identification of differences in cation transport in different patient populations.

The observations summarized here have led us to postulate as a working hypothesis that there is a sub-group of depressed patients who have a genetically determined abnormality in cell membrane properties regulating the movement of electrolytes across the plasma membrane (Mendels and Frazer, 1974). This sub-group of patients may partially overlap with a diagnostic group designated as showing manic-depressive illness, and is likely to have a positive response to treatment with lithium carbonate during the depressive phase.

If the RBC lithium ratio does reflect some inherent properties of the red cell, then it suggests the possibility that lithium may be used as a "marker" substance to detect biological differences among groups of depressed patients: differences which may not be apparent in the absence of the drug.

VI. Depression: A Heterogeneous State

While some workers have argued that the classification of psychiatric patients serves no purpose (Menninger *et al.,* 1963), suggesting that all mental illnesses are essentially the same, differing only in degree and form, there is evidence to suggest that this may be a shortsighted view. Classification has often been an essential step in the development of new concepts of medical disorders and this may apply to psychiatric illness as well. It is important to identify the clinical and biological features which characterize sub-groups of patients as well as those which distinguish between them. The same obviously applies to therapeutic response. In the main, attempts to divide depressed patients on the basis of their response to different anti-depressants has not been marked with particular success (Rush and Mendels, 1974). However, this relative failure in the past should not preclude future efforts.

Certainly our experience with lithium carbonate supports this approach. The controversy which surrounds its clinical effectiveness in depression may in part be due to the fact that investigators have studied different "types" of patients. Further, if our findings of a significant correlation between the RBC lithium: plasma lithium ratio and clinical response are confirmed, it would provide an important link between therapeutic response, a clinically based classification and biological specificity.

Failure to distinguish between meaningful sub-groups of depressed patients incurs the risk of obscuring highly significant findings which may apply to relatively small numbers of patients.

VII. Relationship Between Depression and Mania

If lithium is both an anti-manic and anti-depressant agent, it raises further questions about the current "bipolar" concept of their relationship. Some of these have been discussed earlier (Whybrow and Mendels, 1969; Mendels, 1970; Mendels, 1974), and need only be summarized here. There is evidence that many manic patients have concurrent symptoms usually associated with depression, including actual sadness, pessimism, guilt, self-doubt, crying and suicidal occupation (Winokur et al., 1969; Kotin and Goodwin, 1972; Mendels et al., 1974). The two states seem to show several biological abnormalities, including a reduction in cerebrospinal fluid 5-hydroxyindole-acetic acid (Mendels et al., 1972a); disrupted pattern of cortisol release into plasma (Sachar, 1973); reduced levels of platelet MAO activity (Murphy and Weiss, 1972); reduced erythrocyte catechol-O-methyl-transferase activity (Dunner et al, 1971); increased amplitude response in the cortical evoked potential (Buchsbaum et al., 1971); similar changes in the sleep electro-encephalogram (Mendels and Chernik, 1974); and reduced transfer of Na^{22} from plasma to cerebrospinal fluid (Carroll, 1972). Clearly, there is a need to re-evaluate the significance of these observations.

VIII. Recommendations for Further Investigations

While there has been an upsurge of interest in this area of investigation over the past few years, it is clear that only a small number of depressed patients have been included in systematic, well-controlled studies designed to determine the anti-depressant efficacy of lithium carbonate. This reviewer is of the opinion that there is evidence to support the claim that lithium is an effective anti-depressant agent in selected patients. However, this impression must be evaluated in further large-scale studies. Such studies, if they are to be useful in contributing to the clarification of this important problem should pay attention to the following:

(i) Clear and specific definition and description of the patients included in the study: these criteria should be carefully noted and reported.

(ii) Collection of information about important phenomenological, epide-miological and historical features of the illness: this information should be collected in a systematic, controlled fashion and correlated with response or non-response to lithium carbonate. The variables which need to be considered include pattern of the illness; previous history of depression and or mania; fre-quency of episodes; age of onset; presence of features of aggressive behavior either while depressed or as part of the personality; and family history of affective illness.

(iii) The effectiveness of lithium must be compared with established anti-depressant drugs and with placebo.

(iv) Attention must be paid to the dose of lithium, the duration of treatment and plasma levels. All of these should obviously be sufficient to insure adequate exposure to the drug.

(v) Further evaluation of the suggestion that there is a significant correlation between erythrocyte lithium concentration and clinical response.

(vi) Specific and detailed reports of clinical change using both observer and self-ratings must be included.

Acknowledgements

The preparation of this review and some of the studies summarized in it were supported in part by Research Funds from the Veterans Administration and by NIMH grant #1 RO3-MH16920.

A number of collaborators made valuable contributions to various phases of this work. Particular acknowledgement is due to Alan Frazer, Ph.D. Other co-workers include Elizabeth Dorus, Ph.D., William Dyson, MD, G. Pandey, Ph.D, Steven Secunda, MD and Arthur Schless, MD.

References

Andreani, G., Caselli, G. and Martelli, G. (1958). *G. Psichiat. Neuropatol.* **86,** 273–328.

Aronoff, M. S., Evens, R. G. and Durell, J. (1971). *J. psychiat. Res.* **8,** 139–159.

Baer, L., Durell, J., Bunney, W. E., Jr., Levy, B. S., Murphy, D., Greenspan, K. and Cardon, P. V. (1970). *Archs gen. Psychiat.* **22,** 40–44.

Beilin, L. J., Knight, G. J., Munro-Faure, A. D. and Anderson, J. (1966a). *J. clin. Invest.* **45,** 1817–1825.

Beilin, L. J., Knight, G. J., Munro-Faure, A. D. and Anderson, J. (1966b), *J. gen. Physiol.* **50,** 61–74.

Buchsbaum, M., Goodwin, F., Murphy, D. L. and Borge, G. (1971). *Amer. J. Psychiat.* **128,** 19–25.

Bunney, W. E., Jr. and Davis, J. M. (1965). *Archs gen. Psychiat.* **13,** 483–494.

Cade, J. F. J. (1949). *Med. J. Aust.* **36,** 349–352.

Carroll, B. J. (1972). *In* "Depressive Illness, Some Research Studies" (B. Davies, B. J. Carroll and R. M. Mowbray, eds.), pp. 247–260. Thomas, Springfield.

Chernik, D. A. and Mendels, J. (1972). *In* "Sleep Research" (M. H. Chase, W. C. Stern and P. L. Walter, eds.), Vol. 1, pp. 131. Brain Information Service/Brain Research Institute, University of California, Los Angeles.

Copeland, J. R. M. Cooper, J. E., Kendell, R. E. and Gourlay, A. J. (1971). *Brit. J. Psychiat.* **118,** 629–640.

Davis, J. M., Klerman, G. L. and Schildkraut, J. J. (1968). *In* "Psychopharmacology: A Review of Progress 1957–1967" (D. H. Efron, J. O. Cole, J. Levine and J. R. Wittenborn, eds.), pp. 719–738, U.S. Government Printing Office, Washington, D.C.

Dunner, D. L., Cohn, C. K., Gershon, E. S. and Goodwin, F. K. (1971). *Archs gen. Psychiat.* **25,** 348–353.

Dyson, W. L. and Mendels, J. (1968). *Curr. ther. Res.* **10,** 601–608.

Endicott, J. and Spitzer, R. L. (1972). *J. nerv. ment. Dis.* **154,** 88–104.

Fieve, R. R., Platman, S. R. and Plutchik, R. R. (1968). *Amer. J. Psychiat.* **125,** 487–498.

Frazer, A., Secunda, S. K. and Mendels, J. (1972). *Clinica chim. Acta* **36**, 499–509.
Frazer, A., Mendels, J., Secunda, S. K., Cochrane, C. M. and Bianchi, C. P. (1973). *J. psychiat. Res.* **10**, 1–7.
Garrod, A. B. (1859). "Gout and Rheumatic Gout". Walton and Maberly, London.
Goodwin, F. K., Murphy, D. L. and Bunney, W. E., Jr. (1969). *Archs gen. Psychiat.* **21**, 486–496.
Goodwin, F. K., Murphy, D. L., Dunner, D. L. and Bunney, W. E., Jr. (1972). *Amer. J. Psychiat.* **129**, 44–47.
Hamilton, M. (1960). *J. Neurol. Neurosurg. Psychiat.* **23**, 56–62.
Hansen, C. J., Retboll, K. and Schou, M. Quoted by Schou, M. (1968). *J. psychiat. Res.* **6**, 67–95.
Hartigan, G. P. (1963). *Brit. J. Psychiat.* **109**, 810–814.
Himmelhoch, J. M., Detre, T., Kupfer, D. J., Swartzburg, M. and Byck, R. (1972). *J. nerv. ment. Dis.* **155**, 216–220.
Johnson, G. (1974). *Compreh. Psychiat.* **15**, 43–47.
Klerman, G. (1972). *In* "Disorders of Mood" (J. Zubin and F. A. Freyhan, Eds.), pp. 165–193. John Hopkins Press, Baltimore.
Kotin, J. and Goodwin, F. K. (1972). *Amer. J. Psychiat.* **129**, 679–686.
Kraepelin, E. (1921). "Manic-Depressive Insanity and Paranoia". Translated by M. Barclay, Livingstone, Edinburgh.
Lingjaerde, O., Edlund, A. H., Gormsen, C. A., Gottfries, C. G., Haugstad, A., Hermann, I. L., Hollnagel, P., Mäkimattila, A., Rasmussen, K. E., Remvig, J. and Robak, O. H. (1974). *Brit. J. Psychiat.* Submitted for publication.
Lyttkens, L., Soderberg, U. and Wetterberg, L. (1973). *Lancet* **1**, 40.
Mendels, J. (1968). *Brit. J. Psychiat.* **114**, 1549–1554.
Mendels, J. (1970). "Concepts of Depression", John Wiley and Sons, Inc., New York.
Mendels, J. (1973). *In* "Lithium: Its Role in Psychiatric Research and Treatment" (S. Gershon and B. Shopsin, eds.), pp. 253–267. Plenum, New York.
Mendels, J. (1974). *In* "American Handbook of Psychiatry" (S. Arieti, ed.), pp. 448–479. Basic Books, New York.
Mendels, J. and Chernik, D. A. (1974). *In* "Comprehensive Textbook of Depression" (F. F. Flach and S. Draghi, eds.), in press. John Wiley and Sons, Inc., New York.
Mendels, J. and Cochrane, C. (1968). *Amer. J. Psychiat.* **124**, 1–11.
Mendels, J. and Frazer, A. (1973). *J. psychiat. Res.* **10**, 9–18.
Mendels, J. and Frazer, A. (1974). *Amer. J. Psychiat.* In press.
Mendels, J. and Hawkins, D. R. (1967). *Archs gen. Psychiat.* **16**, 344–354.
Mendels, J. and Hawkins, D. R. (1971). *Archs gen. Psychiat.* **25**, 274–277.
Mendels, J. and Secunda, S. K. (1972). "Lithium. Clinical and Research Aspects". Gordon and Breach, New York.
Mendels, J. and Stinnett, J. (1973). *In* "Biological Psychiatry" (J. Mendels, ed.), pp. 99–131. John Wiley and Sons, Inc., New York.
Mendels, J., Frazer, A., Secunda, S. K. and Stokes, J. W. (1971). *Lancet* **1**, 448–449.
Mendels, J., Frazer, A., Fitzgerald, R. G., Ramsey, T. A. and Stokes, J. W. (1972a). *Science* **175**, 1380–1382.
Mendels, J., Secunda, S. K. and Dyson, W. L. (1972b). *Archs gen. Psychiat.* **26**, 154–157.
Mendels, J., Weinstein, N. and Cochrane, C. (1972c). *Archs gen. Psychiat.* **27**, 649–653.
Mendels, J., Fitzgerald, R. G. and Stern, S. (1974). In preparation.

Mendlewicz, J., Fieve, R. R., Stallone, F. and Fleiss, J. L. (1972). *Lancet* **1**, 599–600.

Menninger, K., Mayman, M. and Pruyser, P. (1963). "The Vital Balance". Viking, New York.

Murphy, D. L. and Weiss, R. (1972). *Amer. J. Psychiat.* **128**, 1351–1357.

Nahunek, K., Svestka, J. and Rodova, A. (1970). *Int. Pharmacopsychiat.* **5**, 249–257.

Noack, C. J. and Trautner, E. M. (1951). *Med. J. Aust.* **38**, 219–222.

Noyes, R., Jr., Ringdahl, I. C. and Andreasen, N. J. C. (1971). *Compreh. Psychiat.* **12**, 337–347.

Noyes, R., Jr., Dempsey, G. N., Blum, A. and Cavanaugh, G. L. (1974). *Compreh. Psychiat.*, in press.

Prange, A. J., Jr. (1964). *Dis. nerv. Sys.* **25**, 217–221.

Robins, E., Munuz, R. A., Martin, S. and Gentry, K. A. (1972). *In* "Disorders of Mood" (J. Zubin and F. A. Freyhan, eds.), pp. 33–45. Johns Hopkins Press, Baltimore.

Rush, J. and Mendels, J. (1974). In preparation.

Sachar, E. Presented at the annual meeting, Psychiatric Research Society, Philadelphia, October, 1973.

Schildkraut, J. J. (1965). *Amer. J. Psychiat.* **122**, 509–522.

Schou, M. (1968). *J. psychiat. Res.* **6**, 67–95.

Serry, M. (1969). *Aust. N.Z. J. Psychiat.* **3**, 390–397.

Smith, E. K. M. (1972). *Clin. Sci.* **42**, 447–453.

Stokes, J. W., Mendels, J., Secunda, S. K. and Dyson, W. L. (1972). *J. nerv. ment. Dis.* **154**, 43–48.

Stokes, P. E., Shamoian, C. A., Stoll, P. M. and Patton, M. J. (1971). *Lancet* **1**, 1319–1325.

Sugita, E. T., Stokes, J. W., Frazer, A., Grof, P. and Mendels, J. (1973). *J. clin. Pharmacol.* **13**, 264–270.

Van der Velde, C. D. (1970). *Am. J. Psychiat.* **127**, 345–351.

Vojtechovsky, M. (1957). *In* "Problemy Psychiatrie v praxi a ve vyskumu", Praha. Quoted by Schou, M. 1968. *J. psychiat. Res.* **6**, 67–95.

Whybrow, P. C. and Mendels, J. (1969). *Amer. J. Psychiat.* **125**, 1491–1500.

Winokur, G., Clayton, P. J. and Reich, T. (1969), "Manic Depressive Illness". C. V. Mosby Company, St. Louis.

Zall, H., Therman, P. O. G. and Myers, J. M. (1968). *Amer. J. Psychiat.* **125**, 549–555.

Zuckerman, M. (1960). *J. consult. Psychol.* **24**, 457–462.

Note Added in Proof

In a recently completed study involving 17 depressed patients treated with lithium carbonate, we have found that the clinical improvement with lithium is significantly correlated with baseline platelet MAO level. Using tyramine as a substrate for the measurement of platelet MAO, we found that the nine patients who improved when treated with lithium had a mean pre-treatment platelet MAO level of $9 \cdot 91 \pm 2 \cdot 31$ (mean $\pm$ SEM) whereas the eight patients who did not improve with lithium had a mean baseline MAO level of $79 \cdot 2 \pm 11 \cdot 08$ (Mann-Whitney U test significant $p < 0 \cdot 001$). What was particularly striking was that there was absolutely no overlap in values between the two groups. Thus, the responders' platelet MAO values ranged between $0 \cdot 0$ and $16 \cdot 5$ and the non-responders' baseline values ranged between $32 \cdot 8$ and $112 \cdot 9$. If these findings are confirmed, then routine estimation of baseline platelet MAO levels may be a valuable method of selecting individual patients for treatment with lithium carbonate (S. Wilson, W. Dyson, J. Mendels, (in preparation)).

5

LITHIUM PROPHYLAXIS OF RECURRENT ENDOGENOUS AFFECTIVE DISORDERS

M. Schou and K. Thomsen

I. Introduction

The development of lithium prophylaxis and the scientific debate it generated have been described elsewhere (Schou, 1973). This chapter aims at reviewing the evidence available today and at comparing the results obtained in different studies. A number of two-group double-blind trials have been completed within recent years, and the results of these studies are discussed in detail. Since valuable information about lithium prophylaxis may be obtained from one-group non-blind trials, the assumptions underlying such studies are discussed, and the results of some of them presented.

In addition to the evidence obtained through systematic trials there is a body of clinical experiences and impressions which is less well documented but which may nevertheless be of theoretical interest and of practical value for the physician who is using lithium for the treatment of individual patients. Problems and observations of this kind are therefore also considered.

Observations dealing with comparisons of lithium and other drugs are reviewed in Chapter 7 and have therefore been omitted here.

II. Definition of Terms

1. *Recurrent endogenous affective disorders*

Prophylactic lithium treatment has been employed mainly for "recurrent endogenous affective disorders". This term as used here includes recurrent manic-depressive disorder of the bipolar type, recurrent or periodic endogenous depressions (the monopolar type), and recurrent schizo-affective disorder.

By the term "endogenous depression" is meant a disorder typified by certain signs and symptoms such as the subjective sensation of depression, diurnal variation of symptoms with nadir early in the morning, impairment of sleep, feelings of self-criticism, and suicidal ideas. The term is used without etiological preconceptions.

There is disagreement among psychiatrists about the concepts of endogenous and reactive depression. Some hold they are separate entities, whereas others regard all depressions as occurring in a continuum. In this chapter "endogenous depression" means the entity endogenous depression or the endogenous end of the depressive continuum.

"Schizo-affective disorder" designates a mixture or an alternation of manic-depressive and schizophrenic symptoms.

2. *The effect of long-term lithium treatment*

The effect of long-term lithium administration in recurrent endogenous affective disorders has been given various names: prophylactic, normothymotic, mood-normalizing, stabilizing, compensatory, regulatory, and it has been discussed whether one or the other term describes the action of lithium more precisely. This question will be dealt with later. When the terms "prophylactic action" and "maintenance treatment" are employed in the following, this is merely for convenience and does not necessarily mean that these are ideal.

3. *Episode and cycle*

"Episode" is used in this chapter synonymously with attack or phase of mania or depression. A "cycle" is the time from the start of one episode to the start of the following episode; it includes one episode and one interval.

III. Prophylactic Lithium Trials

A. Introduction

The prophylactic action of lithium has been established through two different kinds of study. In one, the frequency of manic and depressive episodes before lithium treatment was compared with the frequency during treatment; lithium was administered with the knowledge of patients and observers, i.e. non-blind. In the other kind of study, the frequency of episodes was compared in two groups of patients, one given lithium and the other placebo; in these studies lithium and placebo were given under double-blind conditions. The two-group double-blind studies are dealt with first.

B. Two-group double-blind trials

1. *Materials and methods*

At the present time eight two-group double-blind studies have been carried out. They differ as regards design, presentation of data, and statistical treatment of the results. In this chapter the studies are presented in such a way that their results are comparable. The reviewers have derived new data from those presented originally by the authors and subjected them to independent statistical assessment.

The design and special features of each two-group double-blind trial are shown in Table I, where the studies are listed in chronological order. Two different types of design have been used. In one, here called "the discontinuation design", patients already in lithium maintenance treatment were switched double-blind at a given point to either placebo or continued lithium. In the other design, here called "the start design", patients not previously given lithium prophylactically were allocated randomly to double-blind maintenance treatment with lithium or placebo.

In six of the eight studies, patients were included on the criterion of having suffered affective episodes with a frequency at or above a specified minimum during the years preceding the start of lithium maintenance treatment. In the study of Melia (1970) the patients were selected for not having had a single period of freedom from mood swings longer than nine months during the two years before lithium treatment was started. In the first study of Prien *et al.* (1973a) most of the patients had been hospitalized at least twice during the preceding two years.

In all the studies a mood swing was recorded as an episode when it was severe enough to necessitate either hospitalization or the administration of supplementary treatment.

TABLE I. Two-group double-blind trials: designs and features

Author	Design	Selection criterion	Trial period (months)	Serum lithium (mmoles/litre)
Melia (1970)	Discontinuation	—	24	Not determined
Baastrup et al. (1970)	Discontinuation	$\geqslant 2$ ep./2 years	5	0·6–1·5
Coppen et al. (1971)	Start	$\geqslant 3$ ep./3 years	14	0·7–1·2
Hullin et al. (1972)	Discontinuation	$\geqslant 5$ ep./5 years	6	0·6–1·4
Cundall et al. (1972)	Discontinuation	2 ep./3 years	6	0·5–1·2
Stallone et al. (1973)	Mixed discontinuation and start	$\geqslant 2$ ep./2 years	24–28	0·8–1·3
Prien et al. (1973 a)	Discontinuation	—	24	0·5–1·4
Prien et al. (1973 b)	Discontinuation	$\geqslant 2$ ep./2 years and $\geqslant 3$ ep./5 years	24	0·5–1·4

The trials were terminated according to different designs. In six of the studies, the patients were maintained on trial medication until a predetermined day when the study was terminated for the whole group. In the studies of Melia (1970) and Baastrup et al. (1970), each patient continued in the trial only until the occurrence of an episode. He or she was then taken out of the study, given appropriate antimanic or antidepressive treatment and returned to open lithium maintenance treatment. For the patients who did not relapse, the trial was brought to an end after a pre-fixed duration of two years in the study by Melia (1970). Baastrup et al. (1970) used a sequential analysis design and terminated the trial as soon as the border of significance had been reached ($p < 0.01$). They chose this design for ethical reasons, to reduce morbidity and suicide risk to a minimum.

2. Results

The results of the two-group double-blind trials were expressed in various ways. The one shown in Table II was chosen here because it permits comparison of the studies.

The table shows the total number of patients in each trial, the number who suffered relapse, one or more, during the trial period, and the number who completed the trials without suffering relapse. The total number of patients is counted here as those who entered the trial minus those who dropped out of it for irrelevant reasons: intercurrent disease, pregnancy, etc. Included in the number of patients who relapsed during the trial are those who dropped out because they relapsed, as well as those who completed the trial in spite of one or more relapses.

It appears from the table that fewer patients suffered relapse among those given lithium than among those given placebo. In most instances the difference had a high degree of statistical significance. The studies where differences were not significant or where the significance reached only the 5% level were based on small patient groups or short trial periods. Bipolar and monopolar patients responded equally well to lithium maintenance treatment.

3. Discussion

The outcome of the two-group double-blind trials was influenced by various factors, and it must be examined whether any of these introduced bias in favour of lithium or imposed limitations on the conclusions to be drawn from the studies.

The trials used a double-blind design, and leaks in the blindness involved risk that bias among the clinical assessors might influence the outcome. Data to be presented later in this chapter indicate, however, that possible leaks in the blindness are unlikely to have affected the results of the trials significantly. In agreement with this, Coppen et al. (1971) found no significant differences in

TABLE II. Two-group double-blind trials: patients having relapse and patients not having relapse during trial period.

Author	Diagnostic group	Medication	Total No. of patients[a]	No. of patients who during trial period		Significance[c]
				relapsed[b]	did not relapse	
Melia (1970)	Bipolar + monopolar	Lithium	9	5	4	n.s.
		Placebo	9	7	2	
Baastrup et al. (1970)	Bipolar	Lithium	28	0	28	p <0.001
		Placebo	22	12	10	
	Monopolar	Lithium	17	0	17	P = 0.001
		Placebo	17	9	8	
	Bipolar + monopolar	Lithium	45	0	45	p <0.001
		Placebo	39	21	18	
Coppen et al. (1971)	Bipolar	Lithium	16	3	13	p <0.001
		Placebo	22	21	1	
	Monopolar	Lithium	11	2	9	p = 0.01
		Placebo	14	11	3	
	Bipolar + monopolar	Lithium	27	5	22	p < 0.001
		Placebo	36	32	4	
Hullin et al. (1972)	Bipolar + monopolar	Lithium	18	1	17	p = 0.05
		Placebo	18	6	12	

Cundall et al. (1972)	Bipolar	Lithium	12	4	8	p < 0.05
		Placebo	12	10	2	
	Monopolar	Lithium	4	3	1	n.s.
		Placebo	4	2	2	
	Bipolar + monopolar	Lithium	16	7	9	n.s
		Placebo	16	12	4	
Stallone et al. (1973)	Bipolar	Lithium	19	5	14	p < 0.001
		Placebo	23	21	2	
Prien et al. (1973 a)	Bipolar	Lithium	85	36	49	p < 0.001
		Placebo	86	75	11	
Prien et al. (1973 b)	Bipolar	Lithium	14	5	9	p < 0.05
		Placebo	10	9	1	
	Monopolar	Lithium	23	13	10	p < 0.05
		Placebo	21	19	2	
	Bipolar + monopolar	Lithium	37	18	19	p < 0.001
		Placebo	31	28	3	

[a] Excluding patients who dropped out of the study for irrelevant reasons.
[b] Including patients who dropped out of the study because they relapsed.
[c] One-tailed fourfold table test (Documenta Geigy, 1970) for $N \leqslant 60$; χ^2-test for $N > 60$.

indices of morbidity between patients for whom the assessors guessed correctly whether the medication was lithium or placebo and patients where the guess was wrong.

It has already been mentioned that some of the studies were based on small patient groups or short trial periods; this reduced the chances of demonstrating statistically significant differences between the effects of lithium and placebo. The study of Baastrup *et al.* (1970) had a short trial period and yet achieved a high degree of statistical significance; this is because the patient groups were large.

The studies were carried out with patients suffering from the bipolar and the monopolar type of endogenous affective disorder. Data to be presented later in this chapter show that patients suffering from schizo-affective disorder respond less well to lithium maintenance treatment. Any admixture of the groups with such patients must therefore reduce the chances of demonstrating significant differences between lithium and placebo. In the first study of Prien *et al.* (1973a) six of the patients in the lithium group and two in the placebo group had a previous diagnosis of schizophrenia.

Patients often forget or neglect to take medication prescribed by the physician, and the risk of this is greater with prophylactic than with therapeutic drug administration because the patients over long periods of time are without any signs or symptoms to remind them of the disease and the treatment. In all but one of the two-group double-blind trials, serum lithium concentrations were determined at intervals. The patients accordingly knew they were under control, and this may have stimulated them to take their medication regularly. However, in the studies of Hullin *et al.* (1972) and Cundall *et al.* (1972), some of the patients were found to have serum lithium levels below the specified minimum at the time they relapsed. They were not excluded from the studies, and this reduced the chances of demonstrating significant differences between the effects of lithium and placebo. Moreover, there may have been patients who took their tablets only during the days preceding the control visit and therefore appeared to have been taking the medication as prescribed without actually having done so. Some of the relapses occurring in the group of patients given lithium may have developed as a result of such negligence; this again would reduce the chances of demonstrating a difference between the effects of lithium and placebo.

In Table II, patients were recorded as having relapsed or not having relapsed during the trial period and no respect was paid to the number of relapses each patient suffered. This procedure is adequate for testing the null-hypothesis that lithium exerts no more prophylactic action than placebo, but it leads to an underestimation of the prophylactic efficacy of lithium. In all the studies there were more placebo patients than lithium patients who relapsed. Therefore the lithium patients as a group were exposed for a longer time than the placebo patients to the risk of suffering relapse. In the study of Melia (1970), for example, the lithium patients were in the trial for a mean of 433 days and the placebo patients for a mean of 224 days. In the study of Stallone *et al.* (1973) the corresponding periods were 672 days and 250 days. The number of patients suffering relapse during treatment with lithium and treatment with placebo, respectively, should be seen in the light of this 2–3 times longer exposure period for the lithium patients.

The discontinuation studies were carried out with patient groups who had been in lithium treatment for some time before the trial; these groups may have had an overrepresentation of patients who responded to the treatment. This does not invalidate the trials, which tested the null-hypothesis that there was no difference between lithium and placebo, but it imposes a limitation on the conclusions that can be drawn concerning the quantitative efficacy of lithium treatment in unselected patient groups. Conclusions drawn from studies using the start design have no such limitations.

4. *Conclusions*

The eight two-group double-blind comparisons of lithium and placebo differ in a number of respects: design, duration of trial period, criteria for selection of patients, diagnostic composition of patient samples, etc. In spite of this, and in spite of the factors which reduced the chances of demonstrating a statistically significant difference between the effects of lithium and placebo, the trials show with striking similarity that lithium exerts a prophylactic action against further recurrences of endogenous affective disorder that is clearly superior to that of placebo.

During recent years the assertion has occasionally been made that lithium exerts prophylactic action in bipolar cases and not in monopolar cases. The statement is not supported by the evidence of these trials, which shows that the prophylactic efficacy of lithium is as good in the monopolar type of endogenous affective disorder as in the bipolar type.

C. One-group non-blind trials

The first evidence of a prophylactic action of lithium against not only manic but also depressive recurrences was obtained from trials carried out with one group of patients, studied before and during lithium treatment. They were based on an "open" design, with patients and physicians knowing that lithium was being administered. The one-group non-blind studies add evidence to that of the two-group double-blind studies concerning the prophylactic action of lithium in recurrent bipolar and monopolar affective disorder. Some of them include observations on patients with recurrent schizo-affective disorder and so provide information concerning the value of lithium maintenance treatment in this diagnostic group. They are therefore worth considering, but before they are dealt with, the assumptions underlying one-group non-blind studies will be examined. Recent years have brought evidence bearing on this matter.

1. *The role played by physician and patient attitudes*
It has occasionally been claimed that only studies controlled for the influence of observer bias and the psychological effect of the treatment, i.e. double-blind studies, yield valid information. This is clearly not so under all circumstances. If observer bias and the psychological effect of the treatment are without significance for the outcome of the trial, a non-blind design may yield equally valid information. The non-blind studies on lithium prophylaxis were based on the assumption that observer bias and psychological factors would be unlikely to exert significant influence on the frequency of recurrences in patients suffering from endogenous affective disorders.

Schou *et al.* (1970) determined the quantitative role played by patient and physician attitudes by comparing the rate with which relapse occurred after double-blind and after non-blind discontinuation of lithium maintenance treatment. When lithium was discontinued double-blind, observer bias and psychological factors continued to work at full force. When lithium was discontinued openly, the effect of these factors came to an end. If patient and physician attitudes exerted significant prophylactic action, this should therefore be reflected in a lower rate of relapse in the group of patients given placebo than in the group given no treatment.

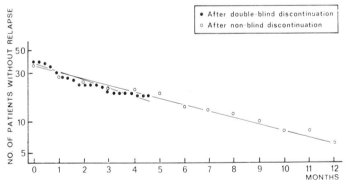

FIG. 1. Comparison of rates of relapse after double-blind and after non-blind discontinuation of lithium; semilogarithmic plot (reproduced by permission from Schou *et al.* (1970)).

The rates of relapse in the two groups were compared by recording the number of patients at the time lithium was discontinued and thereafter recording at short intervals the number of patients who had not yet suffered relapse. As more and more patients relapsed, the number remaining declined. Figure 1 shows a semilogarithmic plot of the observations. It will be noted that the group of patients given placebo and the group of patients given no treatment showed the same rate of relapse: every month the number of those not yet fallen ill was reduced by about 16%.

This study shows that a positively expectant attitude in physicians and patients does not provide effective protection against manic and depressive recurrences. No observations to the contrary have been published. Long-term prophylactic studies of recurrent endogenous affective disorders are consequently not invalidated by being carried out according to a non-blind design.

2. *The prognosis of groups of patients having had frequent affective episodes during recent years*

The one-group studies were carried out with patients selected for having had one or more episodes per year during the two or three years preceding lithium treatment. The studies were based on the assumption that in the absence of prophylactic measures a patient group thus selected would be likely to continue having a high frequency of episodes during the following two or three years.

Ottosson and his associates (Laurell and Ottosson, 1968; Isaksson *et al.*, 1969) studied the course of recurrent manic-depressive disorder in patients admitted to the Psychiatric University Clinic in Umeå in the years 1963–1965. The first admission during this time was used as a dividing point between two 2-year periods: period *a* preceding the admission and period *b* following it. During none of the periods were the patients given prophylactic treatment. A total of 62 patients fulfilled the criterion of having had two or more episodes during period *a* (counted backwards from the start of the admission which resulted in inclusion in the study). The patients suffered 97 episodes during period *a* (the "index" admission being excluded from the calculation), and they suffered 89 episodes during period *b*. This indicates that a group of patients selected for having had frequent episodes during the past two years are likely to have frequent episodes also during the following two years.

Corresponding results were obtained in a similar study from the Psychiatric University Clinic in Zurich (Angst *et al.*, 1969), which was carried out on 37 patients fulfilling the selection criterion and not being given prophylactic treatment. The patients suffered 54 episodes during period *a* and 53 episodes during period *b*.

Schou *et al.* (1970) employed a different approach, using patients in whom prophylactic lithium treatment was discontinued after some time. They compared the rate with which these patients suffered relapse during the period of selection, i.e. before lithium treatment was started, with the rate of relapse after discontinuation of lithium (Fig. 2). The rate of relapse was high during the period of selection and low while the patients were being treated with lithium. After discontinuation of lithium, the rate of relapse rose to the pretreatment level. If the selection procedure had been responsible for the fall during the period of lithium treatment through picking out a patient group with a good prognosis, discontinuation of lithium should not lead to any rise in the rate of relapse. The data in Fig. 2 show that the patients were in fact as prone to suffer relapse after discontinuation of lithium as they had been before lithium treatment started.

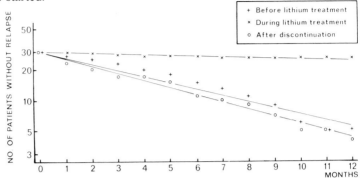

FIG. 2. Comparison of rates of relapse before lithium treatment and after its discontinuation; semilogarithmic plot. A line showing the rate of relapse during lithium administration has been included (reproduced by permission from Schou *et al.* (1970)).

Grof *et al.* (1970) did a similar study and obtained similar results. Their patients had also been selected on the basis of having had two or more episodes within the two years preceding lithium treatment. During a 10-month period prior to lithium treatment, 26 of their 33 patients suffered relapse; during a 10-month period following discontinuation of lithium, 31 of the 33 patients relapsed.

A single study led to results that were radically different from those reported above. From the Psychiatric Register of Camberwell, Saran (1970) selected 32 patients with endogenous depression, manic-depressive psychosis, schizoaffective psychosis, or atypical psychosis, who had been hospitalized at least twice during 1966. For these patients, who were not given prophylactic treatment, the Register showed a total number of 79 episode starts during the two years 1965 and 1966 and only 20 episode starts during the following two years, 1967 and 1968.

With the exception of Saran's study, the evidence indicates that groups of patients selected for having had at least one episode per year during a particular period are likely to have episodes with approximately the same frequency during a later period. Prophylactic studies of recurrent endogenous affective disorders are therefore not invalidated by being based on this assumption.

3. *Results, discussion and conclusions*

One-group non-blind studies of lithium prophylaxis now number close to one-hundred. They differ considerably in documentary value. Some are of high

TABLE III. One-group non-blind trials: number of patients showing a fall, no change, or a rise in relapse frequency during lithium treatment.

Author	Diagnostic group	Mean duration of lithium treatment (months)	No. of patients	No. of patients whose relapse frequency showed			Significances	
				a fall	no change	a rise	Falls vs. rises[a]	Schizo-affective vs. bipolar + polar[b]
Angst et al. (1970)	Bipolar	39	114	76	26	12	p < 0.001	
	Monopolar	27	58	33	20	5	p < 0.001	
	Schizo-affective	28	72	35	25	12	p < 0.01	n.s.
Egli (1971)	Bipolar	24	10	4	5	1	n.s.	
	Monopolar	16	10	7	2	1	p < 0.05	
	Schizo-affective	24	25	16	6	3	p < 0.01	n.s.

[a] One-tailed sign test.
[b] χ^2-test and fourfold table test.

TABLE IV. One-group non-blind trials: number of episodes and mean relapse frequency before and during lithium treatment

Author	Diagnostic group	Mean duration of lithium treatment (months)	No. of patients	No. of episodes and, in parenthesis, mean relapse frequency		Significance	
				Before lithium treatment	During lithium treatment	Before vs. during[a]	Schizo-affective[b] vs. bipolar + monopolar
Angst et al. (1970)	Bipolar	39	114	329 (0·9)	121 (0·3)	p < 0·001	
	Monopolar	27	58	154 (1·2)	42 (0·3)	p < 0·001	
	Schizo-affective	28	72	118 (0·7)	72 (0·4)	p < 0·02	p < 0·001
Egli (1971)	Bipolar	24	10	18 (0·9)	8 (0·4)	n.s.	
	Monopolar	16	10	20 (1·5)	9 (0·7)	n.s.	
	Schizo-affective	24	25	52 (1·0)	21 (0·4)	p < 0·01	n.s.

[a] Wilcoxon's matched-pairs signed-ranks test, calculated by the authors.
[b] χ^2 – test, calculated by the reviewers.

quality, carefully planned and executed and containing valuable clinical observations. Others have serious shortcomings as regards the number of patients studied, the length of the study period, the criteria on which patients were selected, etc.

There is hardly any reason to review all the one-group non-blind studies here. The majority, which includes all systematic studies with large patient groups and long observation periods, show clear-cut prophylactic action of lithium in bipolar and monopolar affective disorder and therefore lend further empirical support to the conclusions drawn from the two-group double-blind studies.

Some one-group non-blind studies contain observations concerning the effect of lithium maintenance treatment in recurrent schizo-affective disorder; those in which the authors explicitly excluded index episodes from their calculations are presented in Tables III and IV. Equally long observation periods before and during lithium treatment were compared for each patient. It appears from both tables that lithium exerts significant prophylactic action in recurrent schizo-affective disorder. According to the study of Angst et al. (1970) the action is less pronounced in this diagnostic group than in bipolar and monopolar affective disorder.

Angst et al. (1970) further examined the actions of lithium in bipolar, monopolar, and schizo-affective disorder by analysing its effect on the duration of episodes and the duration of cycles. Episodes were shortened somewhat during lithium treatment in bipolar patients and of unchanged duration in patients with monopolar and schizo-affective disorder. In contrast to this, the duration of cycles and hence of intervals was markedly prolonged. In bipolar and monopolar patients the cycle prolongations were 61% and 76%, respectively. In schizo-affective patients the prolongation was only 30%. Significance levels for the prolongations were $p < 0.001$, $p < 0.001$, and $p < 0.01$, respectively. It should be noted that these figures underestimate the prophylactic effect of lithium because cycles not concluded at the end of the observation period were counted as if they ended in a relapse at that point.

In assessing observations on schizo-affective patients one should keep in mind that such patients are apt to neglect their medication, especially if it has become part of a paranoid system with ideas of persecution and fear of poisoning. It is, however, questionable whether this alone accounts for the lower prophylactic efficacy of lithium in schizo-affective disorder.

D. Concluding remarks

The systematic studies on the effects of lithium maintenance treatment have borne three important fruits:

(i) The prophylactic action of lithium in recurrent endogenous affective disorders has been confirmed through work carried out by a number of research groups with a variety of experimental designs.

(ii) Evidence has been provided concerning the nature and course of recurrent endogenous affective disorders. It is now known that a positively expectant attitude of physicians and patients does not guard against further manic and depressive recurrences. It is also known that groups of patients having had frequent recurrences within a certain period are likely to have frequent recurrences also during a later period when given no prophylactic treatment.

(iii) Experimental designs for prophylactic trials differ from designs for therapeutic trials. Work with lithium maintenance treatment has led to the development of a number of such prophylactic designs. This may pave the way for further prophylactic trials in psychiatry.

IV. Clinical Problems and Observations

Many aspects of lithium prophylaxis have not been subjected to systematic investigation of the kind described above and therefore remain in the realm of clinical experiences and impressions. This does not mean they are valueless. They may, in fact, be of considerable use in the employment of lithium for treatment of individual patients.

A. Indications for lithium maintenance treatment

1. *Diagnosis*

The studies reviewed in the previous sections showed that lithium treatment exerts its best prophylactic action in the bipolar and monopolar types of endogenous affective disorder but that it also prevents or ameliorates recurrences of schizo-affective disorder to some extent. There is a single study (Prien *et al.*, 1972) which indicates that lithium treatment counteracts both affective and schizophrenic behaviour of schizo-affective patients, at least in mildly active cases. But it is the experience of most authors that whereas lithium may lower the frequency and severity of mood swings and of periods of aggressiveness, it does not exert any significant action on the more typical schizophrenic symptoms such as hallucinations, autism, and delusions. Johnson (1970) even reported that lithium treatment may lead to a worsening of schizophrenic symptoms, but this seems to be an exception rather than a rule.

At the present time it is not possible to give a general answer to whether patients with recurrent schizo-affective disorder should be given lithium maintenance treatment. There is a growing body of clinical experience which indicates that such patients may benefit from long-term treatment with a combination of lithium and a neuroleptic drug.

2. *Frequency and severity of episodes*

In most of the prophylactic trials the patients were selected for having had recurrences of a certain frequency and severity during recent years, for example two or more episodes requiring hospitalization during the last two years. It is important to note that the criteria used for systematic trials cannot be used rigidly for deciding whether individual patients should be given lithium. According to clinical experience, patients with milder and less frequent episodes may also benefit from the treatment. The patients' entire situation as well as the severity of the disease should be taken into account when long-term lithium treatment is being considered.

B. Start of the treatment

Some patients obtain full prophylactic effect from the beginning of the lithium treatment; they suffer no further recurrences of mania or depression. There are other patients in whom the prophylactic action seems to set in gradually so that they have recurrences during the first months of the treatment. In order to reduce the risk of relapse it is therefore important to start prophylactic lithium treatment as soon as possible after the decision about this treatment has been made. That raises the question whether lithium treatment can be started irrespective of whether the patient is in a manic episode, in a depressive episode, or in an interval between episodes.

Starting lithium treatment during an interval or during a mania presents no problems. In the case of mania, the therapeutic and the prophylactic uses of lithium merge. There has been some doubt about the advisability of starting lithium while patients are being treated with tricyclic antidepressants. Lingjærde (1973) has now presented evidence that lithium treatment given together with tricylic antidepressants does not diminish but rather enhances their therapeutic effect.

C. Duration of the treatment

Patients given lithium maintenance therapy understandably often ask how long they must remain in treatment. This question cannot be answered for the individual patient, but evidence pertaining to a group of patients was obtained in the discontinuation study of Baastrup et al. (1970).

Patients who had had one or more episodes per year for at least two years were given lithium maintenance treatment for periods of varying length and were then switched to placebo. After this discontinuation of lithium, the patients who had been in treatment for a long time (4–7 years) relapsed as readily as those having been treated for a shorter time (1–3 years). Continuation of lithium treatment beyond seven years seems accordingly indicated for this group of patients. We do not know whether individual patients in the group might discontinue lithium earlier with impunity. Nor do we know how long lithium should be given to patient groups selected on less stringent criteria. The frequency and severity of the episodes that occurred before lithium treatment must be taken into consideration when patient and physician discuss the advisability of trying to discontinue lithium after it has been given for a number of years.

D. Psychological and social implications of successful lithium prophylaxis

When lithium maintenance treatment changes a life that was previously dominated by frequent and severe manias and depressions to one that is stable month after month, year after year, this is a major event with far-reaching consequences for the patients themselves and for their families and acquaintances (Schou and Baastrup, 1973).

There often develops around a patient with frequent and severe affective episodes a peculiar psycho-social pattern in which patient, spouse, children, friends, and associates all play special roles in a combined effort to mitigate the consequences of the patient's incessant mood changes. This is altered by successful lithium maintenance treatment. Recurrences become few and mild and eventually disappear completely. The patient once more becomes the person he or she was before the disease first started, fear is eventually replaced by confidence in the future, and everybody can breathe a sigh of relief.

However, all is not bliss in every instance. There are patients who feel that lithium treatment makes life "flat" and less colourful, "curbs" their activity, and prevents them from going as fast as they would like (Schlagenhauf *et al.,* 1966; Baastrup and Schou, 1967; Dyson and Mendelson, 1968; Schou, 1968; Vaadal and Robak, 1968; Warick, 1970; Wittrig and Coopwood, 1970). Patients who profited personally or professionally from frequent and long periods of hypomania before lithium treatment may for this reason dislike the effects of the treatment and even reject it (Baastrup and Schou, 1967; Schou, 1968; Böszörményi, 1970; Marshall *et al.,* 1970; Bertagna *et al.,* 1971; Polatin and Fieve, 1971). Some businessmen and executives claim that the hypomanic impetus and energy is necessary for their work and that lithium makes them less capable. Some artists assert that the hypomanic inspiration and indefatigability are essential for both the quality and quantity of their work and that lithium treatment inhibits their creative power. It should be noted, however, that many patients who initially miss the hypomanias eventually get accustomed to the new and stable life course and discover with pleased astonishment that their productivity and creative power are now as good as or better than before lithium treatment started.

For the patients' families and friends a feeling of immense relief is usually the dominant reaction to the results of successful lithium prophylaxis, but sometimes they need time to adjust to the new situation. This is best illustrated by the effect of lithium treatment on marital relations (Dyson and Mendelson, 1968; Mayo, 1970; Demers and Davis, 1971). Successful lithium prophylaxis leads to a radical reshuffling of roles and responsibilities in the family, and the main sufferer under this may be the spouse, whose central role as heroic upholder of home and family is threatened by the patient's re-emergence as a normal person. In these instances, the spouse may become anxious or depressed and be in need of psychiatric assistance during the period of adjustment.

E. Change of recurrences during lithium treatment

Lithium maintenance treatment usually leads to an attenuation of manic or depressive recurrences; sometimes they are only moderately ameliorated, often they disappear completely or appear only in the form of "abortive" attacks. Episodes that are only partially abolished may occur with the same frequency as before lithium treatment. More often they occur less frequently, in some cases their frequency is increased for a shorter or longer period (Michaelis, 1972; Kukopulos and Reginaldi, 1973).

Recurrences of mania and depression which occur during lithium treatment usually present the same symptomatology as the episodes that occurred before lithium treatment was started; the changes produced by lithium are confined solely to frequency and severity. There are, however, instances where the episodes take on a new character during lithium treatment. Dostal (1971) reported the development of "pseudoneurotic" episodes at the time when ordinary affective episodes could have been expected. Arnold (1973) noted the occurrence of mixed manic-depressive conditions, of dysphoria and increased sensitivity, and of narrowing of the emotional range and impoverishment of the quality of affective experiences. Böszörményi (1970) observed transitory confusions or panics, sometimes with compulsive acts and psychomotor unrest; and Krauss and Lauter (1971) saw in some patients persistence of hypomanic restlessness without manic elation, lowered ability to concentrate, and transitory experiences of derealisation ("Entfremdung").

A number of authors have recorded that in some patients the removal of manic-depressive episodes may lead to the appearance of paranoid traits and other personality deviations which previously had been hidden behind the symptoms of the affective disorder (Baastrup and Schou, 1967; Fann et al., 1969; Aronoff and Epstein, 1970; Warick, 1970; Maletzky and Blachly, 1971; Villeneuve et al., 1971).

When manic and depressive episodes are attenuated by lithium maintenance treatment, it becomes increasingly difficult to distinguish between pathological mood changes and changes that are within the normal range of mood variations. It is therefore impossible to give precise data for the frequency with which lithium-treated patients are freed entirely of affective episodes and the frequency with which such episodes occur in mild form and at long intervals. It is the reviewers' impression, supported by experiences reported by others, that most lithium-treated patients occasionally experience abortive episodes or "reminders". These are periods of a few days or a week during which the patients have the feeling that a mania or a depression might be underway without this ever actually happening. Patients in whom the episodes came very regularly before lithium treatment sometimes report that the reminders appear at the time episodes could have been expected.

V. Terminological Reconsiderations

Early in this chapter it was mentioned that the effect of long-term lithium treatment, as well as the treatment itself, have been given several names. We may now consider the proposals in more detail.

Hartigan (1963) first used the term "prophylactic action" because he found lithium of little or no therapeutic value in acute depressive episodes but had promising results when using long-term lithium administration against depressive recurrences. This use of the word has occasionally been criticized on the ground that prophylaxis means the long-term action exerted by a single or a few administrations of a particular procedure, for example vaccination. Defined this narrowly, prophylaxis cannot be used about long-term lithium treatment, which must be continued in order to keep the recurrent affective disorder under control. Prophylaxis may, however, be used in a broader sense.

As pointed out above, lithium may in some instances affect the intensity of recurrences rather than their frequency, and attempts have therefore been made to replace the word "prophylaxis" with a more adequate term: "normo-thymotic" or "mood-normalizing treatment" (Schou, 1963), "stabilizing action" (Baastrup et al., 1970), "compensatory treatment" (Freyhan, 1971), and "regulatory treatment" (Glenn and Reading, 1973). Each of these terms has its advantages; all require the qualification that it is only mood changes of the endogenous type and not mood changes or mental functions in general that are being normalized, stabilized, compensated for, or regulated.

The term "lithium maintenance treatment" has been used frequently in this chapter. It covers maintenance of a normothymic state through lithium treatment in patients with recurrent endogenous affective disorder; it also means treatment given in such a way that an appropriate lithium concentration is maintained in the organism.

We still know so little about what lithium actually does to the patients and their disease that it may be too early to put a definitive name to its effect. Studies on the biochemical mode of action of lithium may lead to deeper insight and more precise terminology.

VI. Summary

Two-group double-blind studies as well as one-group non-blind studies have provided evidence of the ability of long-term lithium administration to prevent or attenuate recurrences of endogenous affective disorder. Lithium prophylaxis appears to be equally effective in bipolar and monopolar cases, less effective in recurrent schizo-affective disorder. Research on lithium prophylaxis has shed light on the nature and course of recurrent endogenous affective disorders. The clinical application of lithium maintenance treatment presents a number of problems concerning indications, start of treatment, duration of treatment, and the psychological and social problems that may arise as a result of successful lithium prophylaxis. Knowledge about these problems is important for full utilization of the treatment.

Acknowledgements

We are indebted to Mrs. Audrey Miller and Dr. D. F. Smith for critical comments on our manuscript.

References

Angst, J., Grof, P. and Schou, M. (1969). *Lancet* 1, 1907.

Angst, J., Weis, P., Grof, P., Baastrup, P. C. and Schou, M. (1970). *Brit. J. Psychiat.* 116, 604–614.

Arnold, O. H. (1973). Paper read at symposium in Nuremburg, October 1973.

Aronoff, M. S. and Epstein, R. S. (1970). *Amer. J. Psychiat.* 127, 472–480.

Baastrup, P. C. and Schou, M. (1967). *Archs gen. Psychiat.* 16, 162–172.

Baastrup, P. C., Poulsen, J. C., Schou, M., Thomsen, K. and Amdisen, A. (1970). *Lancet* 2, 326–330.

Bertagna, L., Peyrouzet, J. -M., Quétin, A. -M. and Dalle, B. (1971). *Rev. Prat. (Paris)* 21, 1743–1757.

Böszörményi, Z. (1970). *Int. Pharmacopsychiat.* 4, 204–209.

Coppen, A., Noguera, R., Bailey, J., Burns, B. H., Swani, M. S., Hare, E. H., Gardner, R. and Maggs, R. (1971). *Lancet* 2, 275–279.

Cundall, R. L., Brooks, P. W. and Murray, L. G. (1972). *Psychol. Med.* 2, 308–311.

Demers, R. G. and Davis, L. S. (1971). *Compreh. Psychiat.* 12, 348–353.

Documenta Geigy (1970). *In* "Scientific Tables", pp. 109–123. J. R. Geigy, Basle.

Dostal, T. (1971). *Activ. nerv. sup. (Praha)* 13, 170–171.

Dyson, W. L. and Mendelson, M. (1968). *Amer. J. Psychiat.* 125, 544–548.

Egli, H. (1971). *Schweiz. med. Wschr.* 101, 157–164.

Fann, W. E., Asher, H. and Luton, F. H. (1969). *Dis. nerv. Syst.* 30, 605–610.

Freyhan, F. A. (1971). *Am. J. Psychiat.* 128, 121–122.

Glen, A. I. M. and Reading, H. W. (1973). *Lancet* 2, 1239–1241.

Grof, P., Cakuls, P. and Dostal, T. (1970). *Int. Pharmacopsychiat.* 5, 162–169.

Hartigan, G. P. (1963). *Brit. J. Psychiat.* 109, 810–814.

Hullin, R. P., McDonald, R. and Allsopp, M. N. E. (1972). *Lancet* 1, 1044–1046.

Isaksson, A., Ottosson, J. -O. and Perris, C. (1969). *In* "Das depressive Syndrom" (H. Hippius and H. Selbac, eds.), pp. 561–574, Schwarzenberg, München, Berlin and Wien.

Johnson, G. (1970). *Dis. nerv. Syst.* 31, 613–615.

Krauss, B. and Lauter, H. (1971). *Nervenarzt* 42, 356–359.

Kukopulos, A. and Reginaldi, D. (1973). *Int. Pharmacopsychiat.* 8, 152–158.

Laurell, B. and Ottosson, J. -O. (1968). *Lancet* 2, 1245–1246.

Lingjærde, O. (1973). *Lancet* 2, 1260.

Maletzky, B. and Blachly, P. H. (1971). "The Use of Lithium in Psychiatry". CRC Press, Cleveland.

Marshall, M. H., Neumann, C. P. and Robinson, M. (1970). *Psychosomatics* **11**, 406–408.

Mayo, J. A. (1970). *Int. Pharmacopsychiat.* **5**, 190–202.

Melia, P. I. (1970). *Brit. J. Psychiat.* **116**, 621–624.

Michaelis, R. (1972). *Nervenarzt* **43**, 437–438.

Polatin, P. and Fieve, R. R. (1971). *J. Amer. med. Assoc.* **218**, 864–866.

Prien, R. F., Caffey, E. M. and Klett, C. J. (1972). *Archs gen. Psychiat.* **27**, 182–189.

Prien, R. F., Caffey, E. M. and Klett, C. J. (1973 a). *Archs gen. Psychiat.* **28**, 337–341.

Prien, R. F., Klett, C. J. and Caffey, E. M. (1973 b). *Archs gen. Psychiat.* **29**, 420–425.

Saran, B. M. (1970). *Int. Pharmacopsychiat.* **5**, 119–131.

Schlagenhauf, G., Tupin, J. and White, R. B. (1966). *Amer. J. Psychiat.* **123**, 201–206.

Schou, M. (1963). *Brit. J. Psychiat.* **109**, 803–809.

Schou, M. (1968). *J. psychiat. Res.* **6**, 67–95.

Schou, M., Thomsen, K. and Baastrup, P. C. (1970). *Int. Pharmacopsychiat.* **5**, 100–106.

Schou, M. (1973). *In* "Lithium. Its Role in Psychiatric Research and Treatment" (S. Gershon and B. Shopsin, eds.), pp. 269–294, Plenum, New York and London.

Schou, M. and Baastrup, P. C. (1973). *In* "Psychopharmacology, Sexual Disorders and Drug Abuse". (T. A. Ban, J. R. Boissier, G. T. Gessa, H. Heinmann, L. Hollister, H. E. Lehmann, I. Munkvad, H. Steinberg, F. Sulser, A. Sundwall and O. Vinař, Eds.), pp. 65–68, North-Holland Publ. Co., Amsterdam and London. Avicenum, Prahue.

Stallone, F., Shelley, E., Mendlewicz, J. and Fieve, R. R. (1973), *Amer. J. Psychiat.* **130**, 1006–1010.

Vaadal, J. M. and Robak, O. H. (1968). *T. norske Laegeforen.* **88**, 1578–1582.

Villeneuve, A., Langlois, M., Chabot, C., Dogan, K., Lachance, R. and Laurent, C. S. (1971). *In* "Advances in Neuro-Psychopharmacology" (O. Vinař, Z. Votava and P. B. Bradley, Eds.), pp. 55–62. North-Holland Publ. Co., Amsterdam.

Warick, L. H. (1970). *Bull. Los Angeles neurol. Soc.* **35**, 169–180.

Wittrig, J. J. and Coopwood, W. E. (1970). *Dis. nerv. Syst.* **31**, 486–489.

6

LITHIUM IN THE TREATMENT OF CONDITIONS OTHER THAN THE AFFECTIVE DISORDERS

N. S. KLINE and G. M. SIMPSON

I. Introduction

The use of lithium in other than affective disorders can be conveniently divided into two categories: (1) those of recurring cyclical or episodic nature and (2) non-episodic conditions. The use of lithium in psychiatry began in the late 19th century, when lithium bromide was used as a sedative and anti-convulsant. Good (1903), in his pioneering experimental studies in lithium, detailed its toxic effects, but also quoted Weir Mitchell as stating that lithium bromide "was as efficient as sodium or potassium bromide, and that its influence over insomnia was greater" (p. 283).

Although a few years later, Squires (1916) was to state, "In epilepsy for rapid action and for soothing purposes, it is the best of the bromides" (p. 844), lithium bromide failed to attain a widespread use. Skin rashes and other toxic side effects of the bromides eventually eliminated their use in medicine and especially so when better substitutes were found.

II. Recurring, Cyclical and Episodic Disorders

A. Epilepsy

Curiously, one of the toxic manifestations of lithium treatment is convulsions, yet lithium carbonate is reported to be an effective anti-convulsant agent. Thus, Erwin *et al.* (1971; 1973) did a 6-week study of lithium carbonate in 17 hospitalized epileptics, 15 poorly controlled, one well controlled and one with an abnormal EEG but without clinical manifestations. One patient had increased seizure activity while ten showed a clear reduction of seizure frequency. James and Reilly (1971) found paroxysmal events in an EEG study were benefited by lithium which they reported as having a "normalizing effect". Of 49 epileptics treated with lithium (and initially with anti-convulsants) Gershon and Yuwiler (1960) report that 60% showed a decrease in seizure frequency and a behaviour improvement between seizures. Jus *et al.* (1973) have reported on the benefits of lithium carbonate in patients with temporal lobe epilepsy. Other writers have also recounted the beneficial effect of lithium in epilepsy: Glesinger (1954); Gershon and Trautner (1956); Williamson (1966); Gershon (1968); and Tupin and Smith (1972).

Isolated case reports, however, relate the onset of status epilepticus in non-epileptic patients as possibly being due to lithium used at dose levels within the normal therapeutic range (Baldessarini and Stephens, 1970). Demers *et al.* (1970) also suggest that "in seizure-prone individuals, lithium may, by some unknown mechanism, induce seizures when serum lithium values are not in the toxic range" (p. 316).

The use of lithium in epilepsy is almost a century old. While the reports are in some ways controversial, the concensus of opinion seems nonetheless to show that lithium has a beneficial effect on epileptics and also on abnormal EEGs. The specific benefits claimed in temporal lobe epilepsy, a difficult condition to treat, certainly warrant further investigation, as does the suggestion that lithium has an overall beneficial effect on all types of epilepsy.

The converse finding that lithium can produce epileptic siezures, requires further investigation particularly as there has been some suggestion that this happened within the therapeutic dose range. That this should be a manifestation of lithium toxicity is not surprising since many drugs can have a reversal of effect in the toxic dose range.

B. Recurring aggression

The reduction of paroxysmal brain activity might in some way be related to the effect of lithium on aggressive behavior was mentioned by Cade in his 1949 study in animals and later confirmed by Weischer (1969) and Sheard (1970). Sheard (1971) was also the first to study this effect in humans. In a study of lithium in prisoners he selected inmates with a previous history of three or more episodes of violent, assaultive crime and with prison behavior characterized by continuing verbal and physical aggressive behavior. The prisoners also had high scores on aggression items of the MMPI and BUSS Rating Scale for Aggression. A self-rating scale with ten items was completed each evening. These included depressive items but also items relating to anger, suspiciousness, and tension. A symptom check-list was completed weekly and the number of incidents of verbal and/or physical aggressiveness were recorded. Likewise, verbal hostility was rated during a clinical interview. A single blind study with drug and placebo given for a four week period in an alternating sequence was then carried out. Serum lithium was maintained between 0·6 mEq/l and 1·5 mEq/l. There was a significant reduction (at the $p < 0.01$ level) in "aggressive affect" associated with a reduction in the number of reprimands for physical or verbal aggression.

Tupin (1972) and Tupin et al., (1973) in a study of 27 male convicts exhibiting violent behavior attempted to replicate the study of Sheard (1971). He selected patients who showed a pattern of frequent violence in and out of prison and a rapid reaction of anger or violence to slight provocation. Diagnoses were schizophrenia, 8; possible schizophrenia, 4; sociopathic personality, 12; others, 3. Previous drugs had been ineffective in controlling their behavior and in this one and a half year study, lithium was given under open conditions with data collected from prison guards and from changes in the patients' security classification as well as by reports from the subjects and observations by the psychiatrist. The mean observation time of prisoners on lithium was 9·9 months. The results showed a significant decrease at the $p < 0.01$ level in the number of disciplinary actions. The subjects felt more in control (which was validated by the observers.)

The problem of aggression is one of intense interest at this moment and obviously covers a wide spectrum of conditions ranging from the normal to extreme pathology. The work in animals (see Chapter 19) strongly suggests that lithium has a beneficial effect on aggressive behavior. The extrapolation from animals to humans is always fraught with danger; nonetheless, the studies in aggressive prisoners carried out by at least two investigators, provide strong supplemental evidence for a lithium effect in this area. The social problems involved and the type of behavior discussed are of such a magnitude that a large-scale controlled study of lithium in this use is urgently needed.

C. Aggressive behavior in children and adolescents

Annell (1969) in an uncontrolled study reported on twelve adolescents of whom only two were diagnosed as suffering from mania. Five cases suffered from attacks resembling periodic catatonia. All illnesses were of a periodic nature. Other diagnoses included a questionable organic syndrome, a post-encephalitic picture and a variety of neurotic states. Many of the patients showed a distinct abnormal personality and indeed, two were admitted to hospital because of delinquency. Eleven of the twelve cases improved. Similarly, Forssman and Wålinder (1969) reported case histories showing that lithium was effective in a variety of atypical conditions. Of the 27 cases reported on, nine cases showed no response and in four of these cases there was evidence of a phasic course which was not, however, described. The diagnosis is not given, but in both confusional states and hyperactive, aggressive states, improvement was noted. Dostal and Zvolsky (1972) reported on 14 severe mentally retarded aggressive adolescents treated for eight months with lithium. Patients were rated once a month, by two independent raters. The trial was uncontrolled, but a statistically significant improvement was noted in aggressiveness, psychomotor activity, restlessness, and undisciplined behavior as well as affectivity. A 65% reduction in outbursts of aggressive behavior was noted throughout the treatment period. In a provocative article, Dyson and Barcai (1970) selected from a group of lithium responding parents, children who had symptoms of hyperactivity, short attention span, low frustration tolerance, explosive anger followed by guilt, sulkiness, depression and poor school performance despite obviously adequate intelligence. One of the two cases reported on, with a diagnosis of "hyperkinetic syndrome" initially responded to amphetamine, but improvement was not maintained. This patient improved on lithium and regressed when it was withdrawn. The second case was not typical of a hyperkinetic syndrome and did respond briefly to amphetamine but responded much better to lithium and also relapsed when it was withdrawn. Many of the symptoms of depression described by Frommer (1968) would fit the hyperkinetic syndrome but no details are given to illustrate the good results claimed with lithium alone or combined with anti-depressants.

Whitehead and Clark (1970) reported on seven children between the ages of 5 and 9 years diagnosed as hyperactive. The children were given lithium carbonate 6–10 mg per pound per day for periods of 4–12 weeks alternating with 4–8 week periods of placebo. Six of the children also received thioridazine in dosages from 0·6 to 1·5 mg per pound per day for a period of 3–6 weeks. Patients were seen weekly and the parents were asked to report activity levels and general behavior. During the last 6 months, a study of each child's activity level was recorded by a "trained observer." No difference between lithium and placebo was noted. Blood levels, though, were not reported in this study so there is a question of whether the dose was adequate. This is particularly pertinent since excretion rates can be very high in children. Gram and Rafaelsen (1972) carried out a double-blind study of 18 psychotic children of mixed diagnoses who had received either lithium or placebo for 6 months and then crossed over to the other drug for the remaining 6 months. The dosages were adjusted to give a therapeutic serum lithium level. Patients were rated by parents and school teachers. After a child's parents were interviewed, a rating scale was used by the teacher to evaluate the patients and was completed daily. The school ratings clearly showed positive effects of lithium treatment.

Lithium and placebo were compared in a double-blind crossover trial in a group of 21 patients with emotionally unstable character disorders, defined by Rifkin et al. (1972) as having chronic maladaptive behavior patterns such as poor acceptance of reasonable authority, truancy, poor work history, manipulativeness, but with co-existing disturbance of depressive and hypomanic mood swings that lasted hours to days. Patients received lithium for 6 weeks and placebo for 6 weeks. There was no time interval between the two administrations. The blood levels of lithium were maintained between 0·6 to 1·5 mEq/l. All patients were free of medication for at least three weeks before entering the study. Statistical analysis showed that lithium carbonate was consistently superior to placebo on the rating scales used.

Campbell et al. (1972) compared chlorpromazine and lithium in a controlled cross-over trial in ten hyperactive, severely disturbed young children, aged 3 to 6 years, six of whom were schizophrenic and one autistic. The patients were matched for motor-activity and prognosis. A 4-week drug-free period separated the cross-over. Lithium was given in therapeutic dosages and chlorpromazine given at 90 mg per day. The authors concluded that, in general, neither lithium nor chlorpromazine were good psychotropic agents for this group. Lithium treatment, however, did produce reduction in explosiveness, aggressiveness, hyperactivity and psychotic speech. The major improvement took place in one well-studied schizophrenic, a boy, who showed auto-aggressive, self-mutilating behavior. Cooper and Fowlie (1973) also reported on the control of self-mutilating behavior in a severely subnormal 20 year old male who received lithium.

In a search for treatment of those hyperactive children who failed to respond to stimulants Greenhill et al. (1973) gave lithium to nine subjects of whom two, with an affective element in their disorder, improved temporarily.

The studies of the effects of lithium on adult aggression have been complemented by the studies on aggressive behavior in children and adolescents. These latter have been mainly of an uncontrolled nature in a very heterogeneous diagnostic grouping ranging from definite organic cases to periodic catatonia, but particularly interesting are the studies on mentally retarded aggressive adolescents, a notoriously difficult group to treat. The positive results obtained in these and in hyperkinetic cases strike the writers as of great potential importance. The presence of a negative study once again highlights the need for further work in this area, though the fact that blood levels were not monitored has already been noted as a criticism of this particular study. Perhaps of more importance is the study of 18 children of mixed diagnoses where a clear lithium effect was shown on their rating at school. The school rating seems to combine both a psychological and a functioning type of evaluation and therefore is perhaps a very sensitive one.

The effect of lithium on self-mutilating behavior is also of interest, particularly as Campbell's case was in a controlled trial. Isolated cases of drug effects in this condition appear from time to time in the literature, but perhaps because of the small number of such patients, no adequate large scale trials have been carried out. The relation of self-aggression to outwardly-directed aggression is one that is poorly understood and the information here, while provocative, is also very preliminary.

D. Aggression in seizure disorders

In a study examining lithium in convulsive disorders, Erwin et al. (1973) reported that lithium not only had an effect on convulsive disorders but also appeared to reduce the level of hostile behavior in patients. In a follow-up study by Morrison et al. (1973), carried out in two parts, 20 inpatients were studied, including 11 with frequent seizures and hyperaggressivity, two with normal EEG's and no seizures but with hyperaggressive behavior, and seven without clinical seizures but with 14 and 6 per second spiking.

Four of these latter showed hyperaggressive behavior. In the second part of the study, 12 patients were referred by the staff because of hyperaggressive behavior and seven were accepted for the study (four of these had received a diagnosis of schizophrenia). They received 3 weeks placebo and 3 weeks lithium treatment. The Buss-Durkee inventory for aggression-hostility was completed at the beginning of the placebo period and at the end of the treatment period. In the first part of the study, 15 patients (as judged by nursing notes and interviews) showed reduction in the frequency of hyperaggressive, assaultive behavior, a decreased tendency to quarrel and greater self-control when provoked. In the second part of the study, the results were mixed with only two patients improving significantly, i.e. scores decreased by more than 25%. In their summary, the number of patients reported on is less than that stated at the beginning and while the results are not conclusive, there would nonetheless appear to be a reduction of hyperaggressive behavior.

If lithium is effective in seizure disorders, then it is perhaps not too surprising that claims have been made for an effect on the behavior associated with seizure disorders. Thus, there are reports on the beneficial effects of lithium in aggression accompanying seizure disorders which might be explained either as the result of the anticonvulsant effect of lithium or as a specific anti-aggressive effect. However, the studies carried out in this area leave much to be desired.

E. Psychopathy and sociopathy

Baastrup (1969) and Jacobsen (1965) report anecdotally on good results in treating psychopathic personalities. Gershon (1971) in his review article also comments on the usefulness of lithium in a sociopathic personality.

F. Mental defectives

In a 2 year double-blind trial of mentally defective inpatients Naylor et al. (1974) evaluated 14 patients subject to recurring affective or behavioral changes. The total number of weeks ill during the year on lithium was significantly less than during the year on placebo. The actual number of episodes was also fewer but not at a statistically significant level. Thus, the major effect was on the duration of the episodes.

G. Schizophrenia

Cade (1949), in his original article, and later Glesinger (1954) and Vartanian (1959) all found lithium useful in schizophrenic patients with excitement. All three studies were uncontrolled as was the study of Mosketi et al. (1963), who gave lithium to 127 patients of mixed diagnostic categories and also reported improvement in schizophrenic patients. Gershon in his 1960 article reported benefit to schizophrenic patients. However, controlled studies on the effects of lithium on acute or chronic schizophrenics yielded opposite results in three studies carried out by the same group (Johnson et al., 1968; Johnson, 1970; Shopsin et al., 1971).

A variety of other authors have treated schizophrenic patients with lithium. They include Gottfries (1968); Zall et al. (1968); Fries (1969); Forssman and Wålinder (1969); Angst et al. (1970); Straker (1970) and Prien et al. (1971). The studies are mostly uncontrolled and present little evidence of the usefulness of lithium in schizophrenia although it might benefit excitement present as part of a schizophrenia picture.

The effect of lithium in schizophrenia requires much further work. It would seem that lithium has a general sedative type of effect and that excited overactive patients of all types might very well gain some benefits from lithium. Certainly there are numerous reports to this effect. However, the few controlled studies have failed to provide confirmation. The problem of schizo-affective psychosis is probably the most perplexing one of all. First of all, this is a diagnosis that is more generously given in North America than in some other countries. It is an ill-defined entity and, certainly to the writers, it seems probable that even in the studies of Johnson et al. (1968), some patients labeled schizo-affective would have been labeled manic-depressive in other countries. Simply because a patient hallucinates is not a reason to label him as schizo-affective as is sometimes done. Many manic-depressive patients hallucinate and are frequently bizarre. It should be noted that Prien *et al.* (1972) found that in schizo-affective patients lithium carbonate was effective. Diagnostic criteria are imprecise but certainly we have a very open mind as to the efficacy of lithium salts in schizo-affective disorders.

H. Periodic catatonia

Annell (1969) reported beneficial effects on adolescent patients who appeared to suffer from periodic catatonia, yet this most cyclical of illnesses did not respond completely in the one case treated by Gjessing (1967).

The small amount of work carried out in periodic catatonia does not allow for any generalization. Certainly it is a rare and fascinating entity which one might have predicted would have responded to lithium.

I. Premenstrual tension

Sletten and Gershon (1966) reported on 8 patients suffering from premenstrual tension, all of whom showed some improvement when treated with lithium. This was an uncontrolled study, as was the study of Fries (1969) who treated 5 patients, 2 of whom gave excellent responses and 3 of whom did not. Tupin (1972) also reported on one patient who showed considerable improvement while receiving lithium. In the only study utilizing placebo controls Singer *et al.* (1974) were unable to confirm this finding.

The studies on premenstrual tension are of considerable interest particularly with regard to the well-known electrolyte and affective components frequently associated with this condition. The positive reports in the uncontrolled studies and the inability to confirm this in the only controlled study leaves this another interesting, but unresolved area.

J. Recurrent alcoholism

Fries (1969) reported one case of alcoholism out of a group of 17 who responded to lithium treatment. However, it transpired that this patient was a periodic alcoholic and may have been suffering from a depressive condition. Most of the other patients stopped taking the drug because it did not have any immediate effect and therefore the trial must be considered inconclusive. Wren *et al.* (1974) studied 73 inpatients requiring detoxification. All were chronic alcoholics; none were suffering from psychotic depression. Seventeen patients were described as habitual excessive drinkers and 56 were alcoholic addicts. Duration of the disease in all cases was 5 years or more. A placebo period of one month preceded the matched group receiving either lithium or placebo. Blood levels were kept at $0 \cdot 6 - 1 \cdot 2$ mEq/l. Placebo was used and identical routines were followed including the collecting of blood for both groups. Forty-three of the 73 patients failed to complete the first period of 48 weeks. There remained 14 patients from the placebo group and 16 from the lithium groups. Twenty-one patients completed 96 weeks of continuous treatment. The criterion rated was disabling drinking, that is, drinking to the point of interference with normal daily life, whether as an inpatient or outpatient, necessitating admission or transfer to special areas for detoxification.

The number of such episodes was the parameter measured. Seventy-three and a half percent of the placebo as against 43·5% of the lithium treated patients had episodes of disabling drinking. this difference was significant at the $p < 0.01$ level. Of the 30 patients maintained on medication for a full 48 weeks, 64% of the placebo group as compared with 25% of the lithium group were involved in such drinking episodes ($p < 0.05$). Thus, in this well controlled study, a statistically significant improvement in drinking habits took place in the group receiving the lithium.

The work on alcoholism by one of the authors and his colleagues is an equally fascinating part of the lithium story. The work was based on the assumption that some alcoholics might be suffering from affective disorders. Like most long-term studies on alcoholism, drop-out rate was very high. Nonetheless, in the patients who continued the follow-up, the beneficial effects of lithium were very convincing indeed, although not apparently related to changes in a depression rating score.

III. Non-Episodic Disorders

A. Tardive dyskinesia, Huntington's Chorea and spasmodic torticollis

One of the non-episodic conditions for which lithium is being used is tardive dyskinesia, a complex and ill defined syndrome produced by neuroleptic drugs of which the bucco-lingual masticatory syndrome (i.e. abnormal mouthing, chewing and tongue movements) plus choreoathetoid movements of limbs and fingers are the main components. An observation made by one of us, (Simpson, 1973a) was that several mis-diagnosed manic patients treated with long-term neuroleptics had developed this condition and improved considerably when they received lithium. Several other non-schizophrenic patients suffering from tardive dyskinesia have also been successfully treated with lithium including a patient whose tardive dyskinesia reappeared when she was withdrawn from lithium and improved when she again received lithium. Simpson (1973b) in an open study of 10 chronically hospitalized patients suffering from severe tardive dyskinesia, gave lithium until blood levels of lithium averaged 1·0 MEq/l. Very little improvement was noted, however, with only a minor improvement in two out of 10 subjects. On the basis of this, we might question the efficacy of lithium in this condition but the poor response may have resulted from the selection of very severe cases. However, since in another case mentioned above we showed improvement on lithium, loss of improvement when lithium was withdrawn and improvement once again when lithium was readministered, we feel that the evidence for the effectiveness of lithium is very strong. Similarly, Prange *et al.*

(1973) reported on 2 patients treated under double-blind conditions with placebo and lithium. Video tapes were taken of both patients at different dose levels of lithium and a placebo; when rated blind by observers, they showed improvement on lithium which was dose related and relapses occurred when placebo was substituted for lithium. Having seen the video tape of one of these patients, one would have to say that the improvement was dramatic. A large controlled trial is planned at our hospital.

The picture of tardive dyskinesia in many cases bears a striking resemblance to Huntington's Chorea. It is of considerable interest that Dalen and Steg (1973) refer not only to the successful treatment of a case of tardive dyskinesia, but report that 3 of 5 cases of Huntington's Chorea showed a striking reduction in hyperkinetic symptoms and improvement of voluntary movement.

Mattsson (1973) claimed improvement in 3 out of 4 cases of Huntington's Chorea treated with lithium. Objective recordings improved by 80% in 2 cases, 40% in 1 and 15% in the fourth patient.

Other writers such as Manyam and Bravo-Fernandez (1973) have also confirmed the effect of lithium in Huntington's Chorea. We, ourselves, have seen a case showing only mental symptoms but with a positive family history and a positive L-dopa test who showed an improved mental state when receiving lithium. However, a controlled study failed to confirm these observations (Aminoff and Marshall, 1974).

It is also of interest that Van Woert and Ambani (1971) implied that lithium was of benefit in the dyskinetic movements produced by L-dopa in Parkinson patients. Dalen (1973) reports on the effect of lithium in reducing the hyperkinetic movements produced by L-dopa.

Couper-Smartt (1973) also reports on the amelioration of spasmodic torticollis in a single case utilizing a placebo controlled technique.

The efficacy of lithium in treating tardive dyskinesia and Huntington's Chorea is another remarkable finding. The fact that three separate groups of investigators claimed beneficial results in tardive dyskinesia despite the small sample sizes and the lack of control in two of them is noteworthy. The dose relatedness in Simpson's case and in the controlled study of Prange makes this even more convincing. The imprecision of what exactly is tardrive dyskinesia and the knowledge that some of the dyskinesias are permanent and, therefore, not amenable to chemical intervention, will have to be kept in mind in evaluating this subject. The same may be said of Huntington's Chorea where beneficial effects are claimed but where disagreement also exists. Similarities in both of these conditions has been noted before and this would be another factor linking them together. The well known effects of lithium on catecholamine metabolism might well be the link and may well represent an explanation of this activity. The implications of the single case report of spasmodic torticollis improving (this again in a placebo controlled situation) remains to be seen.

B. Thyrotoxicosis

In 1968 Schou and associates reported the development of goiter in 15 patients treated with lithium for periods of 5 months to 2 years. Sedvall *et al.* (1969) suggested that inhibition of thyroid iodine release was the basis of the lithium effect. This suggestion has been confirmed by others (Cooper and Simpson, 1969). Burrow *et al.* (1971) and Temple *et al.* (1972a, b) showed that lithium was a potential therapeutic agent in patients in whom a prompt decrease in thyroid hormone level is required. Temple, in a study of ten thyrotoxic patients who were receiving lithium with serum levels of $0 \cdot 6$ to $1 \cdot 2$ mEq/l for 10 days to 3 weeks, noted that I^{131} release was decreased by 30–85% and that an inhibition of peripheral hormone breakdown also occurred. The only other therapeutic agent that inhibits thyroid hormone directly is iodine but its use is limited and interferes with diagnostic tests. This preliminary report would suggest that lithium may be a valuable treatment in this condition. Gerdes *et al.* (1973) using lithium acetate orally in doses of $0 \cdot 5$ to $1 \cdot 5$ g per day confirmed this by producing a prompt decrease in the rate of I^{131} loss from the thyroid. A mean fall of 30% in serum T_4 was observed within a week as the result of this blocking of hormone release.

The usefulness of lithium in treating acute thyrotoxicosis is probably of momentary interest but does attest to the manifold use that lithium has gained.

IV. Concluding Remarks

The slow acceptance of lithium as a therapeutic modality is almost as interesting as the sudden profound interest in lithium in a wide variety of treatment situations. This may seem to fulfill the prophesies that lithium would prove to be a panacea. On the other hand, of course, it has to be remembered that when chlorpromazine was introduced, physicians used it to prevent vomiting, to lower temperatures, and in a variety of other ways until this uniquely interesting drug was evaluated across the board and its special area of utility defined. That this should also be so for lithium is not surprising, particularly since it has the added advantage of being such a simple substance. The widespread nature of its effects and side effects have led it to be used in a variety of conditions and, no doubt, the future will see other conditions added to this list and also the pruning or setting aside of the use of lithium in at least some of the conditions reported here.

References

Aminoff, M. J. and Marshall, J. (1974). *Lancet.* **1**, 107–109.
Angst, J., Weis, P., Grof, P., Baastrup, P. C. and Schou, M. (1970). *Brit. J. Psychiat.* **116**, 599–619.
Annell, A. L. (1969). *Acta psychiat. scand. Suppl.* **207**, 19–30.
Baastrup, P. C. (1969). *Acta psychiat. scand. Suppl.* **207**, 12–18.
Baldessarini, R. and Stephens, J. (1970). *Archs gen. psychiat.* **22**, 72–77.

Burrow, G. N., Burke, W. R., Himmelhoch, J. M., Spencer, R. P. and Hershman, J. M. (1971). *J. clin. Endocr. Metab.* **32,** 647.

Cade, J. F. J. (1949). *Med. J. Aust.* **36,** 349–352.

Campbell, M., Fish, B., Korein, J., Shapiro, T., Collins, P. and Kohn, C. (1972). *J. Autism child. Schiz.* **2,** 234–259.

Cooper, A. F. and Fowlie, H. C. (1973). *Brit. J. Psychiat.* **122,** 245–250.

Cooper, T. B. and Simpson, G. M. (1969). *Curr. ther. Res.* **11,** 603–608.

Couper-Smartt, J. (1973). *Lancet* **2,** 741–742.

Dalen, P. (1973). *Lancet* **1,** 936–937.

Dalen, P. and Steg, G. (1973). *Lancet* **1,** 107–108.

Demers, R., Lukesh, R. and Prichard, J. (1970). *Lancet* **2,** 315–316.

Dostal, T. and Zvolsky, P. (1970). *Int. Pharmacopsychiat.* **5,** 203–207.

Dyson, W. L. and Barcai, A. (1970). *Curr. ther. Res.* **12,** 286–290.

Erwin, C. W., Gerber, C. J. and Morrison, S. D. (1971). Paper read at World Congress of Psychiat, Mexico City.

Erwin, C. W., Gerber, C. J., Morrison, S. D. and James, J. F. (1973). *Archs gen. Psychiat.* **28,** 646–648.

Forssman, M. and Wålinder, J. (1969). *Acta psychiat. scand. Suppl.* **207,** 34–40.

Fries, H. (1969). *Acta psychiat. scand. Suppl.* **207,** 41–43.

Frommer, E. (1968). *Brit. J. Psychiat.* **2,** 117–136.

Gerdes, H., Littmann, K. J. and Mahlstedt, J. (1973). *Deutsche Med. Wochenschr.* **34,** 1551–1554.

Gershon, S. (1968). *Dis. nerv. Syst.* **29,** 51–55.

Gershon, S. (1971). *Rational drug Ther.* **5,** 1–5.

Gershon, S. and Trautner, E. M. (1956). *Med. J. Aust.* **43,** 783–787.

Gershon, S. and Yuwiler, A. (1960). *J. Neuropsychiat.* **1,** 229-241.

Gjessing, L. R. (1967). *Acta psychiat. scand.* **43,** 372–375.

Glesinger, B. (1954). *Med. J. Aust.* **41,** 277–283.

Good, C. A. (1903). *Amer. J. med. Sci.* **125,** 273–284.

Gottfries, C. G. (1968). *Acta psychiat. scand. Suppl.* **44,** 199–204.

Gram, L. F. and Rafaelsen, O. J. (1972). *Acta psychiat. scand. Suppl.* **44,** 199–204.

Greenhill, L. L., Rieder, R. O., Wender, P. H., Buchsbaum, M. and Zahn, T. P. (1973). *Archs gen. Psychiat.* **28,** 636–640.

Jacobsen, J. E. (1965). *Amer. J. Psychiat.* **122,** 295–299.

James, J. F. and Reilly, E. (1971). *Southern med. J.* **64,** 1322–1327.

Johnson, G., Gershon, S. and Hekimian, L. (1968). *Compreh. Psychiat.* **9,** 568–573.

Johnson, G. (1970). *Dis. nerv. Syst.* **31,** 613–615

Jus, A., Villeneuve, A., Gautier, J., Pires, A., Cote, J. M., Jus, K., Villeneuve, R. and Perron, D. (1973). *Canad. psychiat. Assoc. J.* **18,** 67–74.

Manyam, N. V. B. and Bravo-Fernandez, E. (1973). *Lancet* **1,** 1010.

Mattsson, B. (1973). *Lancet* **1,** 718–719.

Morrison, S. D., Erwin, C. W., Gianturco, D. T. and Gerber, C. J. (1973). *Dis. nerv. Syst.* **34,** 186–189.

Mosketi, K. V., Belskaya, G. M. and Nuratova, I. D. (1963). *Zh. Nevropatol. Psihiat: Korsakova* **63,** 92-95.

Naylor, G. J., Donald, J. M., Le Poidevin, D. and Reid, A. H. (1974). *Br. J. Psychiat.* **124,** 52–57.

Prange, A. J., Wilson, I. C., Morris, C. E. and Hall, C. D. (1973). *Psychopharmacol. Bull.* **9,** 36–37.

Prien, R. F., Caffey, E. M. and Klett, C. J. (1971). Cooperative Studies in Psychiatry,

Report No. 89, Central Neuropsychiatric Research Lab., Perry Point, Md.

Prien, R. F., Caffrey, E. M. and Klett, C. J. (1972). *Archs gen. Psychiat.* **27,** 182–189.

Rifkin, A., Quitkin, F., Carillo, C., Blumberg, A. G. and Klein, D. F. (1972). *Archs gen. Psychiat.* **27,** 519–523.

Schou, M., Amdisen, A., Jensen, S. E. and Oisen, T. (1968). *Brit. med. J.* **3,** 710–713.

Sedvall, G., Jannsson, B., Petterson, U. (1969). *Acta psychiat. scand. Suppl.* **207,** 59–66.

Sheard, M. H. (1970). *Nature, Lond.* **228,** 284–285.

Sheard, M. H. (1971). *Nature, Lond.* **230,** 113–114.

Shopsin, B., Kim, S. and Gershon, S. (1971). *Brit. J. Psychiat.* **119,** 435–440.

Simpson, G. M. (1973a). *Br. J. Psychiat.* **122,** 618.

Simpson, G. M. (1973b). Annual Report, Research Center, Rockland State Hospital, Orangeburg, New York.

Singer, K., Cheng, R. and Schou, M. (1974). *Brit. J. Psychiat.* **124,** 50–51.

Sletten, I. W. and Gershon, S. (1966). *Compreh. Psychiat.* **7,** 197–206.

Squires, P. (1916). "Comp. Brit. Pharmacopoeia". 19th Edition. Churchill, London.

Straker, M. (1970). *Can. psychiat. Assoc. J.* **15,** 21–27.

Temple, R., Berman, M., Carlson, H. E. and Robbins, J. (1972a). *Mayo Clinic Proceed.* **47,** 872–878.

Temple, R., Burman, M., Robbins, J. and Wolff, J. (1972b). *J. clin. Invest.* **51,** 2746–2756.

Tupin, J. P. (1972). *Compreh. Psychiat.* **13,** 209–214.

Tupin, J. P. and Smith, D. B. (1972). Paper presented at NIMH Early Clinical Drug Evaluation Units meeting, Catonsville, Maryland.

Tupin, J. P., Smith, D. B., Clanon, T. L., Kim, L. I., Nugent, A. and Groupe, A. (1973). *Compreh. Psychiat.* **14,** 311–317.

Van Woert, M. H. and Ambani, L. M. (1971). *New Engl. J. Med.* **285,** 1326–1327.

Vartanian, M. E. (1959). *Zh. Nevropathol. Psihiat. Korsakova* **59,** 586–589.

Weischer, M. L. (1969). *Psychopharmacologia* **15,** 245–254.

Whitehead, P. L. and Clark, L. D. (1970). *Amer. J. Psychiat.* **127,** 824–825.

Williamson, B. (1966). *Dis nerv. Syst.* **27,** 775–782.

Wren, J. C., Kline, N. S., Cooper, T. B., Varga, E. and Canal, O. (1974). *Clin. Med. J.* **81,** 33–37.

Zail, H., Therman, P. O. G. and Myers, J. M. (1968). *Amer. J. Psychiat.* **125,** 549–555.

7

THE CLINICAL EFFECTIVENESS OF LITHIUM: COMPARISONS WITH OTHER DRUGS

R. F. PRIEN

I. Introduction

Since Cade's serendipitous discovery in 1949, lithium has been used therapeutically and prophylactically in a variety of mood disorders, including mania, recurrent endogenous depression, schizo-affective psychosis, psychotic excitement, neurotic depression, premenstrual tension syndrome, and behavior disorders in children and adolescents. Some of these applications, particularly those dealing with prophylactic treatment, have aroused considerable interest in the clinical community. Previous chapters have examined some of the evidence supporting the use of lithium in these disorders. The purpose of this chapter is to carefully examine the studies comparing lithium with other drugs. These studies are particularly important since they form the basis for the clinician's decision on whether to use lithium in preference to other treatments.

II. Therapeutic Effect in Acute Mania

There are over 75 published reports on the use of lithium in acute mania, involving over 3000 patients in 20 countries. With few exceptions, these reports are enthusiastic in their endorsement of the drug. Most studies report "therapeutic success" in over 80% of lithium-treated patients. Four placebo-controlled studies report that lithium is more effective than placebo (Schou *et al.*, 1954; Maggs, 1963; Bunney *et al.*, 1968; Goodwin *et al.*, 1969). There appears to be little doubt that lithium is an effective antimanic agent. However, there is still some question as to whether lithium is more effective than other treatments.

Except for two small trials comparing lithium with methysergide (a serotonin antagonist), lithium has been compared only with chlorpromazine. These comparative trials involve a total of 334 patients, 75% of them from one study.

The two lithium-methysergide comparisons were prompted by uncontrolled trials advocating the use of antiserotonin agents in mania (Haskovec and Soucek, 1968; Dewhurst, 1969). The first comparison was conducted by Fieve and co-workers (1968a) in six manic patients over a 10 day period. Lithium carbonate and methysergide were administered to each patient in a randomized crossover design. Analyses of clinical scales revealed "significant improvement" on lithium and "no clinical change" on methysergide. It was concluded that lithium was a more promising antimanic treatment than methysergide. This was supported by Grof and Foley (1971) who administered lithium carbonate or methysergide to 20 manic patients over a 28 day period. Eight of 10 patients on lithium improved compared to three of 10 on methysergide. Five of the patients on methysergide and none on lithium showed deterioration of manic symptomatology.

The most favorable report on lithium therapy was by Johnson *et al.* (1968) who treated 28 manic patients with lithium carbonate or chlorpromazine for a three week period and achieved total remission in 78% of the lithium patients and 36% of the chlorpromazine patients. The two drugs also differed in quality of action. Lithium was superior in normalizing ideation and mood while chlorpromazine acted more quickly in controlling motor activity. Lithium had a relatively slow onset of action, averaging eight days. However, once initial improvement occurred, remission was rapid. Chlorpromazine acted more rapidly in reducing hyperactivity and bringing the patient under control but was slower and less consistent in restoring normal behavior. The authors concluded that lithium has "both quantitative and qualitative differences from chlorpromazine which tend to favor it in most circumstances as the drug of choice in acute mania" (Johnson *et al.*, 1971). However, it was acknowledged that in the early stages of lithium administration, patients may require sedation to control motor overactivity. It was also suggested that because of the different time course of action of lithium and chlorpromazine, combined therapy might be more advantageous in severe mania than either drug alone.

Spring and co-workers (1970) treated 12 patients with either lithium carbonate or chlorpromazine for a three week period. Rating scales revealed no significant difference between the two treatments. Six of the seven patients treated with lithium and three of the five treated with chlorpromazine showed complete remission of symptoms. The two chlorpromazine failures were crossed over to lithium and had a complete remission of manic symptoms. The lithium failure was treated with chlorpromazine and failed to respond. Although lithium appeared to be slightly superior, the small sample size prohibited any definitive conclusions regarding the therapeutic efficacy of either drug.

Platman (1970a) treated 13 manic patients with lithium carbonate and 10 with chlorpromazine over a three week period. Although there was no statistically significant difference between the two treatments, lithium carbonate was slightly superior on six parameters selected from objective rating scales (i.e., negativism, grandiosity, somatic complaints, denial, sleep and severity of illness). One criticism of this study is that patients received placebo for two weeks before starting study medication. Seven patients (23% of the sample) were unable to complete two weeks on placebo and were dropped from the study. this may have biased the sample by excluding the most severely ill patients.

The largest study on lithium therapy was a collaborative project sponsored by the Veterans Administration (VA) and the National Institute of Mental Health (NIMH) in which 255 newly admitted manics at 18 hospitals were randomly assigned to lithium carbonate or chlorpromazine for a three week period (Prien et al., 1973a). At admission, patients were classified as highly active (N = 125) or mildly active (N = 130) on the basis of degree of hyperactivity and excitement. Chlorpromazine was significantly superior to lithium with highly active patients. Chlorpromazine rapidly controlled manic behavior, often within three or four days. In contrast, the highly active group on lithium was still acutely manic at the end of the first week. Attempts to achieve early control by pushing lithium dosage to high levels (1·5 mEq/l or more) only resulted in toxic effects. Almost 40% of the highly active patients on lithium were unable to complete three weeks of treatment compared to 8% of the chlorpromazine patients. With the mildly active patients, the difference between treatments was less clearcut. However, lithium appeared to be the better treatment. Both drugs effectively reduced manic symptomatology but lithium produced fewer side effects and left the patients feeling less sluggish and fatigued.

The results from the VA-NIMH study confirm earlier reports by Baastrup (1969), Demers (1971), Schou (1968), and Tupin (1970) that lithium is not the treatment of choice for the highly disturbed manic. Lithium has a relatively slow onset of action (often five days or more) and cannot provide the rapid control of manic behavior required in acute cases. Rapidly acting neuroleptics such as chlorpromazine are preferable to lithium in these cases. Lithium appears to be most effective with the mildly active, hypomanic patient who does not present a management problem.

It has been suggested that the clinical action of lithium is qualitatively different from that of chlorpromazine and other neuroleptics. Schou (1968), Gershon (1970), and others claim that lithium treats the underlying manic process without sedation while chlorpromazine acts through sedation without affecting underlying mood and ideation. The patient is "contained" until the manic episode remits. To quote Strömgren and Schou (1964), "tranquilizing drugs usually succeed in suppressing the more violent manifestations of mania but are without specific action on the fundamental mood change; the patients are drugged rather than relieved of the manic symptoms". This claim was supported by Johnson et al., (1968) who reported that lithium was superior to chlorpromazine in normalizing primary mood and ideation. In the VA–NIMH study, the results were less definitive. Chlorpromazine produced more drowsiness and sluggishness than lithium. However, there was no difference in underlying ideation or mood between treatment groups at the end of three weeks. This does not rule out the possibility that the two drugs acted differentially on the underlying manic process during the early stages of treatment. A self-report mood scale designed to measure underlying affect was of limited value during the first few weeks because of the inability or unwillingness of many patients to complete the scale. The other controlled studies comparing lithium and chlorpromazine (Platman, 1970a; Spring et al., 1970) produced no evidence to support or refute this claim. This is an area requiring further investigation.

Lithium and chlorpromazine are not the only treatments used in acute mania. ECT is still widely employed with severely disturbed patients because of its rapid action. However, ECT has several disadvantages including a relatively high risk of relapse, temporary memory loss, lack of patient acceptance, and inconvenience of administration. Haloperidol is used frequently in the treatment of mania but has not been evaluated in controlled studies. Other neuroleptics such as thioridazine have been employed with varying success but like haloperidol require more systematic evaluation. Some clinicians contend that the best way to treat the acute manic patient is to combine lithium with an antipsychotic such as chlorpromazine or haloperidol, thus gaining the benefit of both drugs (Schou, 1968; Maletzky and Blachly, 1971). The most popular use of these combinations is to administer the antipsychotic drug immediately to control acute manic behavior and then gradually add lithium. Within a week the antipsychotic drug is gradually withdrawn as lithium concentration becomes adequate. Unfortunately, these alternatives are based entirely on clinical impression. Lithium has not been tested in combination with other drugs and has not been compared directly with any treatment other than chlorpromazine.

To summarize, comparative studies suggest that lithium is most beneficial in manic states involving mild levels of hyperactivity and excitation. The major disadvantage of lithium is its slow onset of action. Initial improvement may require six to 10 days. This time lag can be crucial when the patient is highly active or difficult to manage. Control of excited behavior is not as critical with mildly active patients and lithium does well with this subgroup. The major advantage of lithium, according to several investigators, is its effectiveness in normalizing mood without leaving the patient feeling drugged. Although this claim is yet to be verified by quantitative tests in a controlled study, it is supported by a number of clinicians who have had extensive experience with both lithium and antipsychotic agents. In addition, several clinicians report greater patient acceptance with lithium than with other antimanic treatments, due mainly to the absence of sedating effects with lithium (Schlagenhauf et al., 1966; Baastrup, 1969; Wittrig and Coopwood, 1970). Finally, some investigators contend that a major advantage of lithium is its effectiveness in patients who are resistant to phenothiazines (Fieve, 1970). The other side of the coin (the effectiveness of phenothiazines in patients who are resistant to lithium) has not been studied.

III. Therapeutic Effect in Acute Depression

Controlled trials on lithium therapy in acute depression provide conflicting results. there are two studies comparing lithium with a standard antidepressant, one involving a comparison with desipramine, and the other a comparison with imipramine.

Mendels and co-workers (1972) compared lithium carbonate with desipramine in a double-blind study involving 24 acutely depressed patients with a diagnosis of recurrent endogenous depression. Twelve patients were administered lithium and 12 desipramine. Treatments were administered for three weeks. There was "considerable improvement" in both groups with no significant difference between treatments. At the end of three weeks, three patients on lithium and six on desipramine who failed to show at least 50% improvement on clinical rating scales were switched to the other drug. All but one showed significant improvement over a second three week period. The authors concluded that lithium was as effective as desipramine in the treatment of acute depression.

Fieve and colleagues (1968a) compared lithium carbonate with imipramine in 29 patients hospitalized with acute endogenous depression. Treatments were administered under double-blind conditions for two to four weeks. Utilizing a rather complicated series of analyses involving four scales, the authors reported

E

that "lithium showed a mild antidepressant action in contrast to imipramine which showed a moderate to strong antidepressant effect." Since depressed patients may respond positively to any physiologically active substance, the mild antidepressant effect of lithium is difficult to interpret. The one clear finding is that imipramine was associated with the better therapeutic response.

The results from these studies coupled with contradictory findings from uncontrolled trials (Prien *et al.*, 1971) indicate that further study is needed before lithium is used in place of standard antidepressants. In future studies, particular attention should be paid to the selection and diagnosis of depressed patients. Goodwin *et al.* (1972) report that lithium is a more effective antidepressant with bipolar than unipolar patients while Bunney *et al.* (1970) indicate that tricyclic antidepressants are more effective with unipolar patients (patients were classified as bipolar if they had a history of mania with or without depression and unipolar if they had a history of depression without mania). This suggests that the bipolar–unipolar classification of affective illness might have as important an application in the treatment of acute depression as it does in the prophylactic treatment of recurrent mania and depression (Prien *et al.*, 1973b).

Finally, it should be emphasized that the only controlled studies on lithium therapy in acute depression have involved patients with a diagnosis of endogenous depression. The value of lithium in reactive or neurotic depression has not been studied under controlled conditions.

IV. Prophylactic Effect Against Manic and Depressive Relapse

Baastrup and Schou (1967) and Angst and collaborators (1969) presented the first strong evidence for a prophylactic action of lithium in recurrent affective illness. This evidence was based on longitudinal studies which compared the frequency and severity of relapse before lithium therapy with the frequency and severity during lithium therapy. In both studies, relapse frequency was significantly reduced during lithium treatment in both bipolar and unipolar patients. Lithium was effective in averting depressive as well as manic relapses. These studies were severely criticized on methodological grounds (Blackwell and Shepherd, 1968; Saran, 1969) and lithium prophylaxis became a subject of international controversy. Critics contended that the issue of lithium prophylaxis could not be resolved by longitudinal trials and stressed the need for comparisons with placebo and control medication. Subsequently, there have been several comparisons of lithium with placebo (Baastrup *et al.*, 1970; Melia, 1970; Coppen *et al.*, 1971; Cundall *et al.*, 1972; Hullin *et al.*, 1972; Stallone *et al.*, 1972; Prien *et al.*, 1973a). Most show that lithium is significantly more effective than placebo in preventing recurrence of affective episodes. Unfortunately, there is still little information about how lithium compares with other medication.

The first comparison between lithium and another drug was retrospective.

Angst and colleagues (1969) compared the number of relapses before and during lithium treatment with results obtained several years earlier with imipramine. The study was conducted in two clinics in Prague and Zurich. Ninety-one patients were evaluated on lithium and 63 on imipramine. The samples consisted of patients with manic-depressive illness, recurrent endogenous depression, and schizo-affective psychosis. Patients were followed for up to four years. A relapse was recorded when the patient required hospitalization or additional psychopharmacologic medication. In the group treated with lithium, relapses occurred significantly less often during lithium treatment than before. This was true for all three diagnostic categories. In the imipramine group, there was a slight increase in relapse frequency, although hospital admissions were reduced. This led the authors to conclude that lithium is prophylactically effective while imipramine is not. Caution is required in interpreting these results. The lithium and imipramine trials were conducted several years apart under possibly different therapeutic conditions. The two samples were not comparable nor were treatments administered for equal periods of time. These differences make it difficult to draw any firm conclusions regarding the comparative efficacy of the two treatments.

There are only two studies directly comparing lithium with other drugs. Both used imipramine as the comparison drug. A third study comparing lithium and amitriptyline (Laurell and Ottosson, 1968) was aborted after the first few lithium-treated patients showed marked improvement because the investigators felt that it would be unethical to continue administering other treatments.

Platman (1970b) compared lithium with imipramine in 70 patients with recurrent affective disorders: 49 were assigned to lithium and 21 to imipramine. All patients had had at least two manic and/or depressive attacks requiring hospitalization during the previous two years. Each patient's course of illness during treatment was compared with his course of illness before treatment. Although the lithium group showed a somewhat better response than the imipramine group, neither demonstrated a "major prophylactic effect." However, numerous methodological problems make it difficult to interpret results. Patients were not randomly assigned to the two treatments nor were the treatments administered for equal periods of time. There was no breakdown of results for manic and depressive relapses or for bipolar and unipolar types. Finally, the absence of a placebo group makes it difficult to assess the extent of prophylactic action of either treatment.

Fieve et al., (1968b), in an interim report on the above study, analyzed data from 36 lithium patients and 10 imipramine patients who had completed at least 20 weeks of treatment. There was no significant difference between treatments. Seventeen percent of the lithium patients and 10% of the imipramine patients relapsed severely enough to require hospitalization. When relapse was defined in terms of rating scale data, lithium patients had twice as many relapses as imipramine patients. However, the main effect of both treatments was on the intensity rather than the frequency of relapses. Lithium was particularly effective in reducing the severity of manic episodes while imipramine was most effective in reducing depressive states. This was attributed in part to the fact that the investigators were quick to raise dosage or change medication at the first sign of relapse. The adjusted treatment of these subpsychotic shifts may have been responsible for the reduction in severity of relapse.

The other lithium–imipramine comparison was a recently completed study sponsored by the Veterans Administration and the National Institute of Mental Health as part of their multiphasic project on lithium therapy (Prien *et al.*, 1973b). One hundred twenty-two patients with recurrent affective illness in 18 hospitals were randomly assigned to lithium carbonate, imipramine or placebo following hospitalization for acute depression. Treatments were administered for two years. All patients had had at least one affective episode requiring hospitalization within the previous two years and two requiring hospitalization within the previous five years. Diagnoses included manic-depressive psychosis, depressed type, and recurrent endogenous depression. Patients were classified as bipolar or unipolar on the basis of the presence or absence of a history of mania. The sample consisted of 44 bipolar and 78 unipolar patients. With *bipolar* patients, lithium was significantly more effective than imipramine and placebo in preventing affective episodes (i.e. manic or depressive attacks severe enough to require hospitalization or use of nonstudy drugs). Only 28% of the patients on lithium had episodes compared to 77% on imipramine and 77% on placebo. The difference between lithium carbonate and imipramine was due to the high incidence of manic episodes on imipramine. The difference between lithium and placebo was attributable to both manic and depressive episodes. *Unipolar* patients responded equally well to lithium and imipramine; both treatments were significantly more effective than placebo. Episodes occurred in 48% of the lithium patients, 48% of the imipramine patients, and 92% of the placebo patients.

One problem in interpreting results from the VA–NIMH study is that the study was not completely "blind". Major treatment decisions, such as hospitalization, were made by physicians who knew the identity of the patient's treatment. This raises the question of physician bias and its effect on treatment outcome. In discussing this issue, the investigators reported that scales completed by raters who were blind to the patient's treatment agreed with evaluations made by the treatment physician and revealed no evidence of systematic bias in treatment decisions (Prien *et al.*, 1973b, c). However, as Blackwell and Shepherd (1968) point out, in the absence of a completely double-blind design, the possibility of bias cannot be ruled out.

Results from the VA–NIMH study indicate the importance of considering the patient's previous course of illness before selecting a program of maintenance chemotherapy. Patients with a history of manic episodes (i.e. bipolar patients) are not good candidates for a program involving imipramine. The risk of subsequent manic attack is too great. Lithium is a more suitable treatment for these patients. Patients with a history of depression without mania (i.e. unipolar patients) respond equally well to imipramine and lithium. The advantage in using lithium is that it is a broad spectrum drug that is effective with both unipolar and bipolar patients. The clinician does not have to worry about whether the patient has had previous manic episodes before administering treatment. The disadvantage is that lithium involves more laboratory work (and expense) than imipramine because of the periodic serum lithium determinations required to monitor treatment. However, this can also be an advantage in that serum levels can be a useful aid in adjusting dosage and determining whether the patient is actually taking his medication.

The use of lithium as a prophylactic treatment for recurrent affective illness should be tempered by the knowledge that the drug has been compared only with imipramine. It is possible that chlorpromazine and similar agents may be useful with bipolar patients. Similarly, antidepressants other than imipramine may be effective with unipolar patients. For example, several placebo-controlled studies suggest that amitriptyline is effective in preventing depressive episodes (Hordern et al., 1964; Mindham et al., 1973; Paykel et al., 1973). However, none of these studies has extended beyond nine months. so the long-term efficacy of the drug is not known. The combination of lithium and a tricyclic antidepressant is advocated by some investigators (Fieve et al., 1968b; Zall, 1971). There appears to be no contraindication to using lithium in combination with the tricyclics. However, the clinical efficacy of these combinations has not been evaluated in controlled studies. Also, use of these combinations is predicated on the assumption that lithium is ineffective in preventing depressive recurrences. Based on results from the VA–NIMH study and placebo-controlled trials by Baastrup et al. (1970) and Coppen et al. (1971), this is a dubious assumption. The use of other combinations such as lithium and chlorpromazine, and psychotherapy and antidepressants have gained some support but also remain untested in controlled trials. Obviously, further research is necessary before any drug is regarded as the treatment of choice for preventing affective episodes in recurrent affective illness. However, the fact that drugs such as lithium and imipramine can prevent severe relapse in patients with recurrent mood disorders must be regarded as an exciting finding of significant clinical and research importance.

It should be stressed that the term "prophylaxis" as used in this section refers only to the prevention of episodes requiring hospitalization or supplementary drug therapy. This is the criterion of success used in most prophylactic studies. The capacity of lithium or imipramine to prevent less severe episodes and "normalize" the patient has not been established. It is possible that lithium or imipramine have no true preventive action but instead act to dampen or curb the emerging episode and stabilize the patient sufficiently to avoid hospitalization. In other words, it may be the intensity rather than the frequency of episodes that is affected. Even if this is the mode of lithium's "prophylactic" action, its importance should not be minimized. The prevention of disruptive hospitalizations and severe attacks is by itself a significant contribution to the pharmacotherapy of mood disorders. Also, in each of the comparative studies on lithium, including placebo trials, the samples have included only patients with recent hospitalizations for affective illness. Patients with less severe manifestations of mania or depression have not been tested. Any generalizations from lithium studies must take these considerations into account.

V. Therapeutic Effect in Schizo-Affective and Schizophrenic Disorders

Next to manic-depressive disorders and recurrent endogenous depression, the largest number of reports on lithium therapy have dealt with excited schizoaffectives. There are three types of findings reported in the literature: (1) lithium is effective against pathological excitement in schizo-affective illness, but has no effect on schizophrenic behavior; (2) lithium is effective with both the affective and schizophrenic components of schizo-affective psychosis; and (3) lithium is ineffective with both affective and schizophrenic behavior. Results from uncontrolled studies tend to favor the first alternative. However, the evidence is far from conclusive. One problem is that in many of the studies there is lack of sufficient documentation on diagnostic criteria. Some studies even fail to specify duration of lithium treatment or the criteria for assessing treatment outcome. This raises the possibility that misdiagnosis or natural remission may have contributed to the positive results. There are three studies comparing lithium with active medication in schizo-affective or schizophrenic disorders. Johnson and co-workers (1968) compared lithium with chlorpromazine in 14 hospitalized patients with a diagnosis of schizo-affective psychosis, excited state. Chlorpromazine was significantly superior to lithium. Six of the seven patients on lithium developed a toxic confusional state with disorientation, reduced comprehension, and worsening of schizophrenic symptomatology. None of the chlorpromazine patients showed clinical deterioration. The investigators acknowledge that this finding may be related to the study design in which lithium dosage was increased until therapeutic response or toxicity occurred. It is possible that patients might have responded better with a less rigorous schedule. Another interpretation is given by Maletzky and Blachly (1971) who speculate that "as lithium quiets some symptomatology of schizophrenia, more basic thought disorder may emerge," giving the appearance of a toxic confusional state. However, Johnson and co-workers feel that the most likely explanation is that schizo-affectives are more susceptible to lithium neurotoxicity than manics because of preexisting neurological damage or because of differences in lithium retention and excretion.

A somewhat different set of results were reported in a VA-NIMH study (Prien *et al.*, 1972). Eighty-three newly admitted patients with a diagnosis of schizo-affective psychosis, excited state, were randomly assigned to lithium carbonate or chlorpromazine for a three week period. Patients were classified as highly active (N = 42) or mildly active (N = 41) on the basis of degree of hyperactivity shown at admission. Highly active patients responded very poorly to lithium. This was due primarily to the drug's relatively slow onset of action. Lithium was unable to control excited, hostile behavior in the majority of patients. Approximately 60% of the highly active patients on lithium were not able to complete treatment because of unmanageable behavior compared to only 4% of the patients on chlorpromazine. With mildly active patients, there was no major difference between treatments. Both drugs were effective in reducing schizophrenic and affective symptomatology.

The fact that lithium is as effective as chlorpromazine in reducing schizophrenic behavior in mildly active patients raises the possibility that the drug has neuroleptic properties. This is contrary to the popular conception of lithium as a specific antimanic agent (Gershon, 1970). Another possible explanation is that certain schizophrenic thought disruptions are secondary to mood disturbance and disappear when mood is regulated—rather than being modified directly by lithium (Quitkin *et al.*, 1973).

While the results from the VA–NIMH study have intriguing theoretical implications, their practical implications are less impressive. Even though lithium and chlorpromazine are equally effective in treating mildly active patients, chlorpromazine is probably the most practical treatment. Unlike lithium, chlorpromazine is effective with both highly and mildly active patients. The clinician does not have to worry about degree of activity before administering treatment. Also, lithium involves more laboratory work than chlorpromazine because of frequent serum lithium determinations needed to monitor treatment. Finally, chlorpromazine is available in injectible form which allows even more rapid control of acute behavior.

The differential efficacy of lithium in highly active and mildly active states may explain some of the conflicting results reported in the literature. Investigators who have reported that lithium is relatively ineffective in the treatment of schizo-affective illness may have been working predominantly with highly active patients. In contrast, mildly active patients may have constituted the major portion of samples reflecting positive results with lithium therapy.

Some investigators feel that schizo-affectives who respond to lithium are in reality manics and that poor diagnosis may explain much of lithium's therapeutic success (Lipkin *et al.*, 1970; Meiers, 1970). In the VA–NIMH study, special care was taken to obtain an accurate diagnosis. Patients were independently diagnosed by two psychiatrists at admission according to criteria presented in Mayer-Gross *et al.* (1967) and the American Psychiatric Association's Diagnostic and Statistical Manual of Mental Disorders (1968). In addition, patients were rediagnosed at the time of discharge. Those who were diagnosed as manic-depressive or schizophrenic at discharge were dropped from the sample (this included approximately 6% of the patients in each treatment group).

The VA–NIMH results pertain only to schizo-affectives, not to schizophrenics in general. It should not be assumed that lithium has an antipsychotic effect with nonaffective schizophrenics simply because it has this effect with mildly active schizo-affectives. The literature indicates that the presence of affective factors increases the probability of improvement in schizophrenia (Beck, 1969; Klein and Davis, 1969). There is one controlled trial on lithium therapy in schizophrenia. Shopsin and co-workers (1971) compared lithium with chlorpromazine in 21 newly admitted acute schizophrenics over a three week period. Chlorpromazine was significantly superior to lithium in reducing schizophrenic symptoms. Lithium had little effect on the schizophrenic process and in several cases aggravated baseline pathology. Six of the eleven patients treated with lithium developed toxic confusion similar to that described by Johnson *et al.* (1971). It was concluded that lithium is an ineffective treatment for the schizophrenic patient.

To summarize, the few comparative studies on lithium therapy in schizo-affective and schizophrenic disorders give no justification for using lithium in place of antipsychotic agents such as chlorpromazine. In fact, with highly active patients, lithium is clearly an inferior treatment. It is possible that a combination of lithium and an antipsychotic could prove useful in schizo-affective illness, but this has not been evaluated under controlled conditions. Also, lithium has not been evaluated in schizo-affectives with depressive symptomatology. However, there is no reason to believe that the drug is any more effective with these patients than with excited schizo-affectives.

VI. Effect in Other Disorders

The success with lithium in mania has led to therapeutic trials in a wide range of disorders characterized by strong affective components or undulating course. Lithium has been tested in psychotic excitement, phobic reactions, obsessive-compulsive neuroses, psychomotor epilepsy, toxic psychosis, puerperal psychosis, periodic alcoholism, premenstrual tension syndrome, unstable aggressive personality, and hyperkinesis and other behavioral disorders in children and adolescents. Most of the studies evaluating lithium in these disorders consist of uncontrolled, anecdotal reports. Some success is reported but the scarcity of well controlled studies makes it difficult to assess the contribution of lithium.

There are only two studies comparing lithium with active medication in the above disorders. Rimón and Räkköläien (1968) evaluated lithium iodide in 30 patients with severe confusional states who were not manic or organically impaired. Patients were paired on the basis of age and sex; one of each pair received intravenous lithium while the other received oral chlorpromazine or perphenazine. Patients were treated for seven days. The antipsychotic drugs proved superior in 13 of the 15 pairs. In nine patients lithium had no effect on the illness. In four others, the effect was minimal. It was concluded that lithium is less effective than chlorpromazine and perphenazine in treating confusional states. One reservation about this study concerns the length of the treatment period. Seven days would not appear adequate for evaluating the efficacy of lithium therapy, even with intravenous administration.

Whitehead and Clark (1970) alternated lithium carbonate with thioridazine and placebo in seven hyperactive children. In addition to hyperactivity, four of the children showed neurotic behavior traits and two were diagnosed as psychotic. Each treatment was administered for periods of 4 to 12 weeks. Objective measures revealed no significant difference between lithium and placebo in reduction of activity. Both treatments produced only a marginal benefit. Thioridazine reduced activity in all cases, although the reduction was "not marked." There was no comparison between thioridazine and lithium or thioridazine and placebo nor was there any breakdown of results by diagnostic group.

To summarize, the two studies comparing lithium with other drugs do not suggest any strong therapeutic effect. However, the small number of cases in each diagnostic group and the limited number of disorders studied makes it difficult to draw any firm conclusions about the comparative efficacy of lithium.

VII. Conclusion

When one considers that lithium has been employed as a psychopharmacologic agent for 25 years and has been investigated in hundreds of studies, it is surprising to find that there are only about a dozen trials comparing the drug with active medication. Lithium has been compared with chlorpromazine and methysergide in acute mania, imipramine and desipramine in acute depression, imipramine in recurrent mania and depression (prophylaxis), chlorpromazine in schizo-affective and schizophrenic illness, and chlorpromazine, perphenazine, and thioridazine in other disorders. These comparisons suggest that lithium is more effective than chlorpromazine in the therapeutic treatment of mildly severe mania and is superior to imipramine in the prophylactic treatment of bipolar affective illness. Otherwise, the comparative studies indicate no major advantage to using lithium in place of other treatments. However, it should be remembered that lithium has been compared with only a few drugs in generally small sample trials.

Why then is lithium considered by some clinicians to be the "treatment of choice" in the therapeutic treatment of acute mania and prophylactic treatment of recurrent mania or depression? The main basis for these claims are retrospective comparisons by investigators who have used lithium and other treatments at different times and have found lithium to be superior. Only well controlled trials will indicate whether these impressions are valid. Thus far the evidence is fragmentary. Lithium promises much to the field of pharmacotherapy but requires more extensive evaluation to define its advantages and disadvantages with regard to other available treatments.

References

Angst, J., Dittrich, A. and Grof, P. (1969). *Int. Pharmacopsychiat.* **2**, 1–11.

Baastrup, P. C. (1969). *Acta psychiat. scand. Suppl.* **203**, 149–152.

Baastrup, P. C., Poulsen, J. C., Schou, M., Thomsen, K. and Amdisen, A. (1970). *Lancet* **2**, 326–330.

Baastrup, P. C. and Schou, M. (1967). *Archs gen. Psychiat.* **16**, 162–172.

Beck, A. T. (1969). "Depression: Clinical, Experimental, and Theoretical Aspects". Harper and Row Publishers Inc., New York.

Blackwell, B. and Shepherd, M. (1968). *Lancet* **1**, 968–971.

Bunney, W. E., Brodie, H. K. and Murphy, D. L. (1970). Paper presented at the 78th Annual Meeting of the American Psychological Association, Miami.

Bunney, W. E., Goodwin, F. K., Davis, J. and Fawcett, J. (1968). *Amer. J. Psychiat.* **125**, 499–511.

Cade, J. F. J. (1949). *Med. J. Aust.* **36**, 349–352.

Coppen, A., Noguera, R., Bailey, J., Burns, B. H., Swani, M. S., Hare, E. H., Gardner, R. and Maggs, R. (1971). *Lancet* **2**, 275–279.

Cundall, R. L., Brooks, P. W. and Murray, L. G. (1972). *Psychol. Med.* **3**, 308–311.

"Diagnostic and Statistical Manual of Mental Disorders". (1968). American Psychiatric Association, Washington, D.C.

Demers, R. G. (1971). *Dis. nerv. Syst.* **32**, 249–254.

Dewhurst, W. G. (1969). *Lancet* **1**, 624–625.

Fieve, R. R. (1970). *Int. J. Psychiat.* **10**, 375–412.

Fieve, R. R., Platman, S. R. and Fleiss, J. L. (1969). *Psychopharmacologia* **15**, 425–427.

Fieve, R. R., Platman, S. R. and Plutchik, R. R. (1968a). *Am. J. Psychiat.* **125**, 487–491.

Fieve, R. R., Platman, S. R. and Plutchik, R. R. (1968b). *Am. J. Psychiat.* **125**, 492–498.

Gershon, S. (1970). *Clin. Pharmac. Ther.* **11**, 168–187.

Goodwin, F. K., Murphy, D. L. and Bunney, W. E. (1969). *Archs gen. Psychiat.* **21**, 486–496.

Goodwin, F. K., Murphy, D. L., Dunner, D. L. and Bunney, W. E. (1972). *Am. J. Psychiat.* **129**, 76–79.

Grof, P. and Foley, P. (1971). *Am. J. Psychiat.* **127**, 1573–1574.

Haskovec, L. and Soucek, K. (1968). *Nature, Lond.* **219**, 507–508.

Hordern, A., Burt, C. G., Gordon, W. F. and Holt, N. F. (1964). *Br. J. Psychiat.* **110**, 641–647.

Hullin, R. P., McDonald, R. and Allsopp, M. N. (1972). *Lancet* **1**, 1044–1046.

Johnson, G., Gershon, S., Burdock, E., Floyd, A. and Hekimian, L. (1971). *Brit. J. Psychiat.* **119**, 267–276.

Johnson, G., Gershon, S. and Hekimian, L. (1968). *Compreh. Psychiat.* **9**, 563–573.

Klein, D. F. and Davis, J. M. (1969). "Diagnosis and Drug Treatment of Psychiatric Disorders". Williams and Wilkins Co., Baltimore.

Laurell, B. and Ottosson, J. O. (1968). *Lancet* **2**, 1245.

Lipkin, K. M., Dyrud, J. and Meyer, C. G. (1970). *Archs gen. Psychiat.* **22**, 262–266.

Maggs, R. (1963). *Br. J. Psychiat.* **109**, 56–65.

Maletzky, B. and Blachly, P. (1971). "The Use of Lithium in Psychiatry". CRC Press, Cleveland.

Mayer–Gross, W., Slater, E. and Roth, M. (1967). "Clinical Psychiatry". Williams and Wilkins Co., Baltimore.

Meiers, R. L. (1970). *Schizophrenia* **2**, 87–91.

Melia, P. I. (1970). *Brit. J. Psychiat.* **116**, 621–624.

Mendels, J., Secunda, S. K. and Dyson, W. L. (1972). *Archs gen. Psychiat.* **26**, 154–157.

Mindham, R. H., Howland, C. and Shepherd, M. (1973). *Psychol. Med.* **3**, 5–17.

Paykel, E. S., Klerman, G. L., DiMascio, A., Weissman, M. M. and Prusoff, B. A. (1973). *In* "Psychopathology and Psychopharmacology" (J. O. Cole, ed.), pp. 205–218. Johns Hopkins Press, Baltimore.

Platman, S. R. (1970a). *Amer. J. Psychiat.* **127**, 351–353.

Platman, S. R. (1970b). *Dis. nerv. Syst.* **31**, 132–134.

Prien, R. F., Caffey, E. M., Jr. and Klett, C. J. (1971). *Dis. nerv. Syst.* **32**, 521–531.

Prien, R. F., Caffey, E. M., Jr. and Klett, C. J. (1972). *Archs gen. Psychiat.* **27**, 182–189.

Prien, R. F., Caffey, E. M., Jr. and Klett, C. J. (1973a). *Archs gen. Psychiat.* **28**, 337–341.

Prien, R. F., Caffey, E. M., Jr. and Klett, C. J. (1973b). *Archs gen. Psychiat.* (in press).

Prien, R. F., Caffey, E. M., Jr. and Klett, C. J. (1973c). Paper presented at American Psychiatric Association Meeting, Hawaii.

Quitkin, F. M., Rifkin, A. and Klein, D. F. (1973). *In* "Lithium: Its Role in Psychiatric Research and Treatment". (S. Gershon and B. Shopsin, eds.), Plenum, New York.

Rimón, R. and Räkköläinen, V. (1968). *Brit. J. Psychiat.* **114**, 109–110.

Saran, B. M. (1969). *Lancet* **1**, 1208–1209.

Schlagenhauf, G., Tupin, J. and White, R. B. (1966). *Amer. J. Psychiat.* **123**, 201–207.

Schou, M. (1968). *J. psychiat. Res.* **6**, 67–95.

Schou. M., Juel-Nielsen, N., Strömgren, E. and Voldby, H. (1954). *J. Neurol. Neurosurg. Psychiat.* **17**, 250–260.

Shopsin, B., Kim, S. S. and Gershon, S. (1971). *Brit. J. Psychiat.* **119**, 435–440.

Spring, G., Schweid, D., Gray, G., Steinberg, J. and Horwitz, M. (1970). *Amer. J. Psychiat.* **126**, 1306–1309.

Stallone, F., Shelley, E., Mendlewicz, J. and Fieve, R. R. (1972). Paper presented at Collegium Internationale Neuropsychopharmacologicum Meeting, Copenhagen.

Strömgren, E. and Schou, M. (1964). *Postgrad. Med.* **35**, 83–86.

Tupin, J. (1970). *Hosp. comm. Psychiat.* **21**, 73–80.

Whitehead, P. L. and Clark, L. D. (1970). *Amer. J. Psychiat.* **127**, 824–825.

Wittrig, J. and Coopwood, W. E. (1970). *Dis. nerv. Syst.* **31**, 486–489.

Zall, H. (1971). *Amer. J. Psychiat.* **127**, 1400–1403.

8

METHODOLOGICAL ISSUES IN RESEARCH ON LITHIUM THERAPY

E. S. PAYKEL

I. Introduction: Standard Assessment Procedures

The clinical assessment of lithium efficacy has introduced a number of method-ological problems, and has necessitated adaptations of previously standard procedures for the evaluation of psychotropic drugs. These difficulties arise primarily from certain special features involved in the use of lithium. This chapter will review these methodological difficulties and the controversies surrounding them will be reviewed.

Before discussing the specific issues of lithium therapy we should recall some of the general issues of assessment of drug efficacy in psychiatry. Animal models in psychiatry are still sparse and their validity is often open to question. Assessment therefore depends heavily on human experimentation. However, the effects of psychotropic drugs in normal humans are often much less impressive and different in quality to those in illness. Hence assessment depends primarily on studies of ill patients. The standard assessment procedure of drug efficacy in clinical psychiatry, as in other branches of clinical medicine, has established itself firmly in the last 30 years. It is the double blind controlled clinical trial with random assignment of patients to treatment conditions, appropriate assessment measures and statistical analysis including testing of significance. The commonest variant of this design in psychiatry is the two group comparison with either placebo or a standard drug.

This somewhat cumbersome set of procedures is particularly necessary in psychiatry for a number of reasons. The spontaneous course of psychiatric illnesses is highly variable so that single remissions are often due to chance. Non-specific factors associated with treatment, including the patient's expectations of treatment outcome, may have potent effects. Concurrent environmental measures, such as admission to hospital, may induce marked improvement. Assessment may involve subtle judgements of outcome which are much prone to bias. A variety of precautions incorporated in standard designs is aimed at overcoming these problems.

The most central of these measures is the provision of a control group of patients, in whom all the other effects except that of specific treatment may be expected to operate. Most of these could be controlled for by a group treated in all respects the same but receiving no tablet. Two effects would not be controlled for: non-specific effects of tablet taking, and observer bias. Adequate control for these requires in addition a further precaution, that of double blindness, and this can only retained if an identical tablet is administered to the control group. Double blindness may not always be essential or feasible in clinical trials; it is an additional method of eliminating bias based on the experimenter's expectations. The experimenter must, however, present strong evidence that these are unimportant if he is to dispense with this precaution. This is particularly difficult in psychiatry, where effects of expectations are so strong that uncontrolled studies tend to produce much higher estimates of drug efficacy than do adequately controlled trials (Foulds, 1958).

A third precaution in clinical trials is that of random assignment of patients to treatments. It is necessary to avoid introducing systematic bias between treatment groups based on research preconceptions. It is important that the assignment should be truly random. Alternate assignment to different treatments may readily be penetrated by an astute rater intent on cracking the double blind. This may lead to biased rating, and also to biased assignment whereby patients thought likely to do badly on the less favoured treatment are saved for the better treatment. Random assignment by itself does not, however, guarantee comparability of treatment groups which must therefore be checked separately.

A related issue is that of sampling of trial subjects from the patient population. Two alternative aims might be advanced: one that the sampling be representative, the second that it enable potentially responsive subjects to be included. These two aims are not usually reconcilable, and the second is often the more important. Representative sampling is impeded by the many factors controlling referral to drug trials. Where effective drugs are readily available, patients included in clinical trials are often biased towards chronicity and failure of previous treatment. This may not favour a responsive sample; nor does representative sampling if the responsive subgroup is small. The appropriate group is often difficult to define in the early stages of drug evaluation. Leff (1973) has suggested that drug-placebo differences will be greatest if both patients with good spontaneous prognosis and those with very poor prognosis are excluded from study samples.

Adequate evaluation also requires the use of appropriate assessment measures. The increasing sophistication of psychiatric drug trials has been accompanied by the application of quantitative rating scales for assessment, which, although prone to considerable unreliability and invalidity, provide extra precision. The greatest proportion of drug trials has been in schizophrenia and depression, and, not surprisingly, rating scales for symptoms in these two areas are best developed. Symptom scales for assessing mania have received less attention, as have non-symptomatic areas such as social adjustment and satisfactions. Outcomes may be multiple and different measures do not necessarily parallel each other.

The outcome measures also require appropriate analysis, and intelligent use of tests of statistical significance. One advantage of quantitative rating scales is their suitability for sensitive parametric statistical techniques, including regressional and covariance analyses and sophisticated analyses of variance. Their conformity to parametric assumptions cannot however be assumed.

A final issue concerns reporting. It is important that drug trials be reported in sufficient detail for the reader to judge whether their methodologies are adequate. The exigencies of journal space and pressures of editors do not always further this aim. Lionel and Herxheimer (1970) have described a checklist for assessing reports of therapeutic trials.

The value of the standard controlled trial has been criticised by some authors on a number of grounds (Barsa, 1963; Cromie, 1963). These include the risk of compromising double blindness by side effects, use of fixed rather than flexible doses, use of too short a treatment period, inappropriate or insensitive assessment measures, swamping of responsive by unresponsive subjects, artificial insistence on apparently objective assessments which turn out to be heavily subjective, and contamination by extraneous environmental changes. It is noteworthy that most of these criticisms concern flaws in current practice in designing trials, rather than faults in the basic validity of the method itself.

The established principles of drug evaluation have run into some special problems in connection with lithium. These include problems of experimenter tolerance of concurrent controls, issues of sampling, difficulties in preserving blindness, problems of control of mania, and the design requirements of long term prophylactic studies.

II. Use of Controls: The Retrospective Study Controversy

The use of retrospective controls for studying the prophylactic effect of lithium has been the subject of a vigorous debate. Initial statements were provided by the retrospective report from Baastrup and Schou (1967), and by the critical rejoinder from Blackwell and Shepherd (1968). A counterblast followed from Baastrup and Schou (1968) and a sporadic but spirited correspondence ensued in the pages of the Lancet.

In their initial report Baastrup and Schou studied 88 female patients suffering from recurrent depression or mania and compared their experience of relapse while on maintenance lithium with their prior experience before lithium had been started. Frequency of relapse and time spent in a psychotic state were significantly lower in the lithium maintenance period. Angst *et al.* (1970) in a collaborative study of cases from Switzerland, Czechoslovakia, and Denmark, extended the findings to 244 patients. During the period on lithium therapy the frequencies of episodes and of hospital admissions were reduced and lengths of cycles were increased. The improvements were of considerable magnitude, the experience of patients on lithium being at least twice as favourable as that prior to treatment.

Although the debate concerned prophylactic efficacy, the same issues arise in acute studies, and they really concern the use of controls. It is generally conceded that some kind of control is necessary. The issue for debate is what kinds of controls are acceptable. In general three types of controls have been utilized in lithium studies (Klerman and Paykel, 1970). (A) retrospective historical controls (B) prospective within-patient controls (C) concurrent between-patient controls.

A. Retrospective historical controls

The studies cited used retrospective historical controls. It should be noted that the designs involved comparisons with previous experience in the same patients. An alternative strategy would use data from treatments of the disease as reported in the literature or as documented in other patient groups in the same clinic, all prior to the introduction of lithium. Such a design would be notably inferior however since systematic differences in the characteristics of the samples might markedly affect the prognoses.

The retrospective technique has an apparent advantage: it does not involve withholding a new drug which the investigators believe to be effective. However this design also has crucial disadvantages. First, it cannot be double blind. It thus does not control for non-specific placebo effects of tablet taking or for observer bias. It has been argued that their effects on the course of recurrent affective disorders is slight (Grof *et al.*, 1970). This may be so; there is certainly some evidence that withdrawal from amitriptyline overtly in recovered depressives produces a degree of symptom recrudescence no different from withdrawal to placebo double blind (Paykel *et al.*, 1974). On the other hand, this may not apply in the reverse situation of the introduction of a new medication. At present the amount of evidence available on the effects of non-specific factors in this situation is too limited for the double blind condition to be confidently dispensed with.

Secondly, these designs involve non-random treatment assignments: the control periods always precede lithium periods. A variety of other temporal changes may obtrude and obscure trends. For instance, manic depressives tend to have more frequent episodes as they grow older (Angst and Weiss, 1967), and this might obscure therapeutic results. Moreover, close clinical observations of patients on lithium may lead to the detection of transient or minor episodes which might have been missed during the earlier period when the patients were not on maintenance treatment (Fieve *et al.*, 1968). There may be changes in other treatments given at the same time or in general patterns of management. Moderately ill patients are probably less likely to be admitted to hospital nowadays so that studies which compare retrospective and present hospital admission rates are suspect. Some of these factors can be dealt with. Angst *et al.* (1970) included age at first episode and number of previous episodes as predictor variables in a multiple regression analysis so as to control for the tendency of episodes to become more frequent as time elapsed. However it is difficult to control in this design for all factors, and the suspicion will remain of undocumented ones which may have effects in either direction.

Thirdly, sampling problems may lead to bias. Prophylactic treatment is more likely to be commenced at a time when the patient has had several episodes close together. The studies of both Baastrup and Schou (1967) and Angst *et al.* (1970) in fact specified in selection criteria that subjects must have had at least two episodes in the last two years. Even if the criteria had not specified recurrent illnesses, referral would clearly be more likely in such cases. Although the occurrence of illness episodes in a group may be entirely random, some individual patients will experience episodes more frequently at one time than another. If a drug is commenced in the latter part of a frequent period following a cluster of episodes, the subsequent period is likely on the average to show fewer episodes.

Saran (1970) demonstrated this effect in following up patients not treated by lithium, although some received other medications. However, Prien *et al.* (1973a) attempted a similar analysis in a controlled study of lithium prophylaxis. They found a reduction in episode frequency compared with that prior to treatment only in patients on lithium and not in those on placebo. Baastrup and Schou (1967) attempted to deal with this issue in a subsidiary analysis by omitting the year prior to the start of lithium therapy; Angst *et al.* (1970) excluded the last episode. It is debatable in either case whether this would be adequate.

Blackwell and Shepherd (1968) also suggested two lesser potential flaws in this design. The follow up period may be too short for adequate relapse experience. Total length of symptomatic illness in the period under observation may be a measure of therapeutic rather than prophylactic effect; this would not apply to the length of time from one onset to the next.

The combined results from the summation of all these factors must remain highly uncertain. These were major studies carried out carefully. The magnitude of the effects found was so large as to render their causation solely by supervening factors unlikely. However, by themselves restrospective studies will always be vulnerable to criticisms which only studies using concurrent controls can silence.

B. Within-patient prospective controls

Moving beyond retrospective controls, a second possible design employs the patient as his own control in a prospective fashion. Chassan (1967) and Bellack *et al.* (1961) have advocated the use of single patient intra-individual designs in psychiatric studies. Patients can be selected for whom the drug appears most appropriate, and it can then be given and withdrawn repeatedly. This design differs importantly from the retrospective within-patient control, since the drug can be administered in double blind fashion and the treatment periods can be randomised so as to balance effects of other temporal changes. Provided a sufficient number of periods on and off the drug are used, this type of design will provide a valid test, and appropriate statistics are available (Chassan, 1967). The findings are, however, valid only for the single patient, so that in the long run, the investigators must study a sufficient number of patients to render the combined experience equivalent to a multi-patient crossover study. Moreover, if a true picture is to be obtained, it is important that negative as well as positive studies be published. Unfortunately the natural enthusiasms of investigators, the space exigencies of journals, and the interests of readers are such that negative studies of small numbers of patients are less liable to be published.

This design is not suitable for maintenance studies of lithium. Multiple discontinuation and reinstitution of treatment are ruled out by the lengthy time involved and the serious social consequences of multiple episodes for well patients in the community. A single crossover maintenance study of lithium has been reported (Cundall *et al.,* 1972). True within-patient designs are, however, well suited, and have been used for acute treatment of mania, since responses to commencement and withdrawal of treatment are moderately rapid and patients with the illness are relatively uncommon. The design has been used most effectively by Bunney, Goodwin and colleagues (Bunney *et al.,* 1968; Goodwin *et al.*, 1969) who, in their second report noted findings in 12 manic patients and 18 depressives. Unfortunately it is not clear if treatment and withdrawal periods were truly random in these studies. Published charts suggest intermittent brief periods of withdrawal on schedules which were not far from regular. The authors did not use intra-individual statistics to evaluate findings, possibly because withdrawal periods were relatively infrequent. It is doubtful if the usual clinical situation provides opportunities for a sufficient number of repeated trials for a proper intra-individual analysis to be applied. This design may not be suitable for acute treatment of depression if, as clinical experience suggests, improvement from depression is a slow and delayed but frequently once-and-for-all phenomenon. In general the intra-individual design, although it has been more suitable for lithium than for some other drugs, has been useful at a pilot and hypothesis-generating level rather than as a method for definitive studies.

C. Concurrent between-patient controls

The third type of controlled design is the concurrent between-patient study. This has become the standard for definitive assessment of therapeutic efficacy. Its merits have already been discussed. It is well suited to application of double blind techniques, random assignment, and factorial designs. The concurrent nature of the controls provides an ideal method of controlling for biasing factors. It enables the clinical researcher to approximate as far as he can to the experimental laboratory ideal.

The arguments against the concurrent between-patient design have been on two grounds: methodological and ethical. The methodological objections have already been discussed. They concern imperfections of some studies, rather than basic flaws in the design.

The ethical objections have been several. One set concerns informed consent: there is little doubt that at one time not enough attention was given to this issue, although, at least in the U.K and the U.S.A., safeguards are now adequate. Another ethical objection asks how far it is justified to expose a subject to a new, untried treatment. If present treatments are ineffective and the new treatment appears promising and has been demonstrated to be safe, this argument carries little conviction. If effective treatments are already available the argument is more valid; it may be difficult to justify comparison with a placebo. Comparison with the prevailing standard treatment will, however, be strongly indicated. Basically, this objection is not to the controlled trial but to the introduction of the drug. If it is to be introduced it is better that the comparison be in the form of a controlled trial rather than uncontrolled, since the former method is likely to give a conclusive answer much earlier and with fewer subjects.

Paradoxically a third objection against undertaking a concomitant controlled trial, and the one which has been advanced most commonly with regard to lithium, is the opposite one that patients will suffer from the withholding of an effective therapy. This argument is circular and begs the question: it depends on the prior demonstration of efficacy. It is only in the most exceptionally efficacious treatments that cure is so dramatic as to carry universal conviction. Such treatments are very uncommon in psychiatry. On the other hand the list of ultimately discarded treatments which were previously regarded as effective is too long to stand recapitulation.

The major disadvantages of controlled trials are perhaps the practical ones. Undoubtedly they involve considerable effort and expense to carry out. Usually it takes a surprisingly long time to accumulate an adequate sample although the evolution, in the last 15 years, of the multi-centre trial has alleviated this problem.

The passage of a few years has enabled the original controversy over retrospective studies of lithium prophylaxis to be set in context. Both sets of protagonists can be seen to have proved their points. Concurrent between-patient trials have now been carried out and found to be eminently feasible. They are reviewed in a later section. In the long run only their findings have carried ultimate conviction. They have, however, shown major prophylactic effects for lithium, of the same order as those shown by retrospective studies, justifying the original claims and suggesting that biasing factors were not in fact of major importance in this particular context.

III. Classification and Sampling

Affective disorders span a wide range of clinical pictures. Since the late nineteenth century there has been an active debate among psychiatrists as to the significance of this diversity. One issue concerns the nature of depression itself. When Kraepelin delineated the foundations of modern psychiatric nosology by separating manic-depressive insanity from schizophrenia, he regarded the former as a disease entity based on a medical, neurological model, with specific biological organic aetiology and pathology (Kraepelin, 1921). However, at the same time as Kraepelin and others were classifying psychiatric disorders in terms of illness, another growing school of European psychiatrists, the psychoanalysts, was developing a very different approach. Freud (1917) and Abraham (1924) related depression to actual symbolic losses of a love object. Here was a theory regarding the origin of most, if not all, depressions as psychogenic.

These philosophical issues influence research methodology. Those who view depression as a psychologically induced disorder of living are likely to emphasise the potential influence on outcome of such factors as expectations, enthusiasm, rater set, and the psychotherapeutic relationship. Such investigators will feel the need to control for these factors by placebo groups and double blind designs. On the other hand investigators who view affective disorders as biologically caused illnesses tend to feel that non-specific factors can have only minor and transitory effects on course and outcome. The positions taken by various protagonists in the retrospective control controversy show some evidence of having been coloured in this way by underlying views of the nature of affective disorders.

There has been vigorous controversy for forty years as to whether the heterogeneity of depression can be encompassed within a single disorder or can be further divided. The unitary position of a single disorder derives particularly from the views of Meyer and his psychobiological school that organic and psychological, genetic and environmental aetiology may combine in the same or different individuals to produce the same disorder (Meyer, 1922). In England this view of depression has been associated particularly with Aubrey Lewis (Lewis, 1934). Opposed to it is the view of depression as comprising two separate entities variously termed as endogenous and reactive, psychotic and neurotic (Gillespie, 1929; Carney et al., 1965). An intermediate position suggests that the two polar types are extremes on a continuum, rather than being clearly separable (Kendell, 1968).

The literature on this classificatory controversy came predominately in two bursts, one in the 1930's, the second in the 1960's. There is little doubt that the reawakening of interest was a consequence of the development of antidepressant medications and of hints that tricyclic antidepressants and E.C.T. might be particularly effective in endogenous depressives.

A similar heuristic consequence, with a different emphasis, has accompanied the introduction of lithium, which was initially used in the treatment of mania and other states of excitement, and later extended to the prophylaxis of recurrent mania and depression. This consequence is the marked increase in research interest in manic depressive illness, and the presentation of evidence that bipolar depressions can be separated from other depressive disorders (Perris, 1966; Winokur et al., 1969; Goodwin, 1973). As with the earlier classificatory studies, one important aim of this research is that of predicting who responds best to treatment. The relationship of the bipolar–unipolar dichotomy to the earlier classification has so far been left unclear, although most would probably regard bipolar depression as one subtype of endogenous depression.

The question of sampling is particularly important in depression, because of its heterogeneity in terms of type of clinical picture, severity, and previous history. The label "depression" is inadequate for precise description, and a detailed account of criteria, sampling methods and sample characteristics is desirable. Moreover the place of any subgroup in the total clinical picture must be kept in mind. Over the last fifty years there has been a well documented change in the characteristics of depressed patients under psychiatric treatment. Today's patients tend to be younger, less severely ill, and more commonly neurotic than do those of previous generations (Rosenthal, 1966). They are also more likely to be treated outside hospital. These changes probably result from a number of factors, including the efficacy of modern treatments in alleviating depression; the tendency for patients to receive treatment earlier; the willingness to come for treatment of patients who might not previously have accepted their milder disorders as psychiatric; and, possibly, actual changes in clinical characteristics and epidemiology of the illness.

The result of these changes is that descriptive and therapeutic stereotypes developed from severely ill patients admitted to hospital may no longer apply. A study of depressives sampled from a representative range of treatment facilities in New Haven, Connecticut illustrates this (Paykel *et al.,* 1970). In this study it was found that a substantial proportion of the depressives receiving psychiatric treatment were outpatients. The majority of episodes were reactive or neurotic: endogeneous depressives comprised only about 15% of the total. Bipolar depressions in terms of previous manic episodes were quite uncommon, comprising only 3% of the total. It is important to remember that treatments directed primarily to bipolar depressives, or even to unipolar endogenous depressives will make a limited impact on the total problem of depression.

There is in addition a complex sorting process of referral which determines the type of patient to be found in each treatment setting. Findings from the New Haven survey illustrated this. Overall, depression was diagnosed in about 30% of patients, but the prevalence in different treatment units varied widely from 14% to 50% of patients admitted. More importantly, different clinical pictures tended to be found in different settings. There was, as might be expected, a gradient of severity: mildly ill patients were treated as outpatients, more severely ill patients admitted to hospital. There was also a qualitative difference in the type of clinical picture. Outpatients included many young patients whose depression occurred on a background of disturbed interpersonal relationships suggesting personality disorders. Day hospital patients included a high proportion of recurrent or chronic depressives with a strong admixture of anxiety; severe psychotic or endogenous depressives, and bipolar depressives were found most commonly among inpatients, particularly those admitted to a biological research ward (Paykel, 1971). The type of patient sampled, and thus the outcome of a therapeutic study, might depend heavily on the kind of treatment setting in which the study was conducted.

Problems of sampling are probably less important in the case of mania, although they have not been adequately studied. Most manics are admitted to hospital. It has not so far been suggested that there are fundamentally different types of manic disorder. The difference between mania and excited schizoaffective disorder has, however, been recognised, and has an important influence on findings in acute studies of lithium. Moreover, the overall frequency of mania is much lower than that of depression.

The problem of recurrence is an important one in sample selection for prophylactic studies in mania and depression. Both conditions are commonly recurrent, or followed by chronic morbidity. Winokur *et al.* (1969) found in an eighteen month follow-up of manic-depressives that approximately one-third had fresh episodes and another third had chronic symptoms. However a moderate proportion of depressives probably experience only one episode in their lives. Patients who show frequent recurrence of mania or depression, and are thus the prime targets for long term maintenance studies, comprise only a relatively small proportion of the total.

A last sampling problem concerns the collaborative studies carried out by the Veterans Administration group of workers in the U.S.A., in collaboration with the National Institute of Mental Health, and reported by Prien *et al.* (1972a, b; 1973a, b). These studies have in many respects been model ones, leading the field in methodology and in quality of reporting. They do, however, suffer from one disadvantage derived from the nature of the Veterans Administration Hospitals which comprise the main contributing resources. The patients of these hospitals tend to be a special population biased towards males, with chronic and recurrent disorders, sometimes with the suspicion of secondary gain in the demonstration of a disability related to military service.

IV. Blindness and Toxicity

A particular problem in the evaluation of lithium lies in its narrow dose range of therapeutic efficacy. Lithium has a smaller range between therapeutic effects and seriously toxic side effects than any other commonly used psychotropic drug. The side effects are distinctive and different from those of many comparison drugs. It is unique in psychopharmacology in that monitoring of serum levels is moderately easy and has been regarded, at least in recent years, as mandatory for adequate therapeutic control.

This raises a number of problems in controlled trials. The first is that the distinctive pattern of side effects may compromise blindness. Thus, as will be detailed in subsequent sections, a number of studies have found significant differences between reports of side effects by patients on lithium and those in placebo or other drug control groups. However only the more careful studies report side effects: it cannot be assumed that they were absent or not important potential biases in the others.

Side effects are also potential consquences of placebo administration. In one acute study, Maggs (1963) found that, except for two toxic reactions, minor side effects were infrequent and occurred in both lithium and placebo groups. In a maintenance study Prien *et al.* (1973b) found side effects, mainly anorexia, dry mouth, constipation and somnolence, in 49% of placebo patients. These and similar effects, however, occurred in 69% of patients on lithium.

Baastrup and Schou (1970), in a maintenance study using previously stabilised patients who were withdrawn from drug onto a placebo with an alkaline-bitter taste, found to their surprise no detectable change in side effects on withdrawal.

The problem of side effects probably occurs in controlled trials of many drugs and is often missed because side effects are not recorded, or not included in reports of the research. The degree of biasing effect may not always be large.

A more unique and important problem arises from the need to monitor serum levels, and to adjust the dose accordingly. This means that it is difficult to keep treating psychiatrists in ignorance of the nature of the medication, a requisite for the true double blind condition. This problem has led to several different types of compromise. The issues behind them and their adequacy have rarely been made explicit. Thus some studies have been single blind, open to psychiatrists, blind to patients. This level of blindness is not acceptable, except for pilot studies.

The commonest method of coping with this problem has been to separate treating psychiatrists and raters: treating pscyhiatrists then know the contents of the tablets, but patients, raters and other staff do not. This procedure is often claimed to be double blind. In fact, as usually employed, it is not; at most it may be regarded as "one and a half blind". The crucial flaw is that someone who knows the real nature of the treatment has both contact with the patient and an influence on treatment decisions. He may communicate his knowledge and expectations covertly to the patient or allow it to bias decisions, such as that of withdrawl from the study. The raters are, however, blind and at least their bias cannot directly affect ratings.

Important improvement can be built into this design by preventing the person who knows the blood levels, and thus the treatment, from having contact with the patients. His potential communication with the patient is thus avoided, although the effects of bias on treatment decisions may not be (Mendels *et al.*, 1972; Cundall *et al.*, 1972).

The purest and most satisfying designs were those accomplished in two maintenance studies, reported by Baastrup *et al.* (1972) and Stallone *et al.* (1973). They arranged for fictitious blood levels to be assigned by the laboratory for placebo patients: treating psychiatrists could thus be kept blind and they could also be raters. In the Baastrup study, the laboratory was also distant from the site of treatment. An equally satisfactory procedure from the point of view of blindness, although not from that of clinical use, would be to dispense with blood levels. Only one maintenance study appears to have done this, in a sample of patients previously well stabilised (Melia, 1970).

An important element in all these designs, even for the single blind state, is that blood samples should be taken from the control group. It is also important that dose alterations should be made in this group to parallel those resulting from blood levels in the lithium group. These points are obvious ones and have probably been met in most studies. Unfortunately explicit statements to this effect are frequently lacking in published reports, leading to unnecessary demands on the critic's faith.

V. Acute Treatment Studies

There have now been a number of concurrent between-patient controlled trials of lithium in acute treatment. Table I summarises methodological details of nine studies, all employing levels of blindness better than the single blind state. Five were in manic patients, two in schizophrenics (one of the manic studies also included a group of schizoaffectives). One study was in depressives, and another in patients with emotionally unstable character disorder. Only the last study and one of the studies of mania employed a placebo control group. In all the remainder the control group received chlorpromazine, except for the depressive study, in which desipramine was used.

Some reports fail to specify sufficient details to assure the critical reader that methodological difficulties have been met. The table does not deal with sampling. On the whole, the reports specify their selection criteria explicitly. They vary a good deal in the degree to which they describe referral procedures, representative sampling, sample characteristics, and their comparability between treatment groups. The study in depression employed relatively severe depressives of psychotic or endogeneous type (Mendels, *et al.*, 1972). On the other hand randomisation was well handled. All reports except that of Johnson *et al.* (1971) contain explicit statements that drug treatment assignment was random.

Serum lithium levels were obtained in all the studies. Only Maggs (1963) and Mendels *et al.* (1972) make explicit statements that blood samples were also taken from the control groups. In coping with the problem of dose regulation most of these studies compromised their blindness. Only Mendels *et al.* (1972) explicitly describe a better than one-and-a-half blind state in which the psychiatrist who regulated the dose had no contact with the patients. Four studies used a technique in which a treating psychiatrist had access to information about dose levels, but raters did not (Prien *et al.*, 1972a, b; Spring *et al.*, 1970; Shopsin *et al.*, 1971).

The reports by Rifkin *et al.* (1972), Johnson *et al.* (1971), Platman (1970) do not contain enough information to allow the reader to judge which of the above two models they followed. Maggs (1963) was both treating psychiatrist and rater in his study, the biochemist informing him if serum levels arose above 2 mEq/l. He does not make it clear how often this happened; he hints that such patients may have been withdrawn from the study. Notably however, this was one of the earliest of lithium studies and had to pioneer some of the methodological problems. None of the reports make it explicitly clear that blindness was preserved by having the physician who adjusted the dose make

TABLE I Acute studies of lithium treatment

Authors	Prien et al. (1972a)	Johnson et al. (1971)	Platman (1970)	Spring et al. (1970)
Subject Group	Mania	Mania (also included schizoaffectives)	Mania	Mania
Comparison drug	Chlorpromazine	Chlorpromazine	Chlorpromazine	Chlorpromazine
Randomized assignment	Yes	Not stated	Yes	Yes
Blood levels				
Lithium group	Yes	Yes	Yes	Yes
Control group	Not stated	Not stated	Not stated	Not stated
Blindness				
Raters blind	Yes	Yes	Yes	Yes
Treating doctors in contact with patients blind	No	Not stated	Not stated	No
Side effects more in lithium group	Yes	Yes	Not stated	No (?)
Early terminations	21%; end point analysis	15%; analysis of completers only	Not stated	32%; analysis of completers only
Findings	Highly active— lithium superior Mildly active— equal	Mania—lithium superior Schizoaffective— lithium inferior (Both ns)	Lithium superior (ns)	Equal

...ggs (1963)	Prien et al. (1972b)	Shopsin et al. (1971)	Mendels et al. (1972)	Rifkin et al. (1962)
...nia	Schizoaffective	Schizophrenia	Depression	Emotionally unstable character disorder
...cebo	Chlorpromazine	Chlorpromazine	Desipramine	Placebo
	Yes	Yes	Yes	Yes
	Yes	Yes	Yes	Yes
	Not stated	Not stated	Yes	Not stated
	Yes	Yes	Yes	Yes
...t in some cases	No	No	Yes	Not stated
...(?)	Yes	Yes	Not stated	Not stated
...; analysis of ...ompleters only	End point analysis	Not stated	Not stated	Not stated
...ium superior	Highly active— lithium inferior Mildly active— equal	Lithium inferior	Equal	Lithium superior

occasional alterations in placebo dose as though based on blood levels. However, Rifkin *et al.* (1972) cleverly obviated the need for this by using a constant daily number of capsules and altering the amount of lithium in each capsule.

Subsequent analysis of side effects showed significant differences between lithium and control groups in one study (Prien *et al.*, 1972a), and probably significant differences in three other studies (Johnson *et al.*, 1971; Prien *et al.*, 1972b; Shopsin *et al.*, 1971). Spring *et al.* (1970) suggested that side effects were comparable in the two groups but did not report frequencies. Maggs (1963) found side effects similar, apart from two cases of severe toxicity in the lithium group. Side effects were not described at all in three other studies. Thus blindness did tend to be compromised by side effects. However all the descriptions suggest considerable overlap in side effects so that this difference may not have been important and, as previously discussed, similar criticisms could probably be levelled at studies of many other drugs in which authors have not systematically recorded the presence of side effects.

Acute studies of lithium present an additional set of problems which has not so far been discussed. This arises from the use of manic patients. For one thing, mania is a relatively rare condition: series may take a long time to accumulate, forcing compromise in design, and pressures on the experimenter (Platman, 1970). Moreover, problems of controlling severely disturbed behaviour may overwhelm the best planned research study via refusal to take oral medicine, and the need for additional sedation to control behaviour. This may produce high levels of dropout.

One flaw in four of these studies is failure to describe the number of early terminations. It is not clear whether there were no dropouts, which seems unlikely, or whether reported findings are based only on study completers, which may be misleading. It is highly probable that the treatment failures will be more common in the less effective treatments, and if dropout rates are high those left at the end of the study will tend to be treatment successes, so that real differences in efficacy may be obscured. Five studies reported dropout rates, which varied from 15% to 35%. The former level is highly acceptable, the latter near the margin of acceptability. Two studies dealt elegantly with the problem by carrying out end point analyses which included early dropouts rated at the time of termination (Prien *et al.*, 1972a, b).

The efficacy of lithium in these studies is discussed elsewhere in this volume, but findings are summarised briefly in the table. A weakness of the studies is that only two, one in mania and one in emotionally unstable character disorder, employed placebo controls. In both lithium was superior. The remaining studies might suggest that lithium is about as effective as chlorpromazine in mania but less effective in schizophrenics and schizoaffectives. However, the finding that one drug is equal to another does not, without a placebo comparison, necessarily indicate that either had any effect in the particular patient sample under study. Authors of some studies assume that because significant improvement occurred from commencement to termination, this must be due to the drug rather than to milieu effect or a spontaneous remission. Milieu effects may be less in mania and schizophrenia than depression, although this is not proven; spontaneous remission may certainly occur.

VI. Maintenance Studies

Techniques for controlled trials of acute treatment are well established in psychopharmacology. For maintenance studies, however, the situation is different. The earliest studies of psychotropic drugs were in the acute frame. Only subsequently were long-term trials undertaken, first with phenothiazines in schizophrenia, more recently with antidepressants and lithium in affective disorders. Long term prophylactic studies raise new methodological problems which have required new solutions.

One set of problems has concerned ethics and experimenter resistance in various guises. These have already been discussed. The retrospective control controversy arose over long term maintenance treatment. Long term studies do involve longer exposure of patients and of experimenter to the constraints of a research design with random treatment assignment and double blind conditions. The length of time required to carry them out also renders them logistically more difficult and may involve a lengthy commitment by a research team.

Selection criteria are again important. It is reasonable to select patients with recurrent illnesses since in clinical practice they are logical candidates for prophylactic treatment. This procedure also increases the likelihood of further episodes occurring during the experimental period so that treatment effect can be demonstrated. It must, however, be kept in mind that recurrent illnesses may be atypical and comprise only a small proportion of the total spectrum.

Sampling issues obtrude in a special way into maintenance designs. It is uncommon that maintenance studies involve starting new treatments in well subjects. More commonly the design involves drug withdrawal. Withdrawal studies may be carried out in two ways: all patients may be started on a substance and then withdrawn, or patients may be included in the study only if they have been successfully maintained on the substance in the past. Both designs are likely to involve some selection of patients. The first design need not do so if the patient sample is well when the drug is started. More often this design has been used in maintenance studies of tricyclic antidepressants in which depressed patients are treated with the antidepressant and those who respond included in a trial of early withdrawal versus continuation. This use of the design clearly biases the study in favour of drug responders to acute treatment. It is, however, appropriate to the clinical question being asked, namely that of how long treatment should be continued. This design would be appropriate to lithium treatment of mania, but not depression, since lithium is not usually employed as a definitive acute treatment. More often a different design has been used in lithium maintenance. Patients attending a lithium clinic and being successfully maintained are randomised and some are withdrawn from the drug. In this case there is a bias in favour of patients who respond to lithium maintenance: unsuccessful cases will already have been withdrawn from treatment. Once again, this is not inappropriate to demonstrating therapeutic effects of lithium, provided the process of selection is realised so the results are not automatically generalised to a wider or less selective patient population.

The maintenance withdrawal design has another advantage with respect to lithium. It is possible to stabilise doses beforehand so that the need for frequent dose changes dictated by blood levels, and the occurrence of side effects which may compromise blindness, are minimised. There is, however, the risk that withdrawal may result in withdrawal symptoms on a basis of previous physiological tolerance and dependence. Little attention has been paid to this possibility with respect to lithium (Blackwell, 1970).

Maintenance studies of affective disorders, since they involve well patients, are almost always conducted in outpatients. This results in additional problems of cooperation. Outpatients are more easily lost to treatment by failure to attend, or by moving elsewhere. Moderate attrition rates must be expected. Moreover outpatients show a well documented tendency not to take the tablets which are prescribed for them (Willcox *et al.,* 1965). Some form of monitoring of drug taking is necessary. For lithium this is usually provided by serum levels. This measure does not ensure that patients on placebo take their medication and it may render lithium patients subject to greater exhortation to tablet taking.

The aims and criteria used in evaluating efficacy of long term treatment are multiple and different from those which apply to acute treatment. Reduction of the mortality associated with suicide is a major aim in treating affective disorders, but most maintenance studies are too short for suicide rates to form effective outcome criteria. The usual criteria are the prevention of relapse and of further episodes. These may be measured by reduction in rates of readmission to hospital. This criterion is relatively easily judged and readily quantifiable. However cases requiring hospitalisation occur less frequently than minor symptom recrudescences which do not require admission. Methods for the detection and characterisation of such milder relapses have not been well worked out, and the judgemental criteria used are not necessarily reliable.

There is also an unresolved question surrounding medication-induced recovery from an acute episode. Can this be regarded as an all-or-none cure, or is it a process of symptom suppression which must be continued until spontaneous recovery occurs? It may be useful to distinguish relapses, occurring early after treatment and possibly reflecting recrudescences of the original episode, from recurrences, occurring later due to new episodes. The two maintenance studies reported by Prien *et al.*, (1973a, b) were among the few to use this distinction.

However, the goals of long term treatment extend beyond the prevention of overt relapse and reccurrence. They include relief from persistent minor symptoms, enhancement of personal adjustment including social and vocational adaptation, and increase in the patient's satisfactions with life. Interview symptom rating scales for measuring severe degrees of pathology may be less suitable for characterising persisting minor pathology, or minor relapses. Self report scales may be of greater value, and may also tap satisfactions (Paykel *et al.*, 1974). Assessment of social adjustment and adaption require rating scales specifically designed for this purpose. Such scales are less well developed than symptom scales, but some are available (Paykel *et al.*, 1971).

Table II summarises methodological issues in eight concurrent between-patient controlled maintenance trials of lithium, employing levels of blindness better than single blind. All studies incorporated placebo control groups; one study included in addition a group maintained on imipramine.

Samples were on the whole specified clearly. All studies except one (Prien *et al.*, 1973a) required patients to have recurrent episodes. Subjects in three studies had previously been hospitalised (Hullin *et al.*, 1972; Prien *et al.*, 1973a, b). Subjects in one study were limited to manics (Prien *et al.*, 1973a) and in two studies were limited to depressives (Baastrup *et al.*, 1970; Prien *et al.*, 1972b). The remaining studies included both manic and depressive patients.

All studies employing depressives found it useful to make a distinction between unipolar and bipolar depressives but the endogenous–reactive or psychotic–neurotic designations were rarely utilised. In four studies the design involved withdrawal to placebo of patients successfully maintained on lithium so that lithium responders were selectively favoured. Some subjects in a fifth study also fell into this category (Stallone *et al.*, 1973). A further study included manic patients many of whom had received lithium as acute treatment (Prien *et al.*, 1973a). Initial treatment experience was variable in the remaining two studies.

The length of these studies was on the whole adequate, varying from five months to two years. Once again random assignment was well documented; it was explicitly stated to have occurred in all studies. All studies except one in previously well stabilised patients (Melia, 1970) utilised serum levels. Reports of five studies explicitly state that blood was also taken from the control group. This improvement on the acute studies probably reflects the fact that the maintenance studies were on the whole more recent. Studies were also better designed to achieve blindness than were the acute studies. The study which did not use blood levels was double blind in the orthodox manner.

Three additional studies achieved double blindness by having treating psy-

TABLE II Maintenance studies of lithium

Authors	Baastrup et al. (1970)	Coppen et al. (1971)	Melia (1970)
Comparison drug	Placebo	Placebo	Placebo
Sample	Unipolar and bipolar depressives. Recurrent. Female	Manics, unipolar and bipolar depressives. Recurrent	Manics, unipolar and bipolar depressives.
Withdrawal of previously successful lithium maintainance	Yes	No	Yes
Length of trial	5 months	Variable to 26 months	24 months
Randomized assignment	Yes	Yes	Yes

Blood levels
  Lithium group
  Control group
	Yes
	Yes
		Yes
		Yes
			No
			No

Blindness
  Raters blind
  Treating psychia-
  trist in contact
  with patient
  blind
	Yes
	Yes
		Yes
		Uncertain
			Yes
			Yes

Side effects more in lithium group	No	Not stated	Yes
Non relapse early terminations	6%	11%	Uncertain
Fate of relapsers	Withdrawn from study	Treated and retained in study	Withdrawn from study
Other assessments	No	Global assessment	No
Findings	Lithium superior in unipolar and bipolar	Lithium superior in unipolar and bipolar	Lithium superior ($p < 0.10$)

llone et al. (1973)	Cundall et al. (1972)	Hullin et al. (1972)	Prien et al. (1973a)	Prien et al. (1973b)
acebo	Placebo	Placebo	Placebo	Placebo and imipramine
polar manic-depressives. Recurrent	Bipolar manic-depressives. Unipolar depressives. Recurrent	Manics, unipolar and bipolar depressives and schizoaffectives. Recurrent. Hospitalized	Manics. Hospitalized	Unipolar and bipolar depressives. Recurrent. Hospitalized
me patients	Yes	Yes	No	No
riable to 28 months	12 months (cross-over study)	6 months	24 months	24 months
s	Yes	Yes	Yes	Yes
es	Yes	Yes	Yes	Yes
es	Not stated	Yes	Yes	Not stated
es	Yes	Yes	Yes	Yes
es	Yes	Yes	No	No
ot stated	Not stated	No	Yes	Yes
%	17%	Uncertain	16%	25%
eated and retained in study	Treated and retained in study	Withdrawn from study	Treated and retained in study	Treated and retained in study
mptom ratings	Overall preference	No	Global assessments also reported	Global assessments also reported
thium superior	Lithium superior in bipolar	Lithium superior	Lithium superior	In bipolar, lithium superior to placebo and imipramine. In unipolar, lithium superior to placebo but inferior to imipramine

F

chiatrists rate the patients while serum levels were supplied by the laboratory, including fictitious levels for placebo patients (Baastrup *et al.*, 1970; Stallone *et al.*, 1973; Cundall *et al.*, 1973). Another study arranged to have blood levels divulged only if they were very high, and found in practice that none had to be (Hullin *et al.*, 1972). In two studies raters were blind but treating physicians had access to serum levels (Prien *et al.*, 1973a, b). In another study treating psychiatrists rated the patient and another physician had access to serum levels and regulated the dose; the report does not make it clear whether or not he had contact with the patient (Coppen *et al.*, 1971). For two reports there are explicit statements that dosage changes were also made in patients on placebo (Coppen *et al.*, 1971; Cundall *et al.*, 1972); in two more studies the design suggests that this occurred (Baastrup *et al.*, 1970; Melia, 1970).

Side effects may, however, have compromised blindness. They occurred more frequently in lithium than in placebo groups in three studies. They did not do so in two other studies, both withdrawal studies. The withdrawal design allows stabilisation prior to the study. Once again, not all studies took the precaution of examining side effects.

As discussed earlier, dropouts may pose a particular problem in long term studies. It is important to separate those due to relapse, which comprises an important outcome criterion, from those due to other causes, mainly non-cooperation. The latter ranged from a low of 6% in a five month study, to a high of 25% in a 24 month study. These levels are acceptable.

The studies handled the question of relapse in two different ways. In three studies subjects who relapsed were withdrawn from the study. Withdrawal on account of relapse was a crucial outcome criterion. In the remaining five studies patients who relapsed were treated by appropriate means and retained in the study, the total number of episodes and total time spent ill being used as outcome measures. This procedure is less satisfactory. Introduction of additional treatments may compromise blindness. Use of length of time spent ill as an outcome measure entails measuring the effects of lithium as a treatment for acute episodes rather than a prophylactic treatment, and also measures the effects of additional treatments. In fact even those studies following this pattern showed substantial rates of dropout due to relapse.

A weakness of all these studies is their dependence on relapse as an outcome measure. Four studies also used global evaluation of status. One study used symptom ratings. The one study which incorporated an assessment of social adjustment did not report findings on it (Prien *et al.*, 1973a).

By and large, the maintenance studies reviewed here were of high quality and methodological problems, although they existed, were relatively minor. All the studies found lithium superior to placebo, although in one study imipramine was suggestively better than lithium in unipolar depressives. Since other evidence exists that maintenance tricyclic antidepressants reduce early return of symptoms in unipolar depressives (Paykel *et al.*, 1974) further comparisons would be of interest. Overall these studies provide much more striking evidence for the efficacy of lithium as a maintenance treatment than is available for it as an acute treatment.

VII. Conclusions

The aim of this review has been to highlight certain methodological problems inherent in the evaluation of lithium. It should be clear from what has gone before that these comments are not intended to be destructive. It is easier to criticise studies than to design them. Assessment of lithium has involved working on the edge of the established procedures, and adapting new techniques to overcome problems that had not presented before. No study can entirely avoid methodological flaws. Compromise is always necessary and the precautions which avoid one problem will often expose the design to another. For the most part the studies reviewed have been well designed major contributions by established and eminent investigators.

The greatest controversy in the past has surrounded the use of retrospective control periods rather than concurrent between-patient controls. In retrospect, claims of both sets of protagonists can be reconciled. Concurrent between-patient controlled trials have proved to be readily feasible, and in the long run only their findings carry the full weight of scientific proof. They have, however, shown major prophylactic effects for lithium, justifying the claims originally made from retrospective studies.

The advent of lithium has impinged on to long-argued issues as to the nature of affective disorders and has contributed substantially to the revival of interest in the postulated disease entity of bipolar manic depressive illness. Studies of lithium therapy share the sampling problems inherent in the diversity of clinical pictures subsumed under affective disorder. Acute studies have all been concerned with severe hospitalised illnesses, which may be appropriate for the focus on mania. Maintenance studies have been restricted almost entirely to recurrent illnesses. More importantly they have been biased towards previous lithium successes. The applicability of findings to the general run of depressives is the main unresolved issue in the recent maintenance studies.

Perhaps the major problem which lithium presents to the therapeutic investigator still remains in the area of blindness. The necessity to control the dose by blood levels, the narrow range between therapeutic and toxic levels, and the distinctive pattern of side effects have made the complete double state difficult to attain. Contamination of blindness may however occur with many other drugs where a characteristic pattern of side effects exists, even though many of these may be mimicked by placebos. Most of the issues which concern lithium have a wider generality in psychopharmacology. This problem has particularly occurred in acute studies of lithium where high blood levels are desired for maximum therapeutic effect. Because the findings have been weak, and there is a dearth of placebo controlled studies, the methodological criticisms must be given weight. Some doubts must therefore remain as to the degree to which lithium is effective in acute mania.

The prophylactic studies of lithium maintenance have on the whole been conducted with rigorous methodology. The unanimity of their positive findings is buttressed by their methodological adequacy. The problems of blindness and dose control are more easily overcome when there has been an opportunity for previous stabilisation. Solutions had been found to some of the earlier problems by the time interest moved from acute studies to maintenance treatment. However maintenance studies present new methodological problems. Maintenance treatment is likely to become of increasing importance in many conditions as the emphasis shifts from the treatment of acute disturbance in hospital to maintenance of well-being in the community. The solutions to problems of design which have been worked out in recent years in relation to maintenance treatment with lithium and other drugs comprise important contributions to the methodology of psychopharmacology for the future.

References

Abraham, K. (1924). *In* "Selected Papers on Psychoanalysis" Hogarth Press London.
Angst, J. and Weis, P. (1967). *Excerpta medica,* **129** *International Conference Series,* 703–710.
Angst, J., Weis, P., Grof, P., Baastrup, P. C. and Schou, M. (1970). *Brit. J. Psychiat.* **116,** 604–614.
Baastrup, P. C. and Schou, M. (1967). *Archs gen. Psychiat.* **16,** 162–172.
Baastrup, P. C. and Schou, M. (1968). *Lancet* **1,** 1419–1422.
Baastrup, P. C., Poulsen, J. C., Schou M., Thomsen, K. and Amdisen, A. (1970). *Lancet* **2,** 326–330.
Barsa, J. A. (1963). *Amer. J. Psychiat.* **119,** 1174–1175.
Bellak, L., Sack, L. and Rosenham, D. (1961). *J. nerv. ment. Dis.* **132,** 531–538.
Blackwell, B. (1970). *Lancet* **2,** 875.
Blackwell, B. and Shepherd, M. (1968). *Lancet* **1,** 968–971.
Bunney, W. E., Goodwin, F. K., Davis, J. M. and Fawcett, J. A. (1968). *Amer. J. Psychiat.* **125,** 499–511.
Carney, M. W. P., Roth, M. and Garside, R. F. (1965). *Brit. J. Psychiat.* **111,** 659–674.
Chassan, J. C. (1967). "Research Design in Clinical Psychology and Psychiatry" Appleton-Century-Crofts. New York.
Coppen, A., Noguera, R., Bailey, J., Burns, B. H., Swani, M. S., Hare, E. H. and Gardener, R. (1971). *Lancet* **2,** 275–279.
Cromie, B. W. (1936). *Lancet* **2,** 996–997.
Cundall, R. L., Brooks, P. W. and Murray, L. G. (1972). *Psychol. Med.* **2,** 308–311.
Fieve, R. R. Platman, S. R. and Plutchik, R. R. (1968). *Amer. J. Psychiat.* **125,** 492–498.
Foulds (1958). *J. ment. Sci.* **104,** 259–265.

Freud, S. (1917). *In* "Collected Papers" Vol. 4. pp 152–173. Hogarth Press, London (1950).

Gillespie, R. D. (1929). *Guy's Hospital Reports* **79**, 306–344.

Goodwin, F. K. (1973) Paper read before the 18th Annual Conference of Veterans Administration Studies in Mental Health and Behavioural Sciences, New Orleans.

Goodwin, F. K., Murphy, D. L. and Bunney, W. E. (1969). *Archs gen. Psychiat.* **21**, 486–496.

Grof, P., Schou, M., Angst, J., Baastrup, P. C. and Weiss, P.. (1970). *Brit. J. Psychiat.* **116**, 599–603.

Hullin, R. P., McDonald, R. and Allsopp, M. N. E. (1972). *Lancet* **1**, 1044–1046.

Johnson, G., Gershon, S., Burdock, E. I., Floyd, F. and Hekimian, L. (1971) *Brit. J. Psychiat.* **119**, 267–276.

Kendell, R. E. (1968). "The Classification of Depressive Illnesses". Maudsley Monograph No. 18. Oxford University Press, London.

Klerman, G. L. and Paykel, E. S. (1970). *Int. Pharmacopsychiat.* **5**, 80–99.

Kraepelin, E. (1913). "Manic-depressive Insanity and Paranoia" (trans. R. M. Barclay 1921) 8th Ed. Edinburgh.

Leff, J. P. (1973). *Brit. med. J.* **4**, 156–158.

Lewis, A. J. (1934). *J. ment. Sci.* **80**, 277–378.

Lionel, N. D. W. and Herxheimer, A. (1970). *Brit. med. J.* **3**, 637–640.

Maggs, R. (1963). *Brit. J. Psychiat.* **109**, 56–65.

Melia, P. (1970). *Brit. J. Psychiat.* **116**, 621–624.

Mendels, J., Secunda, S. and Dyson, W. L. (1972). *Archs gen. Psychiat.* **26**, 154–157.

Meyer, A. (1922). *Archs Neurol. Psychiat.* **8**, 111–121.

Paykel, E. S. (1971). *Archs gen. Psychiat.* **27**, 203–210.

Paykel, E. S., Dimascio, A., Haskell, D. and Prusoff, B. A. (1974). *Psychol. Med.* (in press).

Paykel, E. S.., Klerman, G. L. and Prusoff, B. A. (1970). *Archs gen. Psychiat.* **22**, 11–21.

Paykel, E. S., Weissman, M. M., Prusoff, B. A. and Tonks, C. M. (1971). *J. nerv. ment. Dis.* **152**, 158–172.

Perris, C. (1966). *Acta. psychiat. scand*, **42**, Supp. 194.

Platman, S. (1970). *Amer. J. Psychiat.* **127**, 351–353.

Prien, R. F., Caffey, E. M. and Klett, C. J. (1972a), *Archs gen. Psychiat.* **26**, 146–153.

Prien, R. F., Caffey, E. M. and Klett, C. J. (1972b). *Archs gen. Psychiat.* **27**, 182–189.

Prien, R. F., Caffey, E. M. and Klett, C. J. (1973a). *Archs gen. Psychiat.* **28**, 337–341.

Prien, R. F., Klett, C. J. and Caffey, E. M. (1973b). *Archs gen. Psychiat.* **29**, 420–425.

Rifkin, A., Quitkin, F., Carillo, C., Blumberg, A. G. and Klein, D. F. (1972). *Archs gen. Psychiat.* **27**, 519–523.

Rosenthal, S. H. (1966). *Amer. J. Psychiat.* **123**, 671–681.

Saran, B. M. (1970). *Int. Pharmacopsychiat.* **5**, 119–131.

Shopsin, B., Kim, S. S. and Gershon, S. (1971). *Brit. J. Psychiat.* **119**, 435–440.

Spring, G., Schweid, D., Gray, C., Steinberg, J. and Horwitz, M. (1970). *Amer. J. Psychiat.* **126**, 1306–1310.

Stallone, F., Shelley, R., Mendlewicz, J. and Fieve, R. R. (1973). *Amer. J. Psychiat.* **130**, 1006–1010.

Willcox, D. R. C., Gillian, R. and Hare, E. H. (1965). *Brit. med. J.* **2**, 790–792.

Winokur, G., Clayton, P. J. and Reich, T. (1969). "Manic-depressive Illness". C. V. Mosby Co. St. Louis.

PART I

SECTION C
PATIENT MANAGEMENT:
PRACTICE AND PROBLEMS

9

THE MANAGEMENT OF PATIENTS RECEIVING LITHIUM TREATMENT

R. J. KERRY

I. Introduction: Pre-treatment Considerations

A. Circumstances under which lithium treatment is considered

Lithium does not occur in nature as the pure metal and the term "lithium" in psychiatry refers either to the lithium ion or one of its salts.

Lithium is generally prescribed under three sets of circumstances.

1. Its use in the treatment of acute mania is now established. Although it is occasionally used in depression, it is not the treatment of choice for this condition;

TABLE I. Lithium preparations (already marketed or likely to become available)

	Tablet or capsule Li⁺ content (mmoles):	Amount of salt in tablet or capsule (mg):	Product name	Manufacturer or supplier
I. SUSTAINED RELEASE PREPARATIONS:				
A. Lithium carbonate	12·2	450	Quilonum retard	Penicillin-Ges. Dauelsberg, West Germany
	10·8	400	Hypnorex	Chodel, West Germany
	10·8	400	Plenur	Lasa, Spain
	10·8	400	Priadel	Delandale, England
	8·1	300	Lithium Oral Carrier (Phasal)	Pharmax, England
B. Lithium citrate	6·0	564	Litarex	Dumex, Denmark
C. Lithium sulphate	6·0	330	Lithionit Duretter	Hässle, Sweden
	6·0	330	Lithium Duriles	Pharma-Stern, West Germany
II. ORDINARY PREPARATIONS:				
A. Lithium acetate (anhydrous)	8·1	536	Quilonum	Penicillin-Ges. Dauelsberg, West Germany
B. Lithium adipate	4·1	630	Lithium Scharffenberg	Scharffenberg, East Germany
C. Lithium carbonate	8·1	300	Carbolith	Winley-Morris, Canada
	8·1	300	Eskalith	Smith, Kline and French, U.S.A.
	8·1	300	Licarb	Gilcross, Canada
	8·1	300	Lithane	Roerig, U.S.A
	8·1	300	Litheum	Valdecasas, Mexico
	8·1	300	Lithium Carbonate DHA	Drug Houses of Australia, Australia

8·1	300	Lithium Carbonicum Spofa	Spofa, Czechoslovakia
8·1	300	Lithizine	Paul Maney, Canada
8·1	300	Litho-Carb	Noco, Canada
8·1	300	Lithonate	Rowell, U.S.A.
8·1	300	Liticar	Medica, Finland
8·1	300	Litin Capsule	Yurtoglu, Turkey
8·1	300	Litio Carbonato	Ist. Farmacol. Ital., Italy
8·1	300	Litu	Orion, Finland
8·1	300	Neurolepsin	Kwizda, Austria
8·1	300	Tabl. lithii carbonatis DAK	DAK, Denmark
6·8	250	Lithea	Protea, Australia
6·8	250	Camcolit	Camden, England
6·8	250	Theralite	Théraplix, France
5·4	200	Limanie	Taisho, Japan
5·4	200	Lithium Carbonas	Brocades, Holland
4·0	150	Lithizine	Paul Maney, Canada
4·0	150	Litho-Carb	Noco, Canada
8·1	763	Demalit	Leiras, Finland
5·3	500	Tabl. lithii citratis Ph.N.	Pharmacop. Nord. 1963, Scandinavia

D. Lithium citrate

E. Lithium glutamate (mono)

3·9	600	Lithium Negroni	Negroni, Italy

III. SOLUTION:

A. Lithium gluconate	5·0 in 5 ml 1,000 in 5 ml	Neurolithium	Labcatal, France

Information provided by M. Schou.

2. It is employed prophylactically in manic depressive illness, either preventing the occurrence of both manic and depressive episodes, or reducing their duration and intensity

3. It is occasionally used in other psychiatric conditions where its value is less well known but it is sometimes of benefit.

B. Choice of a lithium preparation

It has been found that, for prescribing purposes, the carbonate is the most convenient salt and it has now been used for over 20 years without presenting any real difficulties. Some of the other lithium salts create problems; the chloride, for example, is one of the most deliquescent substances known, while the citrate is a little bulky for convenient use. Nevertheless the sulphate, citrate, glutamate, gluconate, adipate and acetate are available commercially. The differential advantages of these salts are probably marginal, being related mainly to manufacturing and marketing pressures rather than therapeutic benefits, or to considerations of administration, such as the following:

1. The citrate is very soluble and of acceptable taste; a syrup is to be available soon (Rowell Laboratories, U.S.A.) for those patients who will not take tablets or perhaps hide them for later disposal;

2. The sulphate has been found useful in the manufacture of one form of slow release tablet (Lithionit, Duretter);

3. The acetate is better because it is more quickly absorbed, in the experience of some prescribers (e.g. Quilonum);

4. The carbonate has gained almost universal acceptance because its high molecular ratio of lithium allows the smallest weight of the drug to be prescribed and its extensive use has shown it to be associated with very few problems.

The dose of each tablet or capsule should be checked for lithium content and it is also helpful to bear this dose in mind expressed in milliequivalents or mmol. when calculating the daily dose to be prescribed. Until the last few years lithium was always prescribed as one of the standard preparations but more recently sustained-release forms of lithium have become available. They allow the daily lithium requirements to be taken in one or two doses with reduced likelihood of "peaks" in the serum lithium concentration which may be associated with mild but unpleasant and unwanted side effects. My experience with some of the earlier "long-acting" forms of lithium led me to believe that manufacturing improvements were needed. Some of the original tablets were friable and crumbled in their containers, and some did not have satisfactory absorption characteristics, as their absorption curves varied from person to person and in the same person from time to time. These problems now appear to have been overcome by most manufacturers. Several sustained-release preparations which are now commercially available are satisfactory and often more acceptable to the patient than ordinary preparations. Sustained-release preparations of lithium are described in Chapter 12.

When choosing between a short-acting (or standard) form of lithium and a sustained-release preparation, the prescriber should remember that with the former, the "apparent" serum lithium concentration will depend on the time interval between the tablet being taken and the blood sample being taken. The latter has a more constant level of serum lithium throughout the day. The prescriber should bear this in mind when changing a patient from one preparation to another. Table I lists the available lithium preparations.

C. Physical examination of the patient

The lithium ion is toxic and potentially dangerous if reasonable care is not taken over the clinical examination of the patients before they receive treatment. In particular, it is essential to bear in mind the special risks undergone by patients with poor cardiovascular or renal function. Personal experience, and the experience of psychiatrists generally, suggests that patients who are physically fit when examined medically are not likely to be at risk when treated with lithium.

Where there are special risks, yet the danger of continuing manic depressive illness is high, we have found that smaller doses give sufficiently high therapeutic serum lithium concentrations (e.g. $0 \cdot 8$–$1 \cdot 0$ mEq/l) and treatment has been safe for many years. We have, for example, treated a 55 year old lady for 10 years with 500 mg of lithium carbonate daily, which has produced a serum concentration of about $0 \cdot 6$–$0 \cdot 9$ mEq/l. Before lithium treatment was started, she was severely hypertensive and had poor renal function. She has remained psychiatrically well since, although in her last year before starting lithium she had made two serious suicidal attempts during depressive illnesses.

Other reports suggest that, in physical illness, low maintenance doses may be satisfactory. If the psychiatric indications are very strong but the physical state gives cause for concern, it is justifiable to begin prophylactic lithium with one tablet daily, increasing by one tablet daily after a week or so, having taken daily serum lithium estimations to determine when the serum lithium concentration reaches the lower limits of the desired prophylactic level (about $0 \cdot 6$–$0 \cdot 8$ mEq/l). Obviously such "at risk" patients will usually need a high degree of supervision, at least during the early months of their lithium treatment.

D. Interviews with the patient and his relatives

If a patient who is acutely ill is treated with lithium, then this is the ideal time to plan his eventual treatment with prophylactic lithium. The principles mentioned in Section III B (pp. 156–158) should be planned at this early stage. Briefly, and as far as is compatible with the patient's psychotic state, an explanation should be given about the new type of treatment. It may be important to convey the idea that, although it may be slower than older treatments such as ECT, we are hoping to prevent attacks of illness in the future. Also, explain that the other treatments can be given as well as lithium and that, if they are given, it does not mean lithium will not work. The psychotic patient may not be amenable to discussion and it is very important to gain the confidence of his relatives and to get their co-operation with a new treatment planned on a long-term basis. Relatives sometimes press for a return to older treatments and they often do this by putting pressure on the nursing staff to influence the doctor. Gaining the relatives' confidence averts this manipulation. When treating an acutely psychotic patient, the nursing staff must be trained and supported to carry out the treatment programme. The nursing staff have to bear the stress caused by the psychotic patient and we must ensure that they are genuinely enthusiastic about our treatment plans.

II. Dosage Control in Lithium Treatment

A. Treatment of acute mania

The lithium ion has been used for the treatment of manic attacks since it was first described by Cade in 1949, and this aspect of its therapeutic use is described in detail in Chapter 3. In the actual attack of mania the usual dose range recommended is of the order of 1,000–2,000 mg daily, depending on the body weight of the patient and the need to avoid toxic effects. Certain toxic reactions can be serious and even fatal and treatment can therefore only be justified when given in hospital with adequate clinical and biochemical supervision; it should never be started in the home. The common toxic symptons and signs described in Chapter 13, include diarrhoea, vomiting, thirst, and dry mouth and are an indication for stopping or drastically reducing the dose.

Baastrup and Schou (1967) suggest that the therapeutic dose is approximately 50 mEq of lithium per day, corresponding to 600 mg of lithium carbonate three times a day. It is fairly easy to reach the toxic serum lithium level of 2 mEq/l. It is felt that to obtain a satisfactory response the average serum lithium concentration throughout the day should be about 1·1 mEq/l. Schou and Shaw (1973) feel that there is no therapeutic advantage in using serum lithium levels above 1·3 mEq/l and they recommend a range of 0·7 to 1·3 mEq/l. These concentrations are generally obtained with lithium doses of 25 to 60 mEq per day (equivalent to between 900 and 2,200 mg of lithium carbonate daily).

From the published clinical studies of lithium treatment in mania, it seems that fairly rapid control (within five to ten days) is obtained over the manic state, relapse occurring within about three days if lithium is stopped. During mania the patient tolerates, and indeed requires, higher doses than can be tolerated by normal people without toxic effects. The patient loses his high dose tolerance once the manic attack is under control and his pattern of lithium retention and excretion begins to resemble the normal. At this stage careful biochemical control is of added importance.

In view of the evidence so far ava.'able, certain conclusions about the use of lithium in mania can be drawn. It is not a method of treatment that can be employed outside hospitals with special facilities, and then only after the appropriate examination of the heart and kidneys. Very few psychiatrists would disagree with the view that the acute attack of mania is probably best treated by the established methods of ECT and major tranquilizers such as the phenothiazines. Once the treatment of the acute attack is under way, it is usually appropriate to start lithium prophylactically.

Young people tend to excrete lithium more quickly than old people and consequently the dose required may decrease with the age of the patient. Prien *et al.* (1972) consider that it is difficult to determine from the literature just what constitutes an adequate dose for acutely manic patients, but all clinicians recommend that serum lithium levels do not exceed $2 \cdot 0$ mEq/l. Until the dose of lithium carbonate has been stabilized, it is better to use ordinary short-acting preparations rather than slow release compounds. Short-acting compounds allow quicker effective dose reduction if the serum lithium concentration begins to rise too quickly; stopping a short-acting compound produces a more rapid fall in the concentration than would occur if a long-acting compound were being used.

B. Treatment of acute depression

In spite of an increasing number of enthusiastic reports about the effectiveness in mania, the evidence concerning the action of lithium in the treatment of depression is equivocal, and is reviewed in Chapter 4.

There are certain dangers in giving lithium to depressed patients. For example, Allgén (1969) reports a case in which the serum lithium rose to $3 \cdot 6$ mEq/l without toxic signs being recognised. A poor dietary and fluid intake during a depressive illness is likely to be accompanied by poor urinary excretion and a consequent rising serum lithium concentration. Under these circumstances there are extra dangers should an anaesthetic be given for ECT. The expected signs of lithium toxicity include somnolence, lethargy, muscle weakness and stupor. These signs are also seen with anaesthetic agents such as the barbiturates and an additive effect with lithium may be expected. Jephcott and Kerry (1974) describe an incident when a patient remained unconscious for over two hours following an anaesthetic for ECT although all previous anaesthetics had been, and subsequent anaesthetics were, followed by the normal recovery period of a few minutes. The patient's serum lithium had been monitored every week and was always in the accepted therapeutic range. On this occasion, a serum lithium measurement was made during the period of unconsciousness and found to be $3 \cdot 4$ mEq/l. This suggests that an abnormally raised serum lithium concentration was responsible for this complication. These problems are likely to arise in depressive illness where there is an inadequate diet and, therefore, it is necessary for extra care and extra lithium monitoring to be given before anaesthesia. We now omit lithium treatment during a course of ECT.

C. Treatment of other psychiatric conditions

In view of its success in treating mood disorders where it modifies states of hyperexcitability and produces therapeutic benefit in a disorder which often runs a cyclical course, lithium has been tried in other psychiatric illnesses showing similar features (see Chapter 6). It has been used in such conditions as:

1. Schizophrenia;
2. Childhood psychiatric disorders of a variety of kinds;
3. Hyperactive mentally retarded patients, both children and adults;
4. Patients with mild, but usually almost subclinical mood swings, which cause social difficulties;
5. Periodic psychoses of a non-affective kind;
6. Premenstrual tension;
7. Mood disorders of old age.

Although the results of lithium treatment have been disappointing in many patients with the above conditions, our experience and that of others has been that on a few occasions it has been of limited benefit.

In using lithium treatment with children it is important to relate the initial dose of lithium to the child's body weight. My practice, although my experience is limited, is to suggest a relatively low starting dose with serum lithium estimations about twice a week, gradually increasing the dose weekly until the serum lithium is in the range of 0·8–1·4 mEq/l. Rapid control of psychiatric symptoms is unlikely to be necessary and a regime such as this is safe and unlikely to alarm the child or his parents. The co-operation of the parents is essential and must include regular discussions and briefings along the lines given later in this Chapter.

In elderly patients, particularly where efficient renal clearance may be doubtful, we also start with a small dose, e.g. 250 mg of lithium carbonate twice a day. Daily serum lithium estimations then allow a safe and gradual adjustment to what is often a smaller than usual dose. We have found that, once settled, the dose has remained very constant over several years.

D. Prophylactic treatment of recurrent affective disorders

Many patients will have started prophylactic maintenance treatment with lithium in hospital during recovery from an acute psychotic illness. In the early days of the use of lithium in psychiatry, it was thought best to start treatment in hospital from the point of view of the patients' safety (Cade, 1949), but it is now considered safe to start prophylactic lithium in out-patients (Kerry, 1968; Allgén, 1969). In some areas it is found convenient and economical to have special lithium clinics (rather like diabetic clinics, etc.).

The following general guidelines will be of help in choosing the correct dose of lithium for lithium prophylaxis. A normal healthy adult will need about 20–30 mEq of lithium ion daily to obtain a serum lithium concentration of $0 \cdot 8$–$1 \cdot 4$ mEq/l. This corresponds to about 1,000 mg of lithium carbonate daily ($27 \cdot 2$ mEq/l of lithium ion). Depending on the stated lithium content of the preparation being used, a convenient starting dose expressed in mEq of lithium ion can be selected. Where there is concern about the patient's physical state, about half the usual dose (e.g. 10 mEq of lithium ion) can be chosen initially. In all cases the dose will have to be controlled by serum lithium estimations as one patient may need twice as much lithium as another to maintain the same serum lithium concentration.

There are probably advantages in using ordinary preparations of lithium (rather than sustained release preparations) during the stabilization phase of treatment. With the former, it is easier to produce rapid changes in the serum lithium concentration by varying the dose and, more importantly, it is easier to obtain a rapid excretion of lithium by stopping the tablets or capsules if toxic symptoms or dangerously high serum lithium levels occur. The possibility of employing sustained-release preparations can be considered in each case once the patient is being maintained on a constant dose of lithium. The use of sustained-release preparations is discussed in Chapter 12. Generally, the following principles will be helpful.

1. It will be found that 1,000 mg of ordinary lithium carbonate daily in divided doses will be appropriate for a normal, physically fit adult. As so many preparations of lithium are now available, it may be necessary to calculate a starting dose of the compound being used to give about 20–25 milliequivalents per day of lithium. Smaller starting doses, e.g. 500 mg of lithium carbonate daily (about 10–12 milliequivalents of lithium), should be used where the age or physical state of the patients suggests that the renal lithium clearance may be impaired. Since we are usually instituting prophylactic lithium in a patient who is well at the time of starting, it is obviously safer to begin with a dose that is perhaps too small and then to increase the dose gradually to obtain the correct serum lithium concentration. In practice this procedure is probably more convenient and reliable than placing dependence on any form of test done.

2. If the prescriber is in doubt, the general recommendation of Schou and Baastrup (1967) will prove helpful. They suggest starting with low doses such as 150 mg of lithium carbonate twice a day, and increasing this by 150 mg daily to a total of 900 mg daily. The serum lithium is monitored throughout and the

final dose adjusted to place the serum lithium concentration in the desired range.

3. Some prescribers have found the patient's response to initial test doses to be helpful, but the evidence to support the value of such procedures is still limited. The problems of their interpretation are similar to those involved in the lithium retention test of Serry mentioned later. As a general rule, starting as in 1 or 2 with serum lithium monitoring will be the best way to begin treatment with lithium.

4. The experience of most prescribers is that once the dose of lithium and the serum lithium concentrations have been stabilized for any one individual, they can both be expected to remain remarkably constant over many years unless something (such as the patient's physical circumstances) changes. It should be borne in mind that in exceptional cases there can be sufficient individual variation for one patient to need twice as much lithium as another to attain therapeutic serum lithium concentrations.

5. Serum lithium monitoring is important to make sure that patients are actually taking the proper dose. A large proportion of psychiatric patients do not take their drugs properly (Wilcox *et al.*, 1965). If there is a low serum lithium concentration, the psychiatrist should be able to ascertain the cause in his patient. Fry and Marks (1971), in the context of lithium treatment, stress the need for doctors to use laboratory results in the management of their patients. They believe that more active supervision of patients taking drugs by measuring blood-levels of the therapeutic agent will enable more of them to derive maximum benefit from the drugs they are prescribed. It is perhaps of doubtful value to measure blood levels every few months with a view to avoiding toxicity, but it is probably of considerable value in "persuading" the patient to take his medication regularly.

E. Serum lithium estimations

The laboratory methods of measuring serum lithium are covered in Chapter 10, but the following principles should be observed when treating the patient, whether in hospital or at the out-patient department.

1. An in-patient who is being treated for a psychiatric illness (usually mania) will at first need frequent serum lithium estimations. These should be taken at least three times a week, if not every day. This is because the patient's tolerance for lithium can be expected to change as the clinical condition improves. This frequency of serum lithium estimations is neither necessary nor usually possible in clinically stable out-patients. When starting out-patient treatment with lithium the prescriber will find it useful, as a general principle, to see the patient every week for the first month, then every two weeks for the next month or two. Then, depending on there being a series of satisfactory serum levels, the patient can be seen each month for a further six months. After this, if

progress has been satisfactory, visits and the taking of blood samples every two or three months will be found to be sufficient. Generally, once the dose of lithium has been found to be stable over a period of a few months, the serum lithium concentrations can be expected to remain constant over a period of years, unless the patient's circumstances change, e.g. owing to physical illness.

2. Once the patient has been stabilized on lithium, but only then, it may be necessary to control the treatment without seeing the patient. This often occurs when the distances involved make any other course of action unreasonable. Blood samples may be sent to the lithium clinic or to the laboratory by any convenient transport. The local general practitioner can prescribe the medication with the help of telephoned or written advice from the psychiatrist when the laboratory results are known.

With blood samples from outside practitioners, "technical faults" occurring somewhere between the patient and the laboratory, cause most of the difficulties. These faults are usually of a minor nature and easily avoidable. The laboratory must establish an acceptable means of transport locally with the practitioner taking the blood, who should be advised on the times and procedures suitable for sampling. The correct containers should be specified and the easy way round this problem is to supply the practitioners with labelled containers. It is surprising how many unsatisfactory or unlabelled samples can be received! Personal contact with the patient's practitioner can solve many problems.

3. A method of communicating with the patient should be established in the event of a worrying laboratory result being found. Ideally, results should be to hand before the patient leaves the clinic. It is helpful to explain to the patient that occasionally blood tests need repeating and are not likely to be of serious consequence to the patient—this avoids causing alarm.

III. Principles in the Management of Patients on Prophylactic Lithium

A. Selection of patients

Each patient chosen for prophylactic treatment with lithium will need to be stabilized on his individual dose and then maintained on lithium, presumably for life, rather in the same way that a diabetic patient is stabilized and maintained permanently on the most suitable dose and preparation of insulin. Here also the physician will need to use clinical judgement as to whether stabilization of an individual needs to be carried out as an in-patient or an out-patient.

1. *Indicators of suitability for long-term treatment*

(a) *Physical fitness:* The contra-indications of lithium treatment arising from physical disorders such as hypertension, heart disease, kidney disease and so on, are relative rather than absolute. A patient with, for example, heart disease, may be exposed to a smaller risk owing to lithium toxicity than results from uncontrolled and recurrent attacks of mania. A patient who is physically fit as assessed by an ordinary physical examination is also likely to tolerate lithium treatment. There are, however, special physical circumstances such as glomerulonephritis, pyelonephritis, heart disease and brain damage in which caution needs to be exercised. The occurrence of any of these conditions will be an indication for starting lithium in very low doses.

Whatever the physical state of the patient, the over-riding factor is the avoidance of toxic serum lithium concentrations by controlling both the dose of lithium and its concentration in the blood.

(b) *Frequency, nature and severity of previous psychotic attacks:* The patient most in need of, and likely to benefit from, lithium treatment will have a long history of illness with many attacks. "Psychosis rate" as described by Baastrup and Schou (1967) is a useful concept when considering patients from this standpoint. Any patient who has had two or more manic-depressive episodes during one year, or has had one or more episodes per year during the last two years, is probably sufficiently ill to warrant serious consideration for treatment with lithium. It should also be realized that the frequency of attacks of manic-depressive psychosis is likely to increase rather than decrease as the patient gets older (Angst and Weis, 1967).

The more classical the manic depressive history is, and the more severe the degree of psychotic disturbance shown, the better the patient is likely to respond. A history of more frequent manic than depressive phases also improves the prognosis, though it should be borne in mind that even classical recurrent depressives, if followed up for long enough, are often seen to have some degree of manic illness, and classical unipolar recurrent depressives can still show a good response to lithium.

Atypical features in a patient's history of manic-depressive illness worsen the prognosis for treatment with lithium. Schou (1968) feels that unfavourable prognoses for lithium prophylaxis occur in about one third of manic-depress- ives where the manic picture is tainted with such atypical features as delusions without overt relation to mood, hallucinations of more than episodic character, periods with reticence and contact difficulties, and gross hysterical symptoms, On the other hand, this observation confirms the opinion of most psychiatrists experienced in the use of lithium that such atypical features do not rule out a successful response in many cases. This is especially so in any episodic illness with a strong affective component. In fact, it is probably true to say that the greater the mood swings during the course of a psychiatric illness, the better the chance is of a good response to prophylactic lithium. (Levy, 1968).

(c) *Motivation of the patient and his relatives:* Both the patient and his relatives may reject tablet treatment as the patient may be reluctant to forego what he regards (perhaps mistakenly) as his productive manic epiosdes and the family may enjoy having a hypomanic member. Sometimes the spouse needs to be married to someone who is ill. As with many patients with other illnesses, unless the patient wishes to be cured, lithium treatment is likely to fail.

(d) *Body build:* A high proportion of "lithium responders" have a tendency to be of pyknic build. This is, perhaps, not surprising in view of the accepted association between pyknic build and classical manic depressive illness (Kretschmer, 1952). Nevertheless, it should be remembered that an important minority of patients of asthenic build and with rather atypical features of manic-depressive illness also respond well to prophylactic lithium.

(e) *Age:* The natural history of manic-depressive illness is such that most patients will be approaching middle age by the time they are selected for lithium prophylaxis but the prognosis can nevertheless be equally good in young, middle-aged or elderly patients. Some children have done well, particularly those with behaviour disturbances resembling mania with distractibility and periods of flighty conversation (Frommer, 1968). We have seen such behaviour in some subnormal patients who also subsequently responded to prophylactic lithium.

2. *The concept of lithium responders*

(a) *General principles:* If we accept, as we now must in view of the evidence, that prophylactic lithium is of considerable benefit to a large proportion of psychiatric patients, then identifying those likely to respond to lithium is important. The following guidelines will be found useful:

1. Most psychiatrists will be able to judge clinically those patients who are likely to respond, i.e. those patients possessing a large number of classical or typical features of manic depressive psychosis and a relatively small proportion of features atypical of this illness. As mentioned above, the stronger the affective component in the patient, the better is the prognosis for prophylactic lithium.

2. Even atypical cases should be tried since a small proportion of these do well and remain symptom free. A trial of prophylactic lithium is ultimately the best test to see if a patient is, or is not, a lithium responder and it is the only certain way of separating the "lithium responders" from the "lithium non-responders". This view is now acceptable since experience shows that lithium is a safe long-term treatment. If the clinician feels strongly that the severity and number of psychotic attacks warrant a trial of lithium, it is worth persisting for one or even two years, since the occasional patient responds only after about a year, perhaps having had two or three attacks whilst on lithium. Doctors should remember that the decision *not* to give lithium must often be made after considerable thought.

(b) *Lithium retention and response—Serry's lithium retention test:* It appears that the lithium ion may be differentially retained in body tissues depending on the psychiatric state of the patient, i.e. whether manic, nomothy-mic, or depressed. Unfortunately, at this stage the different reports of the excretion and retention of lithium in various studies are sufficiently controversial to cast doubts on the idea of test doses as a guide to future clinical response (see Chapters 17 and 18). The test most likely to be used is the lithium retention test described by Serry (1969) which is described in Chapter 18. This test, although helpful to some clinicians, is open to certain criticisms. I have had at least one "lithium excretor" who has done very well clinically on lithium carbonate. Schou (1973) feels that there are several reasons that some clini-cians have had difficulty with predictive tests, including the Serry test:

1. The absorption rate from the intestines not only varies from person to person, but also in the same individual from time to time;

2. The rate at which lithium is distributed to the various tissues may vary;

3. The renal lithium clearance will affect the results of such a test.

If there were a reliable predictive test in practice, one would use it, but at the present time one must repeat that the best procedure is to try each patient on lithium who is deemed sufficiently ill to be treated.

B. The interview with the patient and his relatives

It is essential to try to see both the patients and their relatives before starting prophylactic lithium. The importance of the family being involved over the following years of treatment cannot be overstressed. There is no doubt that time spent, and repeatedly spent, with the patients and their relatives is associated with a greater chance of successful treatment. Repeated visits in themselves may be of great importance in obtaining the best response (Kerry, 1968). Extensive experience in psychiatry with lithium has led Schou (1973) to state quite definitely that unless the co-operation and support of the family are secured from the very beginning, lithium treatment is doomed to fail. The interviews can conveniently take the following form:

1. *The patient alone*

Briefly discuss with the patient the nature of his illness. The patient will understand the recurrent nature of his illness if the prescriber goes over his previous episodes with him. It can then be stressed that lithium is going to be prescribed to prevent attacks of illness that may otherwise occur in the future. At this stage it is important to gain his co-operation and for him to say that he is anxious to avoid further illness. Hypomanic illness, particularly if not too severe, is frequently a source of pleasure to the patient rather than a source of distress, and some patients are not, themselves, prepared to give up their future expectations of mild periods of "manic lift". These patients should not be "over persuaded" to undergo treatment and the decisions should be postponed until the patient feels that treatment is worthwhile. Once an agreement about treatment has been reached with the patient, the following issues should be discussed:

(a) *Stressing dosage control:* The precise dose of lithium should be taken exactly as prescribed and the doctor should be told if the routine has been varied, particularly if any tablets have been forgotten. The patient should be made to realise that we rely on this information purely in order to stabilize him on his optimum blood level and that there is no likelihood of the physician being angry with him as long as perfect honesty about his dosage is maintained.

Explain the importance of not "doubling up" the dose if the medication has been missed as this could cause peaks in his blood lithium levels which could produce mildly unpleasant, although not necessarily serious, side effects.

(b) *Dietary advice:* Discuss the importance of maintaining a normal diet, particularly with relation to salt and fluids. Whilst there is no need for any special arrangements he should be advised to avoid any dramatic changes such as going on a diet. Should a special diet become necessary for medical or weight reducing reasons, the patient should be advised to maintain his normal sodium chloride intake (Furlong, 1973).

(c) *Discussions of side effects:* Mild side effects may well be expected in the first few weeks and can be regarded as a normal accompaniment to be expected from this new treatment and they will disappear of their own accord when the body has adjusted to the rising serum lithium levels. These side effects will include a fine tremor, particularly of the hands, mild gastro-intestinal upsets or an occasional loose stool, dryness of the mouth, thirst and urinary frequency.

Symptoms such as persistent nausea, vomiting and diarrhoea, coarse tremors or twitchings, drowsiness, dizziness and ataxia, or slurred speech, are indications for stopping the medication and contacting the physician. How and where to contact the doctor should be explained at this point.

Avoid alarming the patient and say that very few psychiatrists have ever seen a patient with the more serious side effects, such is the safety margin of the treatment with laboratory supervision.

(d) *Explanation of possible weight gain:* Explain the gain in body weight that usually accompanies a successful response to lithium (Kerry *et al.,* 1970). It is important to point out that gain in weight usually accompanies successful treatment with lithium but that after a few months the weight stabilizes at a somewhat higher level. In women, particularly, it is essential to get the patient to accept this as a part of getting better. It is useful to suggest that someone who has had a serious illness for a long time can be expected to weigh less than his peers who have always had good health. The extra weight gained usually brings the patient back to a more average weight for his age. Above all, appetite-suppressing drugs must be avoided and a suggestion might be made that the psychiatrist will ensure that the patient's weight is reasonable in about six months time when weight stabilization should have occurred; dietary advice may be given to ensure that this is the case.

(e) *Further interviews with the patient:* The interview, although detailed enough to cover the above points, needs to be kept fairly brief as patients do tend to forget important items of the programme outline. Gaps can be filled in at subsequent visits and it may help to have some printed advice to give the patient.

2. *The relatives*

The above explanation should be briefly repeated to the relatives. Go into the hopes of successful treatment for the patient, stress the importance of continuing the treatment on a permanent basis and go over some of the reasons frequently given by patients or by relatives for stopping the medication prematurely.

Introduce the idea of a "mood normaliser". The patient will eventually lose the characteristics and consequences of being a psychiatric invalid. It will help if the family is prepared for this change which is usually a happy event but which sometimes may create problems of adjustment in family relationships when the family have to readjust their behaviour to deal with an individual who is now in normal health.

C. Continuing patient and family support in the clinic

It is of value for patients undergoing a long term, and usually successful, treatment to get together and support each other. New patients joining the programme can be favourably influenced by patients who have been free from illness for several years. All the problems of lithium therapy, such as weight gain, can be discussed more successfully on a patient-to-patient basis, and the newcomer persuaded to continue with his treatment.

Secondly, the patient and his family can be helped to cope with the interpersonal problems that sometimes accompany otherwise successful treatment with lithium. When the patient remains well on lithium, it is usually a happy occurrence for all concerned. Unfortunately, in many cases, problems do arise, and can be alleviated by awareness on the part of the doctor. It is worth thinking of the following:

1. The spouse may have need of an ill partner. One female patient, for example, who previously had several hospital admissions a year, has now been well for five years. Her husband was a rather remote individual and coped for many years with his work and domestic responsibilities reasonably well. His wife's recovery increased the social and other demands made upon him; he made a severe suicidal attempt and has now become the psychiatrically ill partner (see Chapter 5).

2. The patient who has probably lacked confidence in forward planning

usually gains in confidence with a lengthening symptom-free period. The spouse and other family members should be aware that the patient will take a renewed and perhaps different interest in his career and spare time activities. Many women patients, for example, will seek employment.

3. The children of manic-depressive patients are usually disturbed and their education may be jeopardized. There is often a happy outcome if the parent's "cure" is anticipated. We have had experience of encouraging headmasters to allow "doubtful" children to proceed to higher education on the grounds that future examination papers might be coped with more adequately. Such experience has made us regard this aspect as being very important when lithium treatment is going to affect a family.

4. In some patients, the mood does not become stable for perhaps about a year. During this time further attacks may occur in which the illness is changed in its amplitude and characteristics. In this respect, it is particularly important to bear in mind that the family and the patient may have to handle a different type of depressive illness. Previously, the patient may have been deeply depressed and dependent. The change often seen is towards a less deeply depressed, and possibly more irritable, individual than formerly.

5. In all cases there has developed a peculiar psycho-social pattern in which patient, spouse, children, friends and associates all play special roles in a combined effort to mitigate the consequences of the patient's incessant mood changes (Schou, personal communication). A degree of psychotherapy, such as that available through a lithium clinic, will probably be the best way of handling the problems raised by the changes brought about by recovery.

D. Additional tests

1. *Biochemical tests*

On all samples of blood from our lithium clinic patients, we also include protein bound iodine and creatinine phosphokinase measurements. These we regard as luxuries which are fortunately easily available to us but not really necessary. Protein bound iodine helps us to monitor thyroid function to some extent and creatinine phosphokinase gives us some idea of continuing psychotic activity, although the patient is stable in mood whilst on, and probably as a result of being on, lithium (Gosling *et al.*, 1972). The continuation of abnormally high peaks of creatinine phosphokinase impresses on the psychiatrist the essentially permanent nature of prophylactic lithium for the patient.

2. *Weighing the patient*

It is useful to weigh the patient at each visit (Kerry *et al.*, 1970), in light clothing which is as standardized as is acceptable to most out-patients. Weighing is useful for two reasons:

1. The patient can be helped to accept the initial weight gain and feel

reassured when his weight becomes stable again. He will have been given an explanation that there is an increase in body weight over the first six months or so, and that this is normal.

2. When his weight becomes stable, he will be reinforced in his ideas that he is well and that he can continue his treatment without any apparent outward effects.

E. Some individual problems with patients on prophylactic lithium

Various circumstances can arise which may interrupt an otherwise smooth programme of lithium maintenance. These should be anticipated by the psychiatrist and they include:

1. *Refusal of further treatment*

The patient may refuse further treatment for one of several reasons:

(a) *Loss of hypomanic periods:* In some individuals mild, but sub-psychotic, hypomania gives them drive and energy which are of considerable personal and professional benefit to them. Many such people have highly productive periods of life associated with periods of mild hypomania. Such patients can still reasonably be advised to start prophylactic lithium. Experience with such patients shows that their long term productivity may be greater, particularly when they are likely to be protected from manic chaos when, although they may think they are doing well, they are nevertheless making a mess of their lives. Such people as I have treated myself over a number of years, do confirm the view that there is a long term improvement of efficiency. In patients with frequent and predominantly depressive mood changes, on the other hand, several months may pass before any relief is experienced and in such patients it is important to persist with lithium and to support them during their depressions, preferably without anti-depressants. Experience with such patients supports the advice given by Schou in his Special Review (1968, p. 88). Briefly, that is to avoid antidepressants in recurrences of moderate depressive episodes which may occur with gradually decreasing amplitude during the first year of prophylactic lithium. Generally, these depressions are of short duration and tricyclic antidepressants do not shorten them further. Occasionally antidepressants may precipitate a swing into mania and generally it is better not to break the relative stability being reached through continuous lithium treatment. Nevertheless, if severe attacks of depression occur during a course of prophylactic lithium, they must be considered for treatment by all available means, including antidepressant drugs.

(b) *Experience of mild side effects:* The mild, unwanted effects of lithium which may be experienced during the early stages of treatment, may, although transient, be sufficient to cause the patient to discontinue taking his tablets, particularly if he is over-concerned about toxicity. Some patients may be able to tolerate sustained-release preparations of lithium more easily. These transient side effects are more commonly complained of by highly skilled people doing fine work and by some professional people who find a fine tremor especially disturbing.

(c) *Stigma of an incurable illness:* The patient may have been well for years as a result of lithium therapy and may therefore decide to stop medication. The relapse rate is then high. Patients are often loath to accept lithium treatment as a life-time need since this suggests permanent commitment to treatment and the stigma of an incurable illness which they prefer to deny by stopping lithium, (Polatin and Fieve, 1971).

(d) *Persuasion by friends and relatives:* Relatives and friends of the patient may persuade him to stop medication. After a few trouble-free years, the patient may be told, "You are well now and you don't need tablets." Again, in this context, relatives often take this opportunity of denying the presence of mental illness in the family and must be warned about the possible danger if treatment is stopped.

(e) *Weight gain:* Weight gain, particularly in women, may cause the patient to stop treatment. This is not so likely if the pattern of an initial gain is to be followed by stabilization at a somewhat higher weight and is explained. Concern about body weight is related to social class and may be handled by either:

1. The patient being encouraged to accept the increased weight accompanied by good health;

2. Calorie control. Appetite suppressants should be avoided as they are psychiatrically undesirable.

2. Occurrence of pregnancy during lithium treatment

This is dealt with in Chapter 15. It should be borne in mind that one would not lightly give psychotropic drugs, including lithium, during the first trimestre of pregnancy. Although teratogenesis in animals has occasionally been reported, the incidence of foetal abnormality in humans so far seems to be no higher than normal. In fact, that the mother is on lithium does not appear to be an indication for the termination of pregnancy (Schou, 1968). The small risk of lithium will have to be weighed against dangers of a manic-depressive attack using the guide-lines outlined in Chapter 15.

3. Lithium in association with medical and surgical conditions

The key factors which should alert the prescriber toward extra care in the use of lithium are states which are likely to disturb the patient's electrolyte (notably sodium) balance. These include:

(a) *Surgical operations involving anaesthetics:* The hazards of giving an anaesthetic with a very high serum lithium level are now recognized (Jephcott and Kerry, 1974). The danger stems from the possible additive effects of lithium and drugs such as the barbiturates.

(b) *Physical illnesses:* Severe and acute illness may cause considerable metabolic upset. Fluid and salt balance may be disturbed. Then, although it may often be possible, and always desirable, to monitor the patient's serum lithium, it is better to stop treatment, for a time at least. The chances of the patient suffering psychiatrically over a short period are statistically remote.

Owing to the possibility of a sudden lowering of renal clearance at these times, there may be a sudden and unexpected variance in the patient's serum lithium concentration. The dangers, if this happens, are high, whereas the dangers of stopping treatment, for perhaps a week or so, are very small. Physical illnesses, including Addison's disease and heart failure, or treatment with diuretics usually contraindicate continued lithium treatment. Any condition accompanied by sweating or diarrhoea could give rise to potentially dangerous increases in the serum lithium concentration.

(c) *Simultaneous administration of other medication:* Apart from the emergency conditions described above, it seems that lithium is safe in combination with all drugs used by medical practitioners. This enables the prescriber to use lithium with confidence when the patient has some non-pyschiatric illness which requires medication. When the doctor is considering the general psychiatric management of the patient, it is desirable that the patient should be encouraged to manage without any other psychotropic drugs—rather he should be helped with psychotherapeutic support during his adjustment to lithium.

4. *Travel undertaken during lithium treatment*

Patients embarking on long journeys should be advised to keep to their dietary pattern. A proper fluid intake is important particularly where time is lost or gained in travelling across time zones.

5. *Strenuous physical exercise*

In a recent series of experiments using rats, Smith (1973) demonstrated that strenuous physical exercise decreased renal lithium clearance. Smith comments that if this finding may be generalized to man, it implies that dosage adjustments may become necessary to avoid side effects or toxic reactions in those patients who, whilst undertaking lithium therapy, engage in physical exercise of an extreme or strenuous nature.

6. *Climatic conditions*

Tropical climates and hot environments may lead to fluid and salt balance changes in patients who may lose both by sweating. In heavy industrial occupations, such as blast furnace work, the patient will be well advised to make sure that he maintains a normal diet. If a normal amount of salt is included in the food, a dietary supplement of salt tablets is unnecessary but it may be useful if mild lithium toxicity occasionally appears. It is more important to realize that frequent serum lithium monitoring in the early days of lithium prophylaxis tends to stabilize such workers at doses of lithium which are somewhat lower than average doses. In these cases alcohol intake should be restricted.

IV. Conclusions

The value of lithium as a prophylactic against manic-depressive illness has been established over a period of nearly twenty years. It is also often of value in other conditions. When lithium is used it is important that the principles described in this chapter are borne in mind so that it may be used safely and to the best advantage. In particular, adequate serum lithium monitoring combined with the continuing psychiatric support of both the patients and relatives will increase the chances of a successful outcome of the treatment. Even though the mechanisms through which lithium treatment works are unknown, it does offer relief to many patients suffering from what would otherwise be crippling psychiatric illnesses.

References

Allgén, L. G. (1969). *Acta. psychiat. scand. suppl.* **207**, 98–105.
Angst, J. and Weis, P. (1967). *In* "Neuro-Psychopharmacology", Amsterdam: Excerpta Medica Foundation, I.C.S. **129**, 703–710.
Baastrup, P. C. and Schou, M. (1967). *Archs gen. Psychiat.* **16**, 162–172.
Cade, J. F. J. (1949). *Med. J. Aust.* **36**, 349–352.
Frommer, E. A. (1968). *In* "Recent Developments in Affective Disorders" (A. Coppen and A. Walk, eds.), *Brit. J. Psychiat., Spec. Pub.,* **2**, 117–136.
Fry, D. E. and Marks V. (1971). *Lancet,* **1**, 886–888.
Furlong, F. W. (1973). *Can. psychiat. Assoc. J.* **18**, 75–76.
Gosling, R., Kerry, R. J. and Owen, G. (1972). *Brit. med. J.* **3**, 327–329.
Jephcott, G. and Kerry, R. J. (1974). *Brit. J. Anaesthes.* (In Press).
Kerry, R. J. (1968). *Brit. med. J.* **4**, 187.
Kerry, R. J., Leibling, L. I. and Owen, G. (1970). *Acta. psychiat. scand.* **46**, 238–243.
Kretschmer, E. (1952). "A Textbook of Medical Psychology", The Hogarth Press, London.
Levy, B. S. (1968). *J. Amer. med. Assoc.* **206**, 1045–1047.
Polatin, P. and Fieve, R. R. (1971). *J. Amer. med. Assoc.* **218**, 864–866.
Prien, R. F., Caffey, E. M. and Klett, C. J. (1972). *Brit. J. Psychiat.* **120**, 409–414.
Serry, N. (1969). *Lancet* **1**, 1267–1268.
Schou, M. (1968). *J. psychiat. Res.* **6**, 67–95.
Schou, M. (1973). *Psychiat. Neurol. Neurochir.* **76**, 511–522.
Schou, M. and Baastrup, P. C. (1967). *J. Amer. med. Assoc.* **201**, 696–698.
Schou, M. and Shaw, D. M. (1973). *Practitioner* **210**, 105–111.
Smith, D. F. (1973). *Int. Pharmacopsychiat.* **8**, 217–220.
Wilcox, D. R. C., Gillan, R. and Hare, E. H. (1965). *Brit. med. J.* **4**, 790–792.

10

METHODS OF SERUM LITHIUM ESTIMATION

The Late H. I. Coombs, R. R. H. Coombs and U. G. Mee

I. Introduction

A dose of lithium that may be inadequate for one patient may be potentially lethal for another. While being no substitute for careful clinical observation, proper management of patients on lithium therapy requires careful control of blood lithium levels as the therapeutic level of lithium is so very close to the toxic level (Koch-Weser, 1972). In addition, very low levels may indicate that the patient is not taking his tablets (Fry and Marks, 1971). This careful control in turn requires a simple and reliable technique for repeated estimation of lithium blood levels but, unfortunately, until very recently the development of practical measuring techniques trailed behind therapeutic hopes.

Not long after the initial discovery of lithium in the mineral petalite by Arfwedson in 1818, Alexander Ure in 1843 suggested using lithium carbonate in the treatment of gout, after observing that uric acid calculi dissolved rapidly in weak solutions of lithium *in vitro* and, by 1866, lithium was actually being used in the treatment of gout by Garrod and others, though this use soon fell into disrepute. Meanwhile, in 1861, Kirchhoff and Bunsen had extended their spectroscopic technique to include analysis for lithium and cited Folwarczny, who was reported to have detected traces of lithium in the blood and muscle of man. Most of the early studies were on the lithium content of minerals, however (Grandeau, 1863), and the spectroscopic techniques were only qualitative (Desgrez and Meunier, 1920). Quantitative measurement necessitated complex extraction procedures followed by precipitation of lithium as lithium phosphate in a strong solution of ammonia to separate off the soluble phosphates of sodium and potassium (Good, 1903).

Attempts were also made to separate lithium from other alkaline metal ions by paper chromatography (Covello and Ciampa, 1965) and a semi-quantitative colorimetric method for detecting lithium in serum using ferric periodate was proposed by Plum (1957).

However, with the advent of a commercially available flame photometer (Collins and Polkinhorne, 1952), the first simple, fully quantitative technique for measuring lithium was developed, initially for inorganic solutions (Stuart *et al.*, 1957). This was soon extended to blood and other biological fluids. More recently, atomic absorption spectrophotometry has also been adapted to serum lithium measurements.

So sensitive are the techniques available today that they can be used to estimate the minute amounts of lithium present in normal people (Woods *et al.*, 1968) and have confirmed early reports that lithium was present in detectable quantities in some normal human blood samples (Bertrand and Bertrand, 1951, Keilholz, 1921). The level is, however, very variable; in pregnant women and people drinking water with a high lithium content, values up to 15 ng/ml are not uncommon (Wittrig *et al.*, 1970). The value of serum lithium levels also varies with the time which has elapsed since the last oral dose and with the preparation used, whether this is one of the ordinary or one of the sustained release type. Figure 1 shows the variation in serum lithium concentrations throughout a 24 hour period in a patient on lithium with three doses a day of ordinary lithium tablets (Amdisen, 1973). The variation with the time of doses is discussed at greater length in Chapter 12. In our experience, variations in serum lithium with the timing of doses has not been much of a problem in the practical management of most patients but a few patients who are difficult to stabilize may require admission to hospital for detailed studies with repeated lithium measurements over a 24 or 48 hour period.

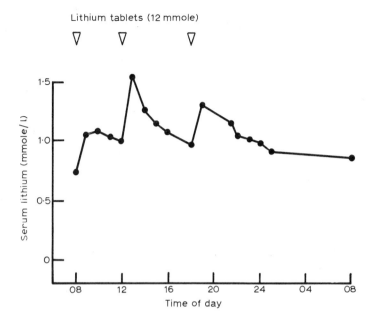

Fig. 1. Serum lithium concentrations throughout 24 hours in a patient on maintenance treatment with lithium, given ordinary tablets at 8 a.m., 12 noon and 6 p.m. (Redrawn from Amdisen, 1973, with permission)

II. Flame Photometry

A. Principles

When an element and, in particular, one of the alkaline metals, sodium, potassium, lithium or calcium, is heated in a flame a proportion of the atoms of that element are excited to higher energy levels. When these atoms return to their original energy level they emit radiation at certain specific wavelengths or colours which are characteristic of the element involved. The intensity of this light at one of the particular wavelengths is then, in most cases, proportional to the amount of the element in the flame at that moment. Modern flame photometers are designed to give a flame that can be maintained with a constant form and temperature. Homogeneous standard and unknown solutions are sprayed in turn in droplet form into the flame at a constant rate with a nebulizer. As serum contains many elements, radiation of one of the wavelengths that is characteristic of the element to be measured must be separated from extraneous

G

emission, and flame photometers incorporate an optical filter or a mono-chromator for this purpose. The intensity of the radiation at the selected wavelength is then proportional to the amount of that element in the original solution. The principle of flame photometry is shown diagrammatically in Fig. 2.

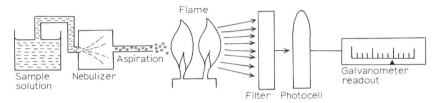

FIG. 2. Diagrammatic representation of flame photometry.

The introduction of flame photometry revolutionised the estimation of sodium and potassium in biological fluids as this is so laborious by classical chemical methods. A little later, serum calcium was measured by the same technique and Baker (1955) used a dilute lithium solution as an internal standard for calcium estimations. The methods for lithium estimation initially described were developed to measure the amounts in mineral samples in which lithium concentrations may be far higher than the therapeutic levels in patients' blood (Stuart *et al.*, 1957; Sykes, 1956). This method has now been adapted to measure lithium concentration in serum as this has become of clinical importance (Barrow, 1960; Helm and Andriesse, 1961; Lang and Herrmann, 1965; Schou, 1958). The following simple technique has been found consistently reliable (Coombs, 1971).

B. Materials and method

1. 2ml of the unknown serum are pipetted into a centrifuge tube. This serum should be free from haemolysis. It can be stored for two weeks or more at 4°C before analysis.

2. 8ml of 0·01 normal hydrochloric acid, which can be prepared from a normal solution by diluting 10 ml to one litre, are added and the sample, which becomes cloudy within a few minutes, is mixed and allowed to stand.

3. The sample is then heated in a simmering water bath for 5 minutes, transferred to a cold water bath, centrifuged when it is cool and the clear supernatant fluid is poured into a cuvette. This removes the protein from the sample.

4. A 0·3 mmol/l standard solution of lithium is prepared by dissolving 0·1919g of lithium sulphate in water and making up to one litre. Because of the

dilution of the serum from 2ml to 10ml, this 0·3 mmol/l standard is effectively equivalent to 1·5 mmol/l in comparison with the undiluted serum sample.

5. The standard solution and the supernatant fluid from the test solution are sprayed in turn and the apparent lithium content of the serum can then be calculated, as shown in the example (see below). An EEL Model 100 flame photometer, as shown in Fig. 3, is very suitable for the estimations but an appropriate lithium filter is essential.

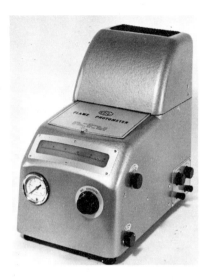

FIG. 3. EEL Model 100 flame photometer. (Evans Electroselenium Ltd., Halstead, Essex, England)

6. To correct for the effects of potassium, sodium, calcium and other ions always present in serum, a sample of pooled serum from several patients who are not on lithium may then be treated in the same way as the test serum. The average value for this pooled normal serum, which is usually approximately equivalent to 0·22 mmol/l of lithium, is then subtracted from the apparent level to give the true level of lithium.

Calculations for Estimating Serum Lithium

Adjust galvanometer to read zero with deionized water.
Set galvanometer to read 50 units with the 0·3 mmol/l standard solution of lithium.

Then read the unknown solution.

Example:
   Unknown solution reads 25 units.
   As the unknown solution is serum which has been diluted 1 in 5 from 2 ml
   to 10 ml, the serum contains an apparent lithium level of

$$0 \cdot 3 \times (25/50) \times 5 = 0 \cdot 75 \text{ mmol}/1.$$

But with pooled normal serum from patients not on lithium the reading is
equivalent to $0 \cdot 22$ mmol/1.
Therefore the true level of lithium in the unknown serum equals

$$\begin{array}{r} 0 \cdot 75 \\ -0 \cdot 22 \\ \hline 0 \cdot 53 \text{ mmol/l} \\ \hline \end{array}$$

Result:
Serum lithium $0 \cdot 53$ mmol/l

C. Problems

1. *Contamination of glassware*
Certain kinds of chemically hardened glassware may produce contamination
sufficient to affect significantly the estimation of serum lithium levels in the
therapeutic range, increasing results by 10–15% and completely invalidating
measurements of endogenous lithium (Wittrig *et al.*, 1969). This glassware
should be avoided.

2. *Serum protein*
Deproteinization increases the accuracy of the method and prevents blockage
of the atomizer. It is most easily achieved by adding hydrochloric acid and
heating. Trichloroacetic acid has also been used as a protein precipitant but it
lowers the readings for lithium by at least 5% and often more and may make the
solution cloudy (Little *et al.*, 1968). 96% Ethanol has also been tried but leads
to high coned flames which may be unsuitable for the apparatus and can cause
considerable variability in the results (Brown and Legg, 1970). Some flame
photometers, for example the Eppendorf photometer, can be used with dilution
of the sample alone and deproteinization of the sample is not essential
(Amdisen, 1967).

3. *Sodium, Potassium and Calcium*
Variation in the concentration of these elements does affect photometer readings with a given level of lithium, as shown in Fig. 4, in which the effect of
different concentrations of sodium, potassium and calcium on the emission at

671 nm of a standard solution of lithium containing 2 mmol/l is demonstrated. A suitable correction may easily be made for these and other ions by using pooled normal serum for the standards, as in the example above. Alternatively, the standard solutions of lithium may be made up to include 140 mmol/l of sodium, 4 mmol/l of potassium and 2·5 mmol/l of calcium, being the concentrations usually found in serum. Slight variations within the biological range then have only a minimal effect on the photometer readings (Amdisen, 1967).

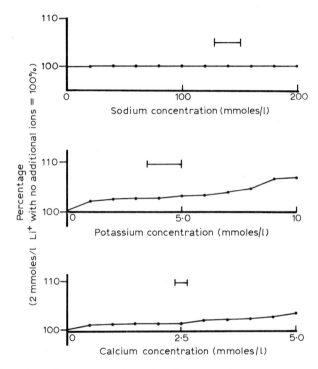

FIG. 4. Effect of varying concentrations of sodium, potassium and calcium on lithium emission as measured with the EEL Model 100 flame photometer. A 2 mmol/l solution of lithium containing no additional ions has been taken as 100% and the effect of increasing concentrations of sodium, potassium and calcium is shown. The bar shows the normal biological range for each ion.

4. Fuel gas

The best results for lithium determination are obtained with the routine use of propane, with its flow controlled by a sensitive regulator. This ensures constancy of fuel composition and freedom from the pressure variations inevitable with fluctuating demands on the town gas supply (Coombs, 1971). Excellent results may, however, be obtained in many areas with town or natural gas and, in areas where fire regulations prohibit the use of heavier-than-air fuel gases, a rotary pump and attached manifold may be used to compress natural gas from the mains, which can then be supplied at a constant pressure to the burner module (Nevius and Lanchantin, 1965). Natural gas when used with the EEL flame photometer may give a low emission with lithium owing to a relatively cold flame. The sensitivity of the method may then be significantly increased by adding acetone to the diluting solution to produce a 15–20% concentration of acetone (Denswil and Detmers, 1972).

5. *Lithium sensitive photocell*
It is essential that a lithium sensitive photocell is used as some recently introduced photocells which give greatly enhanced sensitivity for potassium estimations are quite unsuitable for lithium determinations (Coombs, 1971).

III. Atomic Absorption Spectrophotometry

A. Principles
Atomic absorption spectrophotometers are now available in many laboratories and the technique has certain theoretical advantages in the absolute measure ment of small amounts of a number of elements (Walsh, 1955). If an element is heated in a flame, as well as emitting light at particular wavelengths it will also absorb light at the same wavelengths. If light of specific wavelengths produced by heating an element in a lamp is shone through a flame, the amount of light of these wavelengths absorbed by the flame will vary directly with the amount of that element in the flame. It is this quantitative absorption of specific wave-lengths of light that forms the basis of atomic absorption spectrophotometry, as shown diagrammatically in Fig. 5.

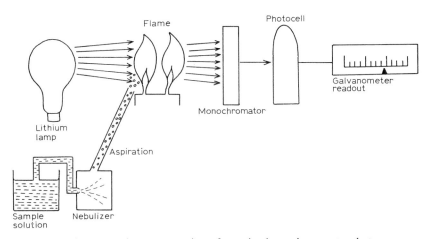

FIG. 5. Diagrammatic representation of atomic absorption spectrophotometry

Atomic absorption spectrophotometry has the advantage of being highly specific though, unfortunately, other substances in the flame may alter the activity of the element under assay and thereby its absorption of the light. In contrast to classical flame photometry, atomic absorption spectrophotometry can be applied to a very wide range of elements, including lead, gold, zinc and copper, which are difficult to estimate by other means. An appropriate lamp for each element is required, to produce light of the various specific wavelengths. An air-acetylene mixture is also required for the burner to produce the high temperatures which give more accurate results.

Despite their considerable cost atomic absorption spectrophotometers are now available in many laboratories and their application to the measurement of a number of elements in serum has been extended to include lithium estimations (Blijenburg and Leijnse, 1968; Bowman, 1967; Hansen, 1968; Lehmann, 1968).

B. Materials and method

1. The serum sample of unknown lithium content is diluted ten times with deionized water.

2. A master standard solution of 5 mmol/l of lithium is prepared by dissolving 0·1847 g of high purity lithium carbonate in the minimum quantity of 5 N hydrochloric acid needed. This solution is then boiled to expel carbon dioxide, cooled, transferred to a litre flask and diluted to the mark with deionized water. Working standards containing 0·025, 0·05 and 0·1 mmol/l of lithium can then be prepared by appropriate dilutions.

3. The standards and sample are then aspirated in turn into the atomic absorption spectrophotometer. This must be adjusted for estimating lithium

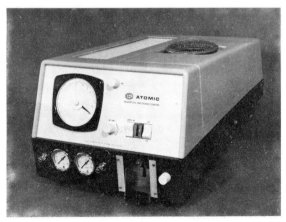

FIG. 6. EEL Model 140 atomic absorption spectrophotometer. (Evans Electroselenium Ltd., Halstead, Essex, England)

with an appropriate lithium hollow cathode lamp. The wavelength for lithium absorption or emission of 670·8 nm must then be set on the machine. A suitable machine for the analysis is the EEL 140, shown in Fig. 6.

4. A calibration curve is constructed from the readings obtained for the standard solutions. The lithium content of the test samples can then be read directly from this graph.

C. Problems

1. *Dilution*

Serum is too viscous and contains too much salt to be sprayed into the flame direct without causing rapid blockage of the burner. The sample is, therefore, best diluted, at least one in five, though this may cause some loss of sensitivity (Bowman, 1967). For research purposes it has, however, been possible to estimate lithium in very small amounts in serum after only a one in one dilution with a detergent solution such as Sterox® or Nonidet® (British Drug Houses, Poole, Dorset, England). Standards should then be prepared from a synthetic serum containing sufficient glycerol to match the viscosity of normal serum (Woods *et al.*, 1968).

2. *Interference by other elements*

In the amounts present in normal serum, calcium and magnesium have little effect on lithium absorption but sodium and potassium at normal serum concentrations have been found to enhance lithium absorption by 3% (Bowman, 1967), or even up to 8% in some studies (Zettner *et al.*, 1968), but sodium in excess of 500 mmol/l depresses lithium absorption (Little *et al.*, 1968). This should be allowed for by making up a standard solution to include similar amounts of sodium and potassium to normal serum, say 140 mmol/l sodium and 4 mmol/l potassium. In contrast, when potassium and sodium levels in standard and test solutions are comparable, minor variations in protein concentration at a dilution of 1:10 seem to have little effect. These effects are discussed in greater detail in the next chapter on the estimation of lithium in urine.

IV. Comparison of Flame Photometry and Atomic Absorption Spectrophotometry

Though the necessary equipment is very expensive, atomic absorption spectrophotometry is far more versatile and specific than flame photometry. The alkaline metals, sodium, potassium and lithium are, however, excited at a temperature lower than most elements and, with the low temperature propane flames of classical flame photometry, other spectra are not excited, minimising spectral interference. In addition, the characteristic wavelengths of the spectra of the alkaline metals are widely separated from each other and from most other

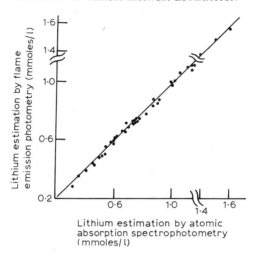

Fɪɢ. 7. Comparison of serum lithium concentrations measured by flame emission spectrophotometry and atomic absorption spectrophotometry (Redrawn from Pybus and Bowers, 1970, with permission).

elements, so that inexpensive optical filters can be used to separate the spectra and more complex monochromators are not essential. For lithium estimations, therefore, the cheap and simple flame photometer remains more than adequate.

In practice both methods have been found to give satisfactory results and when both techniques are applied to the same samples the results are very comparable, as illustrated in Fig. 7 (Pybus and Bowers, 1970; Blijenberg and Leijnse, 1968; Levy and Katz, 1970). Atomic absorption spectrophoto-

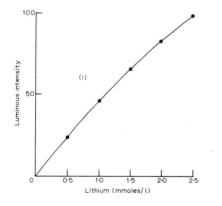
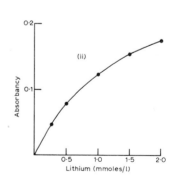

Fɪɢ. 8. Calibration curves for lithium. (i) Flame emission photometry. (ii) Atomic absorption spectrophotometry. (Redrawn from Blijenberg and Leijnse, 1968, with permission).

metry has the theoretical advantage of no spectral interference but, as mentioned, this does not seem to be much of a problem with flame photometry as far as lithium is concerned. Chemical interference with, for example, formation of lithium phosphate, and ionic interference remain theoretical problems with atomic absorption spectrophotometry but, in fact, the effects are negligible at the temperature of the air-acetylene flame. Flame emission photometry also has the advantage of a virtually linear response in the therapeutic range in contrast to atomic absorption spectrophotometry, for which a calibration curve must be constructed, as shown in Figure 8 (Blijenberg and Leijnse. 1968).

Most laboratories have only a few samples to analyse for lithium at one time. As the flame photometer is very widely available, the technique simple and reliable and the method very similar to that already used extensively for sodium and potassium estimation, the flame photometric method seems to be the more useful for lithium (Robertson *et al.*, 1973, Woollen and Wells, 1973). After the serum has been separated, the average technician can easily accomplish 30 lithium estimations within an hour using flame photometry.

In addition, careful comparative studies have shown that, for lithium, flame emission photometry may actually be more sensitive than atomic absorption spectrophotometry (Robertson *et al.*, 1973). Horncastle (1973) reports that in his experience the detection limit for lithium by flame emission photometry is 0·003 micrograms/litre but by atomic absorption spectrophotometry it is 5 micrograms/litre. Both atomic absorption spectrophotometry and flame emission photometry have been adapted to measure serum lithium in fully automated systems but flame photometry has proved much the easier to modify for this purpose (Kallweit and Porter, 1970, and Nevius and Lanchantin, 1965).

V. Special Applications of Analysis for Lithium

A. Capillary blood samples

The techniques using flame photometry have also been extended to the analysis of very small amounts of fingertip capillary blood, avoiding the necessity of venepuncture (Villeneuve *et al.*, 1971). The blood is collected in capillary tubes which are plugged with plasticine and centrifuged. The 0·2 ml samples of serum are then each mixed with 1·8 ml of a metal-free non-ionic detergent (Acatinox—Scientific Products, Division of American Hospital Supply Corp., Evanston, Illinois, U.S.A.). The blank and standard solutions of pooled lithium-free serum and pooled serum with a known added quantity of lithium are also made up with a similar proportion of the detergent and the solutions assayed in the flame photometer in the usual way.

The results of this method have correlated well with those of the usual method using venous blood, the correlation coefficient being 0·99. It is possible to adapt atomic absorption spectrophotometry to measure very small amounts as well but it is technically much more difficult to ensure accuracy.

B. Erythrocytes

A technique to measure lithium concentration in erythrocytes by atomic absorption spectrophotometry has been developed and Frazer *et al.* (1972) showed that in 15 patients with an average plasma lithium concentration of 1·21 mmol/l the average red cell lithium was significantly lower, at 0·72 mmol/l.

For the estimation heparinized venous blood is well mixed and a sample removed for haemoglobin and haematocrit determinations. The volume of the remainder is measured and 1·0 ml of an isosmotic solution of cobalt-EDTA is added. The addition of cobalt-EDTA is a refinement to assess the amount of plasma trapped betwen the red cells during centrifugation. This is essential for measurements of intraerythrocyte sodium levels as the sodium concentration is so much greater in the extracellular fluid, but it is less important for lithium measurements.

The blood sample is then centrifuged at 1600 g for 60 minutes and the plasma, "buffy" coat and the top 5 mm of packed cells are removed. A 1 ml aliquot of packed red cells is then diluted to 50 ml and after complete haemolysis the concentration of lithium is determined by atomic absorption spectrophotometry. Analysis of split sample pairs showed a reproducibility to 1·5% for fifteen samples, a level of accuracy very close to the 1·2% achieved by the same workers for plasma lithium determinations.

C. Cerebrospinal fluid

Lithium can be simply measured in undiluted C.S.F. and for analysis by atomic absorption spectrophotometry should be compared with standards containing equivalent amounts of sodium and potassium, i.e. 140 mmol/l sodium and 3·0 mmol/l potassium (Little *et al.*, 1968).

D. Saliva

Fournis and Chazot (1971) have used flame photometry for estimating lithium concentrations in saliva. They recommend a dilution of 1:20 with demineralised water before analysis.

E. Other organs

Wittrig *et al.*, (1970) have developed a technique for accurately measuring the very small amounts of lithium in normal body organs. The tissue is first vacuum dried overnight and then digested with measured amounts of nitric and sulphuric acids. The samples are then dry ashed overnight at 600°C, reconstituted in water and analysed by atomic absorption spectrophotometry. It was found that in the rabbit, of all the organs analysed, the thyroid contained the greatest amount of endogenous lithium and that human uterine tissue also contained considerable amounts, as shown in Table I.

TABLE I. Lithium in mammalian organs (from Wittrig *et al.* (1970) with permission).

		Number of Samples	Mean Lithium Content (mg/Kg ash weight)
Rabbit			
	Heart	10	2·26
	Striated Muscle	5	1·49
	Thyroid	8	21·25
	Testes	6	1·08
	Ovaries	3	4·72
	Uterine Tissue	4	1·17
Human			
	Uterine Tissue	13	6·50

References

Amdisen, A. (1967). *Scand. J. clin. Lab. Invest.* **20**, 104–108.
Amdisen, A. (1973). *Brit. med. J.* **1**, 240.
Arfwedson, A. (1818). *Fysik, Kemi, Mineral* **6**, 145–176.
Baker, R. W. R. (1955). *Biochem. J.* **59**, 566–571.
Barrow, G. R. J. (1960). *J. med. Lab. Technol.* **17**, 236–238.
Bertrand, G. and Bertrand, D. (1951). *Mikrochemie* **36–37**, 1004–1014.
Blijenberg, B. G. and Leijnse, B. (1968). *Clinica chim. Acta.* **19**, 97–99.
Bowman, J. A. (1967). *Analytica chim. Acta.* **37**, 465–471.
Brown, P. B. and Legg, E. F. (1970). *Ann. clin. Biochem.* **7**, 13–18.
Caldwell, H. C., Westlake, W. J., Connor, S. M. and Flanagan, T. (1971). *J. clin. Pharmacol.* **11**, 349–356.
Collins, G. C. and Polkinhorne, H. (1952). *Analyst, Lond.* **77**, 430–436.
Coombs, H. I. (1971). *Brit. J. Psychiat.* **118**, 225–226.
Covello, M. and Ciampa, G. (1965). *J. Chromat.* **20**, 201–204.
Denswil, E. H. and Detmers, J. P. (1972). *Clinica chim. Acta.* **40**, 129–131.
Desgrez, A. and Meunier, J. (1920). *C. r. hebd. Séanc. Acad. Sci. Paris* **171**, 179–182.
Folwarczny, M. cited by Kirchhoff, G. and Bunsen, R. (1861). *Annls. Chim. Phys.* **62**, 461–464.
Fournis, Y. and Chazot, G. (1971). *Path. Biol., Paris* **19**, 787–795.
Frazer, A., Secunda, S. K. and Mendels, J. (1972). *Clinica chim. Acta* **36**, 499–509.
Fry, D. E. and Marks, V. (1971). *Lancet* **1**, 886–888.
Garrod, A. (1866). *In* "System of Medicine" (J. Reynolds, ed.) Vol. I, 865.
Good, C. A. (1903). *Amer. J. med. Sci.* **125**, 273–284.
Grandeau, M. L. (1863). *Annls. Chim. Phys.* **67**, 155–171.
Hansen, J. L. (1968). *Amer. J. med. Technol.* **34**, 1–9.
Helm, H. J. v. d. and Andriesse. D. (1961). *Clinica chim. Acta* **6**, 747–748.
Horncastle, D. C. J. (1973). *Med. Sci. Law* **13**, 3–22.

Kallweit, E. and Porter, C. J. (1970). *Clin. Chem.* **16**, 528–554.

Keilholz, A. (1921). *Pharm. Weekbl. Ned.* **58**, 1482–1495.

Koch-Weser, J. (1972). *New Engl. J. Med.* **287**, 227–231.

Lang, W. and Herrmann, R. (1965). *Z. ges. exp. Med.* **139**, 200–212.

Lehmann, V. (1968). *Clinica chim. Acta* **20**, 523–525.

Levy, A. L. and Katz, E. M. (1970). *Clin. Chem.* **16**, 840–842.

Little, B. R., Platman, S. R. and Fieve, R. R. (1968). *Clin. Chem.* **14**, 1211–1217.

Nevius, D. B. and Lanchantin, G. F. (1965). *Clin. Chem.* **11**, 633–646.

Plum, C. M. (1957). *Clinica chim. Acta* **2**, 67–69.

Pybus, J. and Bowers, G. N. (1970). *Clin. Chem.* **16**, 139–143.

Robertson, R., Fritze, K. and Grof, P. (1973). *Clinica chim. Acta* **45**, 25–31.

Schou, M. (1958). *Acta pharmacol. tax.* **15**, 70–84.

Stuart, W. A., Simpson, M. and Hardwick, W. H. (1957). *Analyst, Lond.* **82**, 200–203.

Sullivan, J. V. and Walsh, A. (1966). *Spectrochim. Acta* **22**, 1843–1852.

Sykes, P. W. (1956). *Analyst, Lond.* **81**, 283–291.

Ure, A. (1843). *Pharm. J.* **3**, 71–74.

Villeneuve, A., Dery, R. and Genest, P. H. (1971). *Clin. Biochem.* **4**, 194–195.

Walsh, A. (1955). *Spectrochim. Acta.* **7**, 108–117.

Wittrig, J. J., Anthony, E. J., Woods, A. E. and Coates, J. T. (1969). *Clin. Chem.* **15**, 1237–1240.

Wittrig, J. J., Woods, A. E. and Anthony, E. J. (1970). *Dis. nerv. Syst.* **31**, 767–771.

Woods, A. E., Crowder, R. D., Coates, J. T. and Wittrig, J. J. (1968). *Atomic Absorption Newsletter* **7**, 85–86.

Woollen, J. W. and Wells, M. G. (1973). *Ann. clin. Biochem.* **10**, 85–88.

Zettner, A., Rafferty, K. and Jarecki, J. J. (1968). *Atomic Absorption Newsletter* **7**, 32–34.

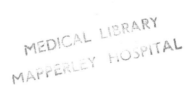

11

THE ESTIMATION OF LITHIUM IN URINE

A. Amdisen

I. Introduction

Flame photometry is the only method feasible for almost all quantitative determinations of the lithium ion when its use as psychotropic drug is concerned.

The present chapter has the limited aim of drawing attention to sources of error often overlooked when this method of analysis is used for the determination of lithium concentration in urine. The quantitative significance of these sources of error may vary from one type of apparatus to another. The problems described in the following might, therefore, to a certain degree be specific to the devices used, and perhaps cannot directly be transferred to other forms of apparatus. The problems might be more critical than suggested below, but they could be less critical too. In any event, they have always to be borne in mind.

II. Sources of Interference in Flame Emission Photometry: General Considerations

The fundamentals of the flame photometric method have already been outlined in Chapter 10, but some further comments having particular relevance to lithium estimation in urine, must be made here.

Final solutions of biological material (i.e. samples pretreated by dilution with water or watery substances), contain substances which, in flame photometry, react in ways which will interfere with the lithium determination. The most important forms of interference which occur during lithium estimation in urine stem from background emission and ion interference.

Background emission: Some of the light emitted by concomitant interfering substances has a wave-length which corresponds to that of the lithium spectral line, and they therefore simulate an additional lithium content in the urine sample.

Ion interference: The ions of the concomitant substances influence the equilibrium between lithium ions and lithium atoms in the flame and thereby introduce an error to the readings of the flame photometer.

In emission flame photometry both the background emission and the ion interference must be taken into account as sources of error. In atomic absorption flame photometry the ion interference only is worrying; the background emission is efficiently counteracted by the technical construction of the measuring devices.

Apart from the relative importance of background emission, the distinctive difference between emission and atomic absorption flame photometry concerns the sensitivity. The atomic absorption devices have a higher sensitivity for determination of, for example, magnesium, zinc and lead, while the emission method has a higher sensitivity to other elements such as sodium, potassium, and calcium; where lithium is concerned, however, the sensitivities of the two methods are almost equal.

It is also a feature of flame photometric methods that final solutions of calibration standards with known concentrations of lithium ion are measured simultaneously with the final solutions of the test samples. This provides an opportunity for making some allowance for the sources of error by supplying the calibration standards with the interfering substances in concentrations corresponding to concentrations of the samples. Another possibility is that the final solutions of both the calibration standards and the samples might be supplied with substances which counteract the differences between them.

III. Special Problems of Urine Determination of Lithium Compared to Determinations in Serum

The most important sources of error in the determination of lithium in serum and urine derive from the presence of sodium, potassium, calcium and phosphate ions. The influence of the latter substance is, however, insignificant for serum determinations. Special problems might instead exist with the protein content of serum (see Chapter 10 and Amdisen, 1967).

In serum, sodium, potassium, and calcium are under homeostatic control and are thus within narrow concentration ranges. Both the background emission and the ion interference can, therefore, be counteracted by supplying the calibration standards with concentrations of these substances corresponding to the normal values of serum. Even pathological deviations from the normal concentrations would not produce errors of significance for the clinical situation (Amdisen, 1967).

The situation is quite different when lithium in urine is concerned. In urine the concentrations may vary from very low values (e.g. in polyuria occurring simultaneously with a low intake of the interfering substances), to extremely high values in concentrated urines. Since increased urine output, even to the extent of true polyuria, is not infrequently seen during lithium treatment, whilst in other patients water diuresis may be normal, the whole concentration range of possible interfering substances must be taken into account: i.e., sodium: 0–400 mmol/l; potassium: 3–400 mmol/l; calcium: 2–100 mmol/l; and phosphate: 2–100 mmol/l. In spite of this variation it would still be rational to adjust the standard solution with these substances to the concentrations most frequently found in the urine of lithium-treated patients. It is, however, obvious that critically greater deviations from the standards will very often be present. Even in atomic absorption flame photometry such greater deviations may be critical as sources of error (Lehmann, 1968; Little *et al.*, 1968; Zettner *et al.*, 1968; Robertson *et al.*, 1973). This problem might be solved for both the atomic absorption and the emission method by preparing particular calibration standards adapted to the particular urine sample. This would involve estimations of the interfering substances of the particular urine sample previous to the preparation of each calibration standard; however, this would undoubtedly be too laborious in most circumstances.

Attempts have been made by the author to provide more detailed information about these disturbing phenomena, and thereby to devise practicable analytical procedures for routine urine analysis. The following is an outline of the progress made to date.

IV. Characterization of the Sources of Error in Urine Lithium Estimation

The great variety of urine types produced by patients was simulated by preparing rows of solutions containing varying amounts of a urine pool without lithium, collected from 35 normal persons. This urine pool was characterized by the following concentrations: sodium, 80 mmol/l; potassium: 44 mmol/l; calcium: 6·4 mmol/l; magnesium: 3·0 mmol/l; phosphate: 12·5 mmol/l; creatinine: 0·8 g/l; and urea: 11·0 g/l.

The analytical procedure under investigation demanded a diluting factor for urine of 10. A solution containing 10% of the urine pool was therefore taken as representing the final solution of an average human urine, while a solution containing 1% of the urine pool corresponded to the final solution of a polyuric urine, and a 30% solution to the final solution of a concentrated urine.

A further simplification as compared to the conditions operating in practice, was that all members of one row of solutions containing either increasing concentrations of the urine pool or increasing concentrations of pure salts were supplied with the same lithium concentration.

The concentrations shown in most of the following figures relate to final solutions; the corresponding concentrations of undiluted, real urine would, therefore, be ten times higher.

The investigations were carried out with an emission flame photometer of the Eppendorf type; the atomic absorption photometer used was a spectrophotometer Zeiss PM Q II with flame attachment.

The burning gas used was an air–acetylene mixture.

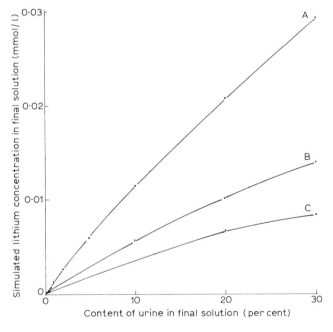

Fig. 1. Background emission of urine. A: urine without pretreatment, apart from dilution with water. B: urine after precipitation of calcium with potassium oxalate. C: urine after precipitation of both calcium and phosphate, the latter with zirconyl chloride. The curves B and C have been corrected for interference by the precipitation media.

A. Emission flame photometry

In emission flame photometry increasing concentrations of lithium-free urine in the final solution produce a gradually increasing background emission (Fig. 1); 30% of urine in the final solution simulates about 0·03 mmol Li^+/l (corresponding to an error of +0·3 mmol/l of a moderately concentrated, real urine).

The background emission of the urine is likely to be almost exclusively caused by its content of calcium, phosphate, potassium and sodium (Fig. 2, and Fig. 1, B and C) with calcium being particularly important in this respect.

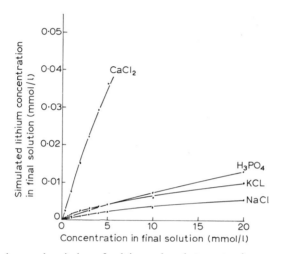

FIG. 2. Background emission of calcium, phosphate, potassium, and sodium.

None of the other substances found in greater amounts in urine, such as magnesium, creatinine, or urea, produce any significant background emission, neither does the zirconyl chloride used for precipitation of phosphate.

It appears from Fig. 3, that the background emission is not the only type of interference in emission flame photometry. At lower lithium levels the presence of very low urine concentrations causes a sudden steep rise in the measured lithium values; with increasing urine concentrations this is followed by a gradual rise caused by the background emission (see also Fig. 1). At a lithium level of about 0·6 mmol/l in the final solution (corresponding to 6·0 mmol/l in undiluted urine) the background can just be discovered on the curve. The curves of 1·5 mmol/l and of higher lithium levels would hardly give rise to any suspicion of the presence of a background emission. These findings are readily understandable in view of the fact that the background emission is independent of the lithium concentration and its percentage significance, therefore, necessarily decreases with increasing lithium concentrations.

In final solutions with a lithium concentration above 0·6 mmol/l the urine influence on the lithium emission is almost exclusively caused by ion interference. Figure 3 further shows that the percentage significance of the ion influence decreases with increasing lithium concentrations.

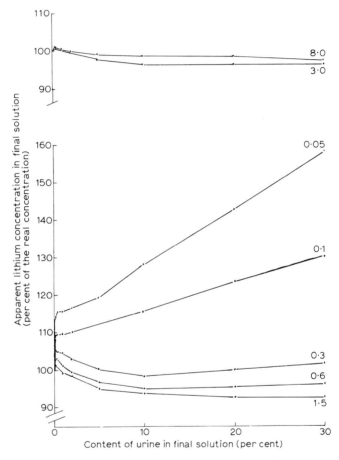

FIG. 3. Interference of varying urine content with the apparent lithium concentration at different actual concentration levels. The figures on the curves show the real lithium concentrations of the final solutions (mmol/l).

When using this artificial and simplified model to provide evaluation of the situation encountered in practice, it must be observed that the calibration standards used in the present study were aqueous solutions of lithium chloride. In the real situation calibration standards would have been adjusted with sodium, potassium, calcium and phosphate to concentrations corresponding to those of the urine pool. Consequently the courses of each of the curves in Fig. 3 should be compared at the point of their 10% urine solution. This reveals that emission flame photometry without any measures other than correction of the calibration standards to counteract the urine interferences, might show the following types of error:

1. Lower lithium concentrations (below 3 mmol Li$^+$/l): Polyuric urines might show concentrations 10 to 15% too low. Decreased renal excretion of water might produce lithium concentrations more than 25% too high.

2. Intermediate lithium concentrations (3 to 10 mmol Li$^+$/l): Polyuria might produce lithium concentrations 5 to 10% too high. Concentrated urines might give values either 5% too high or 5% too low.

3. Higher lithium concentrations (above 10 mmol Li$^+$l): In polyuria, values 3 to 5% too high may be found. The influence of decreased water content of the urine would be insignificant.

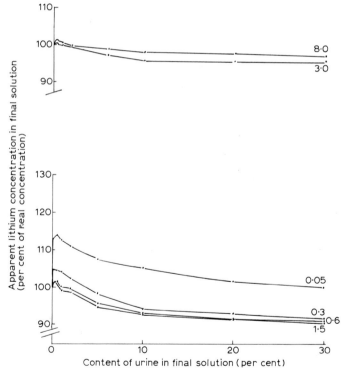

FIG. 4. Ion interference of varying urine content on the apparent lithium concentration at different actual concentration levels. The figures on the curves show the real lithium concentrations of the final solutions (mmol/l). (Curves from Fig. 3, corrected for background interference as shown in Fig. 1).

The ion interference is more clearly demonstrated when the curves of Fig. 3 are corrected for background emission (by subtraction of the values of Fig. 1, A). Figure 4 shows that there is a common trend at different lithium concentration levels: enhancement of the lithium emission produced by low urine contents in the final solutions; depression of the emission caused by increasing content of urine; and a decreasing percentage significance with increasing lithium concentrations. It is further worth remarking that, relatively, the depressive effect decreases with increasing urine concentration at all lithium levels.

When increasing concentrations of pure sodium chloride or potassium chloride are used instead of the urine pool a corresponding ion influence is revealed (Fig. 5).

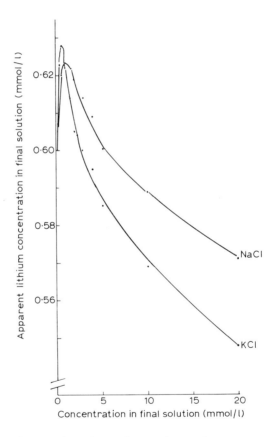

Fig. 5. Ion interference of varying sodium and potassium concentrations on the apparent lithium concentration in final solutions with 0·6 mmol/l of lithium (the curves are corrected for the background interference as shown in Fig. 2).

Compared with sodium, potassium has a stronger enhancing effect as well as a stronger depressive effect on the lithium emission. Other experiments, not described here, have shown that calcium exerts a very weak enhancement and a somewhat weaker depression than sodium. Phosphate and oxalate (the latter used for precipitation of calcium) produce a weak depression only.

Both enhancement and depression of the lithium emission may be partly due to nonspecific cation effects, since the addition of 4 mmol of potassium to the sodium solution neutralizes the enhancement effect of sodium (Fig. 6); further, the depressive effect of sodium on the emission is significantly reduced.

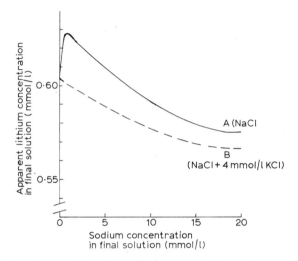

FIG. 6. Ion interference of varying sodium concentration on the apparent lithium concentration in final solutions with 0·594 mmol/l of lithium. A Diluent: Demineralized water. B Diluent: 4 mmol/l potassium chloride.

It has previously been recommended that advantage might be taken of these properties by using a solution of 40 mmol potassium chloride instead of water as a diluent for the ten times dilution of the urine samples and of the standard solutions (Amdisen, 1971). However, later experiences have shown that the resulting high content of dry matter in the final solutions causes trouble with the atomizer and the burner of the flame photometers, and it is now recommended that a more appropriate diluent would be an aqueous solution containing approx. 10 mmol of potassium chloride and approx. 50 mmol of ammonium chloride. The influence of increasing amounts of urine in the final solution after precipitation of calcium and phosphate (see Fig. 1) and following the use of such a diluent is shown in Fig. 7. The evaluation of the significance of this for the real situation again involves comparing the courses of the curves at the points corresponding to their 10% urine content. It appears that:

1. The errors caused by polyuria or by concentration of the urine would now be acceptably small for most purposes even for lithium concentrations as low as

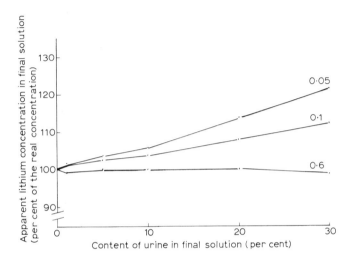

Fig. 7. Interference of varying urine content on the apparent lithium concentration at different levels, after the use of correcting measures. Calcium and phosphate of the urine solutions were precipitated with potassium oxalate and zirconyl chloride, respectively. The calibration standards were furnished with corresponding concentrations of potassium oxalate and zirconyl chloride. Final solutions of both urine and calibration standards were supplemented with potassium chloride and ammonium chloride, 10 and 50 mmol/l, respectively. The figures on the curves show the real lithium concentrations of the final solutions (mmol/l).

about 1 mmol/l (corresponding to the 0·1 curve in Fig. 7) but not for concentrations lower than this.

2. The error introduced by natural variations in the urines would be insignificant at higher lithium concentrations (lithium concentrations higher than 0·6 mmol/l in the final solution are not presented in the figure because they were confluent with the 0·6 curve).

On the basis of the experiences described above, the following procedure has been developed for the emission flame photometer (Eppendorf) used in the present investigations:

Urine: To 10 ml of urine add 0·5 ml of a 1·05 mol/l potassium oxalate solution, mix thoroughly, stand for 10 min. and then centrifuge. To 5 ml of the supernatant add 0·5 ml of a 1·05 mol/l zirconyl chloride solution. Mix thoroughly, stand for 20 min and centrifuge again.

Final solution of urine: To 1·0 ml of the latter supernatant add 10 ml of a 50 mmol/l ammonium chloride solution.

Calibration standards: (Content: 80 mmol/l sodium chloride; 76 mmol/l potassium chloride; 42 mmol/l potassium oxalate; and 0, 2, or 10 mmol/l of lithium chloride). To 5 ml of the standard solution add 0·5 ml of a 1·05 mol/l zirconyl chloride solution. Mix thoroughly, stand for 20 min and centrifuge again.

Final solution of calibration standard: To 1·0 ml of the final supernatant add 10 ml of a 50 mmol/l ammonium chloride solution.

(The procedure involves giving the final solutions of both urine and the standards solutions a surplus concentration of potassium and ammonium chloride of 9·26 and 45·5 mmol/l respectively).

Calculation: Urine lithium (mmol/l) = 1·05 × (R-FU) × (C-CS)/(R-FCS) where (R-FU) is the scale reading of the final solution of the urine; (R-FCS) is the scale reading of the final solution of the calibration standard; and (C-CS) is the lithium concentration of the calibration standard. The calibration curve of this procedure is a straight line only within a lithium concentration range of 0 to about 15 mmol/l. Therefore, urines found to contain more than 15 mmol/l of lithium are redetermined after dilution to a concentration of around 10 mmol/l with a solution containing 80 mmol/l of sodium chloride and 44 mmol/l of potassium chloride.

Lithium recovery of normal urines supplied with lithium chloride to give the following concentrations; 0·5, 2·0, 5·0, 10·0, 30·0, and 60·0 mmol/l of lithium was found to be 98–102%, and the coefficient of variation 0·5–1·6%.

One conclusion to be drawn from the investigations described above is that in spite of its somewhat higher sensitivity, the emission flame photometry method should only with caution be used to determine lithium concentrations in urine if it has been necessary to operate with final solutions containing lithium at a concentration lower than 0·1 mmol/l.

Perhaps even lower lithium concentrations in urine could safely be determined if the oxalate and zirconyl precipitations of calcium and phosphate, respectively, were supplemented with precipitations of sodium and potassium using ethanol and ether as described by Jackman and Balazs (1970).

B. Atomic absorption flame photometry

With the Zeiss PM Q II atomic absorption flame photometer no background emission was found, as expected.

The ion interference produced by increasing amounts of urine in the final solution was closely comparable to results presented in Fig. 4. An exemplifying curve is shown in Fig. 8A.

Addition of 50 mmol/l of ammonium chloride to the final solution does not

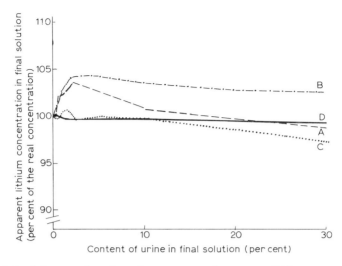

Fig. 8. Ion influence of varying urine content on the apparent lithium concentration
of final solutions with an actual lithium concentration of 0·6 mmol/l.
A: Final solutions of urine without further additions.
B: Final solutions of urine supplemented with 50 mmol/l of ammonium chloride.
C: Final solutions of urine supplemented with 10 mmol/l of potassium chloride.
D: Final solutions of urine supplemented with 50 mmol/l of ammonium chloride
and 10 mmol/l of potassium chloride.

affect the enhancement of the absorption produced by smaller amounts of urine,
but decreases the depressive effect of the higher urine (Fig. 8B).

Furnishing the final solutions with 10 mmol/l of potassium chloride alone,
removes the enhancement, but affects the depression of the atomic absorption
to a minor degree only (Fig. 8C). However, supply of both ammonium chloride
and potassium chloride to the final solutions reduces the ion interference to a
negligible level (Fig. 8D).

The following method was developed for the determination of lithium
concentration in urine using the Zeiss PM Q II atomic absorption apparatus.

Calibration standards: Aqueous solutions of lithium chloride at concentrations of 0, 0·5, 1·0, 2·0, 4·0 and 6·0 mmol/l.

Final solutions of standards: To 1·0 ml of the standard solution add 10 ml of
a diluent containing 11 mmol/l potassium chloride and 55 mmol/l of ammonium chloride.

Urine (final solution of urine): To 1·0 ml of urine are added 10 ml of the
diluent used for dilution of the calibration standards.

$$\text{*Calculation:* Urine lithium (mmol/l)} = \frac{(R-FU) \times (C-CS)}{(R-FCS)}$$

where, (R-FU) is the scale reading of the final solution of urine, (R-FCS) is the scale reading of the standard solution, and (C-CS) is the lithium concentration of the standard solution used.

The calibration curve of the present procedure is a straight line only within a lithium concentration range of 0 to 6 mmol/l. Therefore, urines found to contain more than 6 mmol/l are redetermined after dilution with water to a concentration around 4 mmol/l.

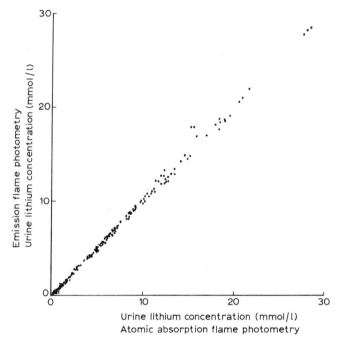

FIG. 9. Correlation between emission flame photometry and atomic absorption flame photometry. Lithium determinations on urines of persons who had taken lithium.

For lithium concentrations at 0·5 mmol/l or higher the reliability and the precision of this method are of the same order of magnitude as found for the emission method of 1·0 mmol/l and above.

The sensitivity of the method allows the determination of lithium concentrations down to about 0·1 to 0·2 mmol/l in urine, though at these low concentrations the accuracy is less (coefficient of variation: 2 to 3%).

It appears from Fig. 9 that there is a very close correlation between the emission method and the atomic absorption method described when used for determinations of lithium in urine sampled from individuals treated with lithium.

However, the deviations between the two methods are unacceptably great at lithium concentrations below 1 mmol/l primarily because of the lower accuracy of the emission method at these concentration levels (Fig. 10).

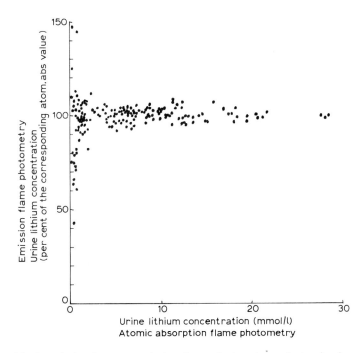

FIG. 10. Correlation between emission flame photometry and atomic absorption flame photometry. The results of the emission method expressed as percentages of the corresponding result of the atomic absorption method (see Fig. 9).

Atomic absorption might be the method of choice for urine estimation because of the simplicity of the procedure, though determinations of lithium concentrations even by this method should be used with caution if it has been necessary to operate with final solutions containing lithium at a lower concentration than 0·05 mmol/l.

V. Conclusion

The great variations which occur in the concentrations of a number of cations in urine might, because of ion interference, be important sources of error in determination of lithium concentrations lower than about 10 mmol/l with both emission and atomic absorption flame photometers. This may, however, be counteracted by straightforward measures such as the addition of potassium and ammonium chlorides to the dilution fluid.

In emission flame photometers the interference effect of the background emission upon lithium estimation creates additional problems for the determination of concentrations lower than 10 mmol/l. These may be counteracted by precipitation of calcium, sodium, potassium, and phosphate from the urine. The analysis is, however, thereby made more complicated, and in spite of the somewhat higher sensitivity of the emission method for lithium determinations, results showing lithium concentrations lower than 0·1 mmol/l in the final solutions should possibly be used with caution.

The atomic absorption method seems preferable for lithium estimations in urine because of the simplicity of the procedure and the higher accuracy at lower concentration levels. However, the results should also be used with caution if it has been necessary to operate with lithium concentrations lower than 0·05 mmol/l in the final solutions, even if ion interference has been counteracted by use of a proper diluent.

Acknowledgements

I am indebted to Mrs. V. Glud-Jensen for valuable suggestions and skilful technical assistance, and to Dr. Odvar Skaug for advice concerning the precipitation procedure with zirconyl chloride.

References

Amisen, A. (1967). *Scand. J. clin. Lab. Invest.* **30,** 104–108.

Amdisen, A. (1971). *In* "Advances in Neuro-Psychopharmacology". (O. Vinař, Z. Votava, P. B. Bradley, eds.) pp. 67–71. North-Holland Publishing Company, Amsterdam.

Jackman, D. A. and Balazs, N. D. H. (1971). *Biochem. Med.* **5,** 97–100.

Lehmann, V. (1968). *Clinica chim. Acta,* **20,** 523–525.

Little, B. R., Platman, S. R. and Fieve, R. R. (1968). *Clin. Chem.* **14,** 1211–1217.

Robertson, R., Fritze, K. and Grof, P. (1973). *Clinica chim. Acta.* **45,** 25–31.

Zettner, A., Rafferty, K. and Jarecki, H. J. (1968). *Atomic Absorption Newsletter* **7,** 32–34.

12

SUSTAINED RELEASE PREPARATIONS OF LITHIUM

A. Amdisen

I. Introduction

The present chapter on the use of sustained release preparations in oral administration of the lithium ion is devoted to the fundamental problems only. Sustained release preparations which are already available and marketed are mentioned only to illustrate the fundamental principles of sustained release. This field of lithium treatment is at present undergoing a rapid evolution: a detailed description of any particular preparation might, therefore, be outdated within a short time.

Ordinary tablets are always designed to release the drug within a few minutes of being placed in water or watery mixtures. If the drug is soluble and does not become bound to the contents already present locally in the alimentary canal, and if it is easily absorbed, the absorption will start immediately upon the release of the drug from the tablets; the full amount of drug ingested will thus pass into the organism within a short time. If the drug readily passes into the blood and extracellular fluid, the blood concentration will show a steep rise, reaching a high peak shortly after the tablet intake. This high peak creates problems during treatment with drugs of a high toxicity and with drugs where the side effects depend on the momentary blood concentration. Special difficulties might partly be counteracted by dividing the daily tablet dosage into several smaller doses given at more frequent intervals. More than two daily doses are, however, always an inconvenience and the intervention of sleeping time necessitates that one longer time interval occurs between tablets every day.

II. Survey of Sustained Release Preparations in General

The following outline of the fundamental properties of sustained release preparations and of the methods by which sustained release may be achieved, is based mainly on a short survey presented by Sjögren (1971).

The special properties of a sustained release product depend on the gradual release of the drug during its passage through the stomach and the intestines. The course of the absorption will thus be extended over a long period of time and the initial peak concentration will be decreased. Maintenance of a relatively constant drug concentration in the body gives a more uniform pharmacological response and may reduce the frequency and intensity of side effects. In particular, drugs irritating the gastrointestinal mucosa may be better tolerated when given in a slow release form. A reduced number of administrations per day may often be achieved; this will be more convenient for the patient and may reduce the risk of dosage errors due to forgetfulness.

If a constant concentration of a drug is to be maintained in the body, the drug has to be absorbed at the same rate as it is eliminated. It is of course practically impossible to make tablets or capsules giving such an absorption because of the great variations in the biological factors involved in drug absorption and elimination. An adequately formulated sustained release preparation, however, gives a more even pattern of blood concentration of the drug.

The transport of a drug in solid dosage form through the gastro-intestinal tract is subject to many variations, such as changes in the speed of propagation and mixing, and in the composition of the stomach and intestinal contents. If the dissolution of the drug from the product is affected by factors such as these, a steady and reproduceable release rate of the drug *in vivo* cannot be expected. Large uncontrolled variations in the rate of solution and absorption are obviously not acceptable for drugs with a narrow margin between the therapeutically effective concentration and the concentration giving side effects or producing a risk of intoxication.

Most drugs appear to be absorbed by a process of passive transport through the gastrointestinal mucosa, but in spite of this the efficiency of absorption in different parts of the gastrointestinal tract may vary considerably. The sustained release product has to be adjusted to the factors influencing the absorption of the particular drug. The product should further be formulated so as to release nearly the whole dose before leaving the gastro-intestinal tract. It is necessary always to be aware of the risk of impairing the absorption of the drug, because sustained release preparations are deliberately formulated to prevent a rapid dissolution.

The earliest products in this field utilized tablets or capsules with slowly disintegrating coatings in order to obtain the desired slow dissolution. Subsequently, a considerable number of sustained release products have been developed in which the sustained release has been based on other principles.

The methods which have most frequently been adopted for obtaining sustained release in drug products include the following:

1. *Decreased solubility.* This is generally achieved by involving the active drug principle in complex formation or salt formation. Some drugs with a limited solubility can give a certain slow release effect without the use of special pharmaceutical formulations. This may be the case with ordinary tablets containing lithium carbonate. However, if the lithium carbonate tablets meet with greater amounts of hydrochloric acid in the stomach, the slow release effect is lost because the carbonate is rapidly converted to the highly soluble lithium chloride (Fig. 2 and Fig. 4A).

2. *Ion-exchange resins.* The drug in an ionized form may be bound to an ion-exchange resin. The complex obtained is insoluble in water but the drug can be released by an exchange with ions from the gastrointestinal fluid. The release is dependent on the availability of such ions, the diffusion characteristics of these ions through the resins and the diffusion of the drug out of the resin.

3. *Embedding the drug in a non-digestible porous carrier.* The inactive matrix in which the drug is embedded is more or less unchanged throughout the entire release process and the drug is released as a result of diffusion of water into the porous structure, and the diffusion of the dissolved drug outwards.

4. *Dispersion of the drug in slowly digestible or slowly disintegrating material.* In contrast to the principle of the former method in which the pharmacologically inert carrier retains its shape, embedding the drug in a digestible or disintegrable matrix leads to the release of the drug by the continuous surface erosion of the tablet or the pellets.

5. *Coatings with controlled disintegration.* Granules used for tablet production or pellets used for capsules may be coated with slowly disintegrating layers. As long as the coating is intact, the drug cannot dissolve. In order to attain a sustained release instead of delayed release, several fractions of the granules or pellets, with coatings of different resistance, are mixed together in the particular tablet or capsule, the initial dose being provided by a non-coated fraction.

6. *Permeable coatings.* Pellets or granules for the tablet production, or the

.H

tablets themselves, are coated with layers sufficiently permeable to permit a slow diffusion of the water and the dissolved drug.

7. *Embedding the drug in a gel.* Such tablets may contain a quantity of a high viscosity hydrophilic gum. In contact with the water the gum turns into a mucilaginous gel which forms around the tablets and the dissolution of the drug is retarded by the slow diffusion of both water and dissolved drug through the gel.

Several more possibilities exist, as some of the methods mentioned above can be combined in a single preparation.

III. Sustained Release Preparations and Lithium Treatment
A. Pharmacokinetics of the lithium ion

The lithium ion can presumably be absorbed everywhere in the gastro-intestinal tract (Fig. 1).

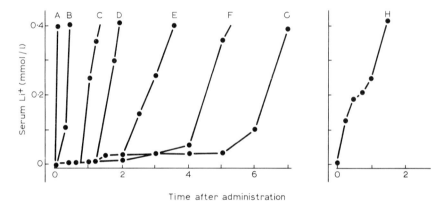

Time after administration

FIG. 1. First part of the serum concentration course in the same person (the author) after administration of: A: ordinary lithium citrate tablets. B: ordinary lithium carbonate tablets. C, D, E, F, and G: enteric coated (*delayed* release) tablets with varying resistance of the coatings. H: lithium citrate rectal suppository. E, F, G, and H provoked, at a point corresponding to the last point of the curves, imperative diarrhoeas preceded by a period of severe abdominal pain. H gave severe abdominal pain immediately after administration which was impossible to withstand for more than about one hour at which point defaecation could no longer be prevented.

When given in a readily absorbed form (for example, as a dilute lithium chloride solution) the absorption of lithium starts immediately after intake. The serum concentration rises rapidly and peaks at a maximum value within about half an hour (Fig. 2). The maximum concentration is high compared to the dosage and body weight. This reveals that most of the dose given is found, temporarily, within a relatively restricted part of the body, presumably in the

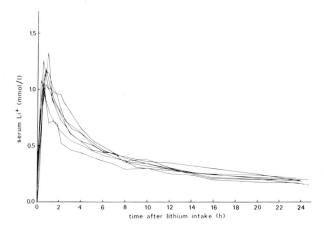

FIG. 2. Serum lithium curves after administration of 24 millimoles of lithium ion as a dilute lithium chloride solution to seven adults (the administration took place at 8 a.m.; the courses from 12–20 h after intake represent the slower decrease during the night, they are not, therefore, comparable to Fig. 3) (Reproduced from Amdisen, 1973b, with permission).

extracellular space, as a result of the rapid absorption of lithium into the extracellular fluid and the somewhat slower distribution of the ion from the extracellular to the intracellular compartment. Following the establishment of a peak serum concentration, there is a fairly quick decrease as a result of the simultaneous operation of renal excretion and the distribution of lithium into

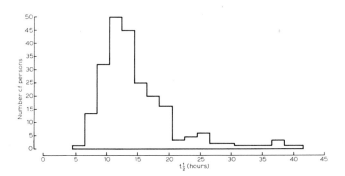

FIG. 3. Distribution of 226 persons according to their serum lithium halftime, $t_{\frac{1}{2}}$, during the interval between 12 and 20 hours after the last intake of lithium. $t_{\frac{1}{2}}$ of each individual patient was determined on the basis of two blood samples, the first drawn at 8 a.m., the second at 3–4 p.m., i.e. the values apply to the decrease in serum concentration during daytime (Reproduced from Amdisen, 1973a, with permission).

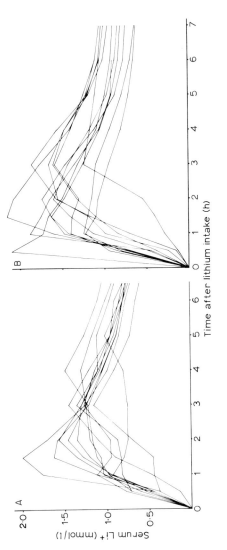

Fig. 4. Serum lithium curves after intake of *ordinary tablets*. A. Eleven volunteers given about 0·70 mmol Li$^+$/kg body weight as ordinary lithium *carbonate* tablets. B. Twelve volunteers given about 0·85 mmol Li$^+$/kg body weight as ordinary lithium *citrate* tablets. (Amdisen, Geisler and Glud-Jensen, unpublished data).

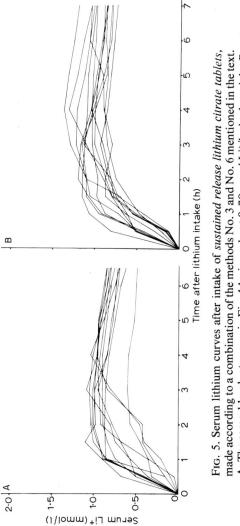

FIG. 5. Serum lithium curves after intake of *sustained release lithium citrate tablets*, made according to a combination of the methods No. 3 and No. 6 mentioned in the text. A. The same 11 volunteers as in Fig. 4A given about 0·70 mmol Li^+/kg body weight. B. The same 12 volunteers as in Fig. 4B given 0·85 mmol Li^+/kg body weight. (Amdisen, Geisler and Glud-Jensen, unpublished data.)

other tissues. Six to eight hours after the intake the decrease has become constant on a pro rate base, i.e. the particular serum concentrations are placed on a straight line on a semilogarithmic graph.

During the daytime the serum lithium curve of this elimination phase falls with a speed corresponding to an average half life for lithium in serum of 8–20 hours in persons with normal renal function (left part of Fig. 3).

When the lithium ion is taken as ordinary tablets the concentration curves become much more variable and unpredictable (Fig. 4). The dissolution from the tablets is obviously strongly affected by the varying conditions in the gastrointestinal tract.

Fig. 5 shows the serum concentration curves of the same persons as in Fig. 4 after the intake of equal amounts of lithium ion in the form of a sustained release preparation. There is a significantly slower rise of the serum concentration; instead of the distinct peak there is now a protracted maximum at a much lower level, and the courses of the serum concentrations are much more uniform. The sustained release preparation used gives a slower absorption than ordinary lithium tablet preparations and it is much less sensitive to the varying conditions of the surroundings during its passage through the stomach and intestines.

These pharmacokinetic properties of the lithium ion draw attention to some practical consequences for treatment procedures in lithium therapy, which might lead to sustained release lithium preparations being used in preference to ordinary preparations.

B. Acute overdosage and sustained release preparations

Among patients undergoing long-term treatment with lithium there will be some who will now and then, in spite of the treatment, suffer from depressive relapses, and the risk of attempted suicide by overdosage of lithium tablets must, therefore, always be taken into account. Further, the well-known situation in which children accidentally take tablets, represents a high risk when lithium tablets are concerned because of the high toxicity of the drug.

The fully developed intoxication syndrome (see Chapter 13 and Chapter 14), revealing that overdosage has taken place, may often be delayed for several hours or even for one or two days (Hanlon *et al.*, 1949; Gaind and Saran, 1970; Amdisen *et al.*, 1973). On the other hand, a high, acute lithium dosage frequently provokes within about an hour both vomiting and long-lasting, vigorous diarrhoea.

If the tablets taken were sustained release instead of ordinary preparations, a higher percentage of the lithium dose taken would probably leave the gastro-intestinal tract as a result of the vomiting and diarrhoea, undissolved in the slow releasing tablets.

C. Sustained release and monitoring of the lithium dosage by serum concentration measurements

To ensure the efficacy of lithium treatment for the majority of patients it is recommended that the lithium dosage should initially be adjusted to give a serum concentration within a narrow range around $1 \cdot 0$ millimoles lithium ion per litre. The limits of this range which have been suggested are $0 \cdot 7$–$1 \cdot 3$, $0 \cdot 7$–$1 \cdot 2$, $0 \cdot 7$–$1 \cdot 1$ or, most recently, $0 \cdot 8$–$1 \cdot 0$ (Schou *et al.*, 1971; Schou and Shaw, 1973; Schou, 1973; Amdisen, 1973b), in a blood sample drawn in the morning before the first dose of the day or, according to an even stricter demand, twelve hours after the evening dose (Amdisen, 1973a, b). However, this has not been generally accepted (e.g Johnson, 1972; Maggs, 1973), possibly because many physicians are overlooking the necessity of bringing under control the many factors influencing the serum concentration (Amdisen, 1973b) and because the concentration-response curve according to which the recommendations are given is based on clinical experiences only (Schou *et al.*, 1971). The very difficult task of systematically mapping out the correlation between serum concentration and clinical response has not yet been undertaken.

It is, however, generally accepted that the dosage necessary to achieve a clinical response in an individual patient is high compared to the dosages which imply a risk of severe side effects and intoxication, and it is therefore necessary to establish procedures for monitoring the drug dosage and to set up control measures to avoid the risk of staggering the treatment. The only way to achieve this degree of safety is to determine a close correlation between the dosage and the concentration used for the initial and later dosage adjustments.

Multiple factors influence the serum concentration of a blood sample drawn between sequential administrations of the drug throughout the day. Some of these factors have a strong influence, e.g., the time interval between last dose and blood drawing, forgetfulness in taking the tablets during the days immediately prior to control of the concentration, and the nature of the dosage schedule; others usually have a weaker influence, but they can occasionally become important by accident, e.g., handling of the blood sample from drawing until it reaches the laboratory, the accuracy of the lithium analysis, *variation of the lithium content of the tablets and variation in dissolution and absorption in the gastrointestinal tract* (Amdisen, 1973b) (Figs. 4 and 5).

Even these weaker influences on serum concentration must be brought under control if a safe monitoring of the lithium treatment is to be achieved, because several factors may by chance influence the serum concentration if they operate simultaneously in the same direction. In this case their conjoint influence may cause undue lurching of the control values.

The general demands on variations of drug content in ordinary preparations, as settled in the pharmacopoeias, permit 20–25% differences between tablets. It would be in the interests of the safety of lithium-treated patients if manufacturers of lithium preparations would guarantee much smaller variations. Further, ordinary tablets often have a low resistance to physical influence; partly broken tablets and powder from the tablets are frequently found in the patients' tablet bottles. Finally, most ordinary tablet preparations and some of the sustained release preparations are sensitive to the varying conditions in the stomach and intestines. This may produce great variations in the course of the serum lithium concentration between dosage administrations (Fig. 4).

These shortcomings imply more or less pronounced unpredictable variations of the blood concentration as determined for the purposes of controlling treatment.

Some of the methods used to obtain slow release will, automatically, give much lower variations than the kind mentioned above, because the process of ensuring the sustained releasing properties demands a very strict accuracy in the amounts of the components used. A very hard and resistant tablet is also an inherent requirement of some of the methods used to produce sustained release products.

The ideal sustained release product should be quite independent of the surroundings in the gastrointestinal tract in its releasing properties, and should give identical courses of the serum concentration between the dose intakes. It is not, in practice, feasible to attain this ideal, but a very close approximation to it is possible (see Fig. 5).

In connection with the safe monitoring of the lithium treatment there are, however, drawbacks involved in the use of sustained release preparations, even if they do fulfil the demands mentioned above; if the release is so protracted that a considerable part of the lithium is not dissolved before the tablets leave the gastrointestinal tract, the amount of absorbed lithium ion will vary from time to time because of the varying gastrointestinal passage rate, and the serum concentration will show corresponding variations (Coppen et al., 1969).

A further requirement of a sustained release lithium preparation, therefore, will be that, on average, the absorption must not be quantitatively lower than that found with ordinary tablets; for example, the total amount of lithium excreted in the urine during 6 to 7 days after a single tablet dose should be equal to that after ordinary tablets. A 100% dissolution should probably be reached within six to nine hours to make a sustained release preparation acceptable for use in lithium treatment (Amdisen and Sjögren, 1968). The releasing time of the product must, therefore, be a compromise; it should be long enough to give a significant reduction of the concentration peaks during the absorptive phase, but sufficiently short to make the absorption quantitatively acceptable.

D. Side effects and sustained release

Some patients suffer from side effects which are so disturbing that they want to stop the lithium treatment; this may especially be seen during the first weeks or

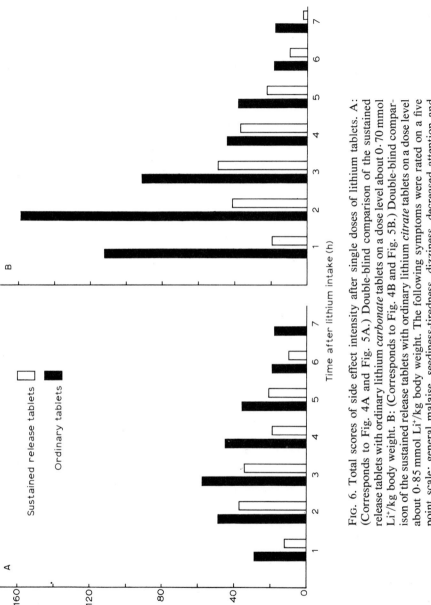

FIG. 6. Total scores of side effect intensity after single doses of lithium tablets. A: (Corresponds to Fig. 4A and Fig. 5A.) Double-blind comparison of the sustained release tablets with ordinary lithium *carbonate* tablets on a dose level about 0·70 mmol Li+/kg body weight. B: (Corresponds to Fig. 4B and Fig. 5B.) Double-blind comparison of the sustained release tablets with ordinary lithium *citrate* tablets on a dose level about 0·85 mmol Li+/kg body weight. The following symptoms were rated on a five point scale: general malaise, seediness-tiredness, dizziness, decreased attention and ability to concentrate, irritability, headache, facial paraesthesias, feeling of heaviness in body and limbs, nausea, and vomiting. (Amdisen, Geisler and Glud-Jensen, unpublished data.)

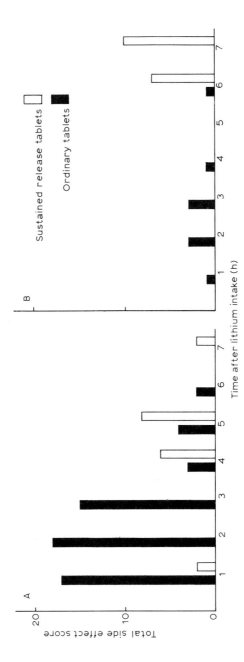

Fig. 7. Total side effect score of the symptoms: abdominal pain, loose stools, and watery stools. Data from the trials mentioned in legend to Fig. 6. (Observe that the ordinates of this figure and Fig. 6 are not alike.) (Amdisen, Geisler and Glud-Jensen, unpublished data.)

few months after start of the treatment. The intensity of the side effects is, however, partly correlated with variations in serum concentration.

Volunteers given a high, single lithium dose show a lower intensity of side effects after a sustained release preparation than after ordinary preparations (Fig. 6). Matussek and v. Hessling (1971) have found corresponding results in patients during lithium treatment, including reduction of hand tremor which is a frequent accompaniment of lithium treatment.

If sustained release preparations were generally used in lithium treatment a reduction in the problems caused by side effects could be expected. Further, most patients could achieve their daily dosage requirement in two doses only; the frequently embarrassing midday dose could then be avoided.

Concerning side effects there may, however, also be certain drawbacks associated with sustained release preparations; abdominal pain, loose stools and diarrhoea, indicating an irritation of the intestines, are often seen during the first few hours after the intake of ordinary lithium preparations. The immediacy of these symptoms is reduced when slow release tablets are used, but corresponding symptoms may still appear several hours after the intake (Fig. 7). Even low concentrations of lithium ion, it would seem, can irritate the distal parts of the intestines (see legend to Fig. 1).

IV. Requirements of Sustained Release Lithium Preparations: Summary

The releasing time should be as long as possible, but not longer than necessary to ensure an absorption quantitatively equal to the absorption from ordinary preparations.

The dissolution of the lithium ion should be as independent as is feasible of the varying conditions of the surroundings in the gastrointestinal tract.

The variation of the lithium content of the tablets should be restricted both between tablets and between production batches.

The preparation should have a high resistance to erosion during storage.

V. Conclusions

A sustained release preparation properly adapted to the demands of lithium treatment might give the acutely over-dosed patient a better chance of survival. It would allow a safer monitoring of the treatment according to the blood concentration, side effects would be reduced, and most patients could use the more agreeable two dose per day scheme instead of the inconvenient three dose regime and thereby avoid the embarrassing midday dose. This would further reduce the risk of dosage errors caused by forgetfulness.

During the present rapid evolution in this field of lithium treatment, the physicians themselves have to ask for documentation from the manufacturer which confirms that the product they intend to use satisfies the requirements of a sustained release preparation, which is formulated to minimise the problems and the dangers inherent in lithium treatment.

References

Amdisen, A. and Sjögren, J. (1968). *Acta Pharmaceut. Suec.* **5,** 465–472.

Amdisen, A. (1963a). *Brit. med. J.* **2,** 240.

Amdisen, A. (1973b). Paper read at Coloque International Théraplix 1973 "Les sels de Lithium en psychiatrie", held in Paris, November 26–27.

Amdisen, A., Gottfries, C. G., Jacobsson, L. and Winblad, B. (1973). *Nord. psych. T.* **27,** 539–549.

Coppen, A., Bailey, J. E. and White, S. G. (1969). *J. clin. Pharmacol.* **9,** 160–163.

Gaind, R. and Saran, B. M. (1970). *Postgrad. med. J.* **46,** 629–631.

Hanlon, L. W., Romaine III, M., Gilroy, F. J. and Deitrick, J. E. (1949). *J. Am. med. Assoc.* **139,** 688–692.

Johnson, D. A. W. (1972). *Clin. Trials J.* **9,** 17–20.

Maggs, R. (1973). *Brit. med. J.* **1,** 416.

Matussek, N. and v. Hessling, P. (1971). *Nervenarzt* **42,** 376–378.

Schou, M., Amdisen, A. and Baastrup, P. C. (1971). *Brit. J. hosp. Med.* **6,** 53–60.

Schou, M. (1972). *Archs. invest. Med.* **3,** 459–471.

Schou, M. (1973). *In* "Lithium. Its Role in Psychiatric Research and Treatment" (S. Gershon and B. Shopsin, eds.), pp. 189–199. Plenum Press, New York.

Schou, M. and Shaw, D. M. (1973). *Practitioner* **210,** 105–111.

Sjögren, J. (1971). *Acta Pharmaceut. Suec* **8,** 153–168.

13

LITHIUM SIDE EFFECTS AND TOXICITY: THE CLINICAL PICTURE

L. VACAFLOR

I. Introduction

This chapter will present a description of the signs and symptoms which characterise lithium side effects and toxic reactions. In addition to outlining the effects which occur and the variability which may be expected in the clinical picture, some attempt will be made to evaluate the degree of seriousness of individual symptoms or groups of symptoms by adopting, wherever this seems feasible, a classification into mild, moderate and severe categories. The major defining criterion for placement within the classification is not the duration of a symptom or the frequency with which it occurs, but the extent to which it impairs or threatens the general functioning of the individual.

Of course this distinction is seldom clear-cut and symptoms placed under one heading may, when they occur in an intensified form or if they are accompanied by other, more serious symptoms, appear also under a different heading.

Factors which may determine the onset and/or modify the clinical course and outcome of side effects are also given brief consideration.

The pathophysiological bases of side effects are dealt with separately in Chapter 32, and Thomsen and Schou, in Chapter 14, discuss the various means by which lithium poisoning may be treated.

For the purposes of the present chapter side effects have been taken as those drug effects which are not obviously related to the major mode of action of the drug in producing its therapeutic action, are fairly readily observed without the use of elaborate biochemical or physiological techniques (routine pathological tests excluded), and are likely to cause some degree of discomfort to the patient, or are suspected as being contrary to the patient's general well-being. Toxic reactions are defined similarly, but with greater emphasis upon the final criterion implying a greater necessity for some form of active intervention on the part of the clinician (F. N. Johnson, personal communication).

II. Side Effects and Toxic Reactions Related to Specific Organ Systems

A. Central nervous and neuromuscular systems

It is now generally agreed that the central nervous system is the principally affected organ of the body under lithium therapy. This realisation represents a change of emphasis resulting from a better understanding of the probable mechanisms of action of lithium, and also from more careful observations of the clinical picture as it appears in the various stages of lithium intoxication. It seems clear that the symptoms directly related to neuromuscular and/or brain dysfunction are present throughout the various stages of lithium side effects and toxic reactions.

1. *Mild effects*

Fine tremor of the hand is by far the most common side effect in this category and is noted in almost all reports which refer to side effects. It is present even when serum lithium levels are well within the acceptable range for therapeutic purposes. It is usually present both when the patient is resting and while movements are being carried out, but it rarely becomes such a problem as to make necessary the discontinuation of therapy, although it may occasionally be advisable for the dose to be adjusted. Unlike some of the side effects produced by major tranquillizers the tremor which occurs in some patients during lithium therapy frequently does not seem to improve by the mere passing of time unless there is an actual decrease of serum concentration, though Schou *et al.,* (1970) showed that whilst about 53% of patients showed lithium tremor within the first week of treatment, another group of patients who had been under treatment for between 1 and 2 years exhibited the symptom with much lower frequency (4%).

In addition to its occurrence in the limbs, tremor may also appear in the lower jaw (Schou, 1959; Strömgren and Schou, 1964; Sikes and Sikes, 1970) and it has been suggested that this is a sign of impending lithium toxicity. Kusumi (1971) notes an eyelid tremor which occurred in one lithium-treated patient.

Muscular weakness has been reported as an accompaniment of lithium therapy (Cleveland, 1913; Hanlon *et al.*, 1949; Waldron, 1949; Radomski *et al.*, 1950; Glesinger, 1954; Fyrö *et al.*, 1970; Sikes and Sikes, 1970), but is, on the whole much less commonly experienced than tremor as a mild side effect and does tend to disappear or show marked improvement after the first few weeks of therapy. Schou *et al.*, (1970) note a drop from 36% of patients reporting weakness one week after the initiation of therapy to a total absence of reports in patients treated for over a year. The subsequent reappearance of such symptoms may simply indicate that there has occurred an undue increase in serum lithium concentration.

2. *Moderate effects*

These include those effects which occur as a result of a worsening of the symptoms described above, and also the appearance of others such as headaches (Baldessarini and Stephens, 1970; Fyrö *et al.*, 1970) and progressively more serious forms of muscular disturbance: trembling (Furlong, 1973); twitchings (Cade, 1949; Stern, 1949; Straker, 1970; Dias and Hocken, 1972; Larson *et al.*, 1972); fasciculations in the limbs (Corcoran *et al.*, 1949; Schou *et al.*, 1968; Van der Velde, 1971) and in the hands and face (Coates *et al.*, 1957); brief facial spasms (Prien *et al.*, 1972) or transient facial paralysis (Schou *et al.*, 1968); tendon jerks (Dias and Hocken, 1972) possibly as a result of hyperactive tendon reflexes and muscular hyperirritability (Corcoran *et al.*, 1949; Stern, 1949; Schou *et al.*, 1968); Parkinsonism or similar symptoms (Duc and Maurel 1953; Shopsin *et al.*, 1970; Kirk *et al.*, 1972); loss of some degree of motor control which may result in stumbling or falling (Furlong, 1973) and which has been described simply as unsteadiness (Waldron, 1949; Greenfield *et al.*, 1950; Rice, 1956) or as mild to serious ataxia (Cade, 1949; Roberts, 1950; Glesinger, 1954; Rice, 1956; Coats *et al.*, 1957; Schou, 1959; Sikes and Sikes, 1970; Straker, 1970; Vacaflor *et al.*, 1970; Rogers and Whybrow, 1971; Prien *et al.*, 1972).

The muscular symptoms are often accompanied by a certain degree of impaired concentration or dullness of sensorium (Schou *et al.*, 1968; Straker, 1970; Levy *et al.*, 1973) which may also include mild disorientation (Van der Velde, 1971; Dias and Hocken, 1972), loss of memory and aphasia (Greenfield *et al.*, 1950; Shopsin *et al.*, 1972). A variety of other unpleasant subjective feelings may also occur, including dizziness or giddiness (Cleaveland, 1913; Cade, 1949; Rice, 1956; Schou, 1959; Strömgren and Schou, 1964; Sikes and

Sikes, 1970; Nahunek *et al.*, 1971), nervousness (Greenfield *et al.*, 1950), faintness (Van der Velde, 1971) or vertigo (Svestka *et al.*, 1970; Vinarova *et al.*, 1972) and there may be minor disturbances of sensory mechanisms resulting in distortions or blurring of vision (Cleaveland, 1913; Corcoran *et al.*, 1949; Waldron, 1949; Greenfield *et al.*, 1950; Schou *et al.*, 1954; Schou, 1959; Sikes and Sikes, 1970; Fyrö *et al.*, 1970; Vinarova *et al.*, 1972) and tinnitus (Baldessarini and Stephens, 1970; Fyrö *et al.*, 1970). With moderate levels of lithium neurotoxicity it is not uncommon for patients to report feeling fatigued, tired, lethargic, apathetic, drowsy or somnolent (Corcoran *et al.*, 1949; Hanlon *et al.*, 1949; Stern, 1949; Glesinger, 1954; Schou *et al.*, 1954; Rice, 1956; Schou, 1959; Maggs, 1963; Fyrö *et al.*, 1970; Straker, 1970; Svestka *et al.*, 1970; Persson, 1971; Rogers and Whybrow, 1971; Van der Velde, 1971; Dias and Hocken, 1972; Ramsey *et al.*, 1972; Vinarova *et al.*, 1972; Levy *et al.*, 1973).

The moderately severe neuromuscular symptoms are usually dose-related, although, as with the mild symptoms, there have been occasional reports of their appearing when patients were receiving acceptable doses and showed consistent serum concentration levels. In such cases it would seem that an unusual sensitivity to lithium is indicated, with consequent increased neurotoxicity (Shopsin *et al.*, 1970). In patients over the age of 50, moderate clouding of the sensorium may develop with relatively low serum lithium concentrations (Vacaflor, unpublished observations; see also the later discussion of age effects).

Muscular incoordination, more extreme ataxias, and other symptoms such as nystagmus (Glesinger, 1954; Schou, 1959; Schou *et al.*, 1968) and slurring of speech (Cade, 1949; Peters, 1949; Glesinger, 1954; Straker, 1970; Vinarova *et al.*, 1972; Levy *et al.*, 1973) are indicative of cerebellar involvement in the moderate side-effect syndrome.

The category of moderate side effects obviously contains a wide range of different symptoms and many of these shade into the category of severe effects. The presence of any of the more disturbing symptoms must direct the attention of the physician to the possibility that the patient is either receiving more lithium than he should, or that other factors are interfering with its adequate excretion.

3. *Severe effects*

The fully developed picture of neural and neuromuscular symptoms during severe lithium intoxication is very striking and not easy to forget. The patient may show any of the symptoms previously mentioned under the heading of mild and moderate and, in addition, presents a progressive impairment of sensorium which passes through states of confusion and mental obfuscation (Peters, 1949; Stern, 1949; Roberts, 1950; Glesinger, 1954; Schou *et al.*,

1954; Sivadon and Chanoit, 1955; Coates *et al.*, 1957; Schou, 1959; Schou *et al.*, 1968; Baldessarini and Stephens, 1970; Shopsin *et al.*, 1970; Vacaflor *et al.*, 1970; Prien *et al.*, 1972) to delirium (Greenfield *et al.*, 1950; Glesinger, 1954), coma (Greenfield *et al.*, 1950; Radomski *et al.*, 1950; Schou, 1959; Schou *et al.*, 1968; Straker, 1970; Vacaflor *et al.*, 1970; Nahunek *et al.*, 1971; Van der Velde, 1971) and eventually death.

At variance with other forms of delirium, hallucinations or other pseudo-perceptions are not prominent, though they have occasionally been reported (Schou, 1959).

In the early stages of severe lithium intoxication there is usually a very marked restlessness (Vinarova *et al.*, 1968) and irritability (Svestka *et al.*, 1970): a growing ataxia and incoordination may prevent the patient completing even simple intentional movements.

In extreme intoxication the patient typically shows severe speech impediment and can only utter grunts; at best, speech is extremely slurred. His whole body is subject to frequent jerky movements involving whole limbs and the fasciculation of groups of muscles. Muscular hypotonus and flaccidity may sometimes occur (Peters, 1949; Roberts, 1950; Coates *et al.*, 1957), whilst in other cases there have been descriptions of rigid cogwheel limb hyperextension (Schou *et al.*, 1968; Lavender *et al.*, 1973). Occasional reports have appeared of lithium-induced choreiform movements (Peters, 1949; Duc and Maurel, 1953; Sivadon and Chanoit, 1955; Coats *et al.*, 1957; Shopsin *et al.*, 1970).

Nystagmus, skin hyperirritability and Parkinson-like symptoms are frequently present and the patient may develop serious difficulties in swallowing even very small quantities of liquid (Stern, 1949; Van der velde, 1971).

Epileptiform seizures, often classified as grand mal, are common (Roberts, 1950; Noack and Trautner, 1951; Glesinger, 1954; Teulie *et al.*, 1955; Schou, 1957, 1959; Wharton and Fieve, 1966; Schou *et al.*, 1968; Baldessarini and Stephens, 1970; Demers *et al.*, 1970; Svestka *et al.*, 1970; Vacaflor *et al.*, 1970; Prien *et al.*, 1972; Shopsin *et al.*, 1972) and the patient may end in status epilepticus (Noack and Trautner, 1951; Teulie *et al.*, 1955). Incontinence of both faeces and urine is usually present even before cerebral convulsions have taken place. The amnesia which may follow severe lithium intoxication and lithium-induced seizures is related to the intensity and duration of the clouding of the sensorium.

4. *Possibility of irreversible brain damage*

It has recently become clear that, in certain rare instances, irreversible brain damage may be produced as a permanent effect of lithium toxcity (Von Hartitzsch *et al.*, 1972) the structures usually involved being the basal ganglia and cerebellum. The damage commonly follows an acute lithium intoxication and becomes clinically visible by symptoms such as ataxia, nystagmus, choreoathetotic movements, and hyperactive deep tendon reflexes.

5. *EEG changes associated with lithium neurotoxicity*

It is usual in cases of suspected neurotoxicity arising from lithium treatment to examine the patient's EEG records. The literature on lithium-induced EEG changes is reviewed in detail in Chapter 31, but some comments are appropriately made here. Shopsin *et al.*, (1970), having reviewed the literature pertinent to lithium neurotoxicity, concluded that the EEG changes were the "most consistent laboratory abnormalities" (p. 177).

The characteristics of the EEG most commonly associated with lithium include:

1. The appearance of generalised slow waves of high voltage (e.g., Corcoran *et al.*, 1949);

2. Decreased alpha activity, with increased theta and delta waves (Schou *et al.*, 1968);

3. A correlation between the severity of EEG changes and the clinical evidence of central nervous impairment, but less correlation with serum lithium levels;

4. An increased likelihood of EEG changes (e.g. focal abnormalities) in individuals that have previously shown existing baseline abnormalities.

B. Gastrointestinal system

Side effects in this system are common and it may be that all patients have, to some degree, gastrointestinal effects during a short period after the initiation of lithium therapy when serum lithium levels are rising rapidly; in the majority of cases, the effects will occur to such a slight extent as to escape attention unless specifically sought. When gastrointestinal irritation does occur it usually subsides fairly rapidly (from 33% incidence to 0% over one to two years, according to Schou *et al.*, 1970) and it seldom reaches a degree of seriousness requiring referral to a clinician.

All the symptoms fall within the mild to moderate category.

The usual picture is of slight disturbances of bowel movement and mild gastric upsets. Reports refer simply to "gastric irritation" (e.g., Talbott, 1950; Prien *et al.*, 1972) and speak of such symptoms as abdominal flutterings, epigastric bloating or stomach pressure (Greenfield *et al.*, 1950; Svestka *et al.*, 1970). Reports of mild abdominal pains do occur (Cade, 1949; Rice, 1956; Svestka *et al.*, 1970; Persson, 1971) though they are not common.

More intense symptoms may be reported including, in particular, nausea (Schou *et al.*, 1954; Baldessarini and Stephens, 1970; Persson, 1971; Furlong, 1973) which may actually lead to vomiting (Cade, 1949; Roberts, 1950; Rice, 1956; Schou, 1959; Strömgren and Schou, 1964; Fyrö *et al.*, 1970; Straker,

1970; Svestka *et al.*, 1970; Van der Velde, 1971; Dias and Hocken, 1972; Vinarova *et al.*, 1972). Anorexia may also be noted to a greater or lesser extent (Cade, 1949; Stern, 1949; Greenfield *et al.*, 1950; Coates *et al.*, 1957; Baldessarini and Stephens, 1970; Dias and Hocken, 1972; Larson *et al.*, 1972). Diarrhoea, characterised by watery or even bloody stools may also be present, though more rarely (Cade, 1949; Strömgren and Schou, 1964; Baldessarini and Stephens, 1970; Fyrö *et al.*, 1970; Straker, 1970; Svestka *et al.*, 1970; Larson *et al.*, 1972; Prien *et al.*, 1972; Vinarova *et al.*, 1972; Lavender *et al.*, 1973). Diarrhoea is the most serious of the toxic effects to be found in the gastrointestinal system and its occurrence may indicate the need for medication to be readjusted; although not serious by itself, diarrhoea can certainly worsen a patient's general condition by contributing to water and sodium loss.

C. Renal system

The fact that lithium is almost totally excreted by the kidneys has led to the belief that very serious or fatal cases of intoxication were due essentially to a primary renal failure. Schou (1957) refers to the kidneys as the *locus minoris resistentiae*. Without denying the very significant role played by the kidneys it is nevertheless clear that the emphasis has been progressively placed on the central nervous system as the principally affected organ in states of lithium toxcity, particularly when this is severe.

1. *Mild effects*

(a) *Increased diuresis and thirst:* Symptoms of polyuria and polydipsia are quite common, particularly at the beginning of lithium therapy, and required no special intervention on the part of the clinician for they are usually spontaneously reversible and cause hardly any discomfort to the patient. As usual, of course, special care has to be taken with elderly patients (in whom these symptoms are more commonly found). The symptoms and their physiological and biochemical bases are discussed in full in Chapter 28.

(b) *Proteinuria:* This too is not a commonly reported symptom but one which is occasionally found when the appropriate tests are carried out (Dias and Hocken, 1972; Lavender *et al.*, 1973).

(c) *Oedema:* The frequency of oedema as a side effect (Baldessarini and Stephens, 1970; Mihovilovic, 1970; Svestka *et al.*, 1970; Vacaflor *et al.*, 1970; Demers and Heninger, 1971) is not well-established. In most instances the oedema is pre-tibial and does not appear to be related to either dose or serum levels. It is usually mild and does not normally call for any active treatment, though in some unusual cases it may become severe enough to lead to a discontinuation of lithium treatment. Reduction of the lithium dose suffices in most instances to reverse the condition. The re-initiation of therapy which has been discontinued because of oedema does not necessarily lead to oedema again, even when the serum lithium levels regain, or even exceed, their original values.

2. Moderate effects

The symptom described as "diabetes insipidus-like" is fully discussed in Chapter 28, it may be regarded as belonging to the category of moderate renal side-effects of lithium. Its frequency is low. It appears either at the beginning of therapy or several months later and is relatively independent of the dose or serum lithium level. In some cases the condition constitutes the only toxic manifestation. In a milder form (as polydipsia and/or polyuria) it occurs in around 60% of patients shortly after treatment and even after more than a year of treatment as many as 23% of patients may still report some symptoms (Schou et al., 1970). Patients showing this particular toxic reaction will urinate a total volume of several litres a day; the urine consistently exhibits a low specific gravity and this remains unaltered despite the administration of pitressin or the infusion of hypertonic saline. Discontinuation of lithium treatment leads to full recovery of the ability of the kidney to concentrate urine. In some instances treatment has been restarted without the recurrence of the diabetes-like syndrome.

3. Severe effects

The most extreme renal reactions to lithium to be noted in the literature concern oliguric renal failure (Dias and Hocken, 1972; Lavender et al., 1973). The condition as it appeared in the few cases reported was clearly related to a general state of serious lithium intoxication where most of the other symptoms of toxicity were present concomitantly or had preceded renal failure by a few days (gastrointestinal disturbances, neural and neuromuscular effects, etc.).

D. Cardiovascular System

The early association of lithium therapy with cardiovascular disorder was understandable in view of the documented cases in the late nineteen-forties and early nineteen-fifties of serious intoxications and occasional deaths occurring in cardiac patients given lithium chloride in taste substitute preparations for common salt (see Chapter 2). These reports resulted in a considerable decrease in the clinical use of lithium and, until quite recently, the available information regarding the relationship between lithium and cardiovascular dysfunction was derived mainly from animal studies. These studies showed that lithium (usually in doses much higher than those adopted for therapeutic purposes in man) led to EKG changes similar to those seen in conditions of hyperkalaemia (QRS widening and T-wave depression) and which eventually led to cardiac arrest (McKusick, 1954).

The findings relating to EKG effects produced by lithium which have so far been reported in the medical literature can be summarised briefly as follows:

1. They are generally mild;

2. They consist of EKG changes similar to those observed in cases of disturbed electrolyte balance (particularly involving potassium);

3. The EKG changes are not noticeably dose-related and their frequency of occurrence varies according to the number of leads which are used for the recording procedure and the frequency with which recordings are taken (Demers and Heninger, 1970, 1971);

4. T-wave depression is the most consistently reported finding (Radomski *et al.*, 1950; Andreani, 1957; Schou, 1959. 1963; Verbov *et al.*, 1965; Schou *et al.*, 1968; Demers and Heninger, 1970, 1971; Larson *et al.*, 1972), though other changes, such as T-wave inversion and amplification (Radomski *et al.*, 1950; Schou, 1959; Verbov *et al.*, 1965; Tangedahl and Gau, 1972) have also been described.

Although most authors claim that the changes are essentially sub-clinical, benign and reversible, there have been occasional reports of actual dysrhythmia (abnormal irritability of the myocardium with frequent extra systoles) (Tangedahl and Gau, 1972) and Dias and Hocken (1972) reported a case of lithium toxicity involving congestive heart failure as a secondary effect of renal damage.

Pfeiffer *et al.*, (1969, 1970) have demonstrated that the average electrical heart activity increases with lithium treatment, though the significance of this finding with respect to the general picture of lithium side effects is not clear.

As interest in the cardiovascular effects of lithium becomes more general we can probably expect an increase in the number of reports of clinical disturbances in this system, although it seems safe to state that serious toxic effects will continue to be rare.

E. Endocrine system

This topic is given full coverage in Chapter 27 and only a few comments need to be made here.

The symptoms associated with pathological change, both structural and functional, which occur in the thyroid gland as a result of lithium treatment, have been reported with increasing frequency. Although there is little agreement regarding the likelihood of occurrence of thyroid dysfunction there is concensus in respect of its generally benign nature when it does occur. There is no general agreement, however, on what mechanisms may be involved in the production of thyroidal symptoms (see Chapter 27).

Lithium given during manic-depression may lead to goitre, with or without associated mechanical problems, as well as to hypothyroidism not accompanied by goitre. From the clinical point of view the disorders are essentially benign and do not normally require discontinuation of lithium therapy. The appearance of thyroidal side effects does not seem to be related to other factors, such as the sex or age of the patient, but the incidence is sometimes held to be higher in subjects with a previous history of thyroid pathology.

The development of exophthalmus in a group of patients was reported by Segal *et al.* (1973) in a study of lithium action which has opened new questions regarding the complex interactions which exist between lithium, the affective disorders, and the hypothalamic–pituitary–thyroidal system. One hundred patients were studied and in 11 of these pathological exophthalmic changes were observed. No significant hormonal abnormalities were detected, and in the six patients in whom thyrotropin levels were measured the values were found to lie within the normal range. The exophthalmic changes were essentially benign and reversible.

Some mention may be made at this point of the sort of time-scale that is involved in the appearance of lithium-induced thyroid effects. Schou *et al.*, (1968) mentioned that the incidence of goitre depended upon when, after commencing lithium therapy, one assessed it; the assessment of 4% incidence reported by Schou and his colleagues was based upon continuous assessment for one year, but they noted that "if there is a latency period for goitre development the incidence becomes higher" (p. 711). Sedvall *et al.*, (1968) showed reductions in serum PBI levels and other changes after as little as 24 hours lithium administration; Cooper and Simpson (1969) and Halmi and Noyes (1972) also showed changes after about the same interval. It is possible that the time of first occurrence of such changes may eventually prove to be useful in warning the physician of impending thyroid trouble.

All the endocrine side effects of lithium may be considered as falling within the mild or moderate categories.

F. Skin

Cutaneous effects have been reported to occur in association with lithium therapy and a few papers have appeared, especially since 1970, which have dealt specifically with these conditions (Callaway *et al.*, 1968; Kusumi, 1971; Carter, 1972; Ruiz-Maldonaldo *et al.*, 1973).

For several reasons it is difficult to make an accurate assessment of the frequency of cutaneous side effects of lithium. To the extent that skin disorders are often found in association with neurotic conditions and may have a psychosomatic component in their aetiology, it might be expected that a given population of psychiatric patients would show a greater incidence of skin disorders than in a normal control group, irrespective of the medication received. Bearing this in mind, it can be stated that:

1. Cutaneous lesions during lithium therapy are relatively uncommon;

2. They are usually of the maculopapular variety, although other variants have been described, including ulcerations (Callaway *et al.*, 1968), pruritic

dermatitis (Nahunek,*et al.*, 1971; Larson *et al.*, 1972), exaccerbation of psoriasis (Carter, 1972) and acneiform reactions (Callaway *et al.*, 1968; Kusumi, 1971; Ruiz-Maldonaldo *et al.*, 1973);

3. Most of the skin reactions occur during the first three or four weeks of therapy (Callaway *et al.*, 1968);

4. The effects do not appear to be dose related, either in frequency of occurrence or in intensity;

5. In some instances lithium has been temporarily discontinued, with the result that the skin lesions disappeared and did not return even when lithium was reinstated (Kusumi, 1971).

In our hospital, two patients were recorded as exhibiting cutaneous reactions to lithium. In one case a generalised maculopapular lesion occurred within hours of the patient's having taken lithium for the first time: it disappeared completely once lithium was discontinued and reappeared when the drug was recommenced. In the second, alopecia areata appeared after 6 months of lithium therapy and progressed to become total (Vacaflor, unpublished observations).

G. Blood

There have been fairly frequent reports of leukocytosis occurring during lithium therapy (Mayfield and Brown, 1966; Freyhan *et al.*, 1970; O'Connell, 1970; Kusumi, 1971; Murphy *et al.*, 1971; Shopsin *et al.*, 1971) and other changes in the blood.

1. *Leukocytosis*

The leukocytosis observed in individuals taking lithium has the following general characteristics:

1. It is relatively common and may, indeed, occur to some degree in the majority of patients on lithium therapy;

2. The actual leukocyte count is usually in the neighbourhood of 10,000 to 14,000/mm³, though it is not surprising to find occasional readings of over 20,000/mm³ (O'Connell, 1970);

3. The increase of white blood cells is mainly neutrophilic in nature, although lymphocytopaenia has been noted to occur to a lesser degree (Mayfield and Brown, 1966; O'Connell, 1970; Shopsin *et al.*, 1971);

4. It is not related to either the dose level of lithium, or the serum lithium concentration (Shopsin *et al.*, 1971);

5. It is reversible and does not, therefore, appear to be caused by permanent changes in the mechanisms of production or destruction of the white cells (Shopsin *et al.*, 1971).

2. *Other blood effects*

A recent report (Hussain *et al.*, 1973) has implicated lithium therapy in the aetiology of a case of aplastic anaemia, but the report concerned a single case and a complicated history of other medications was involved so that the connection of the condition with lithium treatment may not be fully justified. The case is also marked as atypical in that neutrophil counts decreased.

Evidence that lithium may affect red cell aggregation states in *in vitro* studies (Gold *et al.*, 1971) may be important in view of studies on the relationship between erythrocyte aggregation and states of stress (Ecanow *et al.*, 1967) and between red cell settling characteristics and psychotic conditions (Stevens, 1971), but this has yet to be established.

Plasma volumes have been reported to decrease following intravenous loads of lithium chloride in dogs (Butcher, 1969) but no comparable reports are available in the case of humans.

III. Factors Modifying the Nature and Severity of Side Effects

A. Age of the patient

There have been reports of occasional discrepancies between serum lithium levels and the general response of the individual as shown by side effects or signs of toxicity. These discrepancies have usually been noted in elderly patients who, with comparatively low serum lithium readings, developed severe side effects and toxic reactions (Edgell *et al.*, 1970; Van der Velde, 1971). In the three cases reported by Van der Velde, these elderly patients were estuporous, delirious or comatose with serum lithium levels between $1·6$ and $2·2$ mEq/l.

It has been observed in the Montreal General Hospital (Vacaflor, unpublished observations), and it has also been reported in the literature by others (Horowitz and Fisher, 1969), that the less frequent converse phenomenon may also occur, namely the occurrence of very high serum lithium levels without associated signs of toxicity. We have records of three cases, all women aged between 68 and 75, with lithium levels between $2·2$ and $2·9$ mEq/l (assessed in the morning before the first lithium treatment of the day) in whom the only evidence of toxicity was a mild ataxia in one patient.

B. Sodium intake

It is by now well documented that signs of lithium toxicity may sometimes be treated by the administration of sodium chloride to patients (see Chapter 14) and it is also true that a reduced sodium chloride intake may predispose a patient to lithium side effects and toxic reactions. The lowering of the body's salt content could come about by several means, such as the use of diuretics, low salt diets, or even weight-reducing dietary regimes (Furlong, 1973). Whether or not it is advisable to ask patients to add routinely an extra amount of salt to their ordinary food is still, however, a matter of debate.

IV. Summary and Concluding Remarks

An attempt has been made to present a description of the kinds and variety of side effects which accompany lithium therapy, and these have been categorised, as far as possible, into mild, moderate and severe. It is clear that much information still needs to be gathered in order to develop a satisfactory overall clinical picture and the routine use of symptom checklists, such as that provided by Gershon and Shopsin (1973) might be a step towards providing these much needed data.

The study of side effects may well turn out to be important over and above the demands of everyday patient management: the construction of a complete clincial picture which clarifies the frequency and likelihood of each particular symptom occurring and which also indicates the relative severities of the symptoms, would be invaluable in disentangling the many threads of evidence which relate to lithium's site of action.

It has also to be remembered that with our present incomplete understanding of brain functioning, the use of any psychoactive drug treatment which carries even a slight risk of permanent brain damage must be undertaken with considerable caution.

References

Andreani, G. (1957). *J. clin. Med.* **38**, 1759–1775.
Baldessarini, R. J. and Stephens, J. H. (1970). *Archs gen. Psychiat.* **22**, 72–77.
Butcher, H. R. (1969). *J. surg. Res.* **9**, 1–9.
Cade, J. F. J. (1949). *Med. J. Aust.* **36**, 349–352.
Callaway, C. L., Hendrie, H. C. and Luby, E. D. (1968). *Amer. J. Psychiat.* **124**, 1124–1125.
Carter, T. N. (1972). *Psychosomatics* **13**, 325–327.
Cleaveland, S. A. (1913). *J. Amer. med. Assoc.* **60**, 722.
Coates, D. A., Trautner, E. M. and Gershon, S. (1957). *Australas Ann. Med.* **6**, 11–15.
Cooper, T. B. and Simpson, G. M. (1969). *Curr. ther. Res.* **11**, 603–608.
Corcoran, A. C., Taylor, R. D. and Page, I. H. (1949). *J. Amer. med. Assoc.* **139**, 685–688.
Demers, R. G. and Heniger, G. (1970). *Dis. nerv. Syst.* **31**, 667–673.
Demers, R. G. and Heninger, G. (1971). *J. Amer. med. Assoc.* **218**, 381–386.
Demers, R. G., Lukesh, R. and Prichard, J. (1970). *Lancet* **2**, 315–316.
Dias, N. and Hocken, A. G. (1972). *Nephron* **10**, 246–249.
Duc, N. and Maurel, H. (1953). *Concourt Méd.* **75**, 1817–1820.
Ecanow, B. Gold, B. Touquan, S. and Stanaszek, W. (1967). *Dis. nerv. Syst.* **28**, 249–251.
Edgell, P. G., Peterfly, G. and Pinter, E. J. (1970). *Lancet* **1**, 415–416.
Freyham, F. A., O'Connell, R. A. and Mayo, J. A. (1970). *Int. Pharmacopsychiat.* **5**, 137–148.
Furlong, F. W. (1973). *Can. psychiat Assoc. J.* **18**, 75–76.
Fyrö, B., Pettersson, U. and Sedvall, G. (1970). *Pharmacologia Clin.* **2**, 236–240.
Gershon, S. and Shopsin, B. (1973). *In* "Lithium: Its Role in Psychiatric Research and Treatment", (S. Gershon and B. Shopsin, eds.) pp. 107–146. Plenum, New York.

Glesinger, B. (1954). *Med. J. Aust.* **41**, 277–283.

Gold, B., Ecanow, B., Balagot, R. and Levinson, R. (1971). *Dis. nerv. Syst.* **32**, 415–417.

Greenfield, I., Zuger, M., Bleak, R. M. and Bakal, S. F. (1950). *N.Y. State. J. Med.* **50**, 459–560.

Halmi, K. A. and Noyes, R. (1972). *Biol. Psychiat.* **5**, 211–215.

Hanlon, L. W., Romaine, M. Gilroy, F. J. and Dieitrick, J. E. (1949). *J. Amer. med. Assoc.* **139**, 688–692.

Horowitz, L. G. and Fisher, G. U. (1969). *New Eng. J. Med.* **281**, 1369.

Hussain. M. Z., Khan, A. G. and Chaudhry, Z. A. (1973). *Can. med. Assoc. J.* **108**, 724–728.

Kirk, L., Baastrup, P. C. and Schou, M. (1972). *Lancet* **1**, 839.

Kusumi, Y. (1971). *Dis. nerv. Syst.* **32**,853–854.

Larson, C., Kochar, M. S. and Wang, R. I. (1972). *J. clin. Pharmacol.* **12**, 459–464.

Lavender, S., Brown, J. N. and Berrill, W. T. (1973). *Postgrad. med. J.* **49**, 277–279.

Levy, S. T., Forrest, J. N. and Heninger, G. R. (1973). *Amer. J. Psychiat.* **130**, 1014–1018.

Maggs, R. (1963). *Brit. J. Psychiat.* **109**, 56–65.

Mayfield, D. and Brown, R. G. (1966). *J. psychiat Res.* **4**, 207–219.

McKusick, V. A. (1954). *J. clin Invest.* **33**, 598–610.

Mihovilovic, M. (1970). *Int. Pharmacopsychiat.* **5**, 218–220.

Murphy, D. L., Goodwin, F. K. and Bunney, W. E. (1971). *Amer. J. Psychiat.* **127**, 1559–1561.

Nahunek, J. Svestka, J., and Rodova, A. (1971). *Activ. nerv. super.* **13**, 169–170.

Noack, C. H. and Trautner, E. M. (1951). *Med. J. Aust.* **38**, 219–222.

O'Connell, R. A. (1970). *Int. Pharmacopsychiat.* **4**, 30–34.

Pfeiffer, C. G., Singh, M. and Goldstien, L. (1969). *J. clin. Pharmacol.* **9**, 298–307.

Pfeiffer, C. G., Singh, M. and Goldstein, L. (1970). *J. clin. Pharmacol.* **10**, 95-102.

Persson, G. (1971). *Acta. psychiat. scand. Suppl.* **221**, 33–38.

Peters, H. A. (1949). *Wisconsin med. J.* **48**, 1075–1076.

Prien, R. F., Caffey, E. M. and Klett, C. J. (1972). *Brit. J. Psychiat.* **120**, 409–414.

Radomski, J. L., Fuyat, H. N., Nelson, A. A. and Smith, P. K. (1950). *J. Pharmacol. exp. Ther.* **100**, 429–444.

Ramsey, T. A., Mendels, J., Stokes, J. and Fitzgerald, R. (1972). *J. Amer. med. Assoc.* **219**, 1446–1449.

Rice, D. (1956). *J. ment. Sci.* **102**, 604–611.

Roberts, E. L. (1950). *Med. J. Aust.* **37**, 261–262.

Rogers, M. P. and Whybrow, P. C. (1971). *Amer. J. Psychiat.* **128**, 158–163.

Ruiz-Maldonaldo, R., de Francisco, C. P. and Tamayo, L. (1973). *J. Amer. med. Assoc.* **224**, 1534.

Schou, M. (1957). *Pharmacol Rev.* **9**, 17–58.

Schou, M. (1959). *Psychopharmacologia* **1**, 65–78.

Schou, M. (1963). *Acta. psychiat. scand. Suppl.* **169**, 258–259.

Schou, M., Juel-Nielsen, N., Strömgren, E. and Voldby, H. (1954). *J. Neurol. Neurosurg. Psychiat.* **17**, 250–260.

Schou, M., Amdisen, A. and Trap-Jensen, J. (1968). *Amer. J. Psychiat.* **125**, 520–527.

Schou, M. Baastrup, P. C., Grof, P., Weis, P. and Angst, J. (1970). *Brit. J. Psychiat.* **116**, 615–619.

Sedvall, G., Jönsson, B., Petterson, U. and Levin, K. (1968). *Life Sci.* **7**, 1257–1264.

Segal, R. L., Rosenblatt, S. and Eliasoph, I. (1973). *New Engl. J. Med.* **289**, 136–138.
Shopsin, B., Johnson, G. and Gershon, S. (1970). *Int. Pharmacopsychiat.* **5**, 170–182.
Shopsin, B., Friedmann, R. and Gerson, S. (1971). *Clin. Pharmacol. Therapeut.* **12**, 923–928.
Shopsin, B., Stern, S. and Gershon, S. (1972). *Archs gen. psychiat.* **26**, 566–571.
Sikes, J. C. and Sikes, Z. S. (1970) *Dis. nerv. Syst.* **31**, 52–55.
Sivadon, P. and Chanoit, P. (1955). *Ann méd Psychol.* **113**, 790–796.
Stern, R. L. (1949) *J. Amer. Med. Assoc.* **139**, 710–711.
Stevens, J. D. (1971). *Dis. nerv. Syst.* **32**, 554–558.
Straker, M. (1970). *Can. psychiat. Assoc. J.* **15**, 21–27.
Strömgren, E. and Schou, M. (1964). *Postgrad. Med.* **35**, 83–86.
Švestka, J., Nahunek, K. and Radova, A. (1970). *Activ. nerv. super.* **12**, 264–265.
Talbott, J. H. (1950). *Arch. int. Med.* **85**, 1–10.
Tangedahl, T. N. and Gau, G. T. (1972). *New Engl. J. Med.* **287**, 867–869.
Teulié, M., Follin, W. and Bégoin, M. (1955). *Encéphale.* **44**, 266–285.
Vacaflor, L., Lehmann, H. E. and Ban, T. A. (1970). *J. clin. Pharmacol.* **10**, 387–389.
Van der Velde, C. D. (1971) *Amer. J. Psychiat.* **127**, 1075–1077.
Verbov, J. L., Phillips, J. D. and Fife, D. G. (1965). *Postgrad. med. J.* **41**, 190–192.
Vinarova, E., Uhlir, O., Stika, L. and Vinar, O. (1972). *Activ. nerv. super.* **14**, 105–107.
Von Hartizsch, B., Hoenich, N. A., Leigh, R. J., Wilkinson, R., Frost T. H., Wedel, A. and Posen, G. A. (1972). *Brit. med. J.* **4**, 757–759.
Waldron, A. M. (1949). *J. Amer. med. Assoc.* **139**, 733.
Wharton, R. N. and Fieve, R. R. (1966). *Amer. J. Psychiat.* **123**, 706–712.

14

THE TREATMENT OF LITHIUM POISONING

K. Thomsen and M. Schou

I. Introduction

Since the introduction of lithium into medicine, the toxic potential of this drug has been a problem to be faced. Lithium poisoning is dangerous. Deaths have occurred, and there have been cases of permanent neurological aftereffects.

Patients with lithium intoxication have been subjected to a number of treatments, but reliable conclusions about their relative merits cannot be drawn from the literature. In each case, the course and outcome of the intoxication have been influenced by many factors other than the treatment: the severity of the poisoning, the patient's age and general state, the degree of interference with kidney function and with fluid and electrolyte balance, the presence or absence of infection, and, perhaps most important, the time elapsed before treatment was instituted. To be of informative value, comparisons of different treatment procedures would have to be carried out with large numbers of patients, and since lithium intoxications are rare, systematic studies of this kind are not available and are unlikely to become available.

This being so, any proposal concerning treatment of a patient with lithium intoxication must be of a hypothetical nature and to a large extent based on experience gained from experiments with animals and with healthy human subjects. We ask the readers to keep that in mind during their perusal of this chapter.

In a number of respects severe lithium intoxication resembles poisoning with narcotic drugs, and treatment must therefore aim at preventing and counteracting the complications attendant on such conditions. Detoxication is also important. There is no specific antidote against the toxic effects of lithium, and since lithium is not metabolised in the organism, it is primarily its elimination from the body that must be considered. Since lithium is eliminated almost exclusively through the kidneys, we have examined various procedures which might serve to raise the renal lithium clearance when it is normal and when it is lowered. Sometimes lithium cannot be eliminated quickly enough through renal excretion alone; we have therefore studied the effects of peritoneal dialysis and hemodialysis. On the basis of these considerations we present, tentatively, a proposal for how a patient with lithium intoxication might be treated.

II. The Clinical Picture of Impending and of Fully Developed Lithium Intoxication

It is important that a lithium intoxication is diagnosed as early as possible. The intoxication often develops gradually, and the early signs are so undramatic that they may be overlooked or disregarded by patients and physicians. The signs of impending intoxication are: vomiting and diarrhoea, coarse tremor, sluggishness, sleepiness, vertigo, and dysarthria with slurred and indistinct speech. Patients should be instructed that if any of these signs appear, the physician should be contacted immediately for clinical control and determination of the serum lithium concentration.

A patient with fully developed lithium intoxication may be comatose, but often there is only clouding of consciousness, and several instances are known where this led to underestimation of the seriousness of the condition. The intoxication is further characterised by coarse tremor and muscle twitchings, muscular hypertonia with increased and sometimes asymmetrical deep reflexes, epileptiform seizures, attacks of hyperextension of arms and legs, EEG changes, and a greyish hue of the skin (Schou et al., 1968). The intoxication may lead to disturbance of fluid and electrolyte balance, fall in blood pressure, and sometimes shock.

III. General Corrective and Supportive Measures

Death from lithium poisoning may be due to protracted coma, cerebral anoxia, or shock. Lithium poisoning should therefore be given the same corrective and supportive treatment as poisoning with narcotic drugs. This includes frequent determination and careful correction of blood pressure, regular X-ray control of the lungs, preservation of free respiration, frequent change of the patient's position in the bed, physiotherapy of the lungs, and infection prophylaxis. For more detailed information, readers are referred to standard textbooks and treatment manuals.

During lithium intoxication it is particularly important that fluid and electrolyte imbalances are corrected. The patients have often suffered from lithium-induced polyuria, and in the drowsy precomatose state of impending intoxication they may have failed to drink enough. It is also known, from studies on animals, that administration of toxic lithium doses leads to a progressive negative sodium balance; administration of sodium produces a clear-cut improvement in the general state of the animals (Radomski *et al.*, 1950; Thomsen, 1973).

IV. Removal of Lithium from the Organism

Lithium intoxication usually develops when the serum lithium concentration has risen to values above 2 mmol/l; levels as high as 9–10 mmol/l have been seen. Levels lower than 2 mmol/l may also be observed in patients with lithium intoxication if the blood sample is drawn some days after the last intake of lithium. Animal experiments (Thomsen, 1973) as well as clinical experience with lithium-intoxicated patients indicate that the severity of a lithium intoxication is related to the magnitude of the serum lithium concentration; the higher the serum concentration, the more dangerous the intoxication. The evidence further indicates that the severity is related to the length of the period during which the organism is exposed to elevated lithium concentrations (Schou, 1958a); the longer this period, the more dangerous the intoxication. Treatment of lithium intoxication must therefore aim at a rapid removal of lithium from the organism so that patients are exposed to high lithium concentrations only for a short time. This may be accomplished through hemodialysis or peritoneal dialysis, but under certain circumstances a sufficiently rapid removal of lithium can be obtained merely by accelerating the elimination of lithium through the patient's own kidneys. This latter possibility will be examined first.

A. Discontinuation of lithium

Lithium administration should be discontinued as soon as lithium poisoning is suspected. Since the poisoning develops gradually in most cases, severe intoxication can often be avoided if the lithium administration is discontinued at an early stage.

B. Removal through the kidneys

Under most circumstances the renal lithium clearance is about one fifth of the glomerular filtration rate, 15–30 ml/min (Thomsen and Schou, 1968). In patients with lithium intoxication the clearance is often lowered (Schou *et al.*, 1968; Dias and Hocken, 1972; Favarel-Garrigues *et al.*, 1972; Koufen and Consbruch, 1972; Lavender *et al.*, 1973). Clearance of 5 ml/min and less have been observed (Haghfelt *et al.*, 1971). In these cases treatment must aim at normalising the lithium clearance.

1. *Increasing a subnormal lithium clearance*

Procedures for normalising a lithium clearance which is lowered as a result of intoxication are ideally based on knowledge about the underlying mechanism. This is unfortunately not known, but useful information may be obtained from studies on animals, on healthy human subjects, and on patients with kidney disease. These studies show that the lithium clearance can be lowered under a variety of circumstances and that the reversibility of the lowering depends on the circumstances.

(i) In rats, prolonged administration of toxic lithium doses leads to a lowering of the lithium clearance (Thomsen, 1973). The glomerular filtration rate may also fall, but the lithium clearance falls proportionately more. The lowering of the lithium clearance may be prevented by administration of sodium chloride, and sodium chloride may also normalise the clearance if it has already fallen. There is a quantitative relation between the serum lithium concentration of the rats and the quantity of sodium chloride required to prevent the fall of the clearance or to normalise it; the higher the lithium concentration, the more sodium chloride is required.

(ii) A low sodium intake leads to a lowering of the lithium clearance (Schou, 1958b; Thomsen and Schou, 1968). Under these circumstances the lithium clearance is lowered selectively; the glomerular filtration rate remains virtually unaltered. The lowering of the lithium clearance is reversible; administration of sodium chloride leads to normalisation. This may be accomplished with moderate doses of sodium chloride. Thomsen and Schou (1968) studied a healthy human subject who, after having been on a low sodium diet for some time, had a lithium clearance of 5 ml/min. After administration of 100 mmol of sodium chloride, it rose to the normal level of 25 ml/min.

(iii) Long-term administration of thiazides produces a fall of the lithium clearance, possibly through production of a negative sodium balance (Thomsen and Schou, 1973; Petersen *et al.*, 1974). The lowering is reversible; discontinuation of the diuretic leads to normalisation of the clearance.

The three instances described above are characterised by a negative sodium balance, and in all three instances the lowering of the lithium clearance is reversible. The mechanism underlying this phenomenon is probably the following: when the sodium balance is negative, the organism tries to conserve sodium by increasing its reabsorption in the kidney tubules. Lithium is handled like sodium in the proximal tubules (Thomsen and Schou, 1968; Thomsen et al., 1969), and its reabsorption is therefore also increased. This results in a lowering of the clearance. Administration of sodium chloride reverses the process.

(iv) When the glomerular filtration rate is lowered in patients with glomerulonephritis or pyelonephritis, the lithium clearance is lowered proportionately (Thomsen et al., 1969). Under these circumstances administration of even large doses of sodium chloride leads to only a slight rise of the lithium clearance. Only if the glomerular filtration rate becomes normal is there a normalisation of the lithium clearance.

The conclusion to be drawn from these studies is that administration of sodium chloride may lead to normalisation of a lowered lithium clearance when the lowering is due to a negative sodium balance; the procedure is of no value when the lowering is due to kidney disease.

2. Increasing a normal lithium clearance

Attempts have been made to raise a normal lithium clearance to higher values by administration of sodium chloride. The results were disappointing. When the healthy subject studied by Thomsen and Schou (1968) was on a normal diet, his daily sodium intake was about 200 mmol and his lithium clearance 25 ml/min. Administration of additional sodium chloride in massive doses, 500 mmol daily, led to an increase of the lithium clearance to 35 ml/min, a rise of only 40%. In other words, whereas moderate doses of sodium chloride produced a marked rise of the lithium clearance when it was subnormal, the administration of even very large doses of sodium chloride resulted in only a moderate rise of the clearance when it was normal. In the treatment of lithium poisoning, the administration of sodium chloride may be useful for normalising a reversibly lowered lithium clearance; the procedure is of limited value for increasing an already normal clearance.

Thomsen and Schou (1968) also studied whether the administration of diuretic drugs and other procedures might produce an increase in the lithium clearance in healthy human subjects. Water-loading sufficient to produce a tenfold increase of the urine flow did not affect the clearance, nor was the clearance influenced by administration of potassium in doses leading to a threefold increase in the urinary potassium excretion. The lithium clearance was further unaffected by the administration of single large doses of bendroflumethiazide, furosemide, ethacrynic acid, and chlormerodrin, even though administration of these diuretics led to a considerable rise in water and sodium excretion. These procedures, therefore, cannot be recommended for the treatment of lithium poisoning. They may even be contraindicated as prolonged

I

administration of thiazides has been shown to lower the lithium clearance (Thomsen and Schou, 1973; Petersen et al., 1974).

Some diuretics did produce an increase of the lithium clearance (Thomsen and Schou, 1968). After administration of aminophylline, urea, acetazolamide, or sodium bicarbonate, it rose 30–60%. These observations may be accounted for by the hypothesis already referred to, namely that lithium is reabsorbed with sodium in the proximal tubules and reabsorbed only to a small degree or not at all in the distal parts of the nephron (Thomsen and Schou, 1968; Thomsen et al., 1969). Diuretics acting primarily on the proximal tubules increase the lithium clearance; those acting primarily on the distal tubules do not.

On the basis of our observations we proposed using forced diuresis and alkalinisation of the urine for treatment of lithium intoxication (Thomsen and Schou, 1968). The proposal led to therapeutic trials with aminophylline, mannitol, acetazolamide, and sodium lactate (Haghfelt et al., 1971; Shrader, 1972), but whether used singly or in combination, these procedures did not succeed in raising the renal lithium clearance by more than about 50%. We now withdraw this proposal because administration of sodium chloride seems more rational in patients with a reversible lowering of the lithium clearance and dialysis preferable in all other patients needing active treatment.

C. Removal by dialysis

When used correctly, hemodialysis and peritoneal dialysis lead to an effective and speedy removal of lithium from the body. The effect of dialysis is independent of the kidney function, and dialysis supplements the renal elimination of lithium. Dialysis furthermore serves to correct fluid and electrolyte imbalance. The use of dialysis involves a certain, although small, risk for the patients.

1. Peritoneal dialysis

The efficacy of peritoneal dialysis can be estimated by calculating the dialysis clearance, which may amount to 15 ml/min (Wilson et al., 1971; Hartitzsch et al., 1972; Lavender et al., 1973). This is added to the renal clearance.

2. Hemodialysis

During this procedure clearances of about 50 ml/min can be obtained (Amdisen and Skjoldborg, 1969; Hawkins and Dorken, 1969; Hartitzsch et al., 1972; Amdisen et al., 1973). Hemodialysis may be administered for periods of 8–12 hours, depending on the patient's condition; during this period the serum lithium concentration falls rapidly. When the dialysis is discontinued, serum lithium rises as lithium passes from the tissues into the blood. The hemodialysis may then be repreated, but due to the rebound phenomenon the net dialysis clearance will be of the same order as that achieved with peritoneal dialysis. This is added to the renal clearance.

IV. Treatment of Lithium Poisoning: Practical Procedure

The treatments discussed here, administration of sodium chloride and dialysis, may serve to accelerate the elimination of lithium from the organism. We want to emphasize that there is no clinical evidence, i.e. evidence based on comparative trials in patients with lithium intoxication, to show whether these treatments do more good than harm to the patients. However, both clinical and experimental experience indicates that the severity of lithium poisoning increases with the magnitude of the serum lithium concentration and with the length of time the organism is exposed to the elevated lithium level. It is, therefore, reasonable to suppose that the patients' chances of recovery may be improved by employing procedures that accelerate the elimination of lithium.

TABLE I. Proposed Schedule for Treatment of a Patient With Lithium Poisoning.

A patient with lithium poisoning should preferably be treated in a unit for intensive therapy. On admission of a patient with verified or suspected lithium poisoning:

(1) Determine serum lithium.

(2) Institute supportive and corrective measures as in narcotic poisoning.

(3) Start saline infusion, 1–2 litres within the first 6 hours.

Further course of treatment:

(4) If serum lithium is higher than 4 mmol/litre, institute dialysis (hemodialysis or peritoneal dialysis) as soon as possible.

(5) If serum lithium is between 2 and 4 mmol/litre and the patient's clinical condition is poor, institute dialysis as soon as possible.

(6) In all other patients, follow the serum lithium concentration in order to check that lithium is being eliminated rapidly enough from the organism. Determine serum lithium every 3 hours and plot the results on semilogarithmic paper. At 6 hours, draw the line which connects the 3-hour and the 6-hour values and prolong it until it intersects the horizontal line corresponding to serum lithium 0·6 mmol/litre (Fig. 1). Do the same for each successive 3-hour period, using each time the two latest serum lithium values.

(a) If intersection with 0·6 mmol/litre occurs earlier than 36 hours (Fig. 1A), continue treatment with supportive and corrective measures until serum lithium is below 0·6 mmol/litre and the patient's condition is good. Treatment should take place under control of central venous pressure, serum electrolytes, fluid input and output, and urinary excretion of sodium.

(b) If intersection occurs later than 36 hours (Fig. 1B), or if it at any time becomes later than 36 hours (Fig. 1C), institute dialysis.

In the schedule for treatment of lithium poisoning which we here propose, we have tried to weigh the gain of these procedures against the risk involved in their use. Our proposed treatment schedule is shown in Table I.

The schedule is based on the following reasoning.

Some patients with lithium intoxication may have a reversibly lowered

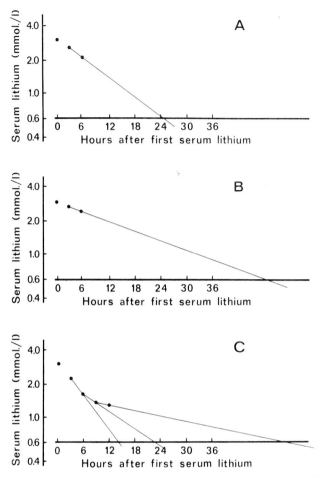

FIG. 1. Diagram illustrating the procedure described in Table I, (6).

lithium clearance. In these patients, the clearance can be normalised by admin-istration of sodium chloride, and since they cannot be recognized in advance, we suggest giving sodium chloride initially to all patients with lithium intoxication. Our suggestion is to give it in a dosage, 150–300 mmol within the first 6 hours, that is sufficiently large to normalise a lowered lithium clearance but not so large that is exposes the patient to the risk of brain and lung edema.

Normalisation of the lithium clearance may sometimes be enough to secure a sufficiently rapid removal of lithium from the organism. Determination of whether this is the case or whether dialysis should be instituted depends on the serum lithium concentration, the patient's general condition, and the rate with which lithium is eliminated through the kidneys. If the serum lithium concentration is high, or if the serum concentration is moderately high and the patient's condition poor, or if the renal elimination of lithium is slow, then the advantages of hemodialysis or peritoneal dialysis are likely to outweigh their risks, and we suggest taking them into use. It should be noted in particular that according to our proposal a high serum lithium concentration is indication for immediate institution of dialysis even if, as is sometimes the case in the beginning with patients having taken a large single overdose of lithium, the clinical condition is relatively unaffected.

The intoxicated patients should under all circumstances be subjected to the general corrective and supportive measures used in the treatment of narcotic poisoning.

VI. Summary

Lithium intoxication is a dangerous condition, which should be treated with the same corrective and supportive measures as narcotic poisoning. One may further consider accelerating the elimination of lithium from the organism. Even though there is no direct clinical proof that this is of benefit to the patients, it seems reasonable to suppose so, and we propose a treatment schedule, which involves administration of sodium chloride and the use of peritoneal dialysis or hemodialysis.

Acknowledgements

We are indebted to Mrs. Audrey Miller and to Drs. A. Amdisen, N. Fjeldborg, H. E. Hansen, O. V. Olesen and D. F. Smith for critical comments on our manuscript.

References

Amdisen, A. and Skjoldborg, H. (1969). *Lancet* **2,** 213.

Amdisen, A., Gottfries, C. G., Jacobsson, L. and Winblad, B. (1973). *Nord. psykiat. T.* **27,** 539–549.

Dias, N. and Hocken, A. G. (1972). *Nephron* **10,** 246–249.

Favarel-Garrigues, B., Favarel-Garrigues, J.–C. and Bourgeois, M. (1972) *Annls méd.-psychol.* **130,** 253–257.

Haghfelt, T., Lund, J. O., Jørgensen, H. E. and Baastrup, P. C. (1971). *Nord. Med.* **86,** 1465–1471.

Hartitzsch, B. von, Hoenich, N. A., Leigh, R. J., Wilkinson, R., Frost, T. H., Weddel, A. and Posen, G. A. (1972). *Brit. med. J.* **4,** 757–759.

Hawkins, J. B. and Dorken, P. R. (1969). *Lancet* **1,** 839–840.

Koufen, H. and Consbruch, U. (1972). *Nervenarzt* **43,** 145–152.

Lavender, S., Brown, J. N. and Berrill, W. T. (1973). *Postgrad. med. J.* **49,** 277–279.

Petersen, V., Hvidt, S., Thomsen, K. and Schou, M. (1974). *Brit. med. J.* **3,** 143–145.

Radomski, J. L., Fuyat, H. N., Nelson, A. A. and Smith, P. K. (1950). *J. Pharmacol. exp. Ther.* **100,** 429–444.

Schou. M. (1958a). *Acta pharmacol. (Kbh.)* **15**, 70–84.

Schou, M. (1958b). *Acta pharmacol. (Kbh.)* **15**, 85–98.

Schou, M., Amdisen, A. and Trap-Jensen, J. (1968). *Amer. J. Psychiat.* **125**, 520–527.

Shrader, D. A. (1972). *J. Kansas. med. Soc.* **73**, 24–30.

Thomsen, K. and Schou, M. (1968). *Amer. J. Physiol.* **215**, 823–827.

Thomsen, K., Schou, M., Steiness, I. and Hansen, H. E. (1969). *Pflügers Arch. Europ. J. Physiol.* **308**, 180–184.

Thomsen, K. (1973). *Acta pharmacol. (Kbh.)* **33**, 92–102.

Thomsen, K. and Schou, M. (1973). *Pharmakopsychiat.* **6**, 264–269.

Wilson, J. H. P., Donker, A. J. M., Hem, G. K. van der and Wientjes, J. (1971). *Brit. med. J.* **2**, 749–750.

15

ADMINISTRATION OF LITHIUM DURING PREGNANCY

M. R. WEINSTEIN and M. D. GOLDFIELD

I. Introduction

A. Scope of the problem

Over the last twenty years substantial evidence has accumulated that lithium is of great value in the prophylaxis of manic episodes and in the prevention of recurrent depressions, and lithium is now the treatment of choice for the acute manic phase of manic-depressive illness. Now that an effective drug is available to treat manic-depressive illness, physicians and others, alerted to recognize these syndromes, diagnose manic-depressive illnesses more often, and schizophrenia perhaps a little less (Taylor and Abrams, 1973). Also, there is a small tendency for women to develop manic-depressive illness more often than men (Spiegel and Bell, 1959), and the age of maximum risk for this illness coincides with the fertile years in women. Taken together, these facts mean that pregnant women will be exposed to lithium, and that the possible teratogenicity and toxicity of lithium in pregnancy will be important for many patients, their families and their physicians. The effectiveness of lithium in reducing the family disruptions produced by untreated manic-depressive illness helps stabilize marriages that earlier might have dissolved. Thus, lithium may contribute to an increased birth rate in families where the mother or father is receiving the drug (Demers and Davis, 1971).

B. Principles of evaluation of lithium studies

In the critical evaluation of studies of lithium toxicity or teratogenicity the following variables need to be considered.

1. *Dose*

Studies of lithium toxicity and teratogenicity which expose the test organisms to extremely high or very low concentrations of the ion may be impossible to evaluate. High enough doses of lithium will be fatal to both mother and embryo; traces of the element occur in the tissues and fluids of most plants and animals, including man (Schou, 1957), and can be ingested indefinitely without apparent effect (Dawson *et al.,* 1970). To be meaningful, studies of teratogenesis must remain within the "teratogenic zone", defined as the dose range which produces tissue levels of a substance sufficient to interfere with embryonic development without *destroying* the embryo (Wilson, 1965). Some of the animal studies analyzed in this chapter used lithium doses so much in excess of the human therapeutic range that we cannot measure or estimate the lower limit of the teratogenic zone in that test animal and extrapolate it to man.

2. *Route of administration*

Routes of administration vary from the simple and direct addition of lithium to the fluid media of developing enbryos to complex systems in which lithium reaches the embryo via a chain including oral ingestion by the mother, intestinal absorption, maternal circulation, transplacental migration and the fetal circulation. Some routes of administration may expose the fetus to transitory "peaks" in the lithium concentrations, and others may produce direct physio-chemical injury to maternal and fetal tissues by high local concentrations of lithium as, for example, with the intraperitoneal (and perhaps perigonadal) injectic lithium in some animal studies.

3. Schedule of administration

In humans lithium is usually taken orally one to four times a day; peak serum levels occur one to four hours after each oral dose (Almy and Taylor, 1973). Lithium crosses the human placenta and achieves equilibrium between the fetal and maternal circulations (Weinstein and Goldfield, 1969; Schou, personal communication). The fetus is therefore exposed to the same concentrations of lithium as the mother, and its exposure waxes and wanes in synchrony with the mother's. It is a defect of some of the animal research to be discussed in this chapter that only the *total* daily dose of lithium is reported, with no apparent concern for the importance of the dose schedule. Administration of the full daily ration of lithium in a single bolus exposes the embryo to higher peak concentrations, and one would expect a greater incidence of teratogenicity from single daily doses than from a regimen using divided doses.

4. Timing of serum concentrations

Because of the rapid clearance of lithium from the serum (Almy and Taylor, 1973), serum levels may be misleading unless one knows the time which has elapsed between the last dose and the sampling of the serum whose concentration is reported.

5. Species used

Extrapolations of experimental results from one species to another is unwarranted and can lead to substantial errors. While evolutionary propinquity may increase the likelihood of concordance of physiological, immunological and other life processes, even species close to one another in regard to some life functions can show striking differences in others. Whether the function under scrutiny (susceptibility to lithium teratogenicity, in the present case) will or will not show a marked comparability in "like" species cannot, unfortunately, be assumed *a priori*, but must be established for each function and with each species pair. In the absence of such evidence, inter-species comparisons should be treated with skepticism; the further apart the species, the more the skepticism is warranted.

6. Genotype

Embryogenesis is controlled chiefly by genotype, and genotypic control of embryogenesis is established at the moment of fertilization. Genetic defects contributed by sperm or ovum can result in fetal malformations, and it is important to distinguish such *genotypic malformations,* in which the defect was present from the moment of conception, from *teratogenic malformations* which are produced by drugs or other noxious agents, after conception. Down's Syndrome, for example, occurring in the child of a lithium-treated woman (or man), should be noted as a genetic (genotypic) anomaly, but not catalogued as evidence of teratogenicity.

Genotype may also have a direct relationship to the frequency of *tetratogenic* malformations because differences among species in their *susceptibility* to a potentially teratogenic agent are genetypically determined (Frasier, 1961).

7. *Embryonic stage at time of exposure*

The stage of embryonic development at which exposure to any potentially teratogenic agent occurs determines which structures, if any, will be disturbed. The earliest stages, such as the *blastula* stage in mammals, are relatively resistant to teratogens (Wilson, 1965), and disturbance of such undifferentiated cells rarely impairs morphogenesis. After cell differentiation occurs and the germ layers form, teratogenic vulnerability increases. This differentiation occurs as early as five days post-conception in the mouse and hamster, nine in the rabbit and eleven in man. At this stage specific areas of the disc develop organ-forming destinies, and the susceptibility to teratongenic effects is at its greatest.

Most organs and systems have definable periods of maximum vulnerability to particular teratogens. However, the more intense the exposure to a teratogen (within limits), the more the period of specific tissue or system vulnerability is prolonged. With further differentiation and organogenesis, susceptibility to teratogenesis again declines. Although in man organogenesis is essentially complete by the 90th day of gestation, the human fetus remains vulnerable to damage from some drugs beyond that stage (Shirkey, 1968).

II. Studies in Pre-mammalian Species

A. Sea urchins

Studies of the effects of lithium on the development and morphogenesis of sub-mammalian forms were begun before 1900; in the interim a very large literature on the subject has accumulated which is outside the scope of this chapter. However, an excellent summary of this work can be found in Schou's (1957) monograph on the biology and pharmacology of lithium; in that monograph Schou refers to reviews of work on invertebrates by Needham (1942) and Lehmann (1945).

The effects of lithium on morphogenesis have been demonstrated and studied in many non-mammalian species; among the sub-mammalian forms whose development is affected by exposure to lithium are ciliates, sponges, planaria, annelids, mollusks, amphibia and teleosts (Runnström and Immers, 1970; DeVincentis and Runnström, 1967; Duvauchelle, 1966; Flickinger *et al.*, 1967; Greenhouse and Hamburgh, 1968; Schou, 1957). Sea urchins have been studied longer and more extensively than any other pre-mammalian organisms since the discovery, almost 80 years ago, of embryonic exogastrulation as a predictable consequence of exposure to lithium.[1] Since then, investigations of the effects of lithium ions on sea urchin eggs have led to the general view that lithium regularly produces an exaggeration of the development of entodermal tissues at the expense of ectoderm ("vegetalization")[2] in the embryo of this invertebrate (Runnström and Immers, 1970; DeVincentis and Runnström, 1967; Schou, 1957). The reversal of lithium's vegetalizing effect, an exaggeration of ectoderm in relation to entoderm, is termed the "animalizing" effect[3] and is produced by pyocyanin, thiocyanate, iodide and depletion of sulfate ions. Potassium may also act as an animalizing influence, countering the effects of lithium in developing sea urchin eggs.

These investigations are summarized in the "double gradient" hypothesis, which holds that the early development of the sea urchin is under the control of two antagonistic morphogenetic influences, vegetalizing and animalizing, localized in the respective vegetal and animal poles of the embryo. The balance between these forces (and the resulting morphogenetic outcome) can be modified by many chemical and physical agents, including lithium which is thought to exert its influence by regulating the development of embryonic mitochondria and RNA synthesis (Berg, 1968).

B. Amphibia

Studies of the effects of lithium on developing *amphibian* eggs have led to the generalization that lithium acts especially on notochord and ectoderm, producing anomalies of the central nervous system and related ectodermal structures such as the eyes (Greenhouse and Hamburgh, 1968; Schou, 1957). Flickinger *et al.* (1967) working with frog embryos, showed that lithium exerts part of its teratogenic effect by inhibiting DNA synthesis, reducing the number of cells in active division, and inducing a redistribution of RNA away from mitochondria and microsomes and towards the soluble phase, dispersed in the cytoplasm. Ficq (1951) demonstrated that lithium was concentrated in the "animal pole" area of developing *axolytl* embryos.

---

[1] *Exogastrulation* is that abnormal process in the development of the embryo in which "the entomesoderm, instead of moving inward beneath the ectoderm, moves in an opposite direction, away from the entoderm". Exogastrulation results in an abnormal gastrula in which entodermal tissue protrudes like a tongue from a single-layered gastrula. (Willier, B. N., *et al.* (1955), p. 235).

[2] *Vegetalization:* "Treatment (of sea urchin eggs) with lithium apparently shifted the boundary between ectodermal and entodermal development above the equator (i.e., prospective ectoderm was converted to entoderm) such that an excessively large gut developed". (Willier, B. N., *et al.* (1955), p. 329).

[3] In animalization "ectodermal differentiations (such as apical tuft cilia in sea urchin embryos) occupy a greater part of the body than normally". (Willier, B. N., *et al.* (1955), p. 330).

C. Birds

Ectodermal structures, and especially the head end of the growing neural tube, were selectively disorganized by lithium in the fluid media of chick embryos cultivated *in vitro* by Duvauchelle (1966). He observed that between 50 and 70% of observed chick blastodiscs developed abnormally, depending on the concentration of lithium used, and that the malformations produced in these chick embryos consisted of micro- or macrocephaly with hypomorphosis of the brain and sensory organs, while endodermal and mesodermal trunk structures were consistently spared. Nicolet (1965) reported that lithium chloride added to chick embryos in concentrations of 2·5 to 25·0 mmol/l chiefly disturbed the development of head and neural structures but had no apparent effects on the vegetal or animal poles.

D. Discussion

Invertebrate embryos (sea urchins, mollusks, etc.) exposed to lithium early in development characteristically show aberrant differentiation of the three primary tissue layers. In non-mammalian vertebrates early exposure to lithium chiefly disorganizes the precursors of the central nervous system, and some structures of the head and neck. While the teratogenic impact of lithium in non-mammalian organisms may tend to group themselves in this way, the bearing of this pattern of malformations on the human use of lithium is not clear. Weighing against a direct extrapolation of pre-mammalian studies to human lithium use are:

1. the great variability of lithium ion concentrations used in such studies, contrasted with the very narrow range of lithium concentrations in maternal and fetal tissues in human use;

2. the absence of information concerning the frequency of spontaneous embryonic abnormalities in many of the non-mammalian forms studied.

III. Mammalian Studies

The requirements for replicable, interpretable and applicable investigations of the effects of lithium in pregnancy, described in Section I.B. of this chapter, have seldom been achieved in studies using laboratory mammals as subjects. Variability of research standards and techniques limits comparability among animal studies, even when the same species are used and the same questions are asked. Because much of this variance seems to stem from differences in dose, route of administration, timing of samples and the species and strains used, we will examine these experiments in detail. Data from these studies are summarized in Table I.

A. Rodents

1. *Mice*

Of three investigations of the teratogenic effects of lithium salts in pregnant mice, one reported no fetal malformations, another reported a very high incidence of development defects and maternal mortality, and a third reported no teratogenic effects when the dose was below levels toxic to the mother.

(a) Bass *et al.*, (1951) used lithium chloride injected intraperitoneally, 2–4 mg per day, in white Albino Farms mice, and in addition they added lithium chloride to the diet in a concentration of 0·5–1·0%. Their animals were treated on days 2 and 3 of gestation in one experiment, on days 6 and 7 in another, and on days 12 and 13 in a third. We estimate that their procedure delivered between 3·6 and 47·6 mEq/kg/day to each animal. Although they observed a small decrease in the number of viable offspring in the groups treated on days 2 and 3 or 6 and 7, Bass *et al.*, reported no fetal malformations resulting from this exposure to lithium.

(b) Szabo (1969, 1970), and Szabo *et al.*, (1970) were the first investigators to report that cleft palate was a specific teratogenic consequence of lithium in mice. These workers gave lithium carbonate in 0·5% tragacanth gel in a single bolus by gavage to Charles River HaM/ICR mice on days 6 to 15 of gestation, in daily doses of 200, 300 and 465 mg/kg, terminating the pregnancies on day 18. At the highest dose, which is equivalent to 27 times the usual human dose (a "Lithium Index" of 27)[4], 30% of the fetuses developed cleft palate, 32% of the fetuses died, and 37% of the pregnant mice died. Only 6% of the fetuses whose mother got 300 mg/kg/day developed cleft palate, and there were no fetal malformations in the 200 mg/kg/day group. Although Szabo labels 465 mg/kg/day the "human equivalent dose" because it produced "a serum lithium level comparable with that of a human therapeutic dose" (Szabo, 1970), he obviously exceeded the upper limit of the tetratogenic zone, as defined in Section I.B.1 of this chapter. His work shows that when sufficient lithium is given to cause severe maternal toxicity and a high incidence of maternal death, fetal deaths and fetal malformations also occur. Szabo's failure to state and take sufficiently into account the interval between oral dose and serum sample might have allowed enormous "pulses" in the serum lithium concentrations to occur and subside *prior* to taking the serum sample, which then seemed to be in the "human range". This would also have encouraged him to consider 465 mg/kg/day a "human equivalent" dose on the basis of such misleading serum

---

[4] We have found it useful when comparing studies to utilize the "Lithium Index". The Lithium Index is the ratio of the total daily dose administered to animals, to the average total daily human oral dose (approximately 0·46 mEq/kg/day). We wish to emphasize, however, that the most important measures of lithium in humans are the *serum lithium concentrations*, as these directly reflect the concentration of lithium to which the maternal and fetal tissues are exposed at any given time. The oral dose may not be a true reflection of the serum lithium concentration.

TABLE I: Effects of lithium in pregnant laboratory animals

Author	Animal/Type	Lithium salt used; Days of administration	Route	Li salt; mg/kg/day	Lithium ion; mEq/kg/day	Plasma or serum concentration, mEq/l	Li index[c]	Defect
(Human)	(Human)	(Carbonate; daily)	(Oral, TID)	(17)	(0·46)	(0·5-1·2)	(1)	(See Tables II, III)
				MICE				
Bass et al. (1951)	Albino Farms white mice	Two daily i.p. doses, LiCl (a) days 2-3 (b) days 6-7 (c) days 12-13; 0·5-1·0% in diet daily	i.p. and diet	150-2000[a]	3·6-47·6[a]	Not given	8-104	No malformations. Decrease in number of viable offspring
Szabo (1969, 1970); Szabo et al. (1970)	HaM/ICR mice	Li$_2$CO$_3$ on days 6-15 of gestation; caesarean day 18	Oral/single dose	465	12·6	1·5[a]	27	Cleft palate 30%
				300	8·1	Not given	18	Cleft palate 6%
				200	5·4	Not given	12	0% cleft palate
Tuchmann–Duplessis and Mercier–Parot (1973)	Swiss albino mice (spontaneous anomaly rate, 1·5%)	LiCl, daily	i.p.	250	6·0[a]	Not given	13	250 mg/kg/day too toxic for pregnancy to continue; other doses produced no increase in anomalies or decrease in fertility
				150	3·6[a]	Not given	8	
				100	2·4[a]	Not given	5	

RATS

Reference	Strain	Dose	Route	(mg)			n	Result
Trautner et al. (1958)	Albino Wistar rats	20 mEq/l LiCl in drinking water; caesarean day 16–18	Drinking water, daily	68[a]	1·6	1·5–2·0	4	No malformations
Johansen and Ulrich (1969)	Wistar rats	Exp. 1: 0·93 mEq/kg/day Exp. 2: 1·78 mEq/kg/day Estimated as LiCl Fetus examined on day 20 of gestation	Diet	39–75[a]	0·93–1·78	0·15–0·5	2–4	No malformations. No abnormalities in size of litter, or weight of fetus, uterus, or placenta
Wright et al. (1970, 1971)	Sprague–Dawley rats	50 mg LiCl on days 1, 4, 7 or 9 of gestation; 20 mg thereafter to day 17 (caesarean)	i.p. single dose	213[a] (average loading dose)	5·1	"In the range observed in human beings;" (4.2 mEq/l "20 min. after initial injection.")	11	Eyes 63%; cleft palate 39%; external ear 45%
Johansen (1971)	Wistar rats	212 mg/kg LiCl on day 4, 7 or 9 of gestation followed by 2 mEq/kg/day to day 19	s.c.[b] / i.p.[b]	212 loading dose; 85 maintenance; in both s.c. and i.p.	5·0 (loading) 2·0 (maintenance)	9–10; (sample drawn 15 minutes post-administration)	11	Bony defects in legs of one fetus (s.c. only); 0·65% incidence. "This may have been spontaneous."

TABLE I—*continued*

Author	Animal/Type	Lithium salt used; Days of administration	Route	Li salt; mg/kg/day	Lithium ion; mEq/kg/day	Plasma or serum concentration, mEq/l	Li index[c]	Defect
		RATS						
Gralla and McIlhenny (1972)	Charles River albino rats	(a) Li_2CO_3 for 14 days before mating; half sacrificed on day 13 of gestation. other half after 21 days of nursing	oral, once daily, gavage	150[a]	4·05	1·4 after 3–5 hrs, 0·9–2·8 after 8 hrs	9	No malformations. Highest dose (4·05 mEq/kg/day) to nursing mothers resulted in less weight gain in pups
				75[a]	2·03	Not given	4	
				25[a]	0·68	Not given	1·5	
		(b) Li_2CO_3 from day 14–21 of gestation	oral, once daily, gavage	150[a]	4·05	See above	9	
				75[a]	2·03	Not given	4	
				25[a]	0·68	Not given	1·5	
		(c) Li_2CO_3 from day 5–15 of gestation, sacrificed day 20	oral, once daily, gavage	150[a]	4·05	See above	9	
				75[a]	2·03	Not given	4	
				25[a]	0·68	Not given	1·5	
Tuchmann-Duplessis and Mercier-Parot (1973)	Wistar rats (spontaneous anomaly rate, zero)	LiCl, daily	i.p.	250	6·0[a]	Not given	13	Occular anomalies in 15% maternal death in 44%
				150–200	3·6–4·8[a]	Not given	8–10	1·0–2·9% occular anomalies; no maternal deaths with lower doses
				100	2·4[a]	Not given	5	No malformations, no maternal deaths

RABBITS

Reference	Animal	Treatment	Route	Dose	Lithium Index	Serum range		Results
Gralla and McIlhenny (1972)	New Zealand albino rabbits	Li$_2$CO$_3$, days 5–18 of pregnancy	oral (capsules), single daily dose	40[a]	1·08	Range 1·5 to 2·4, 1 hour after dose	2	3/10 pregnant animals died; no malformations
				25[a]	0·68		1·5	1/10 pregnant animals died; no malformations

MONKEYS

Reference	Animal	Treatment	Route	Dose	Lithium Index	Serum range		Results
Gralla and McIlhenny (1972)	Rhesus monkeys	Li$_2$CO$_3$, days 14–35 of pregnancy	oral (capsules), single daily dose	25[a]	0·67	Overall range 0·2–1·4; range 0·3–0·4, 24 hrs after dose	1·5	No malformations

[a] Estimated

[b] Experiment #1, s.c. = subcutaneous; Experiment #2, i.p. = intraperitoneal

[c] "Lithium Index" = $\dfrac{\text{mEq/kg/day, animal study}}{\text{mEq/kg/day, human use}}$

concentrations, despite its manifest destructiveness to maternal and fetal tissues.

(c) Tuchmann-Duplessis and Mercier-Parot (1973), in the section of their study using Swiss albino mice with an average weight of 25 g, injected lithium chloride intraperitoneally in doses of 100, 150 and 250 mg/kg/day. They observed a 1·5% incidence of spontaneous fetal anomalies in untreated mice of this strain, and also discovered that the 250 mg/kg/day dose (Lithium Index 13) was too toxic to the mother to permit the pregnancies to continue. They found no increase over the spontaneous incidence of fetal anomalies when 100 or 150 mg/kg/day doses (Lithium Index 5; 8) were used.

2. Pregnant rats

(a) Trautner et al. (1958) carefully designed their studies using Albino Wistar rats to avoid exceeding the teratogenic zone, and to prevent transitory lithium pulses. They gave 20 mEq/l of lithium chloride in the drinking water daily (Lithium Index 4), and achieved stable serum lithium concentrations of 1·5—2·0 mEq/l, equivalent to the highest serum levels advisable in human use. Their technique avoided repeated intraperitoneal injections of lithium-containing solutions which could, in themselves, induce both generalized stress responses and local intraperitoneal tissue damage, including damage to reproductive organs. No malformations were found in the lithium-exposed litters, which also matched untreated controls in size and weight. However, Trautner et al. noted a 15% reduction in the number of corpora lutea in treated females, and concluded that the main effect of lithium given to these animals in sub-toxic doses was on ovulation, and took place before implantation.

(b) In 1969 Johansen and Ulrich reported a study of pregnant Wistar rats given lithium chloride in their diets. Finding that 3·5 mEq/kg/day was toxic to the adult animals they concentrated on animals given 0·93 to 1·78 mEq/kg/day (Lithium Index 2—4) of lithium chloride in the ration, and found no abnormalities of litter size, fetal weight or weight of uteri and placentas at 20 days of gestation. Further, they reported no fetal malformations on gross examination.

(c) In contrast Wright et al., (1970, 1971) using 220—250 g Sprague-Dawley rats, reported malformations of the eyes (63% of fetuses), palate (39%) and external ears (45%) in litters from animals given 50 mg of lithium chloride intraperitoneally on days 1, 4, 7 and 9 of gestation, and followed by 20 mg given each day to day 17, when caesarean sections were done (Lithium Index 11). Eye defects and cleft palates each appeared in 3% of a NaCl-treated control group, while an untreated control group had a zero incidence of both anomalies. In their brief 1970 report Wright et al. state that serum levels were in the range of those "in human beings receiving lithium therapy". However, they show in their more extensive 1971 description of this work that the serum lithium levels in their pregnant animals rose to $4 \cdot 2 \, mEq/l$ "20 minutes after the initial injection", and presumably were in that range after each succeeding dose. In the more complete (1971) report they describe their protocol as employing "maximum sublethal dosages", and they acknowledge that this regimen depressed the appetites of the animals, resulted in a 20% weight loss, and required the use of glucose diet supplements. The occurrence of transitory toxic lithium "pulses", considered a possibility in the discussion of Szabo's work, has clearly occurred in the experiments of Wright *et al.*

(d) In 1971 Johansen attempted to replicate Wright's findings with Wistar rats. He used intraperitoneal doses in one group and subcutaneous injections in a second group. All animals received $212 \, mg/kg$ of lithium chloride on day 4, 7 or 9, followed by daily doses of $85 \, mg/kg$ ($2 \, mEq/kg$) until day 19 when the animals were sacrificed. Johansen, evidently concerned about the phenomenon of lithium "pulses", showed that 15 minutes after either subcutaneous *or* intraperitoneal injection, this schedule produced peak serum values of 9–$10 \, mEq/l$. Despite a Lithium Index of 11, there was only one malformed fetus (bony defects in the legs) among the 152 examined.

(e) In the portion of their work using $230 \, g$ (average weight) Wistar rats, Tuchmann-Duplessis and Mercier-Parot (1973) noted no disturbances in gestation and no anomalies when the animals received $100 \, mg/kg/day$ of lithium chloride (Lithium Index 5). However, when the dose was increased to 150 and $200 \, mg/kg/day$ (Lithium Index 8 and 10), $1 \cdot 0$ and $2 \cdot 9\%$ respectively of the fetuses were found to have ocular anomalies. With the higher dose ($200 \, mg/kg/day$) there was also a small reduction in the number of viable fetuses and a rise in maternal mortality. With a dose of $250 \, mg/kg/day$ (Lithium Index 13) the incidence of fetal anomalies rose to 15%, and 44% of the mothers died. These workers concluded that there is no evident teratogenicity from lithium in rats unless the doses given are frankly toxic to the pregnant females.

3. *Male rats*

(a) There is a theoretical possibility that anomalies might occur in the offspring of lithium-treated males, presumably by alteration of the genetic characteristics of spermatozoa. MacLeod *et al.* (1949) reported that 60 mg/kg to 120 mg/kg of lithium chloride given to adult male rats appears to decrease the capacity of these animals to impregnate fertile fermales, probably by interfering with the anaerobic glycolysis on which spermatic motility in part depends. MacLeod *et al.* found no changes in the sperm morphology of lithium-treated males, however.

(b) Gralla and McIlhenny (1972) pursued the question of the teratogenicity of lithium administered to both male and female rats. They treated female 200–300 g albino Charles River rats with orally-administered lithium carbonate at high (4·05 mEq/kg/day), intermediate (2·03 mEq/kg/day) and low (0·68 mEq/kg/day) doses for 14 days and mated them with males fed 1·35, 0·68 or 0·27 mEq/kg/day for 70 days. High-dose females were mated with high-dose males, etc.; 20 pairs were used at each dose level. The high doses represent a Lithium Index of 9 for the females, 4 for the males. Half the females were sacrificed on 13 day of gestation, the rest 21 days after delivery. In a second study using the same strain and the same doses from days 5–15, and comparing them to a water-dosed control group, the animals were sacrificed on day 20. In concurrent studies of absorption, Gralla and McIlhenny observed that the 4·05 mEq/kg dose (Lithium Index 9) produced a serum level of 1·4 mEq/l after 3 and 5 hours, and 8-hour serum concentrations of 0·9 to 2·8 mEq/l. With regard to the effects of these schedules on fertility and teratogenicity, Gralla and McIlhenny found *no differences* between treated and control groups, except that two female rats treated with 4·05 mEq/kg/day died "unexpectedly", and the average weight of pups nursed by females receiving high-dose lithium carbonate (4·05 mEq/kg/day) was slightly lower than that of the controls.

4. *Rabbits*

Parallel studies by Gralla and McIlhenny of oral lithium carbonate in female New Zealand albino rabbits (3·5–4·5 kg) and in rhesus monkeys (4–6 kg) also showed no interference with pregnancies or evidence of teratogenesis, but again there were several "unexpected" deaths among the rabbits. These authors conclude that "at least three major animal species (rats, rabbits and monkeys) can receive *per os* lithium at various multiples of the clinical dose during pregnancy without affecting the offspring" (our emphasis).

B. Discussion

Lithium salts can be both toxic and teratogenic to rodents if dose, dose schedule and route of administration are arranged to deliver even transiently excessive pulses of high lithium concentration. Enough lithium can kill or weaken the mother; if the mother lives, enough lithium can kill or maim the developing fetus. Table I shows that the likelihood of fetal malformations increases as the dose increases, and is higher when the drug is given in a single daily dose and by parenteral routes. However, it is also clear that when laboratory animals are given lithium by mouth, in the ration, or in several doses per day, and when they are maintained at reasonably *steady* serum concentrations in the range achieved in human use, a Lithium Index as high as 8 or 9 is compatible with continued maternal health, unimpaired fertility, and litters free of anomalies.

IV. Human Studies

A. Chromosome studies

1. In-vitro *experiments*

(a) Friedrick and Nielsen (1969) added lithium at 48 hours to cultures of peripheral leukocytes from a normal 44-year-old man who had never received lithium or other psychotropic agents. They compared the effects of lithium at three concentrations (1·2, 1·8 and 2·4 mEq/l) with control lymphocyte cultures from the same blood sample. At lithium concentrations of 1·2 and 1·8 mEq/l they found no increase in the frequency of gaps, breaks, hypo- or hyperdiploid cells, but at a concentration of 2·4 mEq/l they noted a 2·9% increase in hyperdiploidism compared with the control cultures. Friedrick and Nielsen concluded that toxic effects on human chromosomes seem only to occur at lithium concentrations in the toxic range for man.

(b) Timson and Price (1971) added lithium carbonate to cultures of peripheral lymphocytes at 72 hours of incubation in amounts equivalent to doses of 10·0, 1·0 and 0·1g given to a 70kg man. The cells were from healthy, untreated adults; cells from the same donors were used as controls. Even with the largest lithium doses (equivalent to 7 to 10 times the normal human clinical dose) they found no significant chromosome damage, no change in the mitotic index, and no change in the lymphocyte transformation rate, suggesting that lithium did not effect DNA synthesis or the induction of mitosis in these cells. Timson and Price also emphasized the importance of using simultaneous samples of the subjects' own cells as controls since the mitotic index varies over time, and comparisons of mitotic indices between populations may be misleading.

2. In-vivo *experiments*

(a) Friedrick and Nielsen (1969) also analyzed the chromosomes of three patients treated with lithium, and found in these subjects a significantly increased frequency of breaks and hypodiploidism, but no change in the frequency of gaps or hyperdiploidism. In this study they used as control preparations, peripheral blood samples from *other* subjects matched for age with the lithium-treated patients; they reported the oral doses of lithium given to their subjects but not the serum lithium levels achieved. Serum concentrations are more reliable measures of the intensity of the organism's exposure to lithium than the dose; as noted above there is no simple or reliable relationship between oral dose and serum concentration. Furthermore, the small sample size in the *in vivo* (1 subject) and *in vitro* (3 subjects) parts of the Friedrick and Nielsen study cautions against generalizing from its results.

(b) Sixteen manic-depressive patients treated with lithium for two weeks to two years were studied by Jarvik *et al.,* (1971), who reported no significant differences in the frequency of breaks or hypodiploidy between the lithium-treated subjects and lithium-free controls. Jarvik stressed the marked variability among individuals with regard to gaps, breaks and aneuploidy, and noted the random relationship in her data among serum lithium concentrations, duration of exposure to lithium, and chromosomal abnormalities. She also noted that data from small populations can be misleading: "Had we based our conclusions solely on the placebo group (consisting of four patients), the unusually low level of breaks (less than 1%) in that group would have exaggerated the difference between treated and untreated patients. Even the control group of ten persons is too small to permit definitive conclusions."

(c) Data on 19 manic-depressives treated with lithium were reported by Genest and Villeneuve (1971). They found no differences between these subjects and a control population with respect to chromosomal abnormalities, but noted that the lithium-treated group showed a reduction in the mitotic index.

3. Discussion

The effects of lithium on the chromosomes of peripheral leukocytes, *in vivo* or cultured *in vitro*, vary widely with the specifics of the experimental situation. While the data available are inconclusive, the trend of the report suggests that, in *therapeutic concentrations*, lithium carbonate has no significant effect on chromosomes in man.

B. Teratology and toxicity in human pregnancies

In 1969 the authors treated a woman who conceived while receiving lithium (Weinstein and Goldfield, 1969). Because of the paucity of published information on the teratogenic and other potential hazards of lithium use in human pregnancy, we then established the American Register of Lithium Babies to collect such data. Later, at the suggestion of Dr. M. Schou, this activity was combined with the work of the Scandinavian Register begun earlier by Dr. Schou, and with the Canadian Register, started later by Dr. André Villeneuve. Data from the three sources, the bulk of it reported to Dr. Schou's program, were combined in the International Register of Lithium Babies. In 1973 the Canadian and Scandinavian branches of the International Register ceased collecting this data (Schou et al., 1973b); the American Register continues to solicit reports of lithium treatment in pregnancy. [5]

1. Sources of data

The operation of the Register has been retrospective; its existence and its interest in acquiring reports of "lithium babies" has been announced and

[5] American Register of Lithium Babies, M. R. Weinstein, MD; M. D. Goldfield, MD, The Langley Porter Neuropsychiatric Institute, 401 Parnassus Avenue, San Francisco, California 94143.

reiterated in psychiatric, obstetrical, pediatric and general medical journals, and at professional meetings throughout Europe and in the Western Hemisphere. In addition, the American component of the Register has systematically communicated with departments of psychiatry, pediatrics and obstetrics in North America, describing the Register and asking that a department member be designated to maintain liaison with it. Copies of reporting forms were also distributed to each department. Reports from Scandinavia and Western Europe were stimulated by Dr. Schou's extensive personal contacts with lithium-prescribing physicians, and his identification with the larger issue of lithium treatment.

2. Sources of error

The retrospective approach was chosen because it could give "early warning if the risk of teratogenic effects was as high in women as it was in some of the studies carried out in rats and mice" (Schou et al., 1973b). The chief defect of a retrospective study is the tendency for the sample to be incomplete and selective in ways that may not be apparent. In particular, reports of pathological states and other deviation from normal are more likely to be sent to such a register than are reports of normal babies born to lithium-using women; as one comes closer to a 100% sample of all lithium-exposed pregnancies, this tendency to exaggerate the pathological is reduced. Because the reporting system in Scandinavia was based on Dr. Schou's very close personal contact with lithium-using physicians and clinics, data from Scandinavia almost certainly comes closer to a 100% sample of all pregnancies exposed to lithium than do reports from other parts of the world. However, differences in the incidence of malformations and other abnormal conditions reported from Scandinavia and from all other sources can be examined to estimate and partially control the distortions of the retrospective study.

C. Malformations and other pathology

1. Definitions

In publicizing the operation of the International Register of Lithium Babies we urged physicians to submit reports about *all* babies, normal and abnormal, and *all* pregnancies, complicated or uncomplicated, in which lithium had been used at any point. For purposes of inclusion in the Register, however, the criteria were (a) that the pregnancy had been exposed to lithium *at least* during some part of the first trimester, and (b) that the conceptus had to be available for morphological examination. Congenital malformations were defined as "macroscopic abnormalities of structure attributable to faulty development and present at birth" (Schou et al., 1973b).

TABLE II. International Register of lithium Babies–Malformed Infants**

Case No.	Birth date	Other drugs during pregnancy	Sex and weight (g)	Malformation	Child's fate	Report from:
1	9/3/68*	No information	F. Unknown	Coarctation of the aorta	Malformation corrected with surgery	USA
2	22/5/69	No information	M. 2,800	High intraventricular septal defect	Died on day 4	USA
3	23/8/69†	Chlorpromazine, diuretics	F. 3,080	Stenosis of aqueduct with hydrocephalus, spina bifida with sacral meningomyelocele, bilateral talipes equinovarus with paralysis	Unknown	Canada
4	28/9/69	None used	M. 3,500	Unilateral microtia	Developing normally at age 3, apart from the malformed ear	Denmark
5	?/2/70	Haloperidol, nortriptyline, barbiturates, and others	Unknown, Unknown	Mitral atresia	Died soon after corrective surgery	USA

6	23/2/71	None used	F. 3,050	Cardiac malformation of Ebstein type	Died a few days after birth	USA
7	28/9/71	No information	M. 2,200	Single umbilical artery, bilateral hypoplasia of maxilla	Died five hours after birth	Canada
8	22/2/72	Amitriptyline	F. 3,420	Cardiac malformation of Ebstein type	Died day after birth	Denmark
9	23/5/72	None used	F. 2,200	Atresia of tricuspid valve	Stillborn	Denmark
10	18/1/73	Nortriptyline	F. 3,410	Patent ductus arteriosus and ventricular septal defect; mother 39	Survived 3 months as of report	England

** Adapted from Schou et al. (1973b)
* Reported by Lewis and Suris (1970)
† Reported by Vacaflor et al. (1970)

2. *Malformed infants*

At this time 132 instances of lithium use in pregnancy, meeting the definition noted above, have been collected. Of these, 10 (7·6%) resulted in malformed children. Information about the nature and results of these malformations is shown in Table II. It can be seen that 8 of the 10 malformations involved the cardiovascular system and one each the central nervous system and the external ears. The prominence of head, neck and central nervous system pathology seen in lithium-induced anomalies in other species does not appear to occur in man. Table II also shows that of the 7 instances of malformation in which information about the use of other drugs was obtained, the mother had been treated with antidepressants in three cases and a phenothiazine drug in another.

3. *Stillbirths*

Five of the 132 pregnancies reported to the Register resulted in stillbirths (3·8%). One of these infants (#9, Table II) was also malformed, with atresia of the tricuspid valve. Another was one of twins born at approximately 24 weeks; the other twin died shortly after birth. The mothers of the remaining three still-born infants had received anti-depressant and/or antipsychotic drugs during gestation in addition to lithium.

4. *Down's syndrome*

Two children in the register (1·5%) had Down's Syndrome. In both instances the mother was 38 when she delivered. One of the babies with Down's Syndrome had a normal twin.

D. Discussion

Material reported to the International Register of Lithium Babies cannot be treated as a complete tally or even as a representative sample. Because contacts between the Register and Scandinavian physicians were closer and more complete than such contacts outside Scandinavia, reports from the Scandinavian countries are probably more inclusive and less selective than those from other areas, and less affected by the tendency to over-report pathological states. Table III shows that 3 of the 83 babies (3·6%) reported from Scandinavia were malformed, compared with 7 of the 49 from all other areas (14·3%). In contrast, all 5 of the stillborns reported to the Register came from Scandinavia (3·8% of the total; 6% of the Scandinavian reports). In keeping with the view that Scandinavian physicians have contributed a more nearly complete account of lithium babies than have physicians from other areas, we believe that the Scandinavian figure (6%) is closer to the actual incidence of stillbirths, and that Scandinavian physicians were more thorough than others in reporting lithium babies to the Register when fetal anomalies did *not* occur, but when other problems, including stillbirth, did.

TABLE III. Reports to the International Register of Lithium Babies through January, 1974.

	All Reports		Reports from Scandinavia		Reports from countries outside Scandinavia	
	Number	%	Number	%	Number	%
No. of infants reported	132	100·0	83	100·0	49*	100·0
Liveborn	127	96·1	78	94·0	49	100·0
Stillborn	5†	3·8	5	6·0	0	0·0
Malformed	10	7·6	3	3·6	7	14·3
Down's syndrome	2‡	1·5	0	0·0	2	4·1

* 16 from Europe outside Scandinavia, 26 from USA, 6 from Canada, and 1 from Australia
† One of these was malformed and appears also in that group
‡ Both mothers were 38 years old

It is likely that the overall frequency of congenital anomalies (7·6%) reported to the Register is *higher* than the true incidence of such malformations among the infants of lithium-treated women, and it is quite *unlikely* that it is lower. Even the higher figure for congenital anomalies (7·6%) does not significantly differ from the estimate by Apgar and Stickle (1968) that "at least 7% of live-born—some 250,000 each year—have structural or functional defects of prenatal origin which are detectable during infancy or early childhood."

Although the maximum frequency of congenital malformations reported to the Register (7·6%) does not seem to exceed the expected incidence of such malformations in the general (non-lithium treated) population, it is clearly far lower than the frequencies of congenital malformations reported in lithium-treated laboratory rodents by Szabo and by Wright, *et al.* Thus, while the *true* contribution of lithium to the development of fetal anomalies cannot be learned through retrospective studies such as this, the study offers some reassurance that lithium does not add importantly to the frequency of such anomalies, and it can be said with conviction that the risk of malformations in the infants of lithium-treated women is very much less than that suggested by the most alarming of the animal studies.

V. Recommendations for the Use of Lithium in Pregnancy

A. Risks vs. benefits

Studies of the effects of lithium on the morphogenesis of invertebrates and laboratory animals cannot be extrapolated to guide us in the use of lithium in human pregnancies. However, the results of experiments with lithium in pregnant mammals, while admittedly contradictory in some respects, suggest several principles and precautions which should help minimize the risk of lithium administration to pregnant women. Furthermore, the pooled experiences of many clinicians indicate that the risk from intra-uterine exposure of the fetus to lithium is *minor* when the pregnancy and the lithium are both carefully supervised, and these experiences also suggest certain general principles and cautions.

1. *Informing patients and spouse*

A decision to institute, continue or discontinue lithium administration in a woman for whom pregnancy is a fact or a possibility should be made with the collaboration and informed participation of the patient and her husband. Counselling concerning the risks and advantages of using lithium in fecund or pregnant women should consider the current evidence that pregnancies exposed to lithium do not result in a notably higher-than-usual incidence of fetal abnormalities when lithium dose and serum levels are carefully controlled. It should also weigh the evidence that lithium is an effective treatment and prophylactic in recurrent affective disorders, against the hazards of lithium toxicity in pregnancy and the possibility, however, small, of a teratogenic effect.

B. Reducing risks of lithium use in pregnancy

1. *Selection of patients*

Women in the childbearing years should be treated with lithium *only* if there are very strong indications for its use: these indications may include the treatment of acute manic episodes and the continuing prophylaxis of manic attacks when these have been recurrent and disruptive and not effectively controlled by more conventional therapies such as phenothiazines. On the basis of currently available data it is probably also justifiable to maintain continuous lithium prophylaxis in fecund women with the aim of preventing recurrent severe depressive episodes.

2. *Avoiding conception*

Women treated with lithium should be urged to avoid pregnancy and maintain effective contraception.

3. *Special considerations in the first trimester*

Women receiving continuous lithium prophylaxis should be withdrawn from treatment during the first trimester of pregnancy unless there is convincing historical evidence that withdrawal would seriously endanger the woman or the pregnancy.

4. *Dosage considerations*

When it is found necessary to initiate or continue to administer lithium to a pregnant woman, the dose should be the smallest which will achieve the minimum serum level compatible with desired therapeutic or prophylactic effects: 0·7 to 1·2 mEq/l in most cases. It will therefore be necessary to measure the pregnant woman's serum lithium concentration more frequently than would be indicated were she not pregnant: weekly serum determinations are probably satisfactory in uncomplicated pregnancies.

5. *Avoiding fluctuations in serum lithium concentrations*

In addition to using the smallest amount of lithium adequate for clinical effectiveness, *fluctuations* in maternal serum lithium concentrations should be avoided since they are transmitted directly to the fetus. Such fluctuations, and especially the exposure of the fetus to "pulses" of high lithium concentrations, can be minimized if the following precautions are observed:

(a) Sodium Loss and Diuretics: Major variations in the mother's dietary intake or urinary excretion of *sodium* should be avoided, since sodium loss tends to be associated with increased serum lithium concentration, even with an unchanging lithium intake (Waldron, 1949; Bleiweiss, 1970; Baer, *et al.*, 1971). Therefore, dietary restriction of sodium, use of sodium-depleting diuretics, weight reduction diets which inadvertently restrict dietary sodium, and excessive perspiration, should all be avoided by lithium-treated women. Because fluid retention, ankle edema and weight gain are common problems of pregnancy for which sodium restriction, diuretics, weight reduction and exercise are commonly prescribed, the special consequences of sodium depletion to the lithium-treated woman must be kept in mind. Experience reported to the International Register of Lithium Babies indicates that the use of sodium-depleting diuretics for the alleviation of edema during pregnancy has been a common source of difficulty for mother and infant. *The use of diuretics is contraindicated for anyone taking lithium* (Weinstein and Goldfield, 1970; McKnelly *et al.*, 1970; Goldfield and Weinstein, 1971, 1973).

(b) Timing of Doses and Serum Levels: Maternal serum lithium concentrations are highest one to four hours after a single oral dose and return to baseline values in 12 to 24 hours (Schou, 1968; Almy and Taylor, 1973). The common practice of giving as much as 600 mg of lithium carbonate in a single dose two or three times a day may expose the fetus to a series of lithium "pulses". Whenever lithium carbonate is given to a pregnant woman the individual dose should not exceed 300 mg, given as many times per day as is necessary to maintain the desired serum level; doses should be regularly distributed through the waking hours. For example, a non-pregnant woman who is adequately maintained on a prophylactic program of 1·2 g of lithium carbonate given as 600 mg in the morning and 600 mg in the evening, should be changed, during pregnancy, to a schedule of 300 mg at 9 a.m., 1 p.m., 5 p.m. and 10 p.m., or the like. Lithium carbonate is available in the U.S. only in 300 mg capsules or tablets at this time. However, for women whose daily requirement is 900 mg or less, it would be advisable to prescribe specially compounded capsules of 150 mg, five or six times a day.[6]

C. Special considerations associated with labor

1. *Maternal Toxicity*

(a) Clinical Features of Maternal Lithium Intoxication: Three cases of maternal lithium intoxication closely related to parturition have been reported in the literature, or directly to the International Register of Lithium Babies (Vacaflor *et al.*, 1970; Wilbanks *et al.*, 1970; Barthe, personal communication). Signs of *maternal* intoxication characteristically begin within a few hours of delivery, and include confusion, lethargy, diarrhoea, incontinence, muscle spasms and severe restlessness, sometimes progressing to coma with generalized and/or focal grand mal convulsions. Even with early recognition of the role of lithium in the production of the intoxication and prompt withdrawl of the drug, recovery is typically slow and may require several weeks. Treatment, beyond termination of lithium intake, has been supportive, with careful attention to fluid and electrolyte balance and maintenance of adequate renal function. Urinary excretion of lithium may be accelerated by the administration of urea and aminophylline, and alkalinization of the urine (Thomsen, 1969). See Chapter 13 and 14.

(b) Lithium Clearance in Pregnancy: *Schou et al.*, (1973a) have found that the renal clearance of lithium increases by 50–100% during the course of pregnancy and drops to the pre-pregnancy level at the time of delivery. This change in the renal lithium clearance makes it likely that a pregnant woman receiving lithium will be found to have declining serum lithium concentrations as pregnancy progresses, though her lithium dose is unchanged.

This phasic change in lithium clearance presents the physician with a dual risk: if he increases the lithium dose late in pregnancy to compensate for declining serum lithium levels produced by increased lithium clearance, he may expose the patient and the infant to intoxication at delivery when clearance abruptly falls and maternal serum lithium again rises. If he maintains the dose at the pre-pregnancy or early pregnancy level the patient may "escape" from lithium control into a manic or depressive episode.

As a solution to this problem we recommend close clinical supervision of the patient in the last half of pregnancy to detect early changes in mood or behavior, in conjunction with frequent (weekly or bi-weekly) serum lithium determinations. It is also advisable to reduce the daily lithium dose by 50% in the last week of gestation, to discontinue lithium entirely at the onset of labor, and to reinstitute lithium at the pre-pregnancy dose immediately after delivery.

(c) Sodium Depletion and Lithium Intoxication: It is important to note that

[6] Lithium carbonate *tablets* produced by J. B. Roerig Division, Chas. Pfizer & Company, Inc., U.S.A., are scored and can be broken into fragments of approximately 150 mg.

in two of the three cases discussed above (Vacaflor *et al.*, 1970; Wilbanks *et al.*, 1970) the mother had been salt-restricted and treated with Na-depleting diuretics prior to delivery. Thus, sodium depletion may well have contributed to the development of lithium intoxication as discussed above.

2. *Lithium toxicity in the neonate*

(a) Clinical Features of Neonatal Lithium Toxicity: Because the concentration of lithium in the fetal circulation varies in close parallel to maternal serum concentrations and is essentially identical with that of the mother (Schou *et al.*, 1972), one would expect that maternal lithium intoxication during parturition will be associated with manifestations of neonatal toxicity as well. In fact, in two of the three instances of maternal toxicity cited above (Wilbanks *et al.*, 1970; Barthe, personal communication) there was clear evidence of intoxication of the infant also, and in the third case (Vacaflor *et al.*, 1970), while there is no description of intoxication of the child, the infant was congenitally malformed. In addition, three instances of apparent neonatal toxicity without evidence of maternal intoxication have been reported (Silverman *et al.*, 1971; Tunnessen and Hertz, 1972; Strothers *et al.*, 1973). The descriptions of all five toxic infants emphasize hypotonia or "floppiness", low Apgar scores in the first half-hour, brady- or tachycardia, hypothermia, duskiness and absent Moro reflex. In all instances save one where the information is reported, the serum lithium levels of the toxic infants were well above $1 \cdot 0$ mEq/l shortly after delivery, and had almost certainly been even higher before. Neonatal serum lithium levels dropped steadily over a 1–2 week period and the infants recovered, apparently without residuae of their intoxication, with 1–2 weeks of general supportive care.

(b) Prevention of Neonatal Lithium Intoxication. The human placenta does not modify the effect of maternal lithium concentrations on the fetus; lithium levels are essentially identical on both sides of the placenta. Therefore, all factors which predispose to maternal intoxication likewise predispose to fetal and neonatal intoxication, and prevention of neonatal intoxication requires in effect the avoidance of excessive maternal lithium concentrations as outlined above.

D. Breast feeding by the lithium-treated woman

The lithium concentration in the breast milk of lithium-treated women is from 30% to 100% of that in the mother's serum. Infants breast-fed by lithium-treated women have serum lithium concentrations very close to the concentration of the ingested breast milk (Catz and Giacoia, 1972; Schou and Amdisen, 1973). Renal lithium clearance in infants cannot be assumed to be as effective as that in adults, and transitory disturbances in water and electrolyte balance are common in infants. The physician and the parents together must decide if the benefits of breast-feeding are great enough to warrant the child's exposure to a potentially toxic drug; we believe that breast feeding by lithium-treated women should be discouraged.

Acknowledgements

This work was supported in part by Langley Porter Neuropsychiatric Institute General Research Support Grant FR 72–6, and grants from Smith, Kline and French Laboratories and the J. B. Roerig Division of Chas. Pfizer and Co. Inc.

References

Almy, G. L. and Taylor, M. A. (1973). *Archs gen. Psychiat.* **29**, 232–234.
Apgar, V. and Stickle, G. (1968). *J. Amer. med. Assoc.* **204**, 371–374.
Baer, L. Platman, S. R., Kassir, S. and Fieve, R. R. (1971). *J. psychiat. Res.* **8**, 91–105.
Bass, A. D., Yntema, C. L., Hammond, W. S. and Frazer, M. L. (1951). *J. Pharmacol. exp. Ther.* **101**, 362–367.
Berg, W. E. (1968). *Exp. cell. Res.* **50**, 133–139.
Bleiweiss, H. (1970). *Lancet* **1**, 416.
Catz, C. S. and Giacoia, G. P. (1972). *Pediat. Clins. N. Amer.* **19**, 151–166.
Dawson, E. B., Moore, B. S. and McGanity, W. J. (1970). *Dis. nerv. Syst.* **31**, 811–820.
Demers, R. G. and Davis, L. S. (1971). *Compreh. Psychiat.* **12**, 348–353.
DeVincentis, M. and Runnström, J. (1967). *Expl. Cell. Res.* **45**, 681–689.
Duvauchelle, R. (1966). *Biologica* (Santiago) **39**, 56–67.
Ficq, A. (1951). *C. r. Acad. Sci.* **233**, 1684–1685.
Flickinger, R. A., Miyagi, M. and Moser, C. R. (1967). *Devl. Biol.* **15**, 414–431.
Frasier, F. C. (1961). *In* "Progress in Medical Genetics", pp. 38–80, Grune and Stratton, New York.
Friedrick, V. and Nielsen, J. (1969). *Lancet* **2**, 435–436.
Genest, P. and Villeneuve, A. (1971). *Lancet* **1**, 1132.
Goldfield, M. and Weinstein, M. R. (1971). *Amer. J. Psychiat.* **127**, 64–69.
Goldfield, M. D. and Weinstein, M. R. (1973). *Amer. J. Obstets.-Gynecol.* **116**, 15–22.
Gralla, E. J. and McIlhenny, H. M. (1972). *Toxic appl. Pharmacol.* **21**, 428–433.
Greenhouse, G. and Hamburgh, M. (1968). *Teratol.* **1**, 61–74.
Jarvik, L. F., Bishun, N. P., Bleiweiss, H., Kato, T. and Moralishvili, E. (1971). *Archs. gen. Psychiat,* **24**, 166–168.
Johansen, K. T. and Ulrich, K. (1969). *Acta psychiat. scand. Suppl.* **207**. 91–95.
Johansen, K. T. (1971). *Lancet* **1**, 1026–1027.
Lehmann, F. E. (1945). "Einfürung in die physiologische Embryologie". Birkhaüser, Basel.
Lewis, W. H. and Suris, O. R. (1970). *Texas Med,* **66**, 58.
MacLeod, J., Swan, R. C. and Aitken, G. A. (1949). *Amer. J. Physiol.* **157**, 177–183.
McKnelly, W. V. Jr., Tupin, J. P. and Dunn, M. (1970). *Compreh. Psychiat.* **11**, 279–286.
Needham, J. (1942). "Biochemistry and Morphogenesis". Cambridge University Press, Cambridge.
Nicolet, R. (1965). *Acta Embryol. Morph. Exp.* **8**, 32–85.
Runnström, J. and Immers, J. (1970). *Expl cell Res.* **62**, 228–238.
Schou, M. (1957). *Pharmacol. Rev.* **9**, 17–58.

Schou, M. (1968). *J. psychiat. Res.* **6**, 67–95.

Schou, M. and Amdisen, A. (1973). *Brit. med. J.* **2**, 138.

Schou, M., Amdisen, A. and Steenstrup, O. R. (1972). (Unpublished manuscript).

Schou, M., Amdisen, A. and Steenstrup, O. R. (1973a). *Brit. med. J.* **2**, 137–138.

Schou, M., Goldfield, M. D., Weinstein, M. R. and Villeneuve, A. (1973b). *Brit. med. J.* **2**, 135–136.

Shirkey, H. C. (1968). *In* "Pediatric Therapy, 1966–1967". C. V. Mosby Co., St. Louis.

Silverman, J. A., Winters, R. N. and Strande, C. (1971). *Am. J. Obstets.-Gynecol.* **109**, 934–936.

Spiegel, J. and Bell, N. (1059). *In* "American Handbook of Psychiatry" (S. Arieti, ed.), Vol. 1, pp. 114–149, Basic Books, New York.

Strothers, J. K., Wilson, D. W. and Royston, N. (1973). *Brit. med. J.* **3**, 233–234

Szabo, K. T. (1969). *Lancet* **2**, 8149.

Szabo, K. T. (1970). *Nature* **225**, 73–75.

Szabo, K. T., Hawk, A. M. and Henry, M. (1970). *Toxic. appl. Pharmacol.* **17**, 274–275.

Taylor. M. A. and Abrams, R. (1973). *Archs gen. Psychiat.* **29**, 520–522.

Thomsen, K. (1969). *Acta psychiat. scand. Suppl.* **207**, 83–84.

Timson, J. and Price, D. J. (1971). *Lancet* **2**, 93.

Trautner, E. M., Pennycuik, P. R., Morris, R. J. H., Gershon, S. and Shankly, K. R. (1958). *Aust. J. exp. Biol. med. Sci.* **36**, 305–322.

Tuchmann-Duplessis, H. and Mercier-Parot, L. (1973). *C. r. Seanc. Soc. Biol. et Filiales* **167**, 183–186.

Tunnessen, W. W. Jr. and Hertz, C. G. (1972). *Ped. Pharmacol. Ther.* **81**, 804–807

Vacaflor, L., Lehmann, H. E. and Ban, T. A. (1970). *J. clin. Pharm.* **10**, 387–389.

Waldron, A. M. (1949). *J. Amer. med. Assoc.* **139**, 733.

Weinstein, M. R. and Goldfield, M. (1969). *Dis. nerv. Syst.* **30**, 828–832.

Weinstein, M. R. and Goldfield, M. D. (1970). *J. Amer. med. Assoc.* **214**, 1325–1326.

Wilbanks, G. D., Bressler, B., Peete, C. H. Jr., Cherney, W. B. and London, W. L. (1970). *J. Amer. med. Assoc.* **213**, 865–867.

Willier, B. N., Weiss, P. A. and Hamburger, V. (1955). "Analysis of Development". W. B. Saunders, Philadelphia.

Wilson, J. G. (1965). *In* "Teratology: Principles and Techniques" (J. G. Wilson and J. Warkany, eds.), pp. 251–254, Univ. of Chicago Press, Chicago.

Wright, T. L., Hoffman, L. H. and Davies, J. (1970). *Lancet* **2**, 876.

Wright, T. L., Hoffman, L. H. and Davies, J. (1971). *Tetratol.* **4**, 151–154.

Note Added in Proof

Following completion of this chapter, eleven additional cases were reported to the Register. Two were instances of the rare "Ebstein anomaly"* of the heart and great vessels. Two examples of this malformation (cases six and eight, Table II) were already included in the Register. The eleven new cases also include two reports of major cardiovascular malformations other than the Ebstein type, and seven reports of normal lithium babies.

At this writing (October, 1974), therefore, the Register contains 143 cases. Fourteen (9·8%) show anomalies, and of the fourteen anomalies, twelve are major malformations of the cardiovascular system. All four of the recently reported cardiovascular anomalies

*Nora, J. J., Nora, A. H. and Toews, W. H. (1974). *Lancet* **2**, 594–595.

come from non-Scandinavian countries, exaggerating the previously noted tendency for reports of neo-natal pathology to come disproportionately from sources outside Scandinavia.

However, these new reports produce a relative over-representation of major cardio-vascular malformations in lithium-exposed infants. We can not say with certainty that cardiovascular malformations occur in lithium-exposed infants more often than in non-exposed infants, but it seems likely that they do. The only other ways to understand the occurrence of cardiovascular anomalies in twelve of the fourteen malformed lithium babies reported to the Register would be to assume (1) that there is not only a tendency to report abnormal babies more assiduously than normal infants, but to report dramatic pathology (such as the Ebstein anomaly) more completely than less impressive defects; (2) that lithium exposure *protects* the foetus against *other* kinds of malformation; or, (3) that there is an association between manic-depressive illness and cardiovascular anomalies independent of lithium exposure. There is no evidence to support any of the three possibilities, but the first seems plausible, and the other two merit investigation.

The effect of these additional reports should be to strengthen the cautions expressed in this chapter regarding the exposure of pregnant or potentially pregnant women to lithium.

PART II

PHYSIOLOGICAL, BIOCHEMICAL AND BEHAVIOURAL STUDIES

SECTION A
UPTAKE, DISTRIBUTION AND EXCRETION

16

LITHIUM ABSORPTION AND DISTRIBUTION IN BODY TISSUES

D. K. ANDERSON and L. D. PROCKOP

I. Introduction

Understanding of the fate and metabolism of therapeutically administered lithium ion depends upon knowledge of its distribution in different body tissues. If serum lithium is to be maintained at levels sufficient to be effective in the treatment of manic-depression and other mental illnesses, information on the absorption, tissue distribution, and excretion of this ion is necessary. Since Cade's report stating that lithium salts given to ten manic patients resulted in uniform improvement (Cade, 1949), investigators have extensively studied the pharmacology and biological activity of lithium including the distribution of this ion in body tissues and fluids. Lithium is readily absorbed into blood following either subcutaneous, intraperitoneal, or oral administration and is not bound to plasma proteins (Gershon, 1970). The fact that the lithium concentrations of various organs differ, and the fact that concentration gradients exist across cellular membranes, indicate that this ion is not distributed evenly throughout the water phase (Schou, 1957). The concentration gradients are considerably less than for the other alkali metals, sodium and potassium, indicating that lithium is distributed differently than these ions in extra- and intracellular fluid (Schou, 1957; Gershon, 1970). Schou (1958) reported that although lithium passes into a variety of tissues from the blood, the entry rates vary in different tissues and organs; he suggested that the relatively slow movement of lithium from blood to brain, as compared with the other tissues studied, was due to the low permeability of the blood–brain barrier. Because lithium effects on the central nervous system include those on the electrical activity of nerve cells, on the sodium-potassium transport mechanism of the nerve cell membrane, and on synaptic transmission, it is useful to understand the unique problem the blood–brain barrier and the blood–cerebrospinal fluid (CSF) barrier present to the movement of substances across them.

The initial portion of this chapter will therefore consist of a brief review of the anatomy and physiology of the blood–brain and blood–CSF barriers, with special emphasis on the passage of ions. The main body of the chapter is a detailed discussion of the distribution of lithium in various body tissues along with the mechanisms involved with lithium transport.

II. Blood–Brain and Blood–CSF Barriers

In 1885, Erlich demonstrated that intravenous injection of certain acidic dyes produced a staining of all body tissues except most of the brain, spinal cord and CSF, a finding which led to the concepts of blood–brain and blood–CSF barriers. Because these barriers contribute to physiological, pathophysiological, metabolic and pharmacological aspects of the central nervous system, intensive research has been conducted in various disciplines and, since Erlich's report, several thousand related articles have been published. Many discussions and reviews are available (Barlow, 1964; Dobbing, 1968; Greenspan et al., 1970; Lee, 1971; Prockop, 1973).

A. Anatomy

The morphological locus for the blood–brain barrier is considered to be a property of the various covers encasing cerebral capillaries. Maynard et al. (1957) have published electron micrographs from the rat cerebral cortex which demonstrate that cerebral capillaries consist of a flat uninterrupted endothelial layer resting on a dense continuous basement membrane. These are incompletely invested by a sheath of astrocytic end-feet that cover approximately 85% of the total capillary surface. These neurological processes or "end-feet" are in direct contact with the basement membrane of the capillary and share this membrane with the capillary endothelium so that there is no perivascular space around the cerebral capillaries. Davson (1967) suggested that the astrocytic end-feet, which are a unique feature of cerebral capillaries, might constitute the blood–brain barrier, their cytoplasm and plasma membranes acting like a layer of epithelial cells to slow the passage of molecules from the blood into the cerebral extracellular fluid. Astrocytic processes do not extend to the vessels of the choroid plexus, but the choroidal capillaries are encased by a layer of densely intermeshed and interlocked cuboidal epithelial cells which, in all likelihood, is the functional site of the blood–CSF barrier (Giese, 1973). Figures 1 and 2

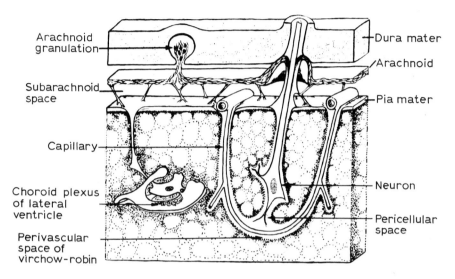

FIG. 1. Diagrammatic representation of the central nervous system with reference to the CSF circulation. Fluid formed within the ventricular system reaches the subarachnoid space to take exit via the arachnoid granulations (villi). Fluid may also interchange with brain extracellular fluid in the pericellular spaces via the perivascular spaces. Fluid may exit along the nerve sheath by means of the periaxonal space. The space between the dura mater and arachnoid is only a potential space and not real as indicated here for schematic purposes. (Drawings for Figs. 1 and 2 by Geraldine Hruska from L. Prockop, Disorders of Cerebrospinal Fluid and Brain Extracellular Fluid, p. 232 and p. 233 "Biology of Brain Dysfunction", G. E. Gaull, ed., Plenum Press, New York, 1973, with permission.)

provide diagrammatic representation of the central nervous system with reference to the CSF circulation and blood-brain barrier.

B. Physiology

The amount of lithium or any other substances within the central nervous system (CNS) is a function of the quantity entering and the amount leaving, i.e., a net amount. For entry into the CNS extra-cellular fluid (ECF) with subsequent access to the intracellular compartment, substances must cross the functionally identical specialized membranes called the blood–brain or blood–

CSF barriers. In addition, it is generally believed that CSF and brain ECF, if not identical, are in equilibrium (Wallace and Brodie, 1940; Cserr, 1965; Katzman *et al.,* 1965; Fencl *et al.,* 1966). Consequently, substances which enter brain ECF from blood will equilibrate with CSF and *vice versa.*

The mechanisms which govern movement of substances into and out of the

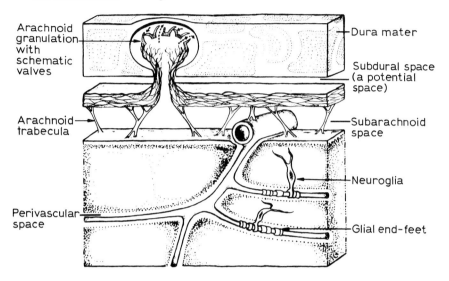

FIG. 2. Diagrammatic representation of elements of the central nervous system with reference to the blood–brain barrier and CSF circulation. The glial end-feet partially enveloping a cerebral capillary are schematically indicated. An arachnoid granulation contains schematic valves. The small solid arrows indicate a situation in which the hydrostatic pressure of the venous blood within the dura mater sinus is higher than that of the CSF within the granulation, with resulting valve closure. This prevents reflux of blood into the CSF compartment. The dashed arrows indicate the reverse, i.e., CSF pressure higher than sagittal sinus venous blood-pressure. The valves are open, with resulting bulk flow of CSF outward into the venous system.

CNS, thereby establishing the net amount within the CNS, are passive diffusion, facilitated diffusion, active transport, and CSF bulk flow.

As will be discussed in detail later, the quantity of lithium within the CNS is probably dependent upon passive diffusion. By this mechanism, substances with a higher degree of lipid solubility, low degree of ionization, and little plasma protein binding move into the brain and CSF readily, attaining equilibrium rapidly. The un-ionized form of a compound penetrates membranes more readily than the ionized forms. Therefore, acidosis or alkalosis can alter drug exchange between blood, brain, and CSF. Further considerations for passive diffusion between blood and CSF are the direction of the concentration and/or electrical gradients, size of the diffusing species (i.e., smaller molecules move faster than large ones), and the fact that anions move more rapidly than cations.

Movement of molecules across membranes separating blood, brain and CSF may not always depend upon passive diffusion, but may involve carrier-mediated transport. When the movement of a molecule across cell membranes requires cellular metabolic energy, can occur against an electrochemical gradient, exhibits saturation kinetics and competitive inhibition, the process is termed active transport; if the transport system exhibits saturation kinetics and competitive inhibition but the transport is not against an electrochemical gradient nor dependent upon cellular metabolic energy, the process is called facilitative diffusion.

For example, facilitative diffusion has been shown to be involved in the movement of glucose from blood to CSF (Bradbury and Davson, 1964; Fishman, 1964) and brain (Crone, 1965). Certain organic acids, e.g., Diodrast and phenolsulfonphthalein, have been demonstrated to be actively cleared from fluid perfusing the brain ventricles (Pappenheimer, *et al.*, 1961). If such organic acids are present in plasma, little or none would be detected in CSF because any amount entering by diffusion would be immediately and rapidly removed.

Another important factor affecting the net concentration of a substance in the CNS is the rapid bulk turnover of CSF. Some substances can exit the CNS by this mechanism. For example, when lactic acid accumulates in brain as the result of hypoxia, it moves from brain ECF to CSF by "sink action" equilibration. Subsequently, it is absorbed into blood with CSF as CSF moves across the arachnoid villi by bulk flow.

Finally, interpretation of ionic distribution and fluxes among blood, brain and CSF requires knowledge of any electrical potential differences existing between these compartments. A potential between blood and CSF represents a potential across both the blood–brain and blood–CSF barriers (Davson, 1967). The potential difference between CSF and blood is between 5 and 7 mV (CSF positive) in a variety of mammals (Mottschall and Leoschke, 1963; Held *et al.*, 1964). Held and his co-workers concluded that the CSF potential must contribute to the exchanges of all charged particles between blood–brain and CSF and must play a role in determining the steady state ionic composition of CSF.

C. Ionic movement across blood–brain and blood–CSF barriers

Studies of the passage of lithium ions across the blood–brain and blood–CSF barriers, and of the distribution of lithium ions amongst body tissues, are best appreciated against the general background of information about related ions.

In one of the first quantitative studies of the movement of ions across the blood–brain and blood–CSF barriers, Wallace and Brodie (1940) found that

CNS and CSF uptake of bromide, iodide and thiocyanate from blood was slow and restricted when compared to uptake by other tissues. Later, Greenburg *et al.* (1943) demonstrated that the rate of increase in concentration of radioactive ions in CSF, following intravascular administration, was in the order: potassium > sodium > bromide > rubidium > strontium > iodide. They indicated that, compared to other tissues, the CNS rate of accumulation of both anions and cations is a slow and selective process.

1. *Sodium*

Sodium movement into brain extracellular fluid is similar to its movement into CSF; it probably enters the CSF largely by way of the choroid plexuses (Davson, 1967). Recently, Wright (1972) demonstrated an active sodium transport from the vascular to ventricular side of plexus cells.

2. *Potassium*

Katzman and Leiderman (1953) found that the rate of equilibration of ^{42}K between the plasma and brain of rats was slow and that despite variations in plasma potassium levels, the potassium flux into brain remained approximately the same. They concluded that potassium movement involved carrier mediation, a finding which was confirmed in a later study (Katzman *et al.*, 1965). Ames and his co-workers oberved that the potassium concentration in freshly formed choroid plexus fluid remained remarkably constant in spite of marked variations in either CSF formation rate (Ames *et al.*, 1965b) or plasma potassium levels (Ames *et al.*, 1965a). This demonstrates some form of regulatory potassium transport system by choroid plexus cells. Wright (1972) found evidence for active potassium transport from the ventricular to serosal side of plexus cells. Cserr (1965) has presented evidence that two separate transport systems are required to explain the movement of potassium from blood to brain and CSF, one located at the choroid plexus and one at the blood–brain barrier. The studies of Bito (1969) indicate that brain extracellular fluid concentrations of potassium (and magnesium) cannot be maintained by the secretory activity of the choroid plexuses and a passive diffusional barrier between blood and brain, but necessitate an active transport system across the blood–brain barrier.

   Using the technique of ventriculocisternal perfusion, Cserr (1965) recovered two thirds of perfused ^{42}K from brain tissue: presumably the remainder entered blood. When ouabain was added to the CSF perfusion fluid, ^{42}K outflux fell to 25% of control values. Since ouabain is known to poison the sodium-potassium transport mechanism, this indicates that 75% of ^{42}K outflux from CSF to brain depends on active transport. Cserr concluded that transependymal potassium exchange is passive and ascribed the active step of ^{42}K outflux to brain cells. Thus, it appeared that ^{42}K in the perfusate was exchanging primarily with brain intracellular potassium pools. Bradbury and Davson (1965), Katzman *et al.* (1965) and Anderson and Heisey (1974) used ventriculocisternal perfusion to demonstrate that ^{42}K outflux from the perfusate did not exhibit saturation kinetics; this finding is consistent with passive diffusion across the ventricular ependyma. Approximately half of the perfused ^{42}K entered the brain. Presumably, the remainder passed into blood. Depression of ^{42}K flux from CSF perfusate under the influence of ouabain was ascribed to a poisoning of the sodium-potassium pump in neurons: this would cause a decreased ^{42}K flux into brain cells and result in a reduction of ^{42}K flux from CSF (Katzman *et al.*, 1965; Bradbury and Davson, 1965).

3. Calcium

Although both active transport and passive diffusion of ^{42}Ca from blood to brain and CSF have been demonstrated (Graziani *et al.*, 1967), no evidence for active calcium transport out of CSF was found by Graziani *et al.* (1965) or Anderson *et al.* (1973). Both groups of investigators concluded that passive diffusion and CSF bulk absorption were responsible for calcium movement from CSF. Approximately 27% (Anderson and Heisey, 1974) to 33% (Graziani *et al.*, 1965) of perfused ^{45}Ca was recovered from brain tissue. The remainder probably entered the blood stream.

III. Lithium Absorption, Distribution and Mechanisms of Transport

Lithium belongs to the alkali metal group which also includes sodium, potassium, rubidium and caesium. Because of its low atomic weight (6·940) it is the lightest metal known and the third lightest element after hydrogen and helium. It has the smallest crystal radius of all the alkali metals, sodium and potassium being 1·3 and 1·7 times larger, respectively. However, lithium goes into solution after therapeutic administration, becoming hydrated. The hydrated radius of lithium is 1·2 and 1·5 times greater than sodium and potassium, respectively. Therefore, lithium ion has the largest effective diameter, lowest diffusion coefficient, and least lipid-solubility, of the alkali metals (Cotton and Wilkinson, 1972; Prockop and Marcus, 1972).[1]

A. Absorption

Ingested lithium is readily absorbed into blood from the gastrointestinal tract as evidenced by studies which demonstrate that 95% of the ingested dose can be recovered in the urine (Trautner *et al.*, 1955) and less than 1% in the faeces (Hullin *et al.*, 1966). Harrison *et al.* (1963) established that lithium was

---

[1] Expressed as mol/l, the solubilities of lithium salts in water at 25° C are: fluoride 0·05, carbonate 0·20, oxalate 0·70, sulphate 3·20, acetate 5·0, hydroxide 5·6, formate 8·0, nitrate 10·5, bromide 18·8, chloride 19·0 and chlorate 48·0.

rapidly absorbed from the duodenum and jejunum of sheep and may be detected in urine within two hours of oral administration. These findings pertain to lithium carbonate administered as a powder or in solution. Commercially, lithium carbonate is available and is frequently administered in capsule form. When administered to patients in this form, plasma levels and urinary excretion also correlates with *in vitro* dissolution rates of the capsules. Dissolution rates of different capsules vary (Sugita *et al.*, 1973).

Further, although lithium is usually given orally as the carbonate in therapy, other forms and routes of administration are available. Lithium chloride given orally to rats is absorbed to a lesser extent than lithium carbonate. Contrawise, lithium chloride is absorbed more rapidly into the blood than lithium carbonate after intraperitoneal (*i.p.*) administration. The patterns of oral and *i.p.* absorption of both compounds are similar (Morrison *et al.*, 1971). Chung *et al.* (1973) found no evidence for active lithium transport across the gastric mucosa of dogs and concluded that lithium transfer out of the gastric lumen was probably passive. Once in the blood-stream, lithium rapidly equilibrates among serum, blood cells, and certain tissues (Gershon, 1970).

B. Distribution

Radomski *et al.*, (1950) found that, generally, ingested lithium was evenly distributed among serum and heart, kidney, muscle, liver, brain and adrenal tissue of dogs. Davenport (1950) demonstrated that one hour after the intra-peritoneal injection of lithium chloride in rats, the lithium concentration in muscle was 43% of that in serum but exceeded the brain lithium concentration by almost five times. However, 24 hours post injection, brain lithium levels exceeded those in both plasma and muscle by approximately 1·5 times. Davenport concluded that bi-directional movement of lithium across the blood–brain barrier was relatively slow compared with its movement into and out of muscle tissue. In a more quantitative study, Schou (1958) injected lithium chloride intravenously into rats and found that lithium entered kidney, liver, bone, muscle, and brain tissue from blood at different rates, decreasing in the order of the listed organs. He demonstrated that the rise in kidney lithium concentration was so rapid that maximum levels were obtained within 15 minutes of injection. In liver, bone and muscle, the rise in lithium levels was somewhat slower, reaching a maximum 1, 3 and 4 hours, respectively, post injection. In brain tissue, maximum lithium concentration was not reached until between 22 and 26 hours after intravenous injection. Schou concluded that this slow movement was the result of the low permeability of the blood–brain barrier.

Morrison *et al.* (1971) confirmed these findings. After oral administration of lithium carbonate to rats, brain levels at one hour were barely detectable and generally rose to a peak at 24 hours. Brain concentrations of lithium were greater than that of plasma between 12 and 24 hours. A similar picture was seen after administration of lithium chloride.

In brain tissue, lithium has been found to concentrate in certain brain-stem structures. Post-mortem examination of the brains of two manic patients treated 3 to 4 days prior to death with lithium carbonate revealed a lithium concentration in the pons which was twice as great as those found in cerebral white and grey tissue or in cerebellar tissue (Francis and Traill, 1970). As judged from studies of evoked potentials from cats, the orbito-frontal cortex is the brain locus first affected by lithium administration (Barratt *et al.*, 1970).

The entrance of lithium into CSF has been repeatedly demonstrated. Hanlon *et al.*, (1949) found that the CSF and serum concentrations of lithium in one case of lithium poisoning were 1·5 and 2·6 mEq/l respectively, yielding a CSF/serum ratio for lithium of 0·58. Similarly, Schou *et al.* (1954) determined that 1 to 2 weeks after the onset of lithium treatment in six cases of manic psychosis, the CSF/serum ratio ranged between 0·33 and 0·67. Gershon and Yuwiler (1960) demonstrated that CSF lithium levels are indefinitely maintained at 40 to 60% of the plasma level in patients to whom lithium had been administered for several weeks. In addition, in animal studies, Gershon (1970) found that two days after lithium administration total lithium brain levels were about 50% of those in plasma. Eight hours following lithium carbonate ingestion, Baker and Winokur (1966) calculated an average CSF/plasma ratio of 0·24, a value which is somewhat lower than those discussed above. Similarly, Platman and Fieve (1968) demonstrated that lithium CSF/serum ratios increased from 0·04 after 2 to 4 hours following ingestion of lithium carbonate, to 0·28, 24 hours post-administration. The lower lithium CSF/serum ratios reported in these last two studies perhaps indicate that lithium does not come into equilibrium among blood, CSF and brain tissues until 24 hours post-administration, even though Platman and Fieve (1968) reported a fixed CSF/plasma ratio as being established 8 hours following lithium administration. Schou's finding that lithium equilibration between brain tissue and serum was not obtained by 48 hours after intravenous injection of lithium chloride in rats is a further indication of a long lithium equilibration time among blood, CSF and brain, resulting from the very slow passage of this ion across the barriers separating the three systems.

Platman *et al.* (1968) found indications that between 2 and 4 hours after oral lithium administration, lithium movement into the CSF of manic patients is more rapid than normal, whereas its movement into the CSF of depressed patients is less rapid than normal. However, 8 hours after administration, Baker and Winokur (1966) could find no significant difference between the CSF lithium levels of manic patients and those of non-manic psychiatric control patients.

Injected lithium has no effect on the CSF sodium or potassium levels in either humans (Platman *et al.*, 1968) or animals (Smith and Balagura, 1972). In addition, injected lithium carbonate does not alter the total sodium or potassium in the brains of rats (Greenspan *et al.*, 1970). Likewise, lithium does not change the sodium transfer rate from blood to brain tissues (Amdisen and Schou, 1968).

C. Mechanisms of lithium transport

1. *Kinetics of entry into the CNS*

Lithium has been shown to enter a variety of tissues from blood. The characteristics governing its kinetics of entry into the central nervous system have not been defined. Because little information is available to explain lithium transport across the membranes of the blood–CNS interface, data concerning lithium movement across other biological membranes should be reviewed. Experiments on lithium flux in frog skin, frog muscle, erythrocytes and mammalian nerve tissue, i.e., non-myelinated C-fibres, have been performed. The flux rate for lithium entry into frog muscle is similar to the passive influx rate of sodium (Keynes and Swan, 1959). Also, lithium and sodium influx permeability coefficients are of the same order of magnitude for erythrocytes (Maizels, 1954). In both tissues, there appears to be no active efflux of lithium comparable to that of sodium, e.g., lithium outflux is only 4 to 10% as fast as that of sodium in frog muscle (Keynes and Swan, 1959). Armett and Richie (1963) found the resting permeability of mammalian non-myelinated C-fibers to lithium was about 70% of that of sodium. Because they did not specifically determine the mode of lithium flux in this neural tissue, they were not able to decide if lithium is actively extruded from the nerve fibers.

Although the data cited above seem to indicate that in the tissues studied active transport of lithium is absent, there is some evidence for active lithium transport in certain epithelial membranes. Herrera *et al.* (1971) demonstrated that lithium flux across toad urinary bladder was inhibited by ouabain. The authors indicate that since ouabain is an inhibitor of the sodium active transport mechanism or pump, their data suggest that lithium moves across the bladder using at least some of the sodium active transport pathway. Zerahn (1955) demonstrated that lithium and sodium competed equally for the same transport pathway in frog skin. Further, he established that frog skin transported lithium against both an electrical and chemical gradient and concluded that the transport process was active in nature. Recently, Candia and Chiarandini (1973) confirmed that under certain conditions lithium was actively transported by frog skin. They found that when sodium was replaced by lithium at the inner surface of the frog skin, the sodium pump was inhibited in a manner similar to that of ouabain. However, lithium was actively transported (by the sodium pump) for several hours when lithium was placed only on the outside of the skin leaving a sodium solution on the inside. These workers concluded that the lithium ion can both inhibit the sodium pump and be actively transported by it, depending on the location of the lithium ion.

Although the above data indicate that certain epithelial membranes are capable of active lithium transport, there is no indication that the same is true of the epithelial membranes separating blood, CSF, and brain tissue (Prockop and Marcus, 1972; Wright, 1972). For example, Wright incubated frog choroid plexus, which is epithelial tissue, *in vitro* in Ringer's solutions containing a variety of test substances, including sodium, potassium, rubidium, caesium, and lithium. He found no evidence of active transport of lithium. In addition, as judged by diffusion potential measurements, lithium has the lowest passive permeability coefficient for choroid plexus tissue among the alkali metals.

2. *Lithium clearance from CSF*

Prockop and Marcus (1972) performed a series of studies to determine whether a specific mechanism, e.g., carrier-mediated transport, maintains CSF lithium levels at 40 to 60% of those in plasma. Because the choroid plexus is an important site for the regulation of water and electrolyte balance of the CSF, *in vitro* rabbit choroid plexus studies were performed. It has been well established that choroid plexus tissue concentrates a variety of substances contained in artificial CSF used as an incubating medium (Welch, 1962; Robinson *et al.*, 1968). In their studies Prockop and Marcus incubated choroid plexus in artificial CSF containing both lithium and iodide (Na ^{131}I). After incubation, the tissue (choroid plexus) to medium (artificial CSF) ratio for iodide was in the range of 30 : 1. Contrawise, lithium was not concentrated. The T:M ratios of less than 1 were compatible with lithium movement into the tissue by simple diffusion (see Table I).

TABLE I. Data from 2 representative *in vitro* studies in which rabbit choroid plexus (tissue) was incubated in artificial CSF (medium) to determine tissue: medium ratios.

TISSUE: MEDIUM RATIOS FOR LITHIUM AND IODIDE IN
2 CHOROID PLEXUS INCUBATIONS

TEST SUBSTANCE	1	2
LITHIUM CARBONATE	0,4	0,9
I ^{131}	31,3	24,0

The same investigators also performed ventriculocisternal perfusion studies in dogs. By this technique, artificial CSF containing test substances was perfused *in vivo* from a lateral ventricle to the cisterna magna. All test substances were cleared from artificial CSF by bulk flow and simple diffusion. Some substances, however, were also cleared by a specialized transport mechanism, e.g., facilitated diffusion or active transport. In their study, Prockop and Marcus found that total lithium clearance could be accounted for by bulk flow and simple diffusion. For example (see Table II), lithium net clearance rate was low, in the same order of magnitude of creatinine for which clearance by simple diffusion has been well defined. These studies indicate that it is likely that bulk flow of lithium into the venous system is the major factor responsible for a normal CSF/plasma lithium ratio of less than unity. Although this work indicates that lithium probably equilibrates between CSF and brain tissue by

TABLE II. Data from *in vivo* studies in dogs in which artificial CSF containing creatinine, lithium carbonate and rose bengal I^{131} was perfused from the lateral cerebral ventricle to the cisterna magna to determine clearance rates, i.e., diffusional permeability coefficients (K_{Dx}).

VENTRICULO-CISTERNAL PERFUSION: CLEARANCE OF
SUBSTANCES FROM ARTIFICIAL CSF

TEST SUBSTANCE	CONCENTRATION IN CSF	CLEARANCE RATE: K_{Dx} (ML/MIN)
CREATININE	3.18 mM	0.041
LITHIUM CARBONATE	3.8 mM	0.053
ROSE BENGAL I 131	TRACER	0.332

passive means, it does not establish the mechanism of lithium entry from blood into CSF and/or brain tissue. Although it is probably a passive process, there are, at present, no studies which quantitate the influx of lithium into CSF or brain tissue from plasma. These studies are in progress in this laboratory.

References

Amdisen, A. and Schou, M. (1968). *Psychopharmacologia* **12**, 236–238.
Ames, A., Higashi, K. and Nesbett, F. B. (1965a). *J. Physiol.* **181**, 506–515.
Ames, A., Higashi, K. and Nesbett, F. B. (1965b). *J. Physiol.* **181**, 516–524.
Anderson, D. K. and Heisey, S. R. (1974). *Amer. J. Physiol.* In press.
Armett, C. J. and Richie, J. M. (1963). *J. Physiol.* **165**, 130–140.
Baker, M. A. and Winokur, G. (1966). *Brit. J. Psychiat.* **112**, 163–165.
Barlow, C. F. (1964). *A. Rev. Med.* **15**, 187–207.
Barratt, E. S., Russell, G., Creson, D. and Tupin, J. (1970). *Dis. nerv. Syst.* **31**, 335–337.
Bito, L. Z. (1969). *Science* **165**, 81–83.

Bradbury, M. W. B. and Davson, H. (1964). *J. Physiol.* **170,** 195–211.
Bradbury, M. W. B. and Davson, H. (1965). *J. Physiol.* **181,** 151–174.
Cade, J. F. J. (1949). *Med. J. Aust* **36,** 349–352.
Candia, O. A. and Chiarandini, D. J. (1973). *Biochim. biophys. Acta* **307,** 578–589.
Chung, R. S. K., Field, M. and Silen, W. (1973). *Gastroenterol.* **64,** 593–598.
Cotton, F. A. and Wilkinson, G. W. (1972). *In* "Advanced Inorganic Chemistry". 3rd Ed. Wiley, New York.
Crone, C. (1965). *J. Physiol.* **181,** 103–113.
Cserr, H. (1965). *Amer. J. Physiol.* **290,** 1219–1226.
Davenport, V. D. (1950). *Amer. J. Physiol.* **163,** 633–641.
Davson, H. (1967). *In* "Physiology of the Cerebrospinal Fluid". Churchill, London.
Dobbing, J. (1968). *In* "Brain Barrier System" (C. A. Lajtha and D. A. Ford, Eds), pp. 417–427. Ekerer, New York.
Fencl, V., Miller, T. B. and Pappenheimer, J. R. (1966). *Amer. J. Physiol.* **210,** 459–472.
Fishman, R. A. (1964). *Am. J. Physiol.* **206,** 836–844.
Francis, R. I. and Traill, M. A. (1970). *Lancet* **2,** 523–524.
Gershon, S. (1970). *Clin. Pharmacol. Ther.* **11,** 168–187.
Gershon, S. and Yuwiler, A. (1960). *J. Neuropsychiat.* **1,** 229–241.
Giese, A. C. (1973). *In* "Cell Physiology". 4th Edition. Saunders, Philadelphia.
Graziani, L., Escriva, A. and Katzman, R. (1965). *Amer. J. Physiol.* **208,** 1058–1064.
Graziani, L., Kaplan, R. K., Escriva, A. and Katzman, R. (1967). *Amer. J. Physiol.* **213,** 629–636.
Greenburg, D. M., Aired, R. B., Boelter, M. D. D., Campbell, W. W., Cohn, W. E. and Murayma, M. M. (1943). *Amer. J. Physiol.* **140,** 47–64.
Greenspan, K., Aronoff, M. S. and Bogdanski, D. F. (1970). *Pharmacol.* **3,** 129–136.
Hanlon, L. W., Romaine, M., Gilroy, F. L. and Deitrick, J. E. (1949). *J. Amer. med. Assoc.* **139,** 688–692.
Harrison, F. A., Hill, K. J. and Mangan, J. L. (1963). *Biochem. J.* **89,** 99P–100P.
Held, D., Fencl, V. and Pappenheimer, J. R. (1964). *J. Neurophysiol.* **27,** 942–959.
Herrera, F. C., Egea, R. and Herrera, A. M. (1971). *Amer. J. Physiol.* **220,** 1501–1508.
Hullin, R. P., McDonald, R. and Dransfield, G. A. (1966). *In* "Proc. IV World. Congr. Psychiat." pp. 1900–1903. Excerpta Medica Foundation, I. C. S. 150.
Katzman, R. and Leiderman, P. H. (1953). *Amer. J. Physiol.* **175,** 263–270.
Katzman, R., Graziani, L., Kaplan, R. and Escriva, A. (1965). *Archs. Neurol.* **13,** 513–524.
Keynes, R. D. and Swan, R. C. (1959). *J. Physiol.* **47,** 626–638.
Lee, J. C. (1971). *In* "Progress in Neuropathology". (H. M. Zimmerman, ed.). pp. 84–145. Grune and Stratton, New York.
Maizels, M. (1954). *Symp. Soc. exp. Biol. Med.* **8,** 202–227.
Maynard, E. A., Schultz, R. L. and Pease, D. C. (1957). *Amer. J. Anat.* **10,** 490–433.
Morrison, J. M., Pritchard, H. D., Brande, M. C. and D'Aguanns, W. (1971). *Proc. Soc. exp. Biol. Med.* **137,** 889–892.
Mottschall, H. J. and Leoschke, H. H. (1963). *Pflug. Archs ges. Physiol.* **277,** 662–670.
Pappenheimer, J. R., Heisey, S. R. and Jordan, E. F. (1961). *Amer. J. Physiol.* **200,** 1–10.
Platman, S. R. and Fieve, R. R. (1968). *Archs gen. Psychiat.* **19,** 659–663.
Platman, S. R., Rohrlich, J. and Fieve, R. R. (1968). *Dis. nerv. Syst.* **29,** 733–738.
Prockop, L. D. (1973). *In* "Biology of Brain Dysfunction" Vol. I. (G. E. Garrett, ed.). pp. 229–263. Plenum Press, New York.
Prockop, L. D. and Marcus, D. J. (1972). *Life Sci.* **11,** 859–868.

Radomski, J. L., Fuyat, H. N., Nelson, A. A. and Smith, P. K. (1950). *J. Pharmacol. exp. Ther.* **100,** 429–444.

Robinson, R. J., Cutler, R. W. P., Lorenzo, A. V. and Barlow, C. F. (1968). *J. Neurochem.* **15,** 1169–1179.

Schou, M. (1957). *Pharmacol. Rev.* **9,** 17–58.

Schou, M. (1958). *Acta Pharmacol.* **15,** 115–124.

Schou, M., Juel-Nielsen, N., Strömgren, E. and Voldby, H. (1954). *J. Neurol. Neurosurg. Psychiat.* **17,** 250–260.

Smith, D. F. and Balagura, S. (1972). *Physiol. Behav.* **9,** 261–262.

Sugita, E. T., Stokes, J. W., Frazer, A., Grof, P., Mendels, J., Goldstein, F. J. and Niebergall, P. J. (1973). *J. Clin. Pharm.* **13,** 264–270.

Trautner, E. M., Morris, R., Noack, C. H. and Gershon, S. (1955). *Med. J. Aust.* **42,** 280–291.

Wallace, G. B. and Brodie, B. B. (1940). *J. Pharmacol. Exp. Ther.* **70,** 418–427.

Welch, K. (1962). *Amer. J. Physiol.* **202,** 757–760.

Wright, E. M. (1972). *J. Physiol.* **226,** 525–571.

Zerahn, K. (1955). *Acta physiol. scand.* **33,** 347–358.

17

TISSUE DISTRIBUTION PATTERNS OF LITHIUM IN THE AFFECTIVE DISORDERS

K. GREENSPAN

I. Background to the Lithium Distribution Studies

In 1955 Noack and Trautner reported that lithium ions were preferentially retained during the manic state (positive lithium balance) and diuresed with recovery (negative lithium balance). They commented:

> "The amount retained by healthy persons varies with the individual, the dosage, the diet (salt and fluid intake) and probably other factors . . . . Maniacal patients appear to retain considerably higher amounts at the beginning of the treatment . . . . Then, quite abruptly, profuse elution starts coincidentally with the reduction in the maniacal symptoms." (p. 220)

and again:

> "The excretion of lithium reflects the clinical state, in so far as maniacal patients tend to retain lithium as long as the mania lasts and begin to excrete it as soon as the maniacal state begins to abate—and possibly retain it again when another maniacal attack is imminent". (p. 220).

Similar findings were also noted by Trautner *et al.* (1955). Initial criticisms of these studies were many, and an attempt by Epstein *et al.* (1965) to replicate the observations, failed to note any difference in 24-hour lithium excretion rates between manic patients and non-manic controls. The author of the present chapter, in collaboration with Dr. Jack Durell, attempted to repeat the work of

281

Trautner and his associates and this chapter is devoted to an outline of the findings of these further investigations, and to some speculations for future research.

It had been assumed by the earlier investigators that both in the acutely manic patient and in the normal control the lithium ion was distributed equally throughout the body's water compartment. Indeed, the over-all body tissue: plasma lithium ratio was thought to approximate unity. Radomski and his associates (1950) and Talso and Clarke (1951), for example, reported that there was little difference between the total body water volume and calculations of the lithium space, and it was suggested that lithium was not differentially distributed amongst the various body organs (Radomski *et al.*, 1950). Other studies also appeared to confirm this general impression. Thus, Bertrand (1951) noted that the erythrocyte and serum levels of naturally-occurring lithium were more or less the same. Schou (1957), however, reviewed a wide range of studies in which various tissue lithium concentrations had been examined under steady state conditions, and drew attention to differences in the rate of uptake of lithium into body organs; he also included his own observations that tissues might differ quite markedly in the manner in which they concentrated lithium—some appeared to do so against a serum-tissue gradient, whereas others, such as cerebrospinal fluid (Schou *et al.*, 1954), had tissue concentrations lower than the simultaneously observed serum concentrations. Schou (1957) concluded that "althouth the lithium concentrations in extracellular and intracellular fluid do not differ greatly, there is for each organ a distinct concentration gradient across the cell wall." (p. 36).

II. The Lithium Distribution Studies in Manic Patients

This background of interesting observations, though not leading to any clearly consistent picture, served as a stimulus for our study of lithium ion retention and distribution patterns in manic-depressive patients. The patients were studied during acutely manic, acutely depressed, and relatively normothymic states, in an effort to clarify the specific patterns of lithium distribution associated with each state.

We were able to study our first patient during an acute manic phase and then, 4 months later, during a relatively normothymic phase. While acutely manic the patient retained 152 mg of lithium ion and then went into a phase of negative lithium balance while being maintained on a constant daily lithium carbonate dosage. On the other hand, when the same dosage of lithium carbonate was administered during the relatively normothymic state the maximum lithium retained was 45 mg and there was no period of appreciable negative lithium balance (Greenspan *et al.*, 1968a). The findings during acute mania thus seemed broadly confirmatory of those of Trautner and his associates.

In collaboration with Bunney and Goodwin, additional manic and normal subjects were studied, with results which were consistent with our initial findings (Greenspan et al., 1968a). In all cases, lithium administered during the manic phase was better retained in the body tissues than when the patients were normothymic. Furthermore, shortly after the commencement of clinical improvement there always occurred a period of negative lithium balance. These effects were, however, only observed after the second day of lithium treatment, and this may explain the negative results reported by Epstein et al. (1965) after only 24 hours lithium treatment.

To clarify further the significance of these findings an apparent lithium space was computed for each patient and compared to the estimated total body water. Rather more than 95% of ingested lithium can be recovered in urine · (Radomski et al., 1950), and the amount retained may be determined by subtracting the quantity recovered in urine from the quantity ingested. The total retained was computed by summing the daily retention values. The apparent lithium space was then calculated by dividing the total lithium retained by the plasma lithium concentration. Total body water space was estimated by referring to Moore's nomogram relating body weight to total body water in normals (Moore et al., 1963). If, as is frequently assumed (Trautner et al., 1955), the lithium ion is distributed equally throughout the body water, the normalized apparent lithium space (apparent lithium space divided by estimated total body water space) should approximate 1·0.

The ratio derived by dividing the apparent lithium space by the mean value of the estimated total body water, and referred to as the normalized maximal apparent lithium space, varied from 1·1 to 1·5 in normothymic patients, whereas in acutely manic patients it varied from 1·7 to 3·1. It thus appears that the assumption of an approximately equal distribution of the lithium ion throughout all body fluids, whilst more or less true for normothymic patients, is not valid for patients in the manic state. The excess lithium retained by manic patients must be stored either in certain intracellular fluids or in extracellular fluids other than plasma.

III. The Lithium Distribution Studies in Depressed Patients

Lithium distribution patterns were also examined in three acutely depressed patients (Greenspan et al., 1968b). All three patients were males, two possessing histories of both manic and depressive states and the third a history of recurrent depression and acute intermittent porphyria. Two patients were maintained on low sodium diets supplemented with salt tablets, whilst the third was on a catechol-free acid ash diet with a controlled salt intake. Clinical status was rated daily, both by the psychiatrist in charge (non-blind) and by a trained rater using the Hamilton Depression Rating Scale (Hamilton. 1960). Both patients and nursing staff were not aware of the time of onset and offset of lithium medication. Two of the patients received 33 mEq lithium ion daily, and the third 49 mEq.

In the three acutely depressed patients studied there was little or no negative lithium balance and normalized maximal apparent lithium spaces were generally less than 1·5. These observations correspond to previous results obtained from normothymic patients. The normalized apparent lithium spaces were plotted against time for the period that each patient was on a constant lithium intake. The first two days' observations were ignored because of their instability and regression equations were then computed for the remaining points. In all cases there was a statistically significant negative slope of the normalized apparent lithium space, the values tending towards unity with continuing lithium treatment. It is interesting that in all threee cases there was a marked decrease in depressive symptoms during the same period.

The data are insufficient for it to be concluded that lithium redistribution was causally related to recovery from depression: it may be simply coincidental. It is necessary to look at lithium redistribution in patients who fail to recover during lithium treatment, and more extensive studies are also required of normothymic patients and normal controls. It must be emphasized that although the lithium distribution changes are statistically significant they are also small in comparison to the much larger redistributions and negative lithium balances observed in manic patients.

The possibility that depressed patients may show similar, though less marked, patterns of lithium ion distribution to those noted in manic patients is interesting, particularly in the light of findings such as those of Coppen *et al.* (1965) of similarities between the two types of patient in sodium ion distribution.

IV. Changes in Saliva Lithium Levels

Shopsin *et al.* (1969) noted that within an hour of the ingestion of lithium carbonate by mouth, lithium could be detected in both serum and saliva, the concentrations in each rising less sharply in manic than in control patients. The relationship between salivary and serum lithium concentrations was expressed as:

Serum Concentration = $(0·46 \times$ Saliva Concentration $- 0·05) \pm 0·34$.

There was found to be an association between lithium concentration in saliva and the onset of recovery from mania. The saliva lithium levels reached peak values about a week after the commencement of lithium treatment: progressive improvement in the patients' clinical status was reported during this time. Decrease in manic symptoms was then followed by a continuous fall in saliva lithium values reminiscent of the massive elution noted by both Trautner *et al.* (1955) and Greenspan *et al.* (1968a, b).

V. Intra-: Extra-Cellular Lithium Ratios; Studies on Erythrocytes

In 1972, Elizur *et al.* examined the relationship between erythrocyte and plasma levels of lithium in psychiatric patients and in hospitalized normal control subjects. They found that both mania and depression were associated with lower erythrocyte lithium concentrations than were noted in either the normal controls or in the manic-depressive patients in their inter-episode periods of normality. There was some suggestion that the effect was more marked during depressive than during manic episodes.

Attention was also directed to this aspect of lithium tissue distribution by Frazer *et al.* (1973) who administered lithium to rats on both chronic and acute schedules. It was found that erythrocyte levels of lithium provided better predictive indices of brain levels than did plasma levels, and it was suggested that if the same were true for humans, then erythrocyte levels might correlate with clinical response to lithium treatment. Mendels and Frazer (1973) subsequently examined the erythrocyte and plasma lithium levels in a number of depressed patients and they reported that the likelihood of clinical improvement was a function of high erythrocyte lithium concentrations and high erythrocyte:plasma lithium ratios. They suggested that their results were indicative of a difference in cell membrane transfer mechanisms in clinical responders and non-responders to lithium therapy.

VI. Conclusions

There is clearly a great need for further studies in the area of lithium tissue distribution, particularly as it may relate to prevailing mood state and to the likely result of lithium therapy. The findings which have been produced to date are undoubtedly intriguing, but they are not sufficiently detailed to allow unequivocal conclusions to be drawn. It will be necessary too to look not only at lithium distributions, but also at concomitant changes in the distribution of other ions, particularly sodium and potassium and possibly also magnesium and calcium, if the full implications of the experimental findings are to become clear.

References

Bertrand, D. (1951). *Bull. Soc. Chim. biol.* **33**, 827–828.
Coppen, A., Malleson, A. and Shaw, D. M. (1965). *Lancet* **1**, 682–683.
Elizur, A., Shopsin, B., Gershon, S. and Ehlenberger, A. (1972). *Clin. Pharmacol. Ther.* **13**, 947–952.
Epstein, R., Grant, L. and Herjanic, M. (1965). *J. Amer. med. Assoc.* **192**, 409–410.
Frazer, A., Mendels, J., Secunda, S. K., Cochrane, C. M. and Bianchi, C. P. (1973). *J. psychiat. Res.* **10**, 1–7.
Greenspan, K., Goodwin, F. K., Bunney, W. E. and Durell, J. (1968a). *Archs gen. Psychiat.* **19**, 664–673.
Greenspan, K., Green, R. and Durell, J. (1968b). *Amer. J. Psychiat.* **125**, 512–519.

Hamilton, M. (1960). *J. Neurol. Neurosurg. Psychiat.* **23,** 56–62.

Mendels, J. and Frazer, A. (1973). *J. psychiat. Res.* **10,** 9–18.

Moore, F. D., Olesen, K. H., McMurrey, J. D., Parker, H. V., Ball, M. R. and Boyden, C. M. (1963). *In* "The Body Cell Mass and Its Supporting Environment". Saunders, Philadelphia.

Noack, C. H. and Trautner, E. M. (1951). *Med. J. Aust.* **38,** 219–222.

Radomski, J. L., Fuyat, H. N., Nelson, A. A. and Smith, P. K. (1950). *J. Pharmacol. exp. Ther.* **100,** 429–444.

Schou, M. (1957). *Pharmacol. Rev.* **9,** 17–58.

Schou, M., Juel-Nielsen, M., Strömgren, E. and Voldby, H. (1954). *J. Neurol. Psychiat.* **17,** 250–260.

Shopsin, B., Gershon, S. and Pinckney, L. (1969). *Int. Pharmacopsychiat.* **2,** 148–169.

18

THE EXCRETION OF LITHIUM

B. Fyrö and G. Sedvall

I. Introduction

Of the total amount of lithium ingested in man more than 98% is excreted in the urine. The remaining fraction is excreted in faeces, sweat and saliva (Kent and

McCance, 1941, Talso and Clarke, 1951). The renal handling of lithium is related to a number of mechanisms, several of which may markedly influence the rate of lithium elimination from the body. The narrow therapeutic range of lithium in man necessitates the maintenance of a serum level between 0·8 and 1·2 mEq/l. Since the elevation of lithium concentrations above this level is rapidly followed by a number of severe toxic symptoms, a detailed knowledge of the renal handling mechanisms for lithium is required. Thus the possibilities of maintaining optimal steady-state levels of lithium in body fluids and of initiating rational treatment of lithium intoxication represent the most important reasons for the detailed discussion on lithium handling in the kidney, which follows below. By its effect on renal elimination of electrolytes, water and organic compounds, lithium may also change a number of homeostatic mechanisms in the organism which may be related to the pathophysiology of affective disorders. Studies on this aspect of the mechanism of action of lithium are closely related to the effect of lithium on renal function and will therefore be considered in this chapter.

II. Renal Function and Electrolyte Metabolism

As discussed in detail in Chapter 21 the physical and chemical characteristics of the lithium ion resemble those of the alkali metals sodium and potassium. Its fate in cells and tissues including those of the kidney is therefore to some extent similar to that of the mentioned cations (Zerahn, 1955; Sexton and Meyer, 1955). Before considering how lithium is handled in the kidney a brief review of modern theories on renal function as regards electrolyte and water transport is necessary.

The most important function of the kidney lies in the homeostatic control of the volume and composition of the body fluids. The kidneys of man have been calculated to contain about 1 million nephrons. A nephron consists of the glomerulus and the tubular system (Fig. 1). Out of the glomerulus, which is a capillary system invaginated in the upper closed end of the epithelial tube of the tubule, fluid and permeable solute ions and molecules are filtered from the plasma into the tubular system. The filtering force is the hydrostatic pressure of the blood; the concentration of the diffusible element is practically the same in the glomerular filtrate as it is in the plasma. Ultrafiltration experiments (Talso and Clarke, 1951; Foulks et al., 1952) have shown that lithium is not protein-bound in body fluids and therefore it diffuses freely from plasma into the tubular system surrounding the glomerulus. The lithium concentration in the primary urine will accordingly approximate that of the plasma. The composition of this primary urine as regards fluid and electrolytes including lithium will be substantially altered during its further passage through the tubular system.

Each tubulus which is about 3–4 cm long forms, during its passage from the glomerulus to the collecting tube, a proximal and a distal convolution. Between

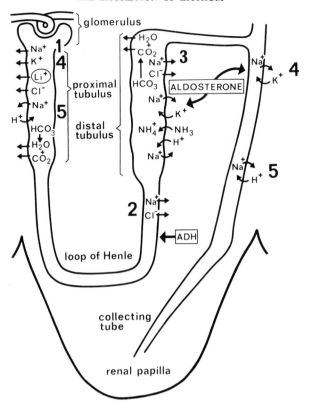

FIG. 1. Schematic illustration of mechanisms for the elimination of electrolytes and fluid from the kidney.

these convolutions the loop of Henle passes towards the papillae. The importance of the reabsorbing function of the renal tubules to the body economy should be emphasized and can be illustrated by a few quantitative considerations. The rate of the glomerular filtration in the healthy adult is about 125 ml/min. In such an individual the extracellular fluid volume is approximately 12·5 litres. Thus a volume equivalent to the total extracellular fluid is filtered across the glomerular capillary bed into the tubules within a period of about 100 minutes. During this time only about 100 ml of urine reaches the bladder. Therefore the tubules normally reabsorb over 99% of the glomerular filtrate. Thus the composition of the tubular absorbate must approximate that of the extra-cellular fluid otherwise severe distortions in the composition of the extracellular fluid would result. The reabsorption of electrolytes of certain molecular species from tubular urine to tubular cells and from those cells to the extracellular fluid is achieved by active transport. For such processes the tubular cells expend large amounts of energy which is derived from metabolic activity. As depicted in Fig. 1 the reabsorption of electrolytes from the tubular system can be divided into several processes.

1. *Proximal reabsorption of sodium*

This process occurs by active cellular transport susceptible to inhibition by pharmacological agents such as diuretics. Under normal conditions this process accounts for the reabsorption of 70 to 80% of the filtered sodium. As discussed in detail below the major fraction of lithium filtered is also reabsorbed by the sodium transport mechanism within this region. The renal epithelium in the proximal tubule is permeable to the diffusion of water so that as solutes are reabsorbed proportional amounts of water diffuse out of the tubule and the tubular fluid remains essentially iso-osmotic with plasma.

2. *Sodium reabsorption from the loop of Henle.*

Here the absorbed quantity may be less significant than that occurring in the proximal tubule but it is of unique importance in determining the final solute concentration of the urine. The descending and ascending thin loops of Henle have different permeabilities to sodium and water. As sodium is absorbed, water does not freely diffuse, so that the solute concentration in the interstitium in the renal medulla becomes hyperosmotic.

3. *Distal reabsorption of sodium*

The absolute amount of sodium reabsorbed in this area is determined not only by the amount filtered but also by the proportion of the filtrate that has already undergone reabsorption at more proximal sites. This distal sodium reabsorption mechanism appears to have discrete sensitivities to the action of adrenocortical hormone and to diuretics. Moreover it seems to have a lower affinity for lithium transport. The permeability of the renal epithelium to water is a function under physiological control. The antidiuretic hormone (ADH), which is an octapeptide (du Vigneaud et al., 1954), has a direct effect on the distal tubules by facilitating water diffusion.

4. *Potassium reabsorption and secretion.*

Potassium undergoes both tubular reabsorption and secretion. Reabsorption occurs largely in the proximal tubule. Secretion is a more distal phenomenon and can be described in terms of a sodium–potassium exchange. The wide variations in the amount of potassium actually excreted are presumably attributable to the secretory mechanism. The amount of sodium in the distal tubule may be an important determinant of the amount of potassium secreted and hence excreted.

5. Sodium-hydrogen exchange.

Pitts and associates demonstrated in 1945 that the amount of acid in the voided urine could not be accounted for by the selective reabsorption of constituents of the glomerular filtrate (Pitts, 1959). This suggested that hydrogen ions were secreted into the urine by tubular cells. Pitts postulated that the source of hydrogen ion secreted by the tubular cell was carbonic acid derived from the hydration of carbon dioxide. The mechanisms involved in tubular hydrogen secretion can be considered in terms of an underlying sodium-hydrogen exchange mechanism.

During physiological conditions the hydration of carbon dioxide proceeds rapidly to supply the amount of hydrogen ion necessary for the exchange reactions. However, this rate can only be achieved if the hydration is catalyzed by the enzyme carbonic anhydrase. Inhibition of this enzyme by drugs like acetazolamide results in excretion of large volumes of alkaline urine.

6. Measurement of glomerular filtration.

The rate of glomerular filtration can be determined in animals and man by measuring the renal excretion of substances that are neither secreted nor reabsorbed by the renal tubule. The technique introduced by Rehberg and elaborated by Homer Smith and his collaborators has contributed substantially to the knowledge of the mechanisms of renal function and it will be briefly described. Certain substances like inulin in man and creatinine in the dog readily pass the glomerular membrane and are not reabsorbed by the tubules. Furthermore they do not gain access to the urine by tubular secretion. Thus the amount of the substance excreted in the urine over a given period of time is a measure of the amount filtered by the glomeruli. It is only necessary to divide this total amount in the urine by the concentration of the substance in the glomerular filtrate to determine the volume of filtrate from which the urine was derived. Since the glomerular filtrate is an ultrafiltrate of plasma the concentration of a substance in glomerular fluid can be ascertained by determining the concentration in plasma. It also follows that the ratio of the concentration of such a substance in plasma and urine provides direct information as to the amount of water reabsorbed by the tubule.

7. Measurement of renal clearance.

Clearance is a concept found useful to describe the renal handling of a substance. It is computed from the formula:

$$C = \frac{U \cdot V}{P}$$

where C = clearance (ml/min); U = concentration of the substance in urine mEq/l; V = urine flow (ml/min); P = concentration of the substance in plasma mEq/ml.

Verbally the clearance for a substance represents the theoretical volume of plasma that is completely cleared of the compound per minute by renal excretion. In healthy men inulin clearance is about 125 ml/min which, as mentioned above, represents the glomerular filtration rate. Compounds which are reabsorbed in the tubules have lower clearance values than inulin whereas compounds with higher clearance values are secreted by the tublar cells into the urine. Some compounds are so efficiently excreted by the tubules that the blood is completely cleared of the compound by a single passage through the kidney. The clearance for such a compound, paraaminohippuric acid (Pah), can accordingly be used for the determination of renal plasma flow, which is in the order of 600 ml/min in the healthy adult human.

III. Mechanisms for Renal Lithium Elimination

A. Lithium clearance

Over the last twenty years, elimination of lithium has been the subject for a number of studies supplying important information. However, lithium excretion is still to a large extent insufficiently understood, especially as regards the molecular mechanisms for its transport in the kidney. Since data from animal experiments indicate substantial species variations the following discussion will mainly cover studies on renal lithium elimination in man.

Ultrafiltration experiments over cellulose membranes (Talso and Clarke, 1951; Foulks et al., 1952) have demonstrated that lithium is not bound to plasma proteins. One must therefore presume that the lithium ion is freely filterable across the glomerular membrane. Micropuncture studies of the tubular system in animals actually proving this assumption do not seem to have been performed. Thomsen and Schou (1968) found that the renal lithium clearance in healthy human subjects is about 20 ml/min. Since the glomerular filtration rate is in the order of 125 ml/min, a major fraction of the lithium ion filtered in the glomerulus must accordingly be reabsorbed actively or passively in the tubules. If the reabsorption of lithium were due to passive back-diffusion the elimination would vary with the rate of water excretion. In experiments on dogs (Talso and Clarke, 1951) and on rats (Schou, 1958) no correlation was found between lithium excretion and the rate of urine flow, nor could Thomsen and Schou (1968) find any significant effect of excessive water loading on lithium clearance in man. Therefore the view suggested by Foulks et al. (1952) that lithium reabsorption may be accomplished by a process of passive back diffusion is unlikely. A reabsorption mediated by active transport seems more in line with the available experimental evidence. This view is also compatible with the occurrence of a mutual interaction of lithium and sodium excretion as discussed below. Studies in dogs and man (Talso and Clarke, 1951; Thomsen and Schou, 1968; Fyrö et al., 1973) have demonstrated that the lithium clearance is largely independent of serum concentrations below the upper therapeutic range. This indicates that lithium transporting mechanisms in the kidney are not saturated at therapeutic lithium concentrations.

B. Relation to Na⁺ excretion

The relation between renal lithium and sodium elimination has been extensively studied both experimentally and clinically. The stimulus to such studies was the early observation of an inverse relation between lithium toxicity and sodium intake (Corcoran *et al.*, 1949; Hanlon *et al.*, 1949; Radomski *et al.*, 1950). Schou (1958) studied the renal lithium elimination in rats. He found that the fraction of filtered lithium excreted in the urine could vary considerably and that it was closely related to both the filtered lithium load and the urinary sodium excretion. A number of studies (Zerahn, 1955; Sexton and Meyer, 1955, and others) have demonstrated that lithium and sodium ions may compete for entrance into, or transport through, animal cells. A similar competition presumably also takes place in the kidney tubules. Thomsen and Schou (1968) studied the effect in man of a sodium-poor and sodium-enriched diet on renal lithium clearance. As demonstrated in Fig. 2 the lithium excretion

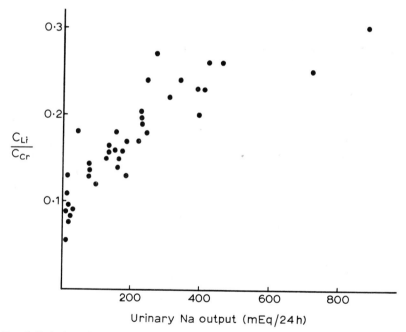

FIG. 2. Relation of lithium excretion fraction (C_{Li}/C_{Cr}) to urinary sodium output under dietary regimens with varying sodium intake. (From Thomsen and Schou, 1968, with permission.)

fraction $C_{Li}/C_{creatinine}$ in the dog was less than 0·1 during sodium deprivation and it rose to about 0·3 during salt loadings. These findings and others are compatible with the view that lithium and sodium ions compete for a transport mechanism within the tubular system. Whereas about 99% of filtered sodium is reabsorbed in the tubules the fraction of reabsorbed lithium is about 80%. Thus the sodium clearance is substantially smaller than that of lithium. Lithium may be transported less efficiently than sodium. It may also be resistant to some of the sodium transporting mechanisms along the tubular systems. The effects of different diuretics on sodium and lithium excretion support the latter possibility as discussed below.

C. Relation to K^+ excretion

Talso and Clarke (1951) found no relation between potassium and lithium excretion in dogs. Foulks et al. (1952) determined lithium clearance during intravenous infusion of hypertonic potassium chloride solutions in dogs and found no appreciable change of the lithium excretion fraction. In man, Thomsen and Schou (1968) administered potassium chloride to healthy subjects causing a 100 to 200% increase of urinary potassium output, but this procedure did not alter lithium excretion. Potassium ions undergo both reabsorption and secretion in the tubules. The absorption occurs largely in the proximal tubules whereas secretion is a distal phenomenon and can be described in terms of a Na^+/K^+ exchange. On the basis of stop-flow experiments in dogs with plasma lithium concentrations of about 20 mEq/l Homer and Solomon (1962) found no evidence of tubular secretion of lithium. Thus, in spite of the fact that lithium is a monovalent cation which enters into cells, it is handled in the kidney in a way which is quite different from that of potassium.

D. Relation to H^+ excretion

Thomsen and Schou (1968) found that a reduction of urinary pH to 4·9–5·6 by administration of ammonium chloride to healthy volunteers left lithium excretion unaffected. Administration of sodium bicarbonate and acetazolamide producing a rise of urinary pH to 7·0–8·0 resulted in a slight rise in the lithium excretion fraction of about 30%. The fact that an increase in the urinary H^+ excretion was without effect on the urinary elimination of lithium contradicts the view that it is pH-dependent. It seems possible, as the authors suggest, that the increase in lithium excretion at high pH values is due to an obligatory excretion of cations with unreabsorbed bicarbonate anion. This interpretation is supported by the data presented by Foulks et al. (1952) who found that infusion of sodium thiosulfate, which also causes an obligatory anion excretion, results in a rise in the excretion of lithium.

IV. Influence of Pharmacological and Hormonal Agents on Renal Lithium Elimination

A. The effect of diuretics

In studies on dogs Foulks *et al.* (1952) found no significant change of the lithium excretion following injection of the mercurial diuretic mercupurin. However, the excretion of sodium was also little affected by the mercupurin. In experiments in man Thomsen and Schou (1968) found that oral intake of chlormerodrine in doses up to 100 mg led to a significant increase of urine flow and sodium output in two of six subjects, but in no case was the excretion of lithium changed. Mercurial diuretics are supposed to interfere with sodium transport in proximal parts of the tubular system (Goldstein *et al.*, 1961) and the studies mentioned above indicate an interaction between sodium and lithium ions in the tubular systems. Therefore, the lack of effect of mercurial diuretics on lithium elimination is unexpected. More experimental data on the effect of other diuretic agents on renal lithium elimination seem required to verify these results. The occurrence of a partially drug-resistant sodium/lithium transporting system in the proximal section of the tubular system cannot be excluded by the experimental evidence available so far.

In an extensive study on the influence of different types of diuretics on urinary lithium elimination Thomsen and Schou (1968) found that furosemide, bendroflumethiazide and ethacrynic acid, which all markedly accelerated the fractional elimination of sodium in acute experiments on healthy subjects, were without significant effect on the lithium excretion. Since all these agents appear to act on the ascending part of Henle's loop (Seldin *et al.*, 1966) it was suggested that lithium is resistant to sodium transporting mechanisms in this part of the tubular system. The compounds that most profoundly increased the lithium excretion fraction were urea and aminophylline. In oral doses of about 80 and 1 g respectively marked increases of the lithium excretion fraction were found. Aminophylline also substantially increased sodium excretion. Since both these agents have been shown to decrease proximal sodium reabsorption (Goldstein *et al.*, 1961; Kleeman *et al.*, 1962) the results obtained are compatible with the view that lithium reabsorption takes place in the proximal tubules.

B. The effect of mineralocorticoids

Aldosterone is the regulatory hormone for sodium–potassium exchange in the distal tubule of the kidney. Administration of the aldosterone inhibitor spironolactone to healthy human subjects (Thomsen and Schou, 1968) was not followed by a significant increase of the lithium excretion fraction but markedly augmented the sodium diuresis. These results were consistent with the effect of DOCA treatment in rats which produced a significant sodium retention but failed to alter external lithium balance (Baer *et al.*, 1971). Subsequent studies

L

by Smith and Thomsen (1973) demonstrated that removal of the adrenal glands in rats leads to a marked sodium loss but a fall in the renal lithium clearance. These findings strongly indicate that the renal transport system which is regulated by adrenal gland hormones can distinguish between sodium and lithium ions. Thus renal lithium handling, unlike sodium handling, appears to be relatively independent of mineralocorticoids.

V. Localization of Lithium Transport in the Kidney

The experimental evidence discussed above, i.e. the data obtained with loading or deprivation of sodium, indicate that some tubular transport mechanisms cannot readily distinguish between sodium and lithium ions. However, as regards sodium reabsorbing mechanisms in the distal parts of the tubular system, the lack of effect of the diuretics which inhibit sodium transport in this area including furosemide, bendroflumethiazide and ethacrynic acid, as well as the aldosterone antagonist spironolactone, indicate that lithium ions are not readily reabsorbed in the ascending loop of Henle and the distal tubule. Homer and Solomon (1962), on the basis of stop-flow studies in dogs, concluded that lithium is reabsorbed at the distal portion of the nephron. It cannot be excluded that such a mechanism exists in the dog, but this view is not incompatible with the assumption that distal reabsorption of lithium under conditions of free urinary flow plays only a minor role when therapeutic lithium concentrations are used.

About 99% of the sodium filtered through the glomerular membrane is reabsorbed in the tubules. During physiological conditions about 80% of the filtered amount is reabsorbed at proximal sites. This mechanism may be regulated by a "third factor", a natriuretic hormone of presumably hypothalamic origin, which inhibits fractional reabsorption of sodium in the proximal tubules (Schulze et al., 1966). Since the lithium reabsorption is about 80% of the filtered amount, which is similar to the proximal reabsorption of sodium, it seems compatible with available evidence that lithium reabsorption takes place mainly at the proximal site, possibly by the same mechanism that is responsible for sodium reabsorption. Thomsen and Schou (1968) and Thomsen et al. (1969) have presented evidence that fractional lithium reabsorption and proximal fractional sodium reabsorption are decreased and increased by the same procedures. They have even suggested that determination of the fractional lithium reabsorption may be a useful tool for the study of proximal sodium reabsorption in intact animals and patients.

Future studies, possibly with micropuncture techniques, seem to be required to establish the relation between lithium and sodium transport in the proximal tubules. Such experiments might also shed light on the question of why mercurial diuretics, which are generally believed to act as proximal sites, have not been shown to influence the renal lithium elimination significantly. So far it also cannot be excluded that the proximal sodium lithium transporting system represents a non-homogeneous mechanism with respect to the action of hormones and drugs.

VI. Interaction of Lithium with the Elimination of Electrolytes and Fluid from the Kidney

A. Electrolytes

Early studies by Trautner et al. (1955) on the effect of lithium on ionic balance in man indicated an augmented excretion of sodium and potassium. A transient increase in the elimination of calcium and magnesium was also found in the urine of healthy subjects. The changes took place only during the first two or three days after the initiation of lithium therapy. These findings were confirmed as regards sodium diuresis by Tupin et al. (1968), Murphy et al. (1969) and Aronoff et al. (1971). On the other hand Tupin et al. (1968) found a decrease in calcium excretion during the first two days of lithium treatment. The increase in magnesium excretion was confirmed by Tupin et al. (1968) and Aronoff et al. (1971). The transient increase of sodium excretion may be due to competition by lithium for proximal sodium reabsorption during the first days of treatment. This presumably results in a reduction of the body pool of sodium, stimulating aldosterone secretion which balances the effect on sodium elimination. The effect on potassium elimination may also be related to the increased aldosterone secretion but also to competition by lithium for potassium reabsorption as suggested from the experiments on stop-flow analysis of lithium handling in the dog by Homer and Solomon (1962). The effects of lithium on calcium and magnesium excretion have not been studied extensively enough to conclude whether renal or extrarenal mechanisms are involved (Nielsen, 1964). As regards magnesium ion balance also, a possible regulation by aldosterone excretion may be involved. The important roles of calcium and magnesium for nerve impulse conduction and transmitter release which may be related to the pathophysiology of manic depressive disorders motivate a future more careful analysis of lithium induced changes in renal handling of these ions. For a detailed discussion of lithium effects on electrolyte balance see Chapter 22.

B. Effect on water excretion

Radomski et al. had, in 1950, already reported polyuria and polydipsia as side effects of lithium treatment in dogs. In his early studies on rats Schou (1958) found that high doses of lithium caused the excretion of a dilute urine which was not concentrated by the administration of vasopressin (ADH). Patients given lithium usually excrete somewhat larger urine volumes during the first days of treatment (Aronoff et al., 1971). Occasionally a severe diabetes insipidus-like state with the excretion of urine volumes of five to ten litres per day are produced (Angrist *et al.*, 1970; Lee *et al.*, 1971; Ramsey *et al.*, 1972). Such very large urine volumes have in most cases appeared several weeks or months after starting lithium carbonate therapy in adequate doses. Those patients fail to concentrate the urine in response to water deprivation, the infusion of hypertonic saline solutions or to injection of antidiuretic hormone. None of the patients with lithium induced diabetes insipidus had a history of pre-existing renal disease or electrolyte imbalance. The polyuria is definitely linked to lithium since the syndrome was completely reversible following the discontinuation of treatment for three weeks (Angrist *et al.*, 1970).

Two mechanisms have been suggested for the diabetes insipidus-like state. Angrist *et al.* (1970) suggested that the lithium induced polyuria was due to hypokalemic nephropathy. However, since the changes in potassium metabolism induced by lithium are usually slight they may hardly explain the very high urine flows observed. The slight changes in potassium metabolism observed may rather be secondary to the polyuria produced. Since the diabetes insipidus-like condition induced by lithium is resistant to the action of ADH it is of renal origin and not due to any deficiency in the production or release of antidiuretic hormone. In studies on isolated hemilobes of neurohypophysis of rats Torp-Pedersen and Thorn (1973) also found that lithium in high concentration did not inhibit the release of antidiuretic hormone induced by potassium incubation. In rats, Harris and Jenner (1969) could suppress the antidiuretic response to exogenous ADH by acute lithium infusion. In experiments on rats fed lithium in their diet (Thomsen, 1970) polyuria did not appear until after some days of lithium administration. Also here the polyuria did not respond to the administration of ADH. The inhibition of the response to vasopressin thus developed gradually and during the first days it was presumably compensated by the normal or possibly increased endogenous production of ADH. It has not been established by which mechanism the kidney is rendered non-responsive to ADH, but high concentrations of lithium have been shown to inhibit the ADH stimulated activity of rabbit kidney adenyl cyclase *in vitro* (Dousa and Hechter, (1970). This enzyme catalyses the conversion of ATP to 3,5-AMP, which mediates the effect of ADH on the tubular cell permeability to water.

The lithium produced polyuria seems to be fully reversible in rat and man. It does not appear to be accompanied by other changes in kidney function. Thus endogenous creatinine clearance and lithium clearance are unchanged in spite of the excretion of large urine volumes. Since Radomski *et al.* (1950) could keep lithium treated dogs in a polyuric state for more than a year and several patients are known to have had a fairly pronounced lithium induced polyuria for several years without secondary effects (Thomsen, 1970), the lithium induced polyuria does not have to be a contraindication for a continued lithium therapy. For a detailed discussion on lithium and polyuria see chapter 28.

VII. Intraindividual Variation in Lithium Elimination

Clinical observations indicate that there is usually little day-to-day and month-to-month variation in lithium elimination. The lithium clearance remains unaffected by procedures of water deprivation or water loading. A low sodium diet, however, leads to a decrease, and high dietary sodium to an increase, in lithium excretion as discussed above. No systematic studies, however, have been performed on intraindividual differences in lithium elimination. Renal lithium clearance was determined at three different serum levels of lithium with a one week interval in a group of healthy volunteers (Table I, Fyrö et al., 1973). No significant differences were found between the renal lithium clearance

TABLE I. Lithium concentrations in serum and calculated clearances of lithium in healthy volunteers at different dose levels of lithium carbonate. (From Fyrö et al., 1973 with permission.)

Dose mEq/day	Serum conc. mEq/l	Clearance ml/min
24·3	0·19 ± 0·01	18·2 ± 1·4
48·6	0·33 ± 0·03	20·5 ± 1·4
72·9	0·49 ± 0·04	21·4 ± 0·7

no. = 7.
Mean ± S. E.

values at the three serum levels. This is in agreement with unpublished data in human subjects by Thomsen and Schou (1968). The lithium clearance was found to be independent of lithium concentrations within a range of 0·05 to 2·0 mEq/l. In experiments on dogs Foulks et al. (1952) infused lithium intravenously and found the excretion fraction to be relatively constant over a range of serum lithium concentrations from 1 to 22 mEq/l.

During pregnancy a significantly higher lithium clearance than after delivery has been reported (Schou et al., 1973). This emphasizes the need for frequent determination of serum lithium concentration and appropriate dosage adjustment in relation to pregnancy and delivery (see Chapter 15).

In old people low values for lithium clearance have been claimed to occur (Schou, 1969). The excretion of lithium will decrease especially when the filtration process is impaired. Intact kidney function must be ascertained during lithium treatment and determination of serum creatinine may be employed for this purpose, since a significant correlation has been found between creatinine and lithium clearance (Geisler et al., 1971, Fyrö et al., 1973). If the glomerular filtration is impaired during the course of lithium treatment, intoxication may occur on a dose of lithium that has previously been appropriate. During lithium intoxication the renal function is affected only moderately and reversibly (Schou *et al.*, 1968).

VIII. Interindividual Variation in Lithium Elimination

Clinical observations indicate that there are large differences in doses required to give therapeutic lithium levels in different patients. Since lithium is excreted almost exclusively through the kidneys, the urinary output is approximately equal to the intake when equilibrium has been established. From one person to another lithium clearance may differ appreciably. Thomsen and Schou (1968) reported lithium clearance values between 19 and 25 ml/min in 6 healthy subjects. They were given 0·6 g of lithium carbonate (16 mEq lithium) about

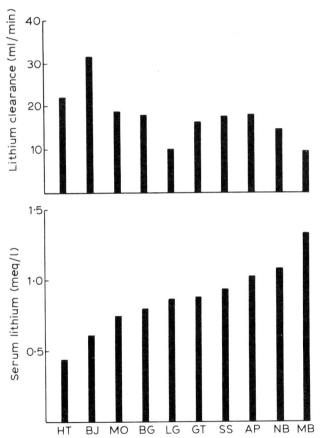

FIG. 3. Renal lithium clearance and morning lithium level in serum of ten healthy subjects following eight days of treatment with lithium carbonate (32 mEq/day). For further explanation see text. (From Sedvall *et al.*, 1970 with permission).

10 hours before the start of 7 hours clearance periods. In old people, lithium clearance values below 10 ml/min have been claimed to occur (Schou, 1969).

Sedvall *et al.* (1970) found lithium clearance values between 9 and 33 ml/min in 10 healthy volunteers who received a fixed dose of lithium for 8 days (Fig. 3). Steady-state levels of morning lithium concentrations were obtained after 5 days and these levels varied up to three-fold between subjects. The lithium levels in serum were significantly inversely correlated with the renal lithium clearance ($p < 0.05$). There was a highly significant inverse correlation ($p < 0.001$) between the steady-state level and the product of lithium clearance and body weight.

Geisler *et al.* (1971) found lithium clearance values between 8 and 35

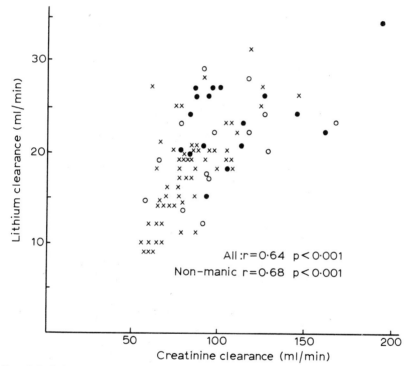

FIG. 4. Relation between lithium clearance and endogenous creatinine clearance. Non-manic patients are indicated by ×, hypomanic patients by ○ and manic patients by ●. (From Geisler *et al.*, 1971 with permission).

ml/min in 45 manic depressive women. A highly significant correlation ($p < 0.001$) was found between lithium and creatinine clearances (Fig. 4), but no difference in clearance was found between patients in manic and non-manic states.

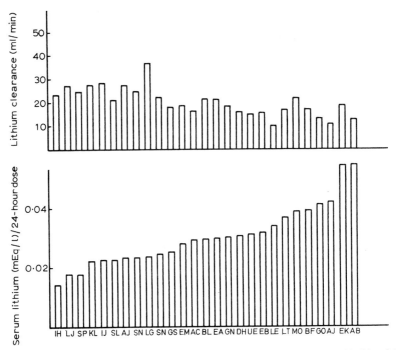

FIG. 5. Renal lithium clearance and morning lithium level in serum divided by daily dose of lithium for 27 manic-depressive patients. For fuller explanation see text. (From Fyrö *et al.*, 1973 with permission.)

The pharmacokinetics of lithium in manic depressive patients was also investigated by Fyrö *et al.* (1973). Here 27 patients with a history of manic-depressive disease were studied. All patients were normothymic at the time of the investigation and had been maintained on lithium daily for three weeks or more. When the ratio between lithium concentration in serum and the daily dose was calculated a four-fold interindividual difference was found. The renal lithium clearance ranged between 10 and 37 ml/min, an almost four-fold interindividual difference (Fig. 5). Clearance values for lithium and endogenous creatinine were significantly correlated with each other (Fig. 6), as earlier shown by Geisler *et al.* (1971). Clearance values for both creatinine and lithium were significantly inversely correlated to lithium levels in serum (Figs 7 and 8). When body weight was taken into account, a still higher correlation coefficient was found for both lithium and creatinine clearance to lithium levels in serum.

In single manic-depressive patients the present authors have observed lithium clearance values up to 56 ml/min. In old people low values of lithium clearance have been claimed to occur (Schou, 1969). In the study of Fyrö *et al.*

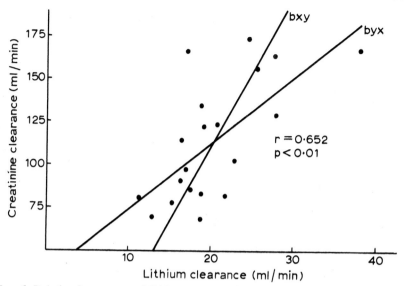

FIG. 6. Relation between renal lithium and creatinine clearance in manic-depressive patients. (From Fyrö *et al.*, 1973 with permission.)

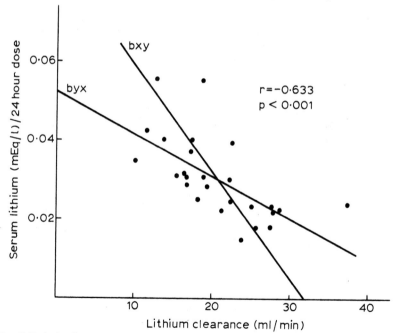

FIG. 7. Relation between the lithium concentration in serum divided by the daily dose of lithium, and lithium clearance. (From Fyrö *et al.*, 1973 with permission.)

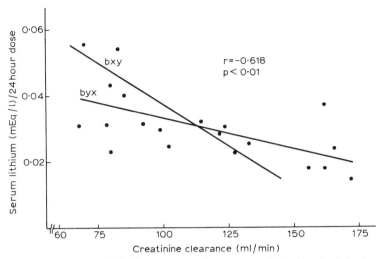

FIG. 8. Relation between the lithium concentration in serum divided by the daily dose of lithium, and creatinine clearance. (From Fyrö *et al.*, 1973 with permission.)

(1973) the age of the patients was 22 to 74 years; no correlation was found between age and lithium or creatinine clearance. None of the patients had any history of a renal disease, which is more common in old age and might influence renal lithium and creatinine clearance.

IX. Renal Lithium Elimination in Manic-Depressive Patients

A. Studies indicating lithium retention in acute manic states

The question of whether lithium is excreted less readily by manic than by other patients has been the subject of a number of studies, which have given inconsistent results. Most of these investigations deal with what is called lithium retention. In reality, however, the authors report on the fraction of an ingested lithium dose excreted in the urine within a particular time period.

Trautner *et al.* (1955) reported that whereas healthy persons excreted 50 to 70% of a lithium dose within 24 hours, manic patients excreted 13 to 19%. Gershon and Yuwiler (1960) noted that healthy individuals excreted 45 to 75% and manic patients 12 to 17% of ingested lithium in the first 24 hours. In these studies control and manic patients received different doses of lithium, however.

The observation that manic patients appear to excrete relatively small amounts of lithium during the initial phase of therapy, coupled with the report of Trautner *et al.* (1955) that a sudden increase occurs in the amount excreted after recovery from mania, gave rise to the suggestion that manics tend to retain lithium. This hypothesis has been tested in several studies. Hullin *et al.* (1968) presented results that are in favour of it. They gave lithium carbonate 0·5 g × 3

(40·5 mEq/day) to 13 manic patients and 10 normal subjects. The patients had a constant dietary intake containing 150 mEq sodium and 2 litres of water per day. No other treatment was given during the study except occasionally haloperidol and sodium amylobarbitone at night. The volunteers consumed an unrestricted and unmeasured diet. The authors state, however, that the lithium balance was essentially similar in these volunteers to those in another group of volunteers who had a standard diet similar to that given to the patients. Only 78 to 79% of the total dose was recovered in the urine for both male and female patients during the first nine days of treatment and the three days following discontinuation of lithium therapy. For the volunteers the mean excretion was approximately 90% of the dose given. The recovery of lithium in the control group was significantly higher than that of the manic group ($p < 0·01$). The retention was calculated as the difference between the oral intake and urinary output of lithium, ignoring other possible routes of loss. The faecal lithium excretion was very low in all patients, amounting to only 0·05–0·2 mEq/day.

Greenspan et al. (1968 a) studied the excretion of lithium in one patient in a manic as well as the normothymic state, another patient during two manic episodes and two patients with history of manic-depressive disease but in normal state at the time of the investigation. Salt and water were given ad libitum; the patients received different doses of lithium and the use of other drugs was not mentioned. The first manic patient retained lithium for 11 days and from the 15th day of treatment there was a negative lithium balance. Clinical evidence of improvement was noted on the ninth day of treatment. During the manic phase this patient retained 152 mEq of lithium. At the height of lithium retention the apparent lithium space was more than twice the estimated volume of total body water. In the normothymic phase this patient retained lithium for only five days, retention was only 45 mEq and the lithium space was the same as total body water. The other manic patient retained 85 mEq of lithium and his lithium space was about twice the total body water. The two non-manic patients reached lithium balance in four days; they retained only 32 mEq of lithium and their lithium spaces were similar to their estimated total body water.

In another report Greenspan et al. (1968 b) studied the excretion of lithium in three depressive patients receiving a diet containing a fixed amount of salt. These patients showed little or no negative lithium balance, corresponding to the previous observations in normothymic patients. The results indicate that lithium metabolism in acutely manic patients differs from that of normothymic and depressed patients.

A source of error in studies on lithium balance is the reliability of urine collections. The apparent increase in the retention of lithium in acutely manic patients can be an artefact if the urine collections were incomplete. Greenspan et al. (1968a) found, however, no significant difference in the creatinine excretion between the periods of positive and negative lithium balance. A strong argument against lithium retention being an artefact is, according to Greenspan *et al.* (1968a), the observation that both manic patients demonstrated a negative lithium balance immediately following the onset of clinical improvement.

Greenspan *et al.* (1968b) also investigated the effect of diet on lithium retention. They found that a decrease in sodium chloride intake resulted in a small increase in lithium retention and an elevation of plasma lithium. The opposite changes occurred when sodium chloride intake was increased. Changes in plasma lithium and lithium retention roughly paralleled each other so that there was no consistent change in the apparent lithium space. The effect of sodium chloride intake was considered to be too small to account for the large differences in lithium ion retention between manic and normothymic patients.

Greenspan *et al.* (1968a) suggested that when lithium is administered to normothymic patients, the amount of lithium retained can be calculated from the plasma lithium level by assuming a roughly equal distribution of lithium throughout the total body water. In acutely manic patients they found a considerably larger amount of lithium ion to be retained than could be computed from this assumption. They suggest that in acutely manic patients lithium ion is stored in the intracellular water of certain tissues or in the extracellular space other than plasma and that during clinical improvement there is an excretion of the retained lithium ion.

Serry (1969a, b) determined the urinary lithium excretion within the first 4 hours after ingestion of 1·2 g lithium carbonate (33 mEq lithium). The patients stayed in bed and were given 1–1·5 litres fluid during the 4 hour period. Intake of food and salt before the experiment was not controlled and some patients received neuroleptics.

Of 51 manic patients studied, 35 excreted less than 1% of the lithium dose within the four hour period, whereas in the control group only 2 of 30 patients did so. Twenty of the manic patients who retained lithium improved within 14 days. Four of the 12 manic patients who excreted more than 1·5% of the ingested dose were treated with lithium but none of them responded to the treatment. Serry also found that 13 of 22 patients with depressed phase of manic-depressive psychosis or recurrent endogenous depression excreted less than 1% of the lithium dose. These patients were treated with ECT and/or antidepressants. Of the 13 patients, 11 became normothymic and lithium excreters, i.e. excreted more than 1·5% of the ingested dose.

The most recent study indicating lithium retention in manic patients is that of Almy and Taylor (1973). They determined lithium excretion during 36 hours after administration of 0·9 g lithium carbonate (24 mEq of lithium) to 10 manic and 10 control patients. No medication was given for 48 hours and nothing by mouth for 8 hours prior to the test. Patients and controls were maintained on the same hospital diet. Salt and fluid intake was not controlled during the experiment. Urine was collected in 6-hour portions. The manic patients retained significantly more lithium than the controls. This difference was apparent at the end of each measured time interval as early as 6 hours after the start of the test. The difference between groups was greatest when the total 36 hour excretion period was compared. Almy and Taylor found a lithium half-life of about 18 hours in normals as compared to more than 36 hours in manic patients. Serum lithium concentrations did not differ significantly between the groups at any time.

The results of Greenspan et al. (1968a), Hullin et al. (1968), Serry (1969a, b) and Almy and Taylor (1973) all indicate that manic patients retain more of an orally administered lithium dose than controls and that this difference is detectable by comparing lithium excretion in the urine. Their findings are compatible with the view that manic patients distribute lithium in the tissues differently from healthy subjects and that the serum concentration does not differentiate lithium-retainers from non-retainers.

B. Studies indicating similarity in lithium excretion in manic and other patients

The urinary excretion of lithium was investigated by Epstein et al. (1965) who gave 1 g lithium carbonate (27 mEq of lithium) to 10 manics and 23 patients with other psychiatric diagnoses. Most patients were on hypnotics, antidepressants and phenothiazines. Intake of food, salt and water was not controlled. The authors found that during 8 hours manic patients excreted 27% of the dose, as compared to 30% for the controls. During the first 24 hours 4 manic patients excreted 64% as compared to 59% in 3 control patients. Neither 8 nor 24 hours lithium excretion as well as differences in concentration of plasma lithium, urine volume or concentration of lithium in urine were statistically different between manics and controls.

Also Platman et al. (1968) studied the excretion of a single lithium dose. For five days before and during the experiment the patients received a regular hospital diet and 3 g sodium chloride per day. Fluid intake was measured but not regulated. In a first group four patients in manic to hypomanic states and three patients in normal to depressed states were given 1·2 g lithium carbonate (32 mEq of lithium) in a single dose. In a second group three patients in manic to hypomanic states and seven patients in normal to depressed states received 0·6 g of lithium carbonate (16 mEq of lithium). The subjects in the second group were fasted from 12 p.m. the day before lithium to 8 a.m. on the day following lithium administration. Patients received 150 ml of water hourly, starting with the administration of lithium and terminating when 2400 ml had been consumed. The excretion of lithium was measured after 12 and 24 hours. No apparent difference was found in excretion in the different clinical states. A wider range and greater variability was found in the first group of patients, which might be due to the irregular fluid intake in this group.

Platman et al. (1968) thus found no difference in lithium excretion between manic and non-manic patients. However, the results indicated an important influence of sodium and fluid intake on lithium excretion. Platman and Fieve (1969) suggested that the inconsistent results concerning lithium excretion during manic and non-manic states found by previous investigators may be explained by diet variability and inadequate urine collection. Sick patients are less co-operative and eat poorly. On recovery they are more co-operative and the diet may improve dramatically; the increase in food intake is probably associated with an increase of salt ingestion and this would cause more lithium to be excreted in the urine.

The experiments of Serry (1969a, b) described above, were repeated by Stokes et al. (1972) in 52 subjects. Thirteen patients were manic or hypomanic and the others were in normothymic or depressed states. Several patients received tranquillizers or antidepressant medication. The subjects were instructed neither to drink nor to eat after midnight before the test. They received an oral dose of 1·2 g lithium carbonate (32 mEq of lithium) and the total urine output was collected over the next four hours. Stokes et al. found only three of 52 patients to be retainers by Serry's criteria, i.e. to excrete less than 1% of the given dose. They found no relation between lithium excretion and gross mood state, or between lithium excretion and subsequent response to lithium therapy.

Both Serry (1969a) and Stokes et al. (1972) reported that several patients changed from retainers to excreters after successful lithium treatment. This was presumably not related to improved absorption, since the lithium concentration in plasma was unchanged. Stokes et al. (1972) speculate as to whether this is due only to the sodium deficiency mechanisms suggested by Platman et al. (1968a) or to some other function of manic-depressive illness as yet not demonstrated.

In order to investigate further the relationship between mood and renal excretion of lithium, Demers and Harris (1972) adopted longitudinal sodium balance studies on three manic-depressive patients. These patients were kept for a minimum of five days on a low sodium diet (69 mEq of sodium per day) before they received a high sodium diet (173 mEq per day). Two patients were treated with chlorpromazine during the whole experiment. All three patients were in a normothymic state when lithium treatment for 15–25 days started. In all cases mean lithium excretion increased during high sodium intake, blood lithium level declined and urine volume increased considerably. The increase in lithium excretion as well as the increase in urine volume was statistically significant in all patients. During high sodium intake, there was a shift in scores towards manic behaviour that was statistically significant in each patient. The data of Demers and Harris (1972) are in agreement with the findings of Platman *et al.* (1968) and Platman and Fieve (1969) that increased sodium intake enhances the lithium excretion when a constant lithium dose is given over a long time period.

In a recent study Geisler *et al.* (1971) examined the amount of lithium excreted in the urine during 11 and 18 hours after oral intake of 0·6 g lithium carbonate (16 mEq of lithium) in 45 manic-depressive women during different phases of the disorder. At the time of the investigation several patients were

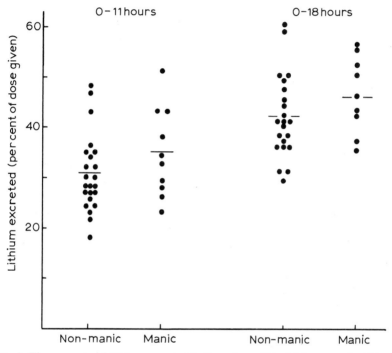

FIG. 9. The amounts of lithium excreted in the urine within 11 hours and within 18 hours after the intake, expressed as a percentage of the dose given. Values are shown for non-manic patients (severely depressed, moderately depressed, and after recovery from mania or depression) and for manic patients. (From Geisler *et al.*, 1971, with permission.)

treated with neuroleptic or antidepressant drugs. During the study caffeine-containing food, drinks or drugs were not administered. The excretion of lithium was found to be similar in manic and other patients. The lithium clearance was positively correlated with creatinine clearance (Fig. 9), sodium excretion, but not with the urine flow. There was no significant difference between the lithium clearance in manic as compared to non-manic patients.

After 20 years of research we still do not know for sure whether lithium is excreted less readily by manic as compared to other patients. Several factors which have been reviewed in this chapter influence lithium excretion. All have to be controlled in both manic and non-manic patients in studies of lithium excretion. For example, in none of the studies where differences in lithium excretion between manic and non-manic patients were found was the intake of sodium chloride determined. There is also an absolute demand that manic and non-manic patients shall receive the same dose of lithium and no other psychoactive medication. It has been reported that chlorpromazine increases the excretion of lithium (Sletten *et al.*, 1966).

The following factors should be controlled in future studies relevant to the problem regarding lithium retention. In future studies aiming at analyzing lithium retention in manic and control patients the following factors should be standardized.

Diet including electrolytes and fluid for at least 5 days before and during experiment.

Dose of lithium used for test.

Time for excretion determination.

Drugs before and during experiment.

The results should be related to clinical condition, motor activity, sex and age.

In no study reported so far have all these factors been considered. Platman *et al.* (1968) did control the intake of sodium before and during their excretion studies and they found no difference in lithium elimination between manic and other patients. Until an extensive study is performed where all the above mentioned factors are controlled before, as well as during, the excretion measurement, there is no significant basis for the view that there is a difference in lithium excretion between manic and non-manic patient categories.

Acknowledgements

This work has been supported by the Swedish Medical Research Council (21X–2291) and the Karolinska Institute.

References

Almy, G. L. and Taylor, M. A. (1973). *Archs gen. Psychiat.* **29**, 232–234.

Angrist, B. M., Gershon, S., Levitan, S. J. and Blumberg, A. G. (1970). *Compreh. Psychiat.* **11**, 141–146.

Aronoff, M. S., Evens, R. G. and Durell, J. (1971). *J. psychiat. Res.* **8**, 139–159.

Baer, L., Platman, S. R., Kassir, S. and Fieve, R. R. (1971). *J. psychiat. Res.* **8**, 91–105.

Corcoran, A. C., Taylor, R. D. and Page, I. (1949). *J. Amer. med. Assoc.* **139**, 685–688.

Demers, R. G. and Harris, R. L. (1972). *Dis. nerv. Syst.* **33**, 372–375.

Dousa, T. and Hechter, O. (1970). *Life Sci.* **9**, 765–770.

du Vigneaud, V., Gish, D. T. and Katsoyannis, P. G. (1954). *J. Amer. chem. Soc.* **76**, 4751–4752.

Epstein, R., Grant, L., Herjanic, M. and Winokur, G. (1965). *J. Amer. med. Assoc.* **192**, 409.

Foulks, J., Mudge, G. H. and Gilman, A. (1952). *Amer. J. Physiol.* **168**, 642–649.

Fyrö, B., Petterson, U. and Sedvall, G. (1973). *Acta psychiat. scand.* **49**, 237–247.

Geisler, A., Schou, M. and Thomsen, K. (1971). *Int. Pharmacopsychiat.* **4**, 149–155.

Gershon, S. and Yuwiler, A. (1960). *J. Neuropsychiat.* **1**, 229–241.

Goldstein, M. H., Levitt, M. F., Hauser, A. D. and Polimeros, D. (1961). *J. clin. Invest.* **40**, 731–742.

Greenspan, K., Goodwin, F. K. and Bunney, W. E. (1968a). *Arch. gen. Psychiat.* **19**, 664–673.

Greenspan, K., Green, R. and Durell, J. (1968b). *Amer. J. Psychiat.* **125**, 512–519.

Hanlon, L. W., Romaine, M., Gilroy, F. J. and Dietrick, S. E. (1949). *J. Amer. med. Assoc.* **139**, 688–692.

Harris, A. C. and Jenner, F. A. (1969). *J. Physiol.* **203**, 73p.

Homer, L. D. and Solomon, S. (1962). *Amer. J. Physiol.* **203**, 897–900.

Hullin, R. P., Swinscoe, J. C., McDonald, R. and Dransfield, G. A. (1968). *Brit. J. Psychiat.* **114**, 1561–1573.

Kent, N. L. and McCance, R. A. (1941). *Biochem. J.* **35**, 837,

Kleeman, C. R., Cutler, R., Maxwell, M. H., Bernstein, L. and Dowling, J. T. (1962). *J. lab. clin. Med.* **60**, 224–244.

Lee, R. V., Jampol, L. M. and Brown, W. V. (1971). *New Eng. J. Med.* **284**, 93–94.

Murphy, D. L., Goodwin, F. K. and Bunney, W. E. (1969). *Lancet* **2**, 458–461.

Nielsen, J. (1964). *Acta psychiat. scand.* **40**, 190–196.

Pitts, R. F. (1959). In "Physiological Basis of Diuretic Therapy". Charles C. Thomas, Springfield, Illinois.

Platman, S. R., Rohrlich, J. and Fieve, R. R. (1968). *Dis. nerv. Syst.* **29**, 733–738.

Platman, S. R. and Fieve, R. R. (1969). *Archs gen. Psychiat.* **20**, 285–289.

Radomski, J. L., Fuyat, H. N., Nelson, A. A. and Smith, P. K. (1950). *J. pharmacol. exp. Ther.* **100**, 429–444.

Ramsey, T. A., Mendels, J., Stokes, J. W. and Fitzgerald, R. G. (1972). *J. Amer. med. Assoc.* **219**, 1446–1449.

Schou, M. (1958). *Acta pharmacol. tox.* **15**, 85–98.

Schou, M., Amdisen, A. and Trop-Jensen, J. (1968). *Amer. J. Psychiat.* **125**, 520–527.

Schou, M. (1969). In "The Present Status of Psychotropic Drugs" (A. Cerletti and F. J. Bové, eds.), pp. 120–122, Excerpta Medica, Amsterdam.

Schou, M., Amdisen, A. and Steenstrup, O. R. (1973). *Br. med. J.* **2**, 137–138.

Schultze, R. G., Slatopolsky, E., Tall, B., Walker, W., Levy, M. and Bricker, N. S. (1966). *Trans. Assoc. Amer. Physicians.* **79**, 322–329.

Sedvall, G., Pettersson, U. and Fyrö, B. (1970). *Pharmacol. Clin.* **2**, 231–235.

Seldin, D. W., Eknoyan, G., Suki, W. N. and Rector, F. C. (1966). *Ann. N.Y. Acad. Sci.* **139**, 328–343.

Serry, M. (1969a). *Aust. N.Z. J. Psychiat.* **3**, 390–397.

Serry, M. (1969b). *Lancet* **1**, 1267–1268.

Sexton, A. W. and Meyer, D. K. (1955). *Fed. Proc.* **14**, 137.

Sletten, I., Pichardo, J., Korol, B. and Gershon, S. (1966). *Curr. ther. Res.* **8**, 441–446.

Smith, D. F. and Thomsen, K. (1973). *Amer. J. Physiol.* **225**, 159–161.

Stokes, J. W., Mendels, J., Secunda, S. K. and Dyson, W. L. (1972). *J. nerv. ment. Dis.* **154**, 43–48.

Talso, P. J. and Clarke, R. W. (1951). *Amer. J. Physiol.* **166**, 202–208.

Thomsen, K. (1970). *Int. Pharmacopsychiat.* **5**, 233–241.

Thomsen, K. and Schou, M. (1968). *Amer. J. Physiol.* **215**, 823–827.
Thomsen, K., Schou, M., Steiness, I. and Hansen, H. E. (1969). *Pflügers Arch.* **308**, 180–184.
Torp-Pedersen, Chr. and Thorn, N. A. (1973). *Acta Endocrinol.* **73**, 665–671.
Trautner, E. M., Morris, R., Noack, C. H. and Gershon, S. (1955). *Med. J. Aust.*, **42**, 280–291.
Tupin, J. P., Schlagenhauf, G. K. and Creson, D. L. (1968). *Amer. J. Psychiat.* **125**, 536–543.
Zerahn, K. (1955). *Acta physiol. scand.* **33**, 347–358.

PART II

SECTION B

BEHAVIOURAL EFFECTS

19

BEHAVIOURAL AND COGNITIVE EFFECTS OF LITHIUM: OBSERVATIONS AND EXPERIMENTS

F. N. JOHNSON

I. Introduction

A. Historical background

The study of the effects of drugs on the behaviour of animals under clearly defined experimental test conditions, has developed, since the early nineteen-fifties, into a distinct scientific discipline with its own specialized terminology and body of techniques. The rise of psychopharmacology paralleled, and indeed received its impetus from, the establishment of the major classes of psychoactive drugs into regular clinical usage: psychopharmacology and pharmacopsychiatry are inextricably linked (Johnson, 1973c). It is, therefore, all

315

the more surprising that lithium should have been subjected to relatively little in the way of thoroughgoing investigation by experimental psychologists. It may be that claims for therapeutic specificity in the case of lithium led investigators to believe that the drug produced its beneficial effects entirely by correcting some metabolic abnormality and that where this abnormality did not exist (as, presumably, in experimental animal subjects) no behavioural effects might be expected to occur. Whatever the reasons, it is not until the last few years that the results of behavioural investigations on lithium have appeared in the literature, and the full picture of this aspect of lithium's effects is still far from being clear. Some general principles may, however, be tentatively discerned, and these may provide appropriate guidelines for future investigations.

B. Some problems with behavioural research on lithium

1. *General problems*

All studies in behavioural pharmacology suffer from certain limitations, whatever the drug under investigation. It is always difficult, for example, to extrapolate from the results of animal studies to the effects produced in humans (and particularly in psychiatric patients). Different investigators use different strains or even species of experimental animals; the experimental test situation may differ along a number of dimensions (e.g., drug dosage size and administration regime, injection times relative to the behavioural test, drug administration route, the behavioural test situation, and so on). There is, in addition, no concensus on the descriptive terms which should be employed in reporting the behavioural effects of drugs. Comparisons between different reports are, therefore, not easy to make, and generalizations about the effects of any drug on behaviour are, under such circumstances, made with caution. Behavioural work with lithium is subject to all of these limitations, and to a few more.

2. *Problems specific to work with lithium*

(a) Comparability of experimental and therapeutic dosage regimes: The most obvious, and most frequently remarked, criticism of lithium studies using animals is that the majority of such studies have employed acute drug administration, or at least administration regimes which fall short of the extended treatment procedures usually associated with lithium therapy (Rees, personal communication; Smith and Smith, 1973; Smith personal communication). The force of such criticisms is clear. There are, however, certain difficulties associated with chronic lithium administration to animals. Many investigators have, for example, shown that lithium chloride ingestion by animals may result in adverse effects (Nachman, 1963a, b) which can operate as aversive stimuli in avoidance conditioning situations (Balagura and Smith, 1970a, b; Cullen, 1970; Nachman, 1970; Nachman et al., 1970; Frumkin, 1971; Boland, 1973; Lehr and Nachman, 1973; Nachman and Ashe, 1973; O'Boyle *et al.*, 1973), and in particular, of course, the animal may learn to avoid drinking lithium chloride solutions (Fregly, 1953; Smith and Balagura, 1969; Smith *et al.*, 1970; Balagura *et al.*, 1972): this complicates any chronic administration regime based on the inclusion of lithium chloride in the animals' food or drinking water.

(b) Choice of an appropriate lithium dose level: It is well known that different animal species are affected unequally by quantitatively equivalent dosage of drugs. This is due partly to variations in metabolic rates which are associated with thermoregulation demands in species with different body sizes, and partly to specific differences in metabolic pathways. Two devices have usually been adopted by investigators: either the actually administered dose has been quantitatively equated with that used in the human treatment situation, appropriately pro-rated for body size differences, or the dose has been adjusted so as to give a serum lithium concentration equal to that achieved during lithium therapy. Of course, neither procedure really overcomes the basic problem of providing direct comparability between human and animal doses, but in the absence of more appropriate rationales they must be regarded as the best that can be achieved at the present time. The matter has not, however, escaped notice and Samuel and Gottesfeld (1973) have recently drawn attention to the complications which are introduced into the problem of understanding the behavioural effects of lithium, not only by the wide range of drug doses, but also by the many variations in administration routes and duration of treatment regimes which have been employed.

(c) Choice of an appropriate placebo: In many cases lithium effects have been compared with those produced by sodium salts in an apparent attempt to minimize the contribution to behavioural change made by disturbances of ionic balance. The decision to employ sodium chloride as the treatment for control subjects when the experiment has involved examining lithium chloride, has usually been predicated upon the assumption that animals cannot discriminate between the chlorides of sodium and lithium. This may well be the case when the drugs are injected intraperitoneally, but oral administration may be complicated by a sodium–lithium discrimination on the part of the animals. Whilst early studies could find no evidence of such a discriminative capacity (e.g., Erikson, 1963), later work with appropriate methodological refinements (Strom *et al.*, 1970) has demonstrated that rats can make the discrimination with relative ease.

(d) Maintenance of drug-placebo blindness in human studies: It is essential for the assessment of drug effects on human behavioural and cognitive processes that the subject's placebo response should be used as the appropriate baseline for comparison. Knowledge on the part of the subject that a drug and not a placebo has been administered makes interpretation of subsequent effects a hazardous business. Unfortunately, maintenance of the subject's ignorance of the drug–placebo distinction is often difficult. For example, Schou (1968) and Schou et al. (1968) reported that when lithium and placebo were given to six student volunteers, two of the subjects correctly identified the lithium treatment periods, even though the experiment was designed to be double-blind. Apparently the frequent slight side effects (such as hand tremor) may be enough to break the double-blind, at least among some normal subjects, and this may invalidate any subjective reports which the subjects make about their mental state whilst under the drug.

(e) Differentiation between primary and secondary drug effects: Schou (1968) and Schou et al. (1968) make the point that feelings of restraint produced by lithium treatment in some manic patients may reflect secondary effects of the removal of manic episodes rather than any direct effect of the lithium per se. This is, of course, a possibility which has always to be borne in mind: the separation of direct (primary) and indirect (secondary) actions of any drug on any behavioural, biochemical or physiological system is never easy.

II. Behavioural Effects

Any attempt to provide a rigorous taxonomy of the behavioural effects produced by lithium is doomed to failure. The information is scattered in the literature and is often presented in the manner of an aside, or as a point tangential to the main argument. The following organization of the material, whilst it serves the present purposes well enough, must inevitably be subject to extensive modification as this whole area of investigation expands.

A. Unconditioned reflexes and responses

Tadano et al. (1972) reported no effects of 600 mg/kg LiCl i.p. on unconditioned responses of mice, though the nature of such responses (apart from the righting reflex) was left unspecified. This negative finding is typical of the majority of reports in this area as far as isolated pieces of the total behavioural repertoire are concerned. Thus Mark and Watts (1971), using between 16·3 and 163 μg LiCl i.c. in chickens, reported that the ability of the animals to peck accurately was not impaired. Similarly, pretreatment with 3 mEq Li$^+$/kg had no effect on the head-dipping behaviour of mice on a hole board (U'Prichard and Steinberg, 1972; Steinberg, 1973).

Vocalization has, however, been mentioned by several investigators as being influenced by lithium, and whilst Harrison Read and Steinberg (1971), using rats, noted that shock-elicited vocalization was unaffected by 2 weeks pretreatment with daily injections of 2 mEq Li$^+$/kg i.p., Tadano et al. (1972) did report that both i.p. (600 mg/kg) and i.c. (80 μg) doses of LiCl inhibited vocalization induced in mice by electric shock. The reports are variable, and contrary to

Tadano's report of lithium-induced suppression of vocalization S. H. Johnson (1971) reported that 2·4 mEq Li$^+$/kg i.p. in rats produced an immediate post-injection syndrome which included the emission of multiple squeaks, whilst Barratt *et al.* (1968) had earlier reported that 7 days of administering 50 mg/kg LiCl i.p. in cats led to various changes in spontaneous behaviour, including hissing on the approach of the experimenter.

B. Activity

Screening tests of new drugs usually include some measures of effects on activity in order to provide a quick assessment of possible sedative properties. In the case of lithium, the information obtained from such tests has proved difficult to interpret. From the time of Cade's original report that lithium produced a reduction in the activity of guinea-pigs (Cade, 1949) many investigators have felt that this was roughly what one might expect of a drug which alleviated manic excitement: confirmation of this expectation has not, however, always been forthcoming. Amdisen (personal communication) has, for example, commented that in spite of a feeling that lithium administered either orally or intraperitoneally to rats and mice really did produce an inhibitory effect on the animals' spontaneous behaviour, activity recordings in vibration cages, activity wheels or photocell devices failed to provide confirmation of this.

The literature and unpublished reports by investigators in this field abound in brief, unsubstantiated comments of the kind made by Amdisen; thus Allison (personal communication) notes that whilst specific behavioural testing was not part of his experimental schedule he did note that rats which received lithium "appeared sedated in that they did not show much spontaneous movement". Corrodi *et al.* (1967) found that rats subjected to doses of 7·5 mEq Li$^+$/kg (isotonic 0·15M LiCl) i.p. exhibited a reduction in spontaneous activity, though again this was a casual observation and no objective activity measurements were provided. Lower doses of lithium were reported to be without effect.

Many reports are either equivocal on the point, or are, for various reasons, difficult to interpret. S. H. Johnson (1971), for example, pretreated rats with daily injections of 2·4 mEq Li$^+$/kg (LiCl) i.p. and noted a decrease in the animals' locomotory activity as compared with saline-treated controls. The difference between the two groups did not, however, reach statistical significance. S. H. Johnson nevertheless felt justified in tentatively concluding that lithium treatment did reduce locomotory activity and that a statistically significant result might have been observed with more subjects in the experimental groups.

Syme and Syme (1973) argued that an appropriate testing situation for lithium effects on behaviour should include the presence of other animals so as to approximate the social situations under which patients receive lithium therapy.

Using an activity platform to record gross activity changes they showed that 3 mEq Li⁺/kg (LiCl) i.p. reduced the activity of rats to a significant degree as compared with saline-treated controls. The effect of the presence of other animals given similar treatment varied according to the time of testing after drug administration: at 20 min post injection the rats were more active when tested individually than when tested in pairs, but the reverse was true 3 h after injection. Interpretation of the results is, however, made difficult by the additional finding that activity differences also occurred in the individually tested saline-treated control rats as a function of the injection–test interval.

Despite all these confusing factors, however, the general feeling had grown by the early nineteen-seventies that lithium did in fact reduce activity: the evidence came from such a variety of sources that, even though it lacked the backing of methodological sophistication, it was difficult to ignore. In 1970 D'Encarnacao and Anderson using photocell activity cage measurements of rats given LiCl i.p. to serum levels of 1·5 mEq Li⁺/l, showed that in the first hour of exposure to the test situation activity counts were depressed as compared with those of a saline-treated control group. Two years later, Johnson and Wormington (1972), working on the assumption that the failure of many earlier experimenters to provide unequivocal demonstrations of the behavioural effects of lithium in animal subjects might have been due to an inappropriate choice of behavioural screening test techniques, employed a measure of activity which was known from previous work to be highly sensitive to drug effects. This test involved monitoring the rearing activity of an animal (i.e. the posture change from the horizontal, or all-fours, to the vertical, or hind-legs only, position). In subsequent experiments (Johnson, 1972a, b) locomotory activity (horizontal movements) was simultaneously monitored. Later investigators have commented on the dissociation between these two types of behaviour. Thiébot *et al.* (1973), for example, showed that staircase step-climbing (essentially a horizontal locomotory component of activity) and rearing were differentially affected by a variety of anxiolytic drugs. Kiseleva and Lapin (1969) had been unable to demonstrate any effect of doses of 100 mg/kg lithium carbonate on the rearing activity of mice, but Johnson and Wormington (1972) reported that, in rats, 2 mEq Li⁺/kg (LiCl) s.c. produced a marked reduction of rearing frequency, although rearing height was unaffected. The reduction of rearing frequency was relatively greater for males than for females. In addition an injection time effect was also noted, the greatest lithium-induced depression of total rearing activity (the product of rearing frequency and rearing height) occurring 20 min after injection. Johnson (1972a) subsequently examined the effect of a larger dose of lithium, 6 mEq Li⁺/kg (LiCl) i.p., and again found rearing activity to be much reduced.

More recently, Smith and Smith (1973) observed the activity of rats in a variety of situations, following chronic lithium administration in the animals' food. In the open field test the lithium-treated rats took longer to reach the wall of the apparatus starting from the centre of the field as compared with control rats, and in a 3-min period the drugged subjects crossed fewer lines in the field. The inhibitory effect on activity increased as the lithium content of the diet was raised. Activity wheel and jiggle cage tests and recordings of spontaneous bar presses in a Skinner box, all confirmed the open field findings of reduced activity under lithium.

The question of lithium effects on general activity cannot, unfortunately, be counted as resolved. There are reports which conflict with those which suggest that activity reduction is the main effect. For example, 120 mg/kg lithium carbonate s.c. was reported by MacLeod *et al.* (1949) to reduce spontaneous movement in a mature rat, but when the same animal was given an increased dosage (180 mg/kg) marked *hyper*activity was noted 22 h later. Similar findings were obtained with two further rats using even higher doses. Männistö and Saarnivaara (1972) subjected mice to chronic administration of LiCl in tap water (200 mg/l) and reported that after 7 days the activity of the animals, as assessed in a photocell activity box, was increased to a significant degree as compared with saline-treated controls. However, the elevation in activity scores recorded following 50 days administration was not statistically significant, and after 90 days the lithium-treated animals showed activity scores identical to those of control subjects. The interpretation to be placed on these findings is obscure.

A group of investigators in London, led by Steinberg, has consistently failed to find effects of lithium on the activity levels of animals except when the activity is raised beforehand by treatment with various drug combinations (see later). Thus, Cox *et al.* (1971) found that neither chronic lithium treatment, 3 mEq Li$^+$/kg (LiCl) i.p. given daily for 15 days, nor acute lithium treatment (a single injection of the same dose level) had any effect on the activity of rats as assessed by the number of entrances made into the arms of a Y-maze in a 5-min period, or on the number of rearing (standing up) responses made in the same period. Harrison-Read (personal communication) notes that, in general, chronic lithium pretreatment (2 mEq Li$^+$/kg per day over 10 days) has little effect on activity in the Y-maze, although in several of his experiments the treatment did lead to a more rapid decline of activity over a 5-min test period. U'Prichard and Steinberg (1972) and Steinberg (1973) reported that 3 mEq Li$^+$/kg did not have any effect on the activity of mice on a hole board.

Clearly, the nature of the response to lithium has yet to be elucidated as far as spontaneous activity is concerned. The variability in the reported findings may reflect differences in animals and techniques, but it is more likely that it is a function of the blanket term "activity" being used to cover what are almost certainly widely different samples from the animals' behavioural repertoires and which, for that reason, respond differentially to drugs.

C. Learning and memory

Whilst the effects of lithium on activity are interesting in themselves, Johnson and Barker (1972) have pointed to the need for close examination of the influences of lithium on more complex psychological functions such as the acquisition, retention and subsequent elicitation and expression of learned responses, which might more directly relate to the kinds of drug-induced changes occurring in the therapeutic situation. One of the first studies in this area was carried out by Wittrig *et al.* (1970) who were, however, unable to demonstrate any effects of lithium on learning acquisition in rats as assessed by errors made in learning a Lashley III maze. Few details of the experiment are given in the report, however, and it is therefore difficult to compare the study with others. The authors made an intriguing comment to the effect that lithium may reduce the errors made by emotional rats and this, in view of claims that lithium may exert a tranquillizing effect, clearly needs amplification.

This work was followed by a well-designed study by Mark and Watts (1971) who used one-day old chicks in a one-trial passive avoidance learning situation to examine the effects of a variety of drugs, including lithium chloride, on the establishment of memory traces. Injection of 0·5 ml LiCl solution (245 μg/ml) in two separate doses, one into each side of the forebrain, produced marked deficits in retention of the learned responses 24 h after the learning experience, but only when the injection was made 5 min before training. Injection 30 or 15 min before the learning trial, though producing some deficit, did not do so to a statistically significant degree. No effect was noted with an injection at a post-injection interval of 10 min. The deficit in retention produced by injection 5 min before training was apparently more-or-less permanent, being detectable 72 h after training. Subsequent experiments demonstrated the memory impairment to be dose-related. A later series of experiments by the same investigators (Watts and Mark, 1971) added further information about the effects of lithium on memory, again using chicks in a one-trial passive avoidance test: the higher the lithium dose, the earlier the memory deficit appeared after training. The authors concluded that lithium exerted a specific inhibitory action on the establishment of short-term traces, possibly via a blocking action on sodium pump mechanisms, and that the effects were not merely the result of a general disruption of brain functioning.

The conclusions drawn by Mark and Watts have recently been challenged by Benowitz and Sperry (1973). These investigators administered 245 μg LiCl in two portions directly to the two cerebral hemispheres of newly-hatched chicks. This was done either 2 or 4 min before, or 10 sec after, subjecting the chicks to a one-trial passive avoidance learning situation. It was found that the drug treatment did not change retention assessed after an interval of 20 min, and hence was presumably without effect on relatively short-term memory processes; however, a severe impairment was noted in retention scores determined

24 hours after training, the effect being greatest with 4 min pre-training and least with 10 sec post-training injections times. The authors suggest that this indicates an effect of lithium on a form of memory trace which, though it does not itself have implications for behaviour within a short period after learning, induces, or acts as a precursor of, a long-term memory trace which is behaviourally active (Benowitz and Magnus, 1973).

Johnson and Barker (1972) examined the effects produced by 3 mEq Li$^+$/kg (LiCl) i.p. on escape-avoidance conditioning in rats. As in the study reported by Wittrig *et al.* (1970) no difference was observed in the rate of acquisition of avoidance responding between the experimental animals and saline-treated controls. However, when the animals were tested 24 h later there was an apparent superiority of the lithium-treated subjects over the controls, reacquisition of the avoidance response being considerably enhanced. When injections preceded the test, rather than the training session, however, the rats given lithium were markedly inferior to the controls in their rate of re-learning, and did in fact show little or no evidence of having previously been trained in the escape-avoidance situation.

Tadano *et al.* (1972) also looked at lithium effects on conditioned avoidance responses in rats. Doses of 600 μg/kg LiCl i.p. inhibited conditioned pole climbing avoidance responses without affecting the unconditioned reactions. Demers and Heninger (1971) excluded memory loss as a side effect of lithium, but Greenfield *et al.* (1950) and Shopsin *et al.* (1972) have made mention of this effect, and Small *et al.* (1972) recorded that it did occur in some normal volunteer subjects to degrees variously recorded as mild, moderate and severe.

The subject of lithium effects on acquisition and retention processes, important though it is for our understanding of the way in which lithium exerts its therapeutic actions, has only begun to be elucidated. Further work in this area is needed to resolve the questions raised by the few studies already to be found in the literature.

D. Social and interpersonal behaviour

Lithium is always administered to patients in a social setting: the beneficial effects which lithium produces are reflected in changed social (and particularly family) relationships. It is therefore important that the precise nature of the interaction between social and lithium influences on behaviour should be clarified. A few studies have gone some way to providing this clarification.

The most obvious of the social relationships likely to be affected as a result of lithium therapy is that between husband and wife, and a few investigators have paid special attention to this. Mayo (1970), for example, reported that lithium stabilized psychosocial adjustment in all categories of patient, and she recorded reports of the patients' spouses to the effect that marked improvement occurred in marital relationships and the quality of family life. Demers and Davis

(1971) examined interpersonal behaviour relationships of 14 manic-depressive patients, all of whom were discharged from hospital on an out-patient basis, having previously received lithium treatment for their illness as in-patients, and who were being maintained on prophylactic lithium. The patients and their spouses were asked to complete two versions of the Marital Partner Attribute Test, one relating to the pre-treatment period and the other to the present situation. Spouses rated the patients as having lost undesirable traits as a result of lithium treatment, though desirable attributes did not increase appreciably in frequency. The patients' mean ratings of their spouses did not differ significantly from the pre-treatment to the in-treatment periods. The results are interesting, but retrospective completion of questionnaires is always unsatisfactory, particularly when the purpose of the questionnaire is as obvious as that of the MPAT; the tendency of subjects to repeat answers on two serially presented forms inevitably reduces the sensitivity of the test.

Syme and Syme, in New Zealand, are the only investigators who have so far attempted an analysis of the social determinants of lithium action in animals. They demonstrated (Syme and Syme, 1973) that the change in activity brought about by lithium chloride (3 mEq Li$^+$/kg i.p.) in rats is a function of the degree of social isolation which occurs between the time of drug administration and subsequent testing. In other studies (Syme and Syme, personal communication) the same investigators used a series of photographs taken every 30 sec over a 10 min period to assess the effects of 3 mEq Li$^+$/kg (LiCl) i.p. on social contact in rats. The animals were examined in groups of seven, 3 h after drug administration, and sociability was indexed as the average distance between the animals with a correction applied for the tendency of the subjects to keep to the periphery of the test arena. Body contact scores were also noted. The investigators found that, in contrast to their expectations, sociability was increased by lithium among the female rats. The male rats showed increased body contact scores but unchanged social distance when the test environment was novel, but showed increased average social distance when the environment was familiar. The results are curious and difficult to interpret, but they are clearly of sufficient interest to justify further work in this area.

Allison (personal communication) observed that his lithium-treated rats spread themselves throughout the cage and did not huddle together after the manner of the controls. Similar findings have been noted in a short study by Johnson and Carroll (unpublished results) in which male rats kept chronically on lithium (10 mM LiCl solution as the drinking water) were housed three to a cage and were scored over a period of 14 days, on two occasions daily, on a four point (0–3) scale according to whether there was no body contact between the animals ($A; B; C$), contact between one pair ($A + B; C$), contact between two pairs ($A + B; B + C$), or contact between all three ($A + B; B + C; A + C$). It was found that, compared with untreated or sodium chloride-treated controls, the lithium-treated rats showed a significantly reduced amount of body contact. This effect seemed greater in the morning than in the afternoon, but the difference failed to attain statistical significance.

The effects of lithium on social behaviour, and the effects of social circumstances on lithium action are two facets of the same problem: they may, in fact, not be separable in experimental situations. The implications of such experimental studies for the post-treatment social readjustment of patients has yet to be assessed.

E. Aggression

Aggression, as a particular form of social interaction, has been defined in many ways. The term is usually used to cover a complex of behavioural and cognitive processes and it is, therefore, all the more remarkable that, as far as human studies are concerned, the majority of reports have been consistent in finding a marked diminution in the number and intensity of agressive acts following lithium administration. The findings using animal subjects are more variable.

1. Aggression in animals

Weischer (1969) was the first to undertake any close examination of lithium effects on intraspecific aggression. She noted that fighting activity in Siamese fighting fish could be eliminated by adding 10 to 30 mEq Li$^+$/l (LiCl) to the water. Fighting was also reduced by lithium in mice and hamsters but returned with the withdrawal of lithium.

In the following year the topic was again taken up, this time by Sheard (1970b) who elicited aggression in pairs of rats by subjecting them to 1-sec pulses of electric shocks administered to their feet at frequencies of 30 shocks per min. The shock period lasted for 1 min; there was then a 2 min interval before the process was repeated. This was continued until five shock periods had been given. After a 5 min interval a further five shock periods were given, this time using a different shock intensity. Six different shock intensities were examined for the lithium-treated rats and (unaccountably) only four for the saline controls. The mean latency to first attack (expressed in seconds for each of the five series of different shock intensities) was significantly increased by lithium at all shock intensities for which saline controls were available. At the two lowest shock intensities no attack behaviour was observed following lithium treatment, the drugged animals apparently being able to withstand higher shocks intensities before reacting aggressively. Sheard eliminated the possibility of a lithium analgesia by showing that neither flinch nor jump responses to shock were affected by the drug.

In another series of experiments Sheard (1970a) observed that p-chlorophenylalanine enhanced the aggressive behaviour of rats. Pretreatment of the animals with 5 mEq Li$^+$/kg (LiCl) i.p. daily for 5 days not only eliminated the aggression but also resulted in a marked increase in resting behaviour.

More recently, Tadano *et al.* (1972) showed that 600 mg/kg LiCl i.p., or 80 μg LiCl i.c., produced an inhibition of the biting and attacking components of electroshock-induced aggression in rats. Other components, such as vocalization and piloerection, were unaffected.

Eichelman and Thoa (1973), in a general examination of the role of monoamines in the control of aggression, reported on the effects of lithium chloride on shock-elicited attack behaviour in high-fighting Long-Evans rats. Administration of 0·8 mEq Li$^+$/kg (LiCl) i.p. daily over a period of 7 days led to a significant decrease in the percentage of attacks produced by 50 electric shocks: a pre-drug score of 38·4% attacks was reduced to a post-drug score of 20·8%, in contrast to scores for sodium chloride-treated controls of 30·7% and 31·5% respectively for pre- and post-drug states. Like Sheard, Eichelman and Thoa reported that jump thresholds were unaffected by lithium. Mouse killing was also unaffected, and this is particularly interesting in that it raises the question of what is the most appropriate index of aggressive behaviour in animals. There may be fundamental differences in the mechanisms underlying elicited aggression and spontaneous aggression, and in consequence, extrapolation from the studies of lithium effects on animal aggression to aggression in humans must be undertaken with added caution.

A few reports have presented findings which fail to confirm that lithium reduces aggression, indicating that there may sometimes be an increase in aggressiveness amongst animals following lithium treatment. It is often difficult, however, to interpret the findings in such cases.

Thus, S. H. Johnson (1971) noted that lithium-induced aggression often occurred in rats as part of the "injection syndrome" which had a duration of 30 to 60 sec after injection. The rat would "attack its cage mates with such fierceness . . . that it became necessary to isolate the subjects in individual cages for the duration of the syndrome" (p. 60). S. H. Johnson recognized that the aggression was unlikely to be a direct effect of lithium on central nervous mechanisms, but was more likely a reaction to pain caused by the injection of lithium chloride. Schreiber *et al.* (1971) noted an increase in aggressive activity between pairs of lithium-treated rats, a finding also reported by Syme and Syme (1973) who, like S. H. Johnson, related it to physical discomfort resulting from drug administration. Thomsen (personal communication) has commented that some of his rats which were given fairly high doses of lithium so that they were more-or-less intoxicated, showed a "somewhat aggressive behaviour", but he suggests that this might have been only an uncharacteristic symptom of lithium intoxication, the animals generally not being in a good healthy condition.

2. *Psychological processes associated with aggression in humans*

Studies of lithium effects on human aggressiveness are fully reviewed in

Chapter 6 by Kline and Simpson. In these and other studies there are several interesting comments relating to psychological processes associated with overt acts of aggression but not themselves aggressive (in the sense of involving combative behaviour).

Barratt et al. (1968), for example, suggested that lithium may act on neural mechanisms determining impulsive behaviour. A reduction in undisciplined behaviour (Dostal and Zvolsky, 1970) and an increase in rule-obeying (Tupin et al., 1973) have been noted as following lithium treatment. Sheard (1971) found that the hostile content of verbal productions was reduced by lithium, a finding which corresponds to reports by Morrison et al. (1973) of lithium-induced suppression of tendencies to quarrel and of expressions of anger and hostility in general. Tupin et al. (1973) also spoke of an increased capacity of subjects to control their feelings of anger under provocation.

A few reports sound dissenting notes. In 1966, Mayfield and Brown reported that one manic patient became progressively more irascible and demonstrated increased hositility under lithium treatment, and occasional irritability and emotional lability was one of the effects noted by Schou (1968) in lithium-treated normal volunteer subjects. More recently, Small et al. (1972) reported that one subject out of 11 normal volunteers quoted irritability as a mild side effect of lithium. These reports are, however, isolated in the literature and in all cases the appropriate comparisons with placebo-treated controls were not-made.

F. Electrical self-stimulation

Arguing that since lithium apparently has marked effects upon the metabolism of brain monoamines it should affect any behaviour mediated by norepinephrine, Ramsey et al. (1972) examined the effect of lithium on just such a behaviour pattern, namely the self-administration by rats of intracranial electric shocks to the medial forebrain bundle. Daily injections of lithium carbonate, 2 mEq Li$^+$/kg i.p., over a period of 9 days, failed to affect self-stimulatory behaviour. The authors concluded that their failure to obtain any effects might be interpreted as showing that any influences of lithium on norepinephrine metabolism did not necessarily carry implications for the *functional* activity of brain norepinephrine, or alternatively that the lithium effect on monoamines might be specific to particular brain regions.

Pick Cassens and Mills (1973), using rats treated with 1 mEq Li$^+$/kg (LiCl) i.p., showed that thresholds for intracranial self-stimulation were elevated at 2 h after injection by 18% and at 24 h by 36%; a further injection 26 h after the first led to as much as a 53% threshold elevation at 48 h as compared with control subjects.

Samuel and Gottesfeld (1973) quote unpublished results by Edelson, Gottesfeld, Samuel and Yuwiler, to the effect that close examination of continous

M

TABLE I. Details of studies on the effects of lithium on drug-induced behaviour.

| Source | Drug-induced behaviour change | | |
	Drug(s) used	Dose levels and administration regime	Behaviour change produced
Matussek and Linsmayer (1968)	desmethylimipramine (DMI) + Ro 4-1284 (a benzoquinolizine)	20 mg/kg DMI + 15 mg/kg Ro 4-1284; i.p.; the Ro 4-1284 given 1 h after the DMI	Hyperactivity, defined as moving at least twice from a 10 cm high cage, and showing typical signs of compulsive behaviour
	amphetamine	6 mg/kg; i.p.	Increased activity (jumping from cage) and stereotyped behaviour
Kiseleva and Lapin (1969)	5-hydroxytrypto-phan ·	250 mg/kg; i.p.	Head twitches
D'Encarnacao and Anderson (1970)	amphetamine	3 mg/kg; i.p.	Increased activity
	desipramine (DMI) + tetrabenazine	20 mg/kg DMI + 20 mg/kg tetrabenazine; i.p.	Increased activity
Sheard (1970a)	p-chlorophenyl-alanine (PCPA)	320 mg/kg; i.p.	Increased sexual and aggressive behaviour

Table 1—*continued*

Lithium effects Lithium salt	Dose levels and administration regime	Serum lithium levels	Effect on drug-induced behaviour	*Animals used*
Chloride	100 mg/kg 17 h before DMI; i.p.	—	None	rats
	100 mg/kg 1 h before DMI; i.p.	—	Reduced % of hyper-active subjects; duration of hyperactivity reduced	
	200 mg/kg 1 h before DMI; i.p.	—	Ditto	
	2 × 100 mg/kg on day before test, then 100 mg/kg 1 h before DMI; i.p.	—	Ditto, but greater effect	
	2 × 200 mg/kg on day before test, then 100 mg/kg 1 h before DMI; i.p.	—	Ditto	
	100 mg/kg daily for 4 days before test, then 100 mg/kg 1 h before DMI; i.p.	—	Complete elimination of drug-induced hyperactivity	
Chloride	100 mg/kg daily for 4 days; i.p.	—	No effect on the drug-induced excitation; stereotyped behaviour prolonged	
Carbonate	1 mg/kg 1 h before 5-HTP; i.p.	—	No effect	mice
	10 mg/kg 1 h before 5-HTP; i.p.	—	Ditto	
	100 mg/kg 1 h before 5-HTP; i.p.	—	Reduced the number of head twitches	
Carbonate	i.p. injections 3 times daily to build up to specified serum lithium level	1·5 mEq Li$^+$/1	Synergistic potentiation of amphetamine effects	rats
Carbonate	Ditto	Ditto	No effect	
Chloride	5 mEq Li$^+$/kg daily for 5 days prior to PCPA, then 2 h before test; i.p.	—	Significant inhibition of both PCPA-induced sexual and aggressive behaviour; resting behaviour increased	rats

Table I—*continued*

Source	Drug-induced behaviour change		
	Drug(s) used	Dose levels and administration regime	Behaviour change produced
Cox *et al.* (1971)	chlordiazepoxide + dexamphetamine	12·5 mg/kg chlordiazepoxide + 1·18 mg/kg dexamphetamine; s.c.	Hyperactivity, defined as the number of entries into arms of a Y-maze in 5 min; high ataxia ratings
S. Johnson (1971)	*dl*-amphetamine	5·0 mg/kg; i.p.	Increased activity (in activity wheel)
	methamphetamine	5·0 mg/kg; i.p.	Ditto
	methylphenidate	10 mg/kg; i.p.	Ditto
		20 mg/kg; i.p.	Ditto
	caffeine	10·0 mg/kg; i.p.	Ditto
	desmethylimipramine + tetrabenazine	20 mg/kg desmethyl-imipramine + 20 mg/kg tetrabenazine; i.p.	Ditto
U'Prichard and Steinberg (1972)	dexamphetamine + chlordiazepoxide	0·5 mg/kg dexamphetamine + 7·5 mg/kg chlordiazepoxide; i.p.	Increased activity on a hole board (head dips)
		1·18 mg/kg dexamphetamine + 12·5 mg/kg chlordiazepoxide; i.p.	Ditto
		2·36 mg/kg dexamphetamine + 25·0 mg/kg chlordiazepoxide; i.p.	Increased activity in a photocell cage
	dexamphetamine only	2·36 mg/kg dexamphetamine; i.p.	Ditto

Table I—*continued*

Lithium effects Lithium salt	Dose levels and administration regime	Serum lithium levels	Effect on drug-induced behaviour	*Animals used*
Chloride	3mEq Li$^+$/kg daily for 15 days, the last dose 3 h before injection of the drug mixture (chronic); i.p.	0·69mEq Li$^+$/l ±0·166 (s.d.)	No effect	rats
	3mEq Li$^+$/kg 3 h before injection of drug mixture (acute); i.p.	1·06mEq Li$^+$/l ±0·258 (s.d.)	Decrease in activity induced by drug mixture; no change in ataxia ratings	
	2mEq Li$^+$/kg 3 h before injection of drug mixture (acute); i.p.	0·67mEq Li$^+$/l ±0·197 (s.d.)	Ditto	
Chloride	2·4mEq Li$^+$/kg daily for 4 days; i.p.	—	Increased activity at first, then reduced it after 90 min	rats
Chloride	Ditto	—	No difference at first then drug-induced activity potentiated after 90 min	
Chloride	Ditto	—	Potentiates the drug-induced activity throughout the test period	
	Ditto	—	Ditto	
Chloride	Ditto	—	Ditto	
Chloride	Ditto	—	Drug mixture-induced activity eliminated	
Chloride	3 meq Li$^+$/kg; i.p.	—	Eliminated increased activity	mice
	Ditto	—	Ditto	
	Ditto	—	No effect	
Chloride	Ditto	—	No effect	

Table I—*continued*

Source	*Drug-induced behaviour change*		
	Drug(s) used	Dose levels and administration regime	Behaviour change produced
Cox and Steinberg (quoted by Steinberg, 1973)	chlordiazepoxide	? dose; + repeated exposure to a novel environment	Increased Y-maze activity
Geyer *et al.* (1973)	yohimbine	0·25 mg/kg i.v.	Mild agitation; decreased response to stimuli; body arching; mild tremor
		0·50 mg/kg i.v.	Ditto
		0·25 mg/kg i.v.	Ditto
		0·50 mg/kg i.v.	

recordings of brain stimulation by lithium-treated animals reveals that a marked diminution in stimulation rate does in fact occur.

III. Effects on Drug-Induced Behaviour

A number of investigators have felt that the effects of lithium on normal behaviour are too elusive to be of great significance and have turned instead to the study of behavioural changes elicited by other drugs. This approach has the added advantage that it may provide information about the biochemical processes by which lithium brings about its behavioural effects. The major studies which have been carried out under this heading are detailed in Table I.

IV. Cognitive Effects

A rigorous study of the cognitive effects of lithium, either in psychiatric patients undergoing treatment with lithium, or in normal volunteer subjects, has not yet been undertaken, and one must rely upon the infrequent comments on the topic which are to be found distributed among the reports in the literature for some indication of what these effects are likely to be. This is, of course, most unsatisfactory. A patient may, for example, report that he *feels* that his ability to concentrate is impaired even though objective tests may demonstrate that this faculty is in fact either unaffected or indeed improved. Awareness of being under the influence of a drug may have more implications than the direct effects of the drug itself for the way in which a patient or volunteer subject makes reports about his thoughts, emotions and other subjective experiences, particularly when the effects of the drug are likely to be subtle.

Table I—*continued*

Lithium effects Lithium salt	Dose levels and administration regime	Serum lithium levels	Effect on drug-induced behaviour	Animals used
Chloride	? dose; ? route	—	Drug-induced activity reduced	mice
Carbonate	50 mg/kg, 1 h before yohimbine (acute); i.p.	1·29 mEq Li$^+$/l	No effect	dogs
	Ditto	Ditto	Ditto	
	600 mg daily for 4–5 days (chronic); oral	1·54 mEq Li$^+$/l	Ditto	
	Ditto	Ditto	Ditto	

A. Cognitive efficiency

The general trend in such reports as are available in the literature seems to indicate that lithium-treated individuals experience a loss of efficiency in performing various classes of mental operation, and this, in its turn, may lead to discernible behavioural changes. Thus an early report by Mayfield and Brown (1966) noted that in one patient lithium treatment led to a deterioration in the organization of verbal productions; this effect may, of course, have been secondary to peripheral impairment of the muscles involved in speech production, but it seems more likely that it was due to some central action of lithium on cognitive integration mechanisms.

In normal volunteers, lithium has been found to lead to reduced intellectual initiative, difficulties in comprehending and integrating information about social situations, and feelings of impaired concentration (Schou, 1968; Schou *et al.*, 1968) and similar findings have been reported by Small *et al.* (1972) in the form of moderate loss of concentration (a relatively rare occurrence), a slowing of mental functions, and some degree of mental confusion (the latter also in lithium-treated manic-depressive patients). In Chapter 13 these symptoms, and others of a more severe nature, are noted as part of the pattern of lithium side effects and toxic reactions.

In three normal volunteer subjects studied by Small *et al.* (1972) lithium produced noticeable signs of impairment in school performance and work efficiency during the second and third weeks of treatment, though these effects lessened considerably in the fourth week. Demers and Heninger (1971) whilst noting some degree of lithium-induced impairment in the cognitive operations associated with a series of visual-motor co-ordination tasks, commented that these cognitive deficits were not accompanied by confusion, and Heninger (personal communication) has suggested that therapeutic doses of lithium may leave logical types of cognitive abilities unchanged.

The cognitive deficits reported under lithium treatment may, as noted earlier, be more apparent than real, and Marshall *et al.* (1970) note that during a manic state a patient often feels a creative urge, the loss of which may frequently lead to lithium therapy being abandoned by the patient. A number of uncontrolled observations have, however, led to the suggestion that lithium therapy may in fact result in a more uniform overall productivity which is of a sounder quality than the sporadic efforts produced during the manic phases.

Tupin *et al.* (1973) noted that when aggressive individuals were treated with lithium, improvement in aggressiveness was sometimes accompanied by some degree of derealization in the first few weeks of treatment, a finding which is interesting in view of the comment by Schou (1968) and Schou *et al.* (1968) that one accompaniment of lithium ingestion in normal volunteers may be the experience of unusually vivid dreams. It is not certain what contribution such effects may make to lithium-induced reduction of cognitive efficiency.

B. Emotions and character traits

Schou (1968) and Schou *et al.* (1968) have reported that lithium is without effect on emotional responses, and this has been broadly confirmed by experiments on animals using behaviour patterns which have been supposed to possess large emotional components. Thus Harrison-Read and Steinberg (1971) found that whilst lithium increased the jump response of rats to electric shocks applied to the animals' feet, the responses commonly regarded as having emotional components (defaecation, vocalization) were unaffected. More recently, Smith and Smith (1973) showed that lithium changes the open field behaviour of rats but concluded that since it had no effect on the length of time for which animals crouched in response to a sudden click stimulus, or upon the amount of open field defaecation, the results "indicate that lithium does not consistently alter emotional reactivity in rats" (p. 87).

Barratt *et al.* (1970) did suggest that lithium might exert differential effects on animals derived from emotional and non-emotional strains, but the comment was not supported by data.

A variety of emotional states which are distributed during affective illness are stabilized by lithium treatment: this is not, of course, to say that lithium acts directly upon the mechanisms responsible for controlling these feelings. Amongst the emotional and character trait effects which have been reported to undergo positive improvements following the institution of lithium therapy are:

endurance and forbearance (Schou, 1968; Schou *et al.*, 1968), enthusiasm (Demers and Davis), self-respect, patience, moodiness, tenseness and self-awareness (Morrison *et al.*, 1973), reflective mood (Tupin *et al.*, 1973) and anxiety (Samuel and Gottesfeld, 1973; Tupin *et al.*, 1973).

V. Concluding Remarks

There is much to say about the behavioural and cognitive effects of lithium but, as yet, little to be concluded. It is clear that much remains to be done in this most interesting area. Future work must certainly pay attention to the problem of extrapolating from the experimental to the clinical context, and appropriate dose levels and regimes and relevant test situations must be used. The emphasis, too, must swing more towards human studies if relevance to lithium therapy is to be preserved and emphasized. Eventually it may be possible to provide a full psychological specification of the psychiatric effects of lithium: that day, unfortunately, seems far away.

References

Balagura, S. and Smith, D. F. (1970a). *Amer. J. Physiol.* **219**, 1231–1234.

Balagura, S. and Smith, D. F. (1970b). *In* "Proc. 87th Ann. Convention APA". 213–214.

Balagura, S., Brophy, J. and Devenport, L. D. (1972). *J. comp. physiol. Psychol.* **81**, 212–219.

Barratt, E. S., Creson, D. L. and Russell, G. (1968). *Amer. J. Psychiat.* **125**, 530–536.

Benowitz, L. and Magnus, J. G. (1973). *Behav. Biol.* **8**, 367–380.

Benowitz, L. I. and Sperry, R. W. (1975). *Expl. Neurol.* **40**, 405–546.

Boland, F. J. (1973). *Anim. Learn. Behav.* **1**, 3–4.

Cade, J. F. J. (1949). *Med. J. Aust.* **36**, 349–352.

Corrodi, H., Fuxe, K., Hökfelt, T. and Schou, M. (1967). *Psychopharmacologia* **11**, 345–353.

Cox, C., Harrison-Read, P. E., Steinberg, H. and TomKiewicz, M. (1971). *Nature* **232**, 336–338.

Cullen, J. W. (1970). *J. comp. physiol. Psychol.* **72**, 79–84.

Demers, R. G. and Davis, L. S. (1971). *Compreh. Psychiat.* **12**, 348–353.

Demers, R. G. and Heninger, G. H. (1971). *J. clin. Pharmacol.* **11**, 274–279.

D'Encarnacao, P. S. and Anderson, K. (1970). *Dis. nerv. Syst.* **31**, 494–496.

Dostal, T. and Zvolsky, P. (1970). *Int. Pharmacopsychiat.* **5**, 203–207.

Eichelman, B. S., Jr. and Thoa, N. B. (1973). *Biol. Psychiat.* **6**, 143–164.

Erikson, R. P. (1963). *In* "Olfaction and Taste" (Y. Zotterman, ed.). Pergamon Press, London.

Fregley, M. J. (1953). *Amer. J. Physiol.* **195**, 645–653.

Frumkin, K. (1971). *J. comp. physiol. Psychol.* **75**, 32–40.

Geyer, H., Sanghvi, I. and Gershon, S. (1973). *Psychopharmacolgia* **28**, 107–113.

Greenfield, I., Zuger, M., Bleak, R. M. and Bakal, S. F. (1950). *N.Y. State J. Med.* **50**, 459–560.

Harrison-Read, P. E. and Steinberg, H. (1971). *Nature New Biology* **232**, 120–121.

Johnson, F. N. (1972a). *Experientia* **28**, 533–535.

Johnson, F. N. (1972b). *Nature* **238**, 333–334.

Johnson, F. N. (1972c). *Psychosomatics* **13**, 203–205.

Johnson, F. N. and Barker, G. (1972). *Dis. nerv. Syst.* **33**, 664–666.

Johnson, F. N. and Wormington, S. (1972). *Nature New Biology* **235**, 159–160.

Johnson, S. H. (1971). Unpublished Ph.D. thesis. University of Tennessee.

Kiseleva, I. P. and Lapin, I. P. (1969). *Pharmacol. res. Commun.* **1**, 108–114.

Lehr, P. P. and Nachman, M. (1973). *Physiol. Behav.* **10**, 79–83.

MacLeod, J.; Swan, R. C. and Aitken, G. A. (1949). *Amer. J. Physiol.* **157**, 177–183.

Männistö, P. T. and Saarnivaara, L. (1972). *Pharmacol.* **8**, 329–335.

Mark, R. F. and Watts, M. E. (1971). *Proc. R. Soc. Lond. B.* **178**, 439–454.

Marshall, M. H.; Neumann, C. P. and Robinson, M. (1970). *Psychosomatics* **11**, 406–408.

Matussek, N. and Linsmayer, M. (1968). *Life Sci.* **7**, 371–375.

Mayfield, D. and Brown, R. G. (1966). *J. psychiat. Res.* **4**, 207–219.

Mayo, J. A. (1970). *Int. Pharmacopsychiat.* **5**, 190–202.

Morrison, S. D., Erwin, C. W., Gianturco, D. T. and Gerber, C. J. (1973). *Dis. nerv. Syst.* **34**, 186–189.

Nachman, M. (1963a). *J. comp. physiol. Psychol.* **56**, 343–349.

Nachman, M. (1963b). *Amer. J. Physiol.* **205**, 219–221.

Nachman, M. (1970). *J. comp. physiol. Psychol.* **73**, 22–30.

Nachman, M. and Ashe, J. H. (1973). *Physiol. Behav.* **10**, 73–78.

Nachman, M.; Lester, D. and Le Magnen, J. (1970). *Science* **168**, 1244–1246.

O'Boyle, M.; Looney, T. A. and Cohen, P. S. (1973). *Bull. Psychon. Soc.* **1**, 250–251.

Pick Cassens, G. and Mills, A. W. (1973). *Psychopharmacologia* **30**, 283–290.

Ramsey, T. A., Mendels, J., Hamilton, C. and Frazer, A. (1972). *Life Sci.* **11**, 773–779.

Samuel, D. and Gottesfeld, Z. (1973). *Endeavour* **32**, 122–128.

Schou, M. (1968). *J. psychiat. Res.* **6**, 67–95.

Schou, M., Amdisen, A. and Thomsen, K. (1968). *In* "De Psychiatria Progrediente" (P. Baudis, E. Petrova and V. Sedivec, eds.) Vol. 2, pp 712–721. Plzen.

Schreiber, V., Rohacova, J. and Pribyl, T. (1971). *Physiol. Bohemoslov.* **20**, 249–254.

Sheard, M. H. (1970a) *Commun. behav. Biol.* **5**, 71–73.

Sheard, M. H. (1970b) *Nature* **228**, 284–285.

Sheard, M. H. (1971). *Nature* **230**, 113–114.

Shopsin, B., Stern, S. and Gershon, S. (1972). *Archs gen. Psychiat.* **26**, 566–571.

Small, J. G., Milstein, V., Perez, H. C., Small, I. F. and Moore, D. F. (1972). *Biol. Psychiat.* **5**, 65–77.

Smith, D. F. and Balagura, S. (1969). *J. comp. physiol. Psychol.* **69**, 308–310.

Smith, D. F. and Smith, H. B. (1973). *Psychopharmacologia* **30**, 83–88.

Smith, D. F., Balagura, S. and Lubram, M. (1970). *Amer. J. Physiol.* **218**, 751–754.

Steinberg, H. (1973). *Biochem. Soc. Trans.* **1**, 38–41.

Strom, C., Lingenfelter, A. and Brody, J. F. (1970). *Psychonom. Sci.* **18**, 209–291.

Syme, L. A. and Syme, G. J. (1973). *Psychopharmacologia* **29**, 85–89.

Tadano, T., Sakurada, S., Nishioka, M. and Kisara, K. (1972). *Jap. J. Pharmacol.* **22**, 96.

Thiébot, M. H., Soubrié, P., Simon, P. and Boissier, J. R. (1973). *Psychopharmacologia* **31**, 77–90.

Tupin, J. P., Smith, D. B., Clanon, T. L., Kim, L. I., Nugent, A. and Groupe, A. (1973). *Compreh. Psychiat.* **14**, 311–317.

U'Prichard, D. C. and Steinberg, H. (1972). *Brit. J. Pharmacol.* **44,** 349P–350P.
Watts, M. E. and Mark, R. F. (1971). *Proc. R. Soc. Lond. B.* **178,** 455–464.
Weischer, M-L. (1969). *Psychopharmacologia* **15,** 245–254.
Wittrig, J., Woods, A. E. and Anthony, E. J. (1970). *Dis. nerv. Syst.* **31,** 767–771.

20

BEHAVIOURAL AND COGNITIVE EFFECTS OF LITHIUM: MECHANISMS

F. N. JOHNSON

I. Introduction

In order to react to its environment, an animal must receive information by way of its sense organs and produce actions using its motor apparatus. Lithium-induced changes in the functioning of either input or output systems will modify behaviour. Having received sensory information the animal must analyse it and make an appropriate response. Sensory analysis implies attaching meaning or significance to the input in the light of memories of past experiences and also with reference to the innate physiological and biochemical demands of the body. Having analysed the input, the animal has to select one response out of its total behavioural repertoire and initiate the execution of that response. Lithium may affect sensory analysis or the executive decision mechanisms (or both) either directly or, via effects on associated processes such as memory and homeostatic feedback systems, indirectly. The available evidence does not allow a definitive choice to be made between these various possibilities, and indeed both conceptually and empirically they may be very difficult to separate; some interesting pointers are, however, provided by the literature.

II. Effects on Sensory Input: Analgesia

Information on this topic is scanty and the few reports of a moderate degree of vision blurring following lithium administration (e.g., Small *et al.*, 1972) are hardly satisfactory evidence of an effect on visual receptors: such effects are almost certainly central and not caused by modification of sense organ functioning. This difficulty which is encountered in distinguishing between peripheral and central influences on sensory processes is particularly evident in interpreting reports of lithium effects on analgesia.

Sheard (1970) found that 5 days pretreatment of rats with 5 mEq Li^+/kg (LiCl) i.p. affected neither the jump nor flinch thresholds to footshock stimulation, indicating that the drug produced no discernible analgesic effect. Indeed, there is some evidence that lithium may produce hypersensitivity to electrical shocks: thus, Weischer and Opitz (1970) reported that 40 mEq Li^+/l concentrations of LiCl in drinking water given over a period of 8 days produced in rodents a lessening of the analgesic effects of various drugs (codeine, dextropropoxylene and glafenine). Whether this represents a pharmacological antagonism to the analgesics or a direct lithium-induced hypersensitivity to pain cannot be determined from this study, though the investigators hypothesised that lithium produced its interference with the analgesics by way of effects on brain monoamines (see Chapter 25). Harrison-Read and Steinberg (1971) found that treatment with lithium chloride for a few days caused rats to become hypersensitive to painful stimulation, such as the insertion of a hypodermic needle or the administration of electric shocks to the animals' feet. Jump response thresholds to footshock were lowered by 10% by 1 mEq Li^+/kg and by 25% by 2 mEq Li^+/kg: this latter was the maximum lowering which could be achieved, however, and higher doses of lithium were reported to lead (occasionally) to lowered sensitivity to shock, possibly as a result of various toxic reactions to the drug. Experiments in which these investigators manipulated 5-hydroxytryptophan metabolism showed that the lithium-induced hypersensitivity could be eliminated by raising 5HT levels (either directly, or by giving imipramine, a drug which may itself enhance the action of 5HT). The authors suggested that a deficit of 5HT might be responsible for the hypersensitivity elicited by lithium. However, Harrison-Read (personal communication) noted that in some experiments he had found that the lithium-induced lowering of footshock thresholds was not very marked, and might indeed be absent. The precise nature of the mechanisms underlying the apparent hypersensitivity to noxious stimulation induced by lithium is obscured by several factors described by Harrison-Read (personal communication). Jump thresholds may be lowered not only by lithium but also by any mild disturbance or slight stress during the pretreatment period (such as a single Y-maze trial, or simply being housed in the same room as that in which the experiments were being conducted). A more marked stress, produced by tumbling the rats in a rotating drum, will also reduce footshock jump thresholds. Mild stress and the more severe stress were, however, found by Harrison-Read to differ in that the threshold lowering was offset by 5HT in the latter case but not in the former. This suggests that the mechanism of threshold lowering may not be unitary and, as Harrison-Read points out, lithium pretreatment may in itself be aversive and produce a mild stress which only secondarily leads to footshock hypersensitivity.

Männistö and Saarnivaara (1972) employed two measures of analgesia in mice: the time taken for a reaction to occur to being placed on a hotplate, and the number of writhing motions made in a 5-min period following an i.p. injection of phenylquinone. Acute administration of doses of 5 and 20 mEq Li^+/kg (LiCl) i.p. (leading to serum levels of $0 \cdot 2$ and $4 \cdot 3$ mEq Li^+/l, respectively) produced no effect on hotplate responses, but the larger dose did significantly reduce the writhing test scores. Chronic administration of lithium chloride in the drinking water (producing serum levels of $0 \cdot 1$ mEq Li^+/l) produced no effect on either analgesic test after 7 or 50 days treatment, but after 90 days the writhing test score was significantly decreased. Lithium treatment potentiated morphine analgesia, but antagonised the antinociceptive effects of tricyclic antidepressants.

The literature relating to lithium effects on analgesia clearly does not, in itself, lead one to conclude anything about the actions which lithium may have upon sensory processes. There is obviously a need for carefully conducted studies to establish whether or not lithium influences such functions as visual and auditory acuity, the sensitivity of pain, heat and touch receptors, etc., and, if so, whether the action is central (as seems likely) or directly upon the sense receptors themselves.

III. Effects on Motor Output

The most extreme effect which lithium can have on motor activity is to induce complete or partial paralysis. Paralysis of the hind limbs has been reported as a toxic reaction to lithium in cats (Good, 1903), rats (MacLeod *et al.,* 1949) and dogs (Neretin, 1959). S. H. Johnson (1971) observed a temporary paralysis of the hind limbs of the rat, frequently resulting in the animal falling over, following i.p. injection of lithium chloride: sodium chloride did not produce this effect, and S. H. Johnson suggested that the mechanism of temporary paralysis in the post-injection syndrome might involve the rapid depolarization of neurones around the injection site.

Rather less extreme types of muscular side-effects are frequently reported to accompany lithium treatment in humans (see Chapter 13): a fine hand tremor is, for example, particularly common in the early stages of treatment. Though most of the observations of tremor have come from studies of human subjects there are a few reports of similar findings in animals. Good (1903) noted the occurrence of limb tremors in some of his lithium-treated cats, an effect also reported by MacLeod *et al.* (1949) in rats and by Neretin (1959) in dogs. To the extent that this effect may occur in animal behaviour studies it may be expected to influence the behavioural outcomes: as yet, however, no satisfactory investigation of lithium-induced tremor has been undertaken using animal subjects and the contribution made by tremor to behavioural effect is therefore uncertain.

Good (1903) also recorded unsteadiness as an effect of high doses of lithium in cats and noted that one of his animals was unable to walk without tottering. However, Cox *et al.* (1971) observed that lithium chloride did not increase ataxia ratings in animals already made slightly ataxic with treatment using other drugs, and whilst Small *et al.* (1972) did note ataxia as a side effect in some lithium-treated patients, the incidence was extremely low and only in one patient could the ataxia be classified as severe. A fuller discussion of the ataxic effects of lithium is to be found in Chapter 13.

Good (1903) and MacLeod *et al.* (1949) reported hind-leg weakness prior to actual paralysis in their lithium-treated animals. Cats receiving 100 mg LiCl/kg daily for a week were reported by Barratt *et al.* (1968) to become very weak at the end of that period. Muscular weakness is, indeed, a frequently reported accompaniment of lithium treatment (see Chapter 13). Self-administration of lithium in prophylactic doses (25 mEq Li$^+$ per day) by Schou and certain of his colleagues (Schou, 1968; Schou *et al.*, 1968) led to feelings of slight muscular weakness during the first week, but thereafter these feelings disappeared. However, higher doses in the therapeutic range (50 mEq Li$^+$ per day) produced no weakness in the muscles.

The posture adopted by animals after lithium administration may also reflect muscular weakness. With high doses, animals frequently crouch in a hunched position (Good, 1903) and dogs receiving daily doses of 150 mg LiCl/kg with their food for 12 months (Neretin, 1959) were observed to spend much of their time lying down.

Demers and Heninger (1971) note that gross alterations of motor function are not usually associated with lithium treatment, but in a study of visual-motor performances of six patients undergoing lithium treatment they noted test performances which were characterized in part by a slowing of motor response. This did not, however, seem to be associated with any discernible problems of muscular co-ordination.

Some investigators have been led to deny that induced muscular weakness plays a significant role in determining lithium's behavioural effects, at least when sub-toxic doses are used (e.g., Cox *et al.*, 1971). Johnson and Wormington (1972), noting that lithium reduced rearing frequency in rats (see Chapter 19), also commented that once a rear had commenced there was no reduction in the height attained and, like Cox and her associates, they held this to indicate that muscular weakness was not one of the behaviourally important effects of lithium. Smith and Smith (1973) have, more recently, confirmed this general impression, reporting that rats fed on lithium-loaded diets were unaffected in the time for which they were able to swim until exhausted.

Under certain circumstances lithium may facilitate motor functioning. Thus, immobility produced in rats as part of an aggressive behaviour complex following electric shock was inhibited by 600 mg/kg LiCl i.p. or 80 μg i.c. Tadano *et al.* (1972). Again, one is forced to conclude that definitive statements about the role of motor effects in determining the behavioural actions of lithium cannot yet be made.

IV. Effects on Sensory Analysis

Johnson (1972a) has suggested that one way in which lithium may produce its behavioural effects is by impairing the animals' ability to analyse and attach significance (i.e., meaning or importance) to stimuli arising from the environment. The evidence for this view comes from many sources.

Cade (1949) in his original report on the effects of lithium, noted marked behavioural changes resulting from large doses of lithium carbonate administered to guinea-pigs; he commented that the animals became "extremely lethargic and unresponsive to stimuli for one to two hours before once again becoming normally active and timid." (p. 350). In a later account of this work, Cade referred to the lithium as producing a state of tranquillization but without producing a concomitant sleepiness, again emphasising that an effect upon responsiveness to stimulation was the most obvious action of the drug (Cade, 1967).

Johnson (1972b) and Johnson and Wormington (1972) demonstrated that lithium reduced rearing activity in rats (see Chapter 19) but that no effect was discernible on horizontal locomotory activity. Rearing activity, under the experimental conditions used by Johnson and his associates, seems to represent a behavioural response to environmental stimulation (Holland *et al.*, 1966; Johnson, 1972b) whilst horizontal activity seems relatively independent of variations in the stimulus configuration of the surroundings (Johnson, 1972b). The view was therefore advanced (Johnson, 1972a) that lithium has a selective action upon activity resulting from a response to stimulation and that any activity of a truly spontaneous and non-reactive nature (the horizontal activity being of this type) would remain unaffected.

This general conclusion finds support from other directions. Johnson (1972b) examined the rearing frequency scores of rats tested for 5 min periods each day over a 6-day period: when given placebo injections the animals reared progressively less frequently each day and it was suggested that they were becoming habituated to the test environment. When given lithium injections for the first 3 days the animals, as expected, reared less frequently: however, when the lithium was withdrawn for the remaining 3 days their rearing scores were significantly higher than those of placebo-treated subjects on equivalent days and not significantly different from the scores shown by the placebo controls during the *first* 3 days. The conclusion was that the lithium prevented the animals from analysing, and therefore from habituating to, the test environment, so that when its influence was withdrawn the animals behaved as though they had never seen the test situation before.

D'Encarnacao and Anderson (1970) reported a lithium-induced "calming effect" on animals placed in activity cages; the high initial activity usually noted in untreated rats, and regarded by the investigators as "arousal activity" as a result of being placed in a novel environment, was markedly reduced by lithium. Cox *et al.* (1971) introduced rats into a novel environment (a Y-maze) after first treating them with a mixture of chlordiazepoxide and dexamphetamine; the exploratory behaviour of the animals (assessed as the number of entries into the arms of the maze) was elevated by the drug treatment, but reduced again by lithium. Cox and her associates did not relate their findings to a lithium effect on stimulus analysis, but it is clearly possible to interpret the data in this way. However, Steinberg (1973), reviewing the work of Cox *et al.* (1971) and other studies of a similar nature, commented that lithium reduced the "spontaneous" activity of the animals and made them "pay more attention to and investigate novel aspects of their environment," (p. 40). This conclusion is clearly opposed to what one would expect if lithium were reducing the animal's awareness of their environment. The kinds of behaviour observed in the experiments to which Steinberg refers are almost certainly not spontaneous in the way that Steinberg seems to employ the term (i.e., as implying a self-generated nature and independence from environmental circumstances); the drug-induced hyperactivity was more likely to be reflecting an increase in *re*activity since Steinberg notes that activity tests in situations similar to the animals' home environments showed less drug-induced hyperactivity and it follows that the drug mixtures must have been producing their effects by increasing the animals' awareness of the differences between home and test situations. A lithium-induced reduction in this hyperactivity is entirely consistent with a lithium effect on stimulus analysis.

Similarly, head-dipping behaviour exhibited by mice on a hole-board is another form of behaviour studied by Steinberg and her colleagues. The form of activity is, almost by definition, environment-directed, and the chlordiazepoxide/amphetamine mixtures used by the investigators increased the frequency of this behaviour—i.e., made the animals respond more frequently to the sight of holes, resulting in extreme stimulus-bound stereotyped responses on occasion. Again, that lithium should reduce head-dipping frequency is predictable if there is a diminution in the significance attached by the animals to the sight of holes on the board.

Steinberg also investigated activity in a Y-maze; this activity which was quite clearly of an exploratory nature, was elevated by pretreatment of the mice with chlordiazepoxide *and* repeated exposure to an open field, this latter procedure serving to enhance the novelty of the "new environment" (p. 40)—i.e., the Y–maze. Lithium, again not unexpectedly on the assumption that it relaxes stimulus control, reduced the Y-maze activity of these mice.

It is not easy to follow Steinberg's argument that the lithium-treated animals were paying more attention to their environment when the drug mixtures used clearly increased the stimulus binding of the animals' behaviour. The lithium effects would, in fact, seem to be better explained in terms of *reduced* attention to the environment, resulting in the animals being freed from the stimulus binding which often led to stereotypy of response patterns.

If lithium does indeed act in this way, as a result of changing central stimulus analysing mechanisms, it ought to be possible to detect variations in the physiological processes which are associated with sensory processing. There is some information on this topic, but not much. Barratt *et al.* (1968) examined the responsiveness of lithium-treated cats to auditory stimuli, using head-turning behavioural responses and evoked cortical responses as behavioural and physiological response indices respectively. Untreated, or placebo-treated, animals produced head-turning responses and evoked cortical responses which both rapidly habituated to repeated presentations of a tone, but treatment of lithium changed the pattern of response in a most interesting manner. Behavioural responses did not occur, or occurred to a markedly reduced degree: cortical evoked responses, however, not only occurred but also *never* habituated. Clearly, since the auditory input reached cortical levels the lithium blockade of the behavioural responses was not mediated by effects on receptors, spinal pathways, or subcortical mechanisms, and it suggests that the action was primarily upon cortical processing. The meaning, or significance, of the stimulus input was, therefore, unassessed and no behavioural response could be initiated. Furthermore, the process of habituation to sensory input implies that new input is analysed and recognized as similar or identical to previous input: a central blocking of analysis explains why the lithium-treated animals never showed habituation to the tone. Similar effects have been found in lithium-treated human subjects, there again being less habituation to stimulus input in the EEG recordings than noted in placebo-treated controls (Barratt *et al.,* 1970).

In addition to exploratory and orienting behaviour there are other behaviour patterns which are elicited and maintained by environmental stimuli. These, too, would be expected to be modified by lithium. Aggression directed towards other animals is clearly under environmental stimulus control and many reports have, indeed, indicated that aggressive behaviour may be dramatically reduced by lithium (see Chapter 19 for full details of these studies).

Some supportive evidence for the hypothesis of stimulus significance reduction by lithium is available from reports made by patients undergoing lithium therapy. Such patients are, for example, frequently quoted as saying that they no longer view as carrying the same importance situations which previously caused them concern or impelled them to some form of action (Bunney *et al.*, 1968; Dyson and Mendelson, 1968): this may, in fact, be a cause for complaint in some patients who previously relied upon situational arousal to provide the stimulus for creative work, and it may lead to the patients' terminating their prophylactic lithium treatment (Polatin and Fieve, 1971).

Schou (1968), reporting on experiences resulting from self-administration of lithium by himself and certain of his colleagues makes the following interesting comment:

> "Psychological effects were, on the whole, subtle and ill-defined . . . . There might be hypersensitivity to sights and sounds. On other occasions responsiveness to environmental stimuli was diminished . . . The subjective experience was primarily one of indifference and slight general malaise. This led to a certain passivity. The subjects often had a feeling of being at a distance from their environment, as if separated from it by a glass wall . . . The subjects . . . found it difficult to comprehend and integrate more than a few elements of a situation." (p. 78).

All of the effects ascribed to lithium, with the exception of the note on occasional hypersensitivity, are clearly quite consistent with the subjects' receiving stimuli but being impaired in their abilities to process and attach significance to the information input.

It would, of course, be useful to have information about the subjective experiences of manic-depressive patients treated with lithium, but as yet there have not been any studies specifically designed to collect the kinds of data which would provide support for, or evidence against, the stimulus significance reduction hypothesis of lithium action. It may be premature to subsume under the terms of such a hypothesis the frequent reports of disorientation, mental confusion and clouding of consciousness which accompany lithium toxicity (see Chapter 13), but this is clearly a possible extension of the hypothesis.

It is also interesting that, on occasion, disorders characterized by obsessionality, or involving phobic reactions, have proved amenable to control by lithium (Forssman and Wålinder, 1969): such conditions may be maintained by extreme forms of stimulus control.

One of the few studies involving human subjects which have direct bearing on the role of lithium in controlling stimulus analysis was performed by Demers and Heninger (1971). These investigators gave three tests of visual-motor function to six patients undergoing treatment with lithium, and also to six matched control subjects. Under lithium treatment there were found to be impaired performances on digit-symbol substitution tests, but Bender-Gestalt test scores were unaffected. The effects were reversible, disappearing on discontinuation of lithium. The results were interpreted as indicating a significant slowing of the rate of information processing (i.e., of the analysis of stimulus input) as a result of lithium administration.

Whilst there are obviously many behavioural effects resulting from lithium administration which do not fit happily into the general framework of the stimulus significance reduction hypothesis, there are many others which not only do so readily, but which are difficult to explain with equal ease on the basis of other models of the drug's action.

V. Effects on the Initiation of Motor Activity

Operationally, it is difficult to distinguish between a lithium-induced impairment of stimulus analysis and a failure of the animal to initiate a response following successful and efficient analysis. Several sources of information suggest that the latter viewpoint may be particularly useful in explaining certain of the drug's behavioural effects, both under experimental circumstances and within the clinical context.

Schou (1968) reported that 50 mEq Li$^+$/day administered to normal volunteer subjects produced effects which can be described as a disturbance of the mechanisms for initiating action. He noted that the subjects "had to overcome a certain resistance against rising and moving and also had the feeling that mental effort was needed to undertake any physical task." (p. 78). That it was initiation and not subsequent execution which was affected is made clear by Schou's next sentence: "Once activity had started the muscles were not weaker than usual, and exercise did not fatigue the subject to any abnormal extent." (p. 78). In the same paper, Schou also referred to the feelings of restraint or internal curbing reported by some patients undergoing lithium therapy, which suggests that the stimuli which initiate activity may be processed but that the activity itself is, in some way, prevented from occurring. This is similar to the claim made by Tupin et al. (1973) that lithium might enhance an individual's self-control, particularly over aggressive impulses, and to the implications of the work by Barratt et al. (1968, 1970) in which the action of lithium is linked to neural mechanisms thought to be involved in impulsive behaviour.

Evidence on the point is also forthcoming from experiments on rats. Johnson and Wormington (1972), commenting on the fact that lithium reduced rearing *frequency* whilst leaving rearing *height* unaffected (Chapter 19) suggested that the drug "impairs the initiation of the response, and not the efficiency of the response once initiated" (p. 160). The parallel with Schou's comment is clear. Smith and Smith (1973) showed that the time for which animals continued to crouch following loud click stimuli was unaffected by lithium, but if it is indeed the case that, in the authors' own words, "lithium inhibits the initiation of voluntary activity in rats" (p. 87) it would seem that it would have been more appropriate to seek an effect of lithium on the *establishment*, rather than upon the *duration*, of responses. This would, of course, involve using stimuli which were not so intense that they could override the undoubtedly subtle actions of lithium. It may be one of the virtues of lithium that it has its action, whether it be on stimulus analysis or upon response initiation, on stimuli of around threshold intensities: this might be sufficient to control the occurrence of abnormal responses without producing a blanket sedating effect upon the wider range of essential activities.

VI. Periodicity

It is possible that lithium exerts some of its effects on behaviour in a more devious manner than by the various mechanisms considered above. It may modify the operation of those behavioural processes which are under the control of oscillatory processes and therefore subject to rhythmic variations.

As Tupin (1972) and Tupin *et al.* (1973) have pointed out, there is some evidence that the therapeutic effectiveness of lithium may extend to the control of non-manic-depressive conditions characterized by periodicity, and this is a view which is developed in Chapter 6. Tupin (1970) had previously reported that, in addition to raising the mean body temperature in a group of manic-depressive patients, lithium carbonate in doses of 300 mg given four times a day, produced a shift in the time of occurrence of the peak daily body temperature from 6 p.m. to 12 noon. There was, however, no change in the period length of the temperature variation cycle.

Support for the view that lithium may directly affect cyclic processes comes from a rather unexpected source. Engelmann (1972) showed that lithium increased the period length of the rhythmic petal movements of *Kalanchoe blossfeldiana* flowers, and commented that this could reflect an action on either the basic oscillator mechanism or on the coupling between the oscillator and the overt rhythm. In later experiments Engelmann (1973) has confirmed the action of lithium in extending period length in *Kalanchoe,* and has demonstrated that the period length is a positive near-linear function of the lithium concentration used in the experiments. In addition, he studied the effects of 2 mg LiCl given in 10 ml drinking water daily over a 15 day period, on the activity cycle of *Meriones crassus* (the desert rat). A slight, but distinct, increase of period length from 23·56 hours to 23·62 hours was reported over a 48 hour period.

Matussek (1971) had previously argued that, in view of the effectiveness of lithium against psychiatric conditions of an essentially cyclic nature, one would expect to find that lithium influenced other cyclic processes in animals. He found, however, that chronic treatment of rats with lithium, producing plasma levels of 0·6 to 0·7 mEq Li^+/kg, had no effect on period length of the activity cycle in these animals. Activity was changed only to the extent that the nocturnal activity scores were reduced as compared with those of control animals.

This area of study is intriguing and may eventually yield valuable information of direct relevance to the understanding of lithium action in recurrent affective disorders.

VII. Concluding Remarks

Understanding the behavioural effects of lithium is not going to be easy: it presents a special challenge to the ingenuity of the experimental psychologist. It may well be that no simple or unitary model will suffice to encompass all the varied effects which lithium produces on behaviour, and it has also to be recognized that a descriptive model which is suitable for the kinds of data which emerge from laboratory experiments may be quite unsuited to the clinical therapeutic situation, and vice versa.

Nothing has been said in this chapter regarding the possible biochemical or physiological bases of lithium's behavioural effects. This reflects in part our ignorance of the organismic bases of behaviour in general, and in part the confusion which presently surrounds the biological effects of lithium in particular.

There is, however, some reason for optimism, and the behavioural observations which are available at the present time, scanty though they may be, do provide a starting point for the establishment of testable hypotheses. The next few years may see those hypotheses being clearly stated, tested, and restated in forms having relevance to the practical issues of lithium therapy.

References

Barratt, E. S., Creson, D. L. and Russell, G. (1968). *Amer. J. Psychiat.* **125**, 530–536.

Barratt, E. S., Russell, G., Creson, D. and Tupin, J. (1970). *Dis. nerv. Syst.* **31**, 335–337.

Bunney, W. E., Goodwin, F. K., Davis, J. M. and Fawcett, J. A. (1968). *Amer. J. Psychiat.* **125**, 499–512.

Cade, J. F. J. (1949). *Med. J. Aust.* **36**, 349–352.

Cade, J. F. J. (1967). *Aust. N.Z. J. Psychiat.* **1**, 61–62.

Cox, C., Harrison-Read, P. E., Steinberg, H. and Tomkiewicz, M. (1971). *Nature* **232**, 336–338.

Demers, R. G. and Heninger, G. R. (1971). *J. clin. Pharmacol.* **11**, 274–279.

D'Encarnacao, P. S. and Anderson, K. (1970). *Dis. nerv. Syst.* **31**, 494–496.

Dyson, W. L. and Mendelson, M. (1968). *Amer. J. Psychiat.* **125**, 544–548.

Engelmann, W. (1972). *Z. Naturf.* **27**, 477.

Engelmann, W. (1973). *Z. Naturf.* **28**, 733–736.

Forssman, H. and Wålinder, J. (1969). *Acta psychiat. scand. Suppl.* **207**, 34–40.

Good, C. A. (1903). *Amer. J. med. Sci.* **125**, 273–284.

Harrison-Read, P. E. and Steinberg, H. (1971). *Nature New Biology* **232**, 120–121.

Holland, H. C., Gupta, B. D. and Weldon, E. (1966). *Activ. nerv. super.* **8**, 140–144.

Johnson, F. N. (1972a). *Dis. nerv. Syst.* **33**, 235–241.

Johnson, F. N. (1972b). *Experientia* **28**, 533–535.

Johnson, F. N. and Wormington, S. (1972). *Nature New Biology* **235**, 159–160.

Johnson, S. H. (1971). Unpublished Ph.D. Thesis; University of Tennessee.

MacLeod, J., Swan, R. C., Aitken, G. A. (1949). *Amer. J. Physiol.* **157**, 177–183.

Männiströ, P. T. and Saarnivaara, L. (1972). *Pharmacol.* **8**, 329–335.

Matussek, N. (1971). *Int. Pharmacopsychiat.* **6**, 170–186.

Neretin, V. IA (1959). *Probl. Haematol. blood. Transfus.* **4**, 36–39.

Polatin, P. and Fieve, R. R. (1971). *J. Amer. med. Assoc.* **218**, 864–866.

Schou, M. (1968). *J. psychiat. Res.* **6**, 67–95.

Schou, M., Amdisen, A. and Thomsen, K. (1968). In "De Psychiatria Progrediente" (P. Baudis, E. Petrova and V. Sedivec, eds). Vol. 2. pp. 712–721. Plzen.

Sheard, M. H. (1970). *Nature* **288**, 284–285.

Small, J. G., Milstein, V., Perez, H. C., Small, I. F. and Moore, D. F. (1972). *Biol. Psychiat.* **5**, 65–77.

Smith, D. F. and Smith, H. B. (1973). *Psychopharmacologia* **30**, 83–88.

Steinberg, H. (1973). *Biochem. Soc. Trans.* **1**, 38–41.

Tadano, T., Sakurada, S., Nishioka, M. and Kisara, K. (1972). *Jap. J. Pharmacol.* **22**, 96.

Tupin, J. P. (1970). *Int. Pharmacopsychiat.* **5**, 227–232.

Tupin, J. P. (1972). *Compreh. Psychiat.* **13**, 209–214.

Tupin, J. P., Smith, D. B., Clanon, T. L., Kim, L. I., Nugent, A. and Groupe, A. (1973). *Compreh. Psychiat.* **14**, 311–317.

Weischer, M-L. and Opitz, K. (1970). *Arzneimittel-Forsch.* **20**, 1046–1048.

PART II

SECTION C

BIOCHEMICAL AND PHYSIOLOGICAL EFFECTS

21

BASIC CHEMISTRY AND BIOLOGICAL EFFECTS OF LITHIUM

E. T. MELLERUP and O. S. JØRGENSEN

I. Introduction

The use of lithium salts against manic-depressive disorders has stimulated research concerning the biology of this ion. The results up to now have clearly indicated that lithium has a wide range of physiological and biochemical actions, but the molecular mechanisms behind these actions have not yet been elucidated. A simple and general explanation might be that lithium replaces other cations in molecules where they are bound, thereby changing the properties of these molecules. It is the purpose of this chapter to compare a few pertinent aspects of lithium chemistry and biology with the chemistry and biology of some other cations in order to illustrate this possibility.

II. Chemistry

Lithium is an element, the third in the periodic system after hydrogen and helium, and the first of the alkali metals: lithium, sodium, potassium, rubidium and cesium. Like the other alkali metals lithium has a single electron in an orbital outside an inert gas core, thereby producing a strong tendency to form a monovalent positive lithium ion.

An important aspect of lithium chemistry is the capacity of the element to form organo-lithium compounds. Such compounds, however, are unstable in water, where, like the pure metal, they will react to form lithium salts. In biological systems the only stable form of lithium is thus the lithium ion.

As an alkali metal, lithium has some properties in common with sodium and potassium, but it is also different from the other alkali metals in a number of ways; in certain respects it is more like the alkaline earth metals, especially magnesium. The main reason for this intermediate position of lithium is the small ionic radius, which results in a high charge density, high hydration energy and high oxidation potential. The chemical bonds in various lithium compounds may also be more covalent than the bonds in similar alkali compounds (Hart and Beumel, 1973).

In Table I it can be seen that the ionic radius of lithium is similar to that of magnesium, and that the charge density is comparable to that of calcium. The similarity between lithium and the alkaline earth metals may be illustrated by the properties of their salts. The chlorides of the alkali metals and of the alkaline earth metals are very soluble, but the chlorides of lithium, magnesium and calcium in particular are so easily hydrated that they deliquesce due to absorption of water from the air. The biologically important anions, carbonate and phosphate, form sparingly soluble salts with lithium, magnesium and calcium, whereas the sodium and potassium salts are very soluble.

In contrast to sodium and potassium, but similarly to magnesium and calcium, lithium forms many salts which are soluble in oxygenated organic liquids such as alcohols and ketones.

As an alkali metal, lithium does not easily form complexes, although the stability constant with, e.g., EDTA (Ethylenediamine-tetra-acetic acid) is placed between the values for sodium/potassium and magnesium/calcium (Martell and Sillén, 1964). Recently, it was found that lithium forms complexes with bidentate ligands (e.g., lithium o-nitrophenolate-(1,10-phenanthroline)) in ethanolic solution, but the stability constants are low compared to those of the alkaline earth metals (Layton et al., 1970). Lithium also forms complexes with macrocyclic polyethers which can be synthesized with variable diameters of the internal hole, so that cations will be bound selectively according to their ionic radius (Pedersen, 1967). Such compounds as well as biologically similar ligands like valinomycin and actinomycin can be considered as potential models for membrane carriers.

III. Biology

Lithium does not normally occur in biological materials, except in trace amounts, and no biochemical or physiological system has been found to be lithium-dependent. Despite this, lithium is tolerated in living systems in considerable amounts compared with other non-biologically occurring metals as, for example, its neighbour in the periodic system, beryllium, which is extremely toxic. This fact may simply reflect the similarity between lithium, sodium, potassium, magnesium and calcium, with respect to such parameters as ionic radius and charge density, whereas these values for beryllium are clearly different from those of the other cations.

TABLE I. Some properties of Group I and Group II elements.

Periodic System Group	Name	Symbol	Atomic number	Atomic weights	Ions	Ionic radii (Å)	Charge density (Coulombs/Å^2)^a	Co-ordination numbers
I (alkali metals)	Lithium	Li	3	6·94	Li$^+$	0·60	0·22	4,6
	Sodium	Na	11	22·99	Na$^+$	0·95	0·088	6
	Potassium	K	19	39·10	K$^+$	1·33	0·045	6
	Rubidium	Rb	37	85·47	Rb$^+$	1·48	0·036	6
	Cesium	Cs	55	132·91	Cs$^+$	1·67	0·029	6,8
II (alkaline earth metals)	Beryllium	Be	4	9·01	Be^{2+}	0·31	1·66	2,4
	Magnesium	Mg	12	24·31	Mg^{2+}	0·65	0·38	6
	Calcium	Ca	20	40·08	Ca^{2+}	0·99	0·16	6,8
	Strontium	Sr	38	87·62	Sr^{2+}	1·13	0·12	6,8
	Barium	Ba	56	137·34	Ba^{2+}	1·35	0·088	6,8
	Radium	Ra	88	226·05	Ra^{2+}	1·43	0·078	—

^{a}Charge density calculated as: Charge on ion (in Coulombs) divided by $4\pi \times$ (ionic radius)^2. Ionic radius expressed in Å.

Most of the cations normally occurring in biological systems are of importance for one or several functions; they may act as enzyme activators, membrane stabilizers, osmotically active substances, charge carriers, etc. Introduction of lithium into an organism should result—at least theoretically—in all functions which depend on a cation being influenced, provided that lithium can replace the "right" cation in position, but not in function. With respect to elements from the transition groups, such as iron, copper, and manganese, it is not likely that lithium will replace any of these ions in proteins, where they are bound in strong complexes, because lithium, as an alkali metal, forms weak complexes with the type of ligands found in proteins.

The concentrations and distribution of lithium are probably determined by its similarity with the alkaline earth metals, e.g., with respect to the solubility of the carbonate and phosphate. The low solubility of the calcium and magnesium salts roughly determines the concentration of these ions in extracellular tissue fluids, namely about 1 mmol/l.

The precipitated calcium and magnesium salts are important constituents of hard structures like bones and teeth. In this connection it is noteworthy that lithium is found in much higher concentrations in bone than in any other tissue, and that lithium remains in bone for long periods after lithium administration has been stopped (Birch and Hullin, 1972).

With respect to complex formation with proteins, lithium may be closer to sodium and potassium than to calcium and magnesium; thus lithium is not protein bound, exchanges rapidly, and does not seriously alter the structure of proteins even when it is present in high concentrations. In isolated systems, it may thus be possible that lithium will be tolerated in concentrations similar to those of sodium and potassium. Examples of such systems are nerve cells *in vitro*, where it is well-known that lithium is the only metal ion which for some length of time is able to replace sodium in the surrounding fluid, maintaining resting as well as action potential. Lithium may also replace sodium in the transport through frog skin. In both cases, however, lithium has additional effects; in nerve cells lithium may, for example, increase the stimulation threshold (Ichiokia, 1955), and in frog skin some of the lithium (in contrast to sodium) may accumulate (Hansen & Zerahn, 1964). Such phenomena may possibly be due to the replacement of some membrane-bound magnesium or calcium by lithium.

An important aspect of cation biology is the uneven distribution which occurs between intra- and extra-cellular phases. This energy-dependent distribution is the physico-chemical basis for membrane potentials, and thereby for the function of nerves and muscles. In most cells sodium and calcium concentrations are much lower than the extracellular concentrations, whereas the opposite is the case for potassium and magnesium. It is interesting that lithium does not show the same degree of uneven distribution as the four other cations, although slight differences between intra- and extracellular concentrations in various tissues may be found. *In vitro* experiments with isolated muscles seem to show that lithium, independent of the initial concentration, reaches the same concentration intra- as well as extracellularly, replacing an equal amount of sodium and potassium (Vinogradova, 1965; Carmeliet, 1962).

Several studies have shown that lithium may be transported into the cell as efficiently as sodium, but that, unlike sodium, it is pumped out of the cell only slowly by the sodium pump (Keynes and Swan, 1959; Wespi, 1969).

The various mechanisms which keep intracellular calcium concentration extremely low do not have a similar effect on lithium. In fact, the distribution of lithium most closely resembles that of ionized magnesium, namely about 1 mmol/l intra- as well as extracellularly. The larger amount of total magnesium intracellularly is due to a larger protein-bound fraction; and as magnesium concentration does not seem to be regulated *per se*, but indirectly depending on the energy state of the cell (Wacker and Williams, 1968), ionized magnesium probably enters and leaves the cell freely. A small magnesium pore or other radius-specific transport mechanism, which effectively excludes sodium, potassium and calcium, would probably allow lithium to penetrate. As lithium is not protein-bound, the concentration may then tend to be the same inside and outside, even if lithium is also transported inward like sodium.

The low concentration of lithium tolerated *in vivo* compared with that of sodium makes it unlikely that lithium should directly influence resting or action potentials. However, the similarities between lithium, magnesium and calcium, both chemically and with respect to concentration range, make it more plausible that lithium may eventually influence such functions as nerve excitability and synaptic transmission, both of which are highly dependent upon magnesium and calcium.

With respect to synaptic and neuromuscular transmission it is well-known that calcium is necessary for the release of several neurotransmitters, whereas magnesium may antagonize the calcium effect. Recently it has been found that lithium *in vitro* is able to stimulate the secretion of acetylcholine in the absence of extracellular calcium (Carmody and Gage, 1973). Such an action of lithium may be explained either by a direct calcium-like effect of lithium or by the release of calcium from intracellular stores due to replacement by lithium.

A special aspect of lithium biology concerns the great number of enzymes reported to be influenced by this ion. Most, if not all, of these enzymes are either activated or inhibited by sodium, potassium, magnesium and calcium. Enzymes which are activated by potassium are often inhibited by lithium, whereas enzymes which are inhibited by calcium may also be inhibited by lithium (like adenyl cyclase from several tissues). Magnesium-activated enzymes are also influenced by lithium, and among these enzymes are several which have ATP as a co-substrate. As ATP in the cells occurs as a Mg-ATP complex it has been suggested that lithium may influence these enzymes via the substrate, namely by forming a Li-ATP complex in competition with magnesium (Balan *et al.*, 1970; Birch, 1973). The influence of lithium on enzymes obviously results in many indirect effects, which would explain why numerous reactions, belonging to all fields of metabolism, are found to be lithium-sensitive.

With respect to the physiological changes lying behind the therapeutic use of lithium, the essential problem will be to single out which among the many effects are the pertinent ones, and not to trace the lithium effects back to a primary cause, which will probably always be a simple replacement of another cation.

References

Balan, G., Cernătescu, D., Trandafirescu, M. and Ababei, L. (1970). 7th Congress CINP, Prague. (Abstracts 1, 19).

Birch, N. J. (1973). *Lancet* **2**, 46.

Birch, N. J. and Hullin, R. P. (1972). *Life Sci.* **11**, 1095–1099.

Carmeliet, E. E. (1962). *Archs int. Physiol.* **70**, 422–423.

Carmody, J. J. and Gage, P. W. (1973). *Brain Res.* **50**, 476–479.

Hansen, H. H. and Zerhan, K. (1964). *Acta physiol. scand.* **60**, 189–196.

Hart, W. A. and Beumel, O. F. (1973). *In* "Comprehensive Inorganic Chemistry". (A. F. Trotman-Dickenson, ed). Vol. 1, pp. 331–367. Pergamon, Oxford.

Ichioka, M. (1955–56). *Jap. J. Physiol.* **5**, 222–230.

Keynes, R. D., and Swan, R. C. (1959). *J. Physiol.* **147**, 591–625.

Layton, A. J., Nyholm, R. S., Banerjee, A. K., Fenton, D. E., Lestas, C. N. and Truter, M. R. (1970). *J. chem. Soc.* (A), 1894–1896.

Martell, A. and Sillén, L. G. (eds) (1964). "Stability Constants", Chemical Society Special Publication No. 17, London.

Pedersen, C. J. (1967). *J. Amer. chem. Soc.* **89**, 7017–7036.

Vinogradova, N. A. (1965). *Citologia* **7**, 247.

Wacker, W. E. C. and Williams, R. J. P. (1968). *J. theoret. Biol.* **20**, 65–78.

Wespi, H. H. (1969). *Pflügers Archs ges. Physiol.* **306**, 262–280.

22

THE EFFECTS OF LITHIUM ON ELECTROLYTE BALANCE AND BODY FLUIDS

R. P. HULLIN

I. Introduction

In view of the known involvement of sodium and potassium ions in both the resting and action potentials of neuronal membranes (Katz, 1966) it is clear that changes in the intracellular:extracellular sodium/potassium ratio across specific membranes within the brain could produce significant variations both

359

N

in cellular excitability and in the magnitude of the action potential. Such changes might be associated with the mood variations which are observed in recurrent affective disorders. It is not surprising, therefore, that, especially during the last twenty years, much attention has been paid to the possible roles of sodium, potassium, and related cations such as calcium and magnesium, in the aetiology and clinical course of manic-depressive psychosis. Associated with electrolyte changes there frequently occur variations in the body's fluid balance, and these have been the subject of investigation in recent years.

Since there are no entirely satisfactory animal analogues of patients suffering from affective disorders, most investigations of electrolyes and body fluid changes in these illnesses have necessarily been carried out on patients, with all the restrictions on methodology which such work imposes. Consequently, the majority of studies have been confined to determinations of electrolyte concentrations in body fluids, electrolyte balance studies, and isotope dilution studies. Results obtained by any of these methods provide only indirect information about what may be happening in the brain itself and interpretation is often difficult since any changes reflect alterations in the metabolism of the whole body, not only those occurring in the central nervous system. No matter how important changes in brain electrolytes might be in the aetiology of affective disorders, available methodology suitable for use in patient studies rarely permits the isolation of brain changes from changes in other organs and tissues. A number of *in vitro* investigations of lithium effects are reported in the literature, but it is often difficult to determine their significance to the clinical therapeutic situation in view of problems of comparability, such as that of equating the doses of lithium used.

II. Electrolyte Metabolism in the Affective Disorders

No really consistent changes in the electrolyte concentrations of body fluids in the affective disorders have been reported (Altschule, 1953). Investigations have included comparisons between diagnostic groups and normal controls and also longitudinal studies in which individual patients with periodic psychiatric illnesses, usually of high frequency, have been studied throughout the pattern of clinical change in an attempt to correlate variations in electrolyte metabolism with changes in psychiatric state. Much of the earlier work has already been adequately reviewed (Gibbons, 1963; Coppen, 1967; Baer *et al.*, 1970c) and only selected studies will be mentioned here.

A. Depression

1. *Sodium*

Sodium retention has frequently been reported to occur in depression, although not all reports are agreed on the matter (Russell, 1960; Baer *et al.*, 1970c)

Schottstaedt et al. (1956a, b) reported periods of sodium and water retention during transient depressions in normal subjects. Particular interest was aroused by several reports (Gibbons, 1960; Coppen et al., 1962) of changes in exchangeable sodium in depression, and Coppen and Shaw (1963) postulated that affective disorder might result from changes in the distribution of sodium across cell membranes. The calculation of intracellular sodium in these studies involved various isotope dilution techniques in which the value for extracellular sodium (derived from the plasma concentration and the extracellular fluid volume) was subtracted from the 24-hour exchangeable sodium, giving the so-called residual sodium value. Since Coppen et al. (1962) considered that the pool of exchangeable sodium in bone (which was a component of residual sodium) was unlikely to change in depression, the results were interpreted as indicating an increase in intracellular sodium in depression.

More recently Cox et al. (1971), examining depressed patients, reported findings which were consistent with the view that sodium moves intracellularly during depression, resulting in a rise of residual sodium. They suggested that this movement of sodium occurred to replace potassium lost from the cell. However, these findings have not always received confirmation (Baer et al., 1970a) and it must be concluded that there are difficulties in the methodology and interpretation of 24-hour isotope distribution volumes. In particular, claims of changes in residual sodium must be treated with caution since the calculation involves subtracting a relatively large extracellular sodium value from a still larger exchangeable sodium value and systematic errors in either determination, particularly in that of the extracellular fluid volume, would seriously invalidate the calculation of residual sodium.

Thus, although the story is incomplete, there are a number of intriguing reports which have associated depression with sodium retention; indeed, our own longitudinal balance studies of bipolar manic-depressive patients on constant dietary intake (Hullin et al., 1968) have frequently indicated a consistently positive sodium balance in depression with the retained sodium being excreted upon recovery or when the patient becomes manic.

Coppen (1960) has also reported alterations in the rate of entrance of radioactive sodium ions into the cerebrospinal fluid in depression, and has claimed that the rate returned to normal only when clinical improvement occurred. This finding was confirmed for a group of patients suffering from severe endogenous depressions (Fotherby et al., 1963) but not for all depressed patients studied. Ueno et al. (1961) found significant but small decreases in the sodium concentration of cerebrospinal fluid of 11 depressed patients. Glen et al. (1968) found that saliva produced by patients with psychotic depression had a higher sodium concentration than controls.

Naylor et al., 1970a,b, 1971) have carried out a series of studies of erythrocyte sodium and potassium metabolism in depression. Using depressed female patients they determined that mean erythrocyte sodium levels in neurotic depressives were lower than those shown by a control group, but no difference was observed between psychotic depressives and controls. An apparent difference in erythrocyte potassium levels disappeared when the data were corrected using the ages of the patients as covariates in an analysis of covariance (Naylor *et al.*, 1970a). In a subsequent study (Naylor *et al.*, 1970b) the investigators showed that active and passive transport of sodium, but not potassium, showed a significant increase on recovery from depression. Even after recovery, however, the patients still showed greater erythrocyte sodium permeability than was exhibited by control subjects. Erythrocyte sodium and potassium concentrations were examined in patients during a depressive illness and again after recovery (Naylor *et al.*, 1971): no change was noted in the concentration values as a result of recovery when all the patients were considered together, but when the patients were classified as either neurotic or psychotic depressives it was noted that a significant erythrocyte sodium decrease did occur on recovery amongst patients in the neurotic group. No potassium changes occurred in either group, however. The neurotic depressives continued to show lowered erythrocyte sodium levels after recovery.

The various reports concerning changes in sodium metabolism and distribution in depression have supported suggestions that a defect in the membrane transport of sodium ions might play an important role in the pathophysiology of depressive illness. Alternatively, however, most of the changes reported could occur secondarily to changes in adrenal steroid secretion, and there is evidence that the secretion of 11-hydroxycorticosteroids increases during depression in many cases (Gibbons and McHugh, 1962; Brooksbank and Coppen, 1967; Hullin *et al.*, 1967c).

2. *Potassium*

No significant changes in potassium metabolism and distribution upon recovery from depression have been reported, although Shaw and Coppen (1966) claimed that when their data on total body potassium were recalculated to take account of changes in body weight and total body water their depressed patients had lower values of total body potassium than those predicted for normals. However, this claim is largely based on total body water values in depressed populations. Furthermore, as Platman *et al.* (1970) point out, the values for normal controls were taken from data collected in a different country and obtained under very different conditions. Platman *et al.* (1970) could not confirm the findings of Coppen and Shaw (1963): whilst depressed patients did generally show some lowering of total body potassium, as compared with their own recovered state, the effects failed to attain statistical significance.

3. *Calcium*

It is not unexpected to find reports that calcium metabolism may undergo changes in a variety of psychiatric conditions, including the affective disorders (Bartter, 1953; Christie-Brown, 1968) since calcium ions are necessary for the metabolic processes involved in the propagation of neural action potentials (Brink, 1954) and in transmitter release at the synapse (Hutter and Kostial, 1954; Rubin, 1970). In addition, calcium stabilises the nerve membrane so that depolarisation is inhibited (Frankenhaeuser and Hodgkin, 1957).

Flach (1964) has discussed the role of calcium metabolism in depressive states and, more recently, Flach and Faragalla (1970) and Faragalla and Flach (1970) have examined what happens to calcium during the recovery from depression brought about by treatment by imipramine or ECT. The general finding of a decreased urinary level of calcium and, in certain patients, of an increased total retention (Flach, 1964) was contrary to reports by Malm (1958) that calcium retention decreased during periods of agitated depression.

The nature of any changes in calcium metabolism in recovery from depression has, indeed, been a matter of some dispute. Malleson *et al.* (1968), for example, were unable to detect any change in calcium levels after modified ECT and they concluded that reports by Flach (1964) of significant decreases in calcium excretion rate and changes in plasma calcium levels after unmodified ECT were due to physical exercise only. Faragalla and Flach (1970), however, subsequently rejected such an interpretation on the grounds that the evidence for increased calcium retention during exercise is scanty and indirect. Faragalla and Flach (1970) noted that when imipramine was used to treat depression calcium uptake into bone was increased; ECT, on the other hand, led to decreased bone uptake. After discussing a variety of possible mechanisms to account for their findings they concluded that variations in calcium metabolism in the affective disorders, probably reflected a general neurohumoral change.

4. *Magnesium*

Magnesium, like calcium, stabilises nerve membranes, but unlike calcium it may inhibit neurotransmitter release at the synapse, and in particular any release of transmitter which depends upon the presence of calcium (Hutter and Kostial, 1954).

Little work has been done on magnesium metabolism in psychiatric disorders since an early report by Weston and Howard (1922) who failed to note any differences between the serum magnesium levels of endogenous depressives and normal controls. Cade (1964) claimed a small, but significant, elevation in plasma magnesium in depressed, but not in manic, patients, but apart from this there is little, if any, firm evidence of any consistent change in serum magnesium in manic-depressive patients (Frizel *et al.*, 1969; Bjørum, 1972; Naylor *et al.*, 1972), although Bjørum *et al.* (1972) did note an increase in urinary magnesium in patients recovering from depression.

B. Mania

Very few studies of electrolyte changes in mania are to be found in the literature. Coppen *et al.* (1966) reported very high values of residual sodium (about twice as high as those in depression) in a group of 13 manic patients. However, these findings are difficult to reconcile with the relatively small weight and body fluid changes and are almost certainly due to the difficulties inherent in residual sodium determinations which have been discussed previously. Baer *et al.* (1970a) found that the values of residual sodium of four manic patients did not approach those quoted by Coppen and his co-workers.

C. Interrelations between electrolytes, adrenocortical steroids, and catecholamines in affective disorders

Maas (1972), after reviewing the experimental evidence, has concluded that adrenocortical steroid hormones regulate ATPase concentrations either directly or by affecting sodium and potassium ion concentrations, and thereby determining the rates of catecholamine transport and synthesis. Maas points out that, on such a hypothesis, any deviation from optimal sodium or potassium ion concentrations, or inhibition of Mg^{++}-dependent $Na^+ + K^+$-activated ATPase, has implications for the brain levels of catecholamine neurotransmitters.

In the light of considerations such as these it is hardly possible to consider the role of electrolytes in the affective disorders in isolation from the concomitant roles played by the pituitary-adrenal axis and the catecholamine transport and synthesis mechanisms in the brain. As Shaw (1971) has said, the electrolyte changes are not to be regarded as providing any unitary or causal hypothesis of the affective disorders

"but as coexisting with other possible aetiological factors. . . . If electrolyte changes are eventually shown to have aetiological significance, these will have to be integrated at some level with other data and in particular with amino acid and amine metabolism". (p. 115).

Interpretation of the effects of lithium on electrolyte balance and the implications which the findings have for our understanding of the mechanisms underlying mood disorders are therefore matters clouded by our relative lack of knowledge about biochemical and physiological interrelationships in the body.

III. Body Fluid Changes in the Affective Disorders

Reports of reduced extracellular water in depression, the abnormality disappearing after recovery, have been fairly consistent (Brown *et al.*, 1963; Hullin *et al.*, 1967a, b; Cox *et al.*, 1971) and it seems reasonable to consider that the evidence for this is strong, although there is no completely satisfactory marker for the extracellular compartment.

Coppen and Shaw (1963) reported that ECT led to an increase in the intracellular body water in just over half of their depressed patients, a decrease occurring in the remainder: a number of patients showed rises in extracellular body water values too. It was reported by Brown *et al.* (1963) that treatment of depressed patients by imipramine led to an increase in extracellular fluid volume which they related to a transfer of water from intra- to extracellular body compartments.

Hullin *et al.* (1967a) noted that, following ECT, the majority of their depressed patients showed an increased extracellular body water compartment, whilst four patients showed elevated levels of intracellular water. These investigators (Hullin *et al.*, 1967b) also observed that, in a group of short-cycle manic-depressive patients, the switch to the depressive from the manic condition was accompanied by a fall in extracellular fluid volume. Allsopp *et al.* (1972) reported a fall in aldosterone production rates in this same transition period and these may be associated with the loss of extracellular fluid.

IV. Lithium Effects on Electrolytes

The resemblance between lithium and sodium, potassium, calcium and magnesium has often been remarked (see Chapter 21) and Schou (1973) has commented that "it is indeed likely that the partial similarity of Li^+ to these four biologically important cations may account for most of the biochemical and physiological effects of lithium salts" (p. 27).

The demonstration that lithium salts are potent anti-manic agents and the evidence that they are also effective prophylactic agents against recurrent affective illness has further stimulated interested in the role of electrolyte metabolism in the aetiology of the affective disorders. Associated with this interest there have been a number of studies undertaken to examine what happens to electrolyte balance during lithium treatment. In a most thorough and detailed report in which they noted a variety of types of ionic disturbances following lithium administration, Trautner *et al.* (1955) laid the foundations for later investigations of lithium-induced changes in ionic balance, but it is only recently, as investigatory techniques have become increasingly sophisticated and the results of *in vitro* experiments have become available, that the full complexity of the picture is emerging.

A. Sodium

In vivo and *in vitro* studies indicate that the passive diffusion of lithium ions resembles sodium ions and that lithium can substitute for both sodium and potassium in some active transport mechanisms (Keynes and Swan, 1959;

McConaghey and Maizels, 1962; Schou, 1957). Once within the cell, lithium ions are extruded less effectively than sodium ions (Keynes and Swan, 1959; Sjodin and Beaugé, 1968; Giacobini and Stepita-Klauco, 1970). Pappano and Volle (1966, 1967) noted that lithium ions do not substitute for sodium ions in synaptic impulse transmission, and when substituted for sodium in muscle cells lithium blocks neuromuscular response (Ghosh and Straub, 1967) but sodium can subsequently be re-substituted without loss of function.

Unlike sodium and potassium, lithium is distributed approximately equally between cells and extracellular fluid (Schou, 1957). Some cells have higher concentrations than serum, others lower, but ratios rarely exceed 2 to 4. However, lithium does not accumulate within the cells at a concentration gradient as high as potassium and hence there must be some outwardly-directed active transport mechanism but one which is relatively less effective than for sodium ions.

There is general agreement that the institution of lithium therapy produces a sodium diuresis which lasts for one or two days (Trautner et al., 1955; Hullin et al., 1968; Tupin et al., 1968; Baer et al., 1970c). Hullin et al. (1968) have reported that, following this period, in a group of manic patients maintained on a constant sodium intake, a decrease then occurred in the urinary excretion of sodium, thus producing a positive sodium balance. Transient increases in the excretion of potassium, calcium and magnesium ions also occurred during the first two days of lithium treatment but these changes were smaller than those for sodium.

Aronoff et al. (1971) suggested that the increase in 24-hour exchangeable sodium which follows the institution of lithium treatment could be secondary either to the retention of exogenous sodium or to the redistribution of existing, but previously metabolically inaccessible, sodium reserves. They do not, from their results, distinguish between these two alternatives.

Whereas Gibbons (1960) and Coppen and Shaw (1963) reported that sodium excretion decreased upon recovery from depression, the findings of Aronoff and his colleagues (Aronoff et al., 1971) suggest that clinical improvement brought about by lithium treatment results in increased sodium excretion. This discrepancy is difficult to explain and Aronoff and his co-workers can only suggest that the time of the studies following the commencement of lithium treatment may be a factor of crucial importance.

Lithium-induced displacement of intracellular sodium has been noted in in vitro studies of kidney slices (Taggart et al., 1953) and in erythrocytes (Flynn and Maizels, 1949; Harris and Maizels, 1951; Harris, 1954; Maizels, 1954).

Amdisen and Schou (1968) were unable to find any effect on the rate at which radioactive sodium was transferred from blood to brain tissue, but there is considerable evidence, from both in vivo and in vitro studies that lithium does result in the transfer of sodium from intracellular to extracellular sites (Ljungberg and Paalzow, 1969; Baer *et al,* 1970b). Baer *et al.* (1970b) found that chronic lithium administration to rats resulted in a significant decrease in brain sodium concentrations. Similar findings were reported by Ho *et al.* (1970): chronic administration of lithium led to an initial rise of lithium and a concomitant decrease in intracellular sodium and potassium in the cerebral cortex. Support for these findings has also come from more recent work by Kjeldsen *et al.* (1973) who report that sodium ion levels in isolated slices of rat brain cortex are lowered when the tissue is maintained in a medium rich in lithium ions. Birch and Jenner (1973) reported an *in vivo* decrease in brain sodium following lithium treatment of rats.

In 1964, Nielsen noted that therapeutic dose levels of lithium did not appear to lead to any change in the concentration of sodium or potassium in serum, and indeed no consistent changes in serum sodium values have been reported since that time. Baer *et al.* (1970a) found that the only significant change in 11 patients treated with lithium was a small increase in the 24-hour exchangeable sodium. This finding was similar to that of Coppen and Shaw (1967) whose results were not statistically significant.

Murphy *et al.* (1969) have suggested that lithium administration to patients with affective disorders produces an elevation of urinary aldosterone. This finding is compatible with the reduced urinary excretion of sodium shown after the first two days of lithium treatment by Hullin *et al.* (1968).

Most pharmacological studies of lithium effects have used higher concentrations of lithium than those employed therapeutically (Schou, 1957). The studies have also tended to be of a relatively short-term nature, whereas it is in the nature of prophylactic lithium therapy that long-term administration is usually involved. It is clear that further work needs to be done in this area, and that laboratory-based studies, particularly those involving *in vitro* techniques, must be designed to approximate more closely to the clinical situation. Even these provisions may not be entirely adequate, however, since the picture of lithium-induced changes in sodium balance is confused to some extent by the fact that the nature of the changes depends upon the clinical response (Baer *et al.,* 1970a).

B. Potassium

Lithium effects in this area are uncertain. In early studies using rats Davenport (1950) found that lithium treatment produced a drop in the potassium levels of skeletal muscles, but in humans a number of investigators have been unable to report much in the way of measurable changes in potassium excretion rates (Trautner *et al.,* 1955; Shaw and Coppen, 1966; Tupin *et al.,* 1968; Murphy *et al.,* 1969; Baer *et al.,* 1970c). Baer *et al.* (1970a) reported a potassium diuresis when lithium was given and suggested that lithium resembled potassium more than sodium and might, therefore, more readily replace the former. However, no systematic effects of lithium on body potassium have been reported (Tupin *et al.*, 1968; Platman *et al.*, 1970) and Platman *et al.* (1970) found no effect of lithium on total body potassium levels in either manic or depressive states.

Murphy and Bunney (1971) suggested that serum and urinary levels of potassium might not provide the most reliable indicators of lithium-induced potassium changes, and they employed instead a whole-body ^{40}K counting technique to measure potassium changes over a two-week period immediately after commencing lithium treatment. These investigators reported that in 12 out of 13 depressed patients total body potassium levels decreased, but that the opposite occurred in manic patients, a rise in body potassium being noted in six out of seven patients. A return to pretreatment potassium levels occurred in some depressed patients who were followed up for a longer period of time, and this may account for some of the findings by other investigators of a lack of effect on potassium produced by lithium. The discrepancy between the results obtained for depressed patients by Murphy and Bunney and those reported by previous workers (e.g., Shaw and Coppen, 1966; Baer *et al.*, 1970c; Platman *et al.*, 1970) may also be related to differences in investigatory techniques.

In the matter of potassium excretion, Murphy and Bunney (1971) noted minimal changes resulting from lithium treatment, a finding which runs counter to results obtained in previous studies (e.g., Radomski *et al.*, 1950; Foulks *et al.*, 1952) and which also has to be squared with the total body potassium loss noted in depressed patients. Murphy and Bunney suggested that this loss might have occurred as a cumulative effect of small undetected increases in urinary excretion, or through faecal or skin loss.

The lithium-induced displacement of potassium from intracellular sites suggested by the work of Murphy and Bunney (1971) finds some support in a number of *in vitro* studies in which lithium-rich media have been used (Flynn and Maizels, 1949; Harris and Maizels, 1951; Taggart *et al.*, 1953; Harris, 1954; Maizels, 1954). Early work by Flynn and Maizels (1949) and by Ponder (1950) established that in incubation media which were relatively rich in lithium and poor in sodium ions, potassium influx into erythrocytes was considerably reduced. Solomon (1952-53) concluded, however, that this was not so much the result of a competition between lithium and potassium as due to the lowered concentration of sodium: a linkage between sodium and potassium active transport was indeed later suggested by Harris (1954).

More recently, Kjeldsen *et al.* (1973) found that the presence of lithium ions in an *in vitro* nutrient medium caused a fall in tissue concentrations of potassium ions in isolated slices of rat brain cortex.

Enzymes which are activated by potassium (such as $Na^+ + K^+$—stimulated ATPase) may be influenced by lithium ions. Skou (1957), for example, reported that lithium enhanced the action of $Na^+ + K^+$—stimulated ATPase, but that the extent of the enhancement was less than that brought about by potassium.

C. Calcium

Lithium has been reported by several investigators as antagonising the actions of calcium ions. Thus the uptake of calcium ions by microsomal preparations from skeletal muscles or from the sarcoplasmic reticulum of heart muscle is inhibited by lithium (Palmer and Posey, 1967; de Meis, 1969, 1971), as is the calcium-induced activation of acetyl phosphates in muscle microsomal fractions (de Meis, 1969) and thiamin diphosphatase in brain (Inoue and Iwata, 1971). Rose and Loewenstein (1971) have shown that calcium-controlled junctional membrane permeabilities are depressed by lithium.

Lithium therapy produces changes in calcium metabolism of patients suffering from affective disorders: serum calcium levels are elevated above normal levels (Mellerup et al., 1970, 1973b; Andreoli et al., 1972), and Tupin et al. (1968) found that for the first 24 to 48 hours after the initiation of lithium treatment there was a decrease in calcium excretion.

Mills et al. (1969) showed that lithium carbonate included in the diet of egg-laying hens resulted in the production of shell-less eggs. Creek et al. (1971). confirming these results, also noted that serum calcium levels were reduced: they reported, however, that soft-shelled eggs appeared before any serum calcium changes were noted, and they concluded that the mechanism of calcium deposition in shells was specifically inhibited, independently of serum changes. This may have some bearing on the effects which lithium produces upon calcium deposition in bone.

The apparent species difference in the effects of lithium on serum calcium levels which is revealed by the work of Creek et al. (1971) clearly needs exploring further, before any conclusions can be drawn upon the interactions between lithium and calcium metabolism in the course of lithium therapy.

D. Magnesium

Lithium antagonises certain actions of magnesium ions. Magnesium is involved in the inhibition of thyroid adenylate cyclase activity and of the activity of DNA polymerase: these inhibitory actions are offset by lithium ions (Wolff et al., 1970; Bishop and Gill, 1971).

Nielsen (1964) reported unpublished observations by Plum and Schou to the effect that serum magnesium levels were elevated following lithium administration to manic patients. In an independent study, Nielsen (1964) produced similar findings, though he was unable to establish any clear correlation between the serum concentrations of magnesium and lithium. No differences in erythrocyte magnesium levels were noted between manic patients and controls.

In rats, lithium apparently leads to a reduction in brain magnesium, but plasma levels were raised (Birch and Jenner, 1973).

Whilst Frizel et al. (1969) found that total plasma magnesium levels were reduced in patients suffering from endogenous depression they also noted that the administration of lithium produced a further drop in these levels. This led Birch (1970) to point to the curious fact that whilst the "non-ionised" fraction of magnesium is, according to Frizel et al. (1969), lowered in depressive states, the result of lithium treatment is further to decrease the magnesium by some 50%: this implies that spontaneous recovery from depression leads to an effect opposite to that of lithium treatment. However, Aronoff et al. (1971) reported results contrary to those of Frizel et al. (1969): they noted that the serum magnesium increased in all but one of their lithium-treated patients, these increases being associated with elevated urinary levels of magnesium. Confirmation of the findings of Aronoff and his co-workers came later from Andreoli et al. (1972) who reported that in lithium-treated rats increases occurred in both serum and urinary magnesium levels, and from Mellerup et al. (1973a) who also recorded a lithium-induced rise of serum magnesium.

There is general agreement on the effects which lithium treatment has upon magnesium excretion levels. For one to two days following the commencement of lithium therapy, Tupin et al. (1968) noted an increase in the excretion of magnesium. Birch (1970) found that daily excretion rates of magnesium were raised as a result of lithium treatment and that the urinary levels returned to near normal upon cessation of the lithium therapy.

V. Lithium Effects on Mineral Metabolism in Bone

Whilst early work on the distribution of lithium in rats and humans after short-term administration has suggested that the metal is fairly uniformly distributed throughout the body (Davenport, 1950; Radomski et al., 1950; Schou, 1957), recent work with rats has demonstrated a high degree of lithium retention in bone following 28 days of treatment (Birch and Jenner, 1973). The retention of lithium in bone during treatment and its subsequent release by bone resorption provides a plausible explanation of the results reported by Hullin et al. (1968), who found that patients on a metabolic balance regimen having previously received lithium for several months showed, after discontinuation of treatment, small amounts of lithium in plasma and urine during discrete periods of 1 to 5 successive days over a period of 14 months: during intervening times the plasma and urine were completely free of the cation. Studies on the distribution of lithium in various tissues of rats maintained for long periods on lithium in the drinking water (Birch and Hullin, 1972) confirmed that lithium was concentrated in bone; investigations of similar tissues six weeks after lithium treatment had been discontinued demonstrated that all tissues investigated, except bone, then contained only traces of lithium. Bone, however, still contained almost

70% of the previous concentration of lithium. This observation has been confirmed in human post-mortem material. A 47-year old male patient, who had been treated with prophylactic lithium for 5 years but who had been off lithium for nine months at the time of death, was found to have a bone lithium concentration in his femur about two and a half times that of a matched control subject who had never received lithium; similar findings have been obtained for two other patients.

Considerations of this kind have led us to investigate the effects of prophylactic lithium on bone metabolism, and it seems that there is a *prima facie* case that lithium treatment over long periods may have an osteoporotic effect in female subjects. To date, each of three bone biopsies of the iliac crest, obtained from patients who had received lithium continuously for at least two years, have shown fairly extensive bone resorption cavities and an increase in the size of the osteoid borders. Similar biopsies obtained from rats kept on lithium in the drinking water for 9 to 12 months also showed evidence of osteolysis.

Studies of hand X-radiographs of 19 randomly-selected patients who had received lithium for at least three years showed that the metacarpal index (Barnett and Nordin, 1960) of five out of 14 female patients was more than two standard deviations below the mean value of this index obtained from a group of normal subjects of similar age and sex. The value of the index was normal for each of the five male patients investigated. The bone biopsies and the determinations of the metacarpal index (which is the percentage of the second metacarpal shaft occupied by compact bone) were carried out by the Medical Research Council Mineral Metabolism Unit at Leeds. The ratio of the metacarpal cortical : total area is considered by Nordin (1971) to represent the degree of osteoporosis in the lower forearm; more extensive studies in this area would be of interest, and are indeed in progress.

That lithium has been found to produce changes in the mineral composition of bone is probably understandable in view of a number of reports linking lithium administration with modifications in inorganic phosphate metabolism (Plenge *et al.,* 1971). Lithium treatment results in decreases in serum levels of phosphate (Plenge *et al.,* 1971; Mellerup *et al.,* 1973a, b), a situation opposite to that noted for calcium and magnesium serum levels in human subjects. In addition, phosphate uptake into bone is reduced by lithium treatment. Jenner and Birch (1973) reported lithium-induced decreases in bone sodium and calcium in rats. Mellerup *et al.* (1970) observed that lithium administration to rats resulted in a decreased uptake of calcium into bones; Mellerup *et al.* (1973a,b) later reported that magnesium uptake into bone was also reduced by lithium, though this was observed only at intervals of 15 min and 2 h after injection of lithium chloride into rats; 18 h after injection the bone levels of magnesium were unaffected by lithium. Under conditions of continuous lithium administration such as occur in the prophylactic situation it is possible that the lithium-induced slowing of magnesium uptake into bone might be maintained, resulting in more-or-less permanent reductions in bone magnesium levels.

VI. Possible Mechanisms of Lithium Effects on Electrolytes

Since lithium ions are not handled exactly like either sodium or potassium, one possible mechanism for the biological actions of lithium is by partial substitution for the normal extracellular or intracellular cations in the physiological processes which determine ion distribution and transfer. However, in view of the physico-chemical relationships between lithium and the cations of sodium, potassium, calcium and magnesium, lithium could also influence the cellular environment as a whole and exert effects upon macromolecules of biological importance. Lithium might, for example, alter the tertiary structure of the macromolecules which comprise cell membranes, hormone receptors or enzyme chains, thereby indirectly affecting the ionic selectivity of membranes as well as cellular responses to hormones or the coupling of energy processes to transport.

Mellerup and Jørgensen, in Chapter 21, have presented the view that many of the physiological and biochemical effects of lithium are a result of the similarities between the lithium ion and other ions in such characteristics as ionic radius and ionisation potential, and Mellerup et al. (1973a,b) suggest that this could provide a possible explanation of the observed lithium-induced changes in mineral metabolism.

As early as 1955, however, Trautner and his co-workers had rejected any simple mechanisms, such as a direct substitution of lithium for sodium, noting that in the initial natriuresis following the commencement of lithium therapy, the excreted sodium exceeded the equivalent of the ingested lithium, a finding which argues in favour of a process of active expulsion of sodium ions.

The reduction of sodium and potassium ion concentrations in rat brain cortex slices, as observed by Kjeldsen et al. (1973) is also not susceptible to any simple explanation based on the substitution of lithium for other ions. The decrease in sodium ion concentrations might, it is suggested, be more consistent with the activation of a $Na^+ + K^+$-activated ATPase at the potassium-sensitive site, together with a specific lithium-induced inhibition of linked potassium and chloride ion uptake (a suggestion which finds support in the decline of chloride ion concentrations in the cortical slices).

Sjodin and Beaugé (1968) suggested that lithium ions directly stimulated sodium pump mechanisms in skeletal muscle, resulting in increased sodium efflux, and in later experiments (Beaugé and Ortiz, 1970) they confirmed this, showing that the stimulating effect which lithium has on sodium efflux is not exhibited by either magnesium or calcium, but is found with other univalent cations which stimulate ATPase.

Baer et al. (1970a) have suggested that sodium and potassium loss from the brain following lithium administration may involve an alteration in mineralo-corticoid secretion. Lithium-induced reduction of aldosterone (Murphy *et al.*, 1969) could provide a mechanism for natriuresis, but it cannot account for all the electrolyte changes such as, for example, kaluresis.

McKusick (1954) claimed that lithium increased serum potassium levels perhaps by displacing potassium from cellular sites, but as for sodium it is more likely that some active extrusion mechanism may be involved.

Nielsen (1964) noted that, apart from lithium treatment, the only other physiological state known to result in elevated magnesium levels is one of renal impairment as a result of disease. However, despite the well-known fact that lithium may result in disturbed kidney functioning, Nielsen suggests that this is not the major cause of lithium-induced serum magnesium elevations. He points out that in renal disease it is a fall in filtration rate resulting from glomerular damage which is responsible for the serum magnesium increase, and that when disease primarily affects the tubules no such rise is observed. Lithium, even in severely intoxicated animals, has been shown to have little effect on the glomeruli (Radomski *et al.*, 1950). Nielsen considered the alternative hypo-thesis that lithium-induced adrenal cortical insufficiency might result in reduced faecal or urinary magnesium excretion, but he rejected this possibility in view of the reports by Radomski *et al.* (1950) that desoxycorticosterone, cortisone, or adrenal cortical extract, failed to reduce serum lithium levels or to protect against lithium intoxication. A possible shift of magnesium from the intra- to the extra-cellular body compartment was ruled out by Nielsen's finding that erythrocyte magnesium levels remained unchanged following lithium administration. Nielsen also rejected the possibility that the therapeutic action of lithium might be linked to a mild magnesium narcosis in view of the fact that such effects occurred to observable degrees only when the magnesium levels were elevated four- or five-fold over the normal: in none of Nielsen's patients did the rise exceed 45%, and indeed averaged only 15%.

Birch (1970) has suggested that lithium, possessing physical and chemical properties which are very similar to those of magnesium, may substitute for the latter in protein molecules in which magnesium is operating in a structural stabilising capacity. This would result in a decrease in the "non-ionised" magnesium fraction, as reported by Frizel *et al.* (1969), and an elevation in serum magnesium levels which would be dealt with either by increased renal excretion of magnesium or by increased magnesium deposition in bone.

Aronoff *et al.* (1971) advanced several possible explanations of their observ-ations that lithium causes elevated sodium and magnesium levels in serum. They rejected any idea that aldosterone might be involved: aldosterone had been thought to stimulate magnesium clearance, but Aronoff and his colleagues noted no relationship between lithium-induced changes in aldosterone output and magnesium clearance values. They suggested instead that a more likely explanation was that lithium mobilised magnesium in bone, causing it to enter a pool of exchangeable magnesium.

Mellerup *et al.* (1973a, b) have put forward the interesting suggestion that the changes in calcium and magnesium metabolism and associated changes in phosphate levels which accompany lithium treatment, may be the secondary effects of lithium-induced modifications in carbohydrate metabolism. They point to the fact that lithium is known to influence over-all carbohydrate and energy metabolism (see Chapter 23) and that this leads to changes in phosphate metabolism—specifically, increased muscle levels of phosphate and decreased uptake of phosphate into serum and bone. Parallel changes may, it is proposed, occur in calcium and magnesium metabolism. In support of this hypothesis Mellerup and his colleagues note that lithium effects on calcium, magnesium and phosphate may be mimicked by insulin (Harrop and Benedict, 1924; Brougher, 1927; Valencia, 1955).

It is clear that the mechanism by which lithium produces its effects on electrolyte balance is still very much an open question. Indeed, it is by no means obvious that only a single mechanism is involved: each of the four cations, sodium, potassium, calcium and magnesium may be affected by different lithium-induced processes. Mechanisms based on simple ionic substitution may be involved—indeed, it would be strange if they were not—but it is obvious that this is not the whole story and that we shall have to look further, possibly to the influence which lithium exerts on various enzymes systems or (via an action on cyclic AMP) on hormonal systems, or to changes brought about in the structural characteristics of membranes, before all the ionic changes elicited by lithium are understood.

VII. Lithium Effects on Body Fluid Distribution

MacNeil and Jenner (Chapter 28) have dealt in detail with the polyuric effects of lithium. In the present chapter, therefore, attention will be directed only towards reports that lithium induces a redistribution of body water between the intra- and extra-cellular body compartments.

There have been consistent reports (Coppen *et al.*, 1965; Coppen and Shaw, 1967; Baer *et al.*, 1970a) that lithium administration produces an increase in total body water. Kerry and Owen (1970) also claimed that lithium treatment reduced the changes in body fluid compartments associated with fluctuating mood swings in manic-depressive patients. Coppen *et al.* (1965) reported a small increase in total body water following one week's treatment with lithium in a group of eight schizophrenic patients. The only significant change in the distribution of electrolytes and water in depressed patients receiving lithium carbonate, was an increase in body water (probably intracellular water) (Coppen and Shaw, 1967) but this could have been a phenomenon seen during recovery from depression, unrelated to lithium treatment (Hullin *et al.*, 1967a).

VIII. Possible Mechanisms of Lithium Effects on Body Fluid Distribution

Shopsin *et al.* (1973) have pointed out that the body fluid changes which follow lithium treatment do not seem to be linked to variations in glomerular filtration rate (Baer *et al.*, 1971). They present data which, they suggest, support the conclusion that the initial changes in water and electrolyte metabolism induced by lithium eventually (after several days) result in the stimulation of renin–aldosterone activity. This activity, it appears, returns to pre-treatment levels after the period of about a week following the initiation of lithium therapy. An increased plasma renin activity, similar to that reported by Shopsin and his colleagues, had previously been noted in lithium treated rats by Gutman *et al.* (1971).

Doubts have, however, been expressed as to whether body fluid changes are directly lithium-induced or whether they are secondary responses associated with clinical improvement. Brown *et al.* (1963) and Hullin *et al.* (1967a) found that recovery from depression was associated with an increase in body water, and Kerry and Owen (1970) noted a correspondence between the body water distribution changes and alterations in the patients' clinical status. Mangoni *et al.* (1970) measured extracellular and total body water volumes in both manic and depressed patients during lithium carbonate treatment, and noted that in both clinical groups recovery was associated with a rise in both body water values. They also reported, however, a similar change in some patients who recovered whilst receiving placebo treatment, and this finding is again in accordance with the view that the body water changes may be more a response to the clinical state than a reaction to the presence of lithium ions *per se*. Shopsin *et al.* (1973) conclude, however, that the sodium–renin–aldosterone response is not attributable to clinical change, but that it is a direct effect of the lithium ion.

Ellman and Gan (1973), noting the reports of lithium effects on body water redistribution, suggested that cerebral mechanisms concerned with the control of water balance were likely to be affected by lithium. They treated rats with lithium chloride in drinking water, and subsequently noted marked depletion of neurosecretory material in the hypophysis and cellular enlargement in the supraoptic nucleus of the hypothalamus. Ellman and Gan concluded that lithium probably influences water balance by affecting the ability of the kidney tubule to react to vasopressin, the enlargement of the supraoptic nucleus cells possibly representing a response to the increased need for vasopressin.

It would appear likely that both direct and indirect effects of the lithium ion are involved in producing body water changes in patients undergoing lithium therapy.

IX. Concluding Remarks

In our attempts to provide biochemical and physiological explanations of the therapeutic actions of lithium, it is of crucial importance that we should come to understand the interactions which occur between the lithium ion and other cations possessing similar physico-chemical characteristics. This will be no easy task, for it is clear that an effect produced by lithium upon one physiological system will have repercussions on many others, and this may lead to secondary effects which are separable only with difficulty from the primary ones. Furthermore, whilst it is understandable and tempting to consider that the anti-manic and prophylactic effects of lithium operate at the same metabolic locus, this is not necessarily so. The time-response relationship for each effect is certainly different and, unlike the anti-manic effect of lithium, the anti-depressive effect, if it exists at all (see Chapter 4) is only mild and marginal.

Future *in vivo* and *in vitro* studies of the effects of lithium on electrolytes and body water may be expected to yield more interesting information which will be invaluable in the elucidation of these complex issues.

References

Allsop, M. N. E., Levell, M. J., Stitch, S. R. and Hullin, R. P. (1972). *Brit. J. Psychiat.* **120**, 399–404.
Altschule, M. D. (1953). In "Bodily Physiology in Mental and Emotional Disorders". p. 156. Grune and Stratton, New York.
Amdisen, A. and Schou, M. (1968). *Psychopharmacologia* **12**, 236–238.
Andreoli, V. M., Villani, F. and Brambilla, G. (1972). *Psychopharmacologia* **25**, 77–85.
Aronoff, M. S., Evens, R. G. and Durrell, J. (1971). *J. psychiat. Res.* **8**, 139–159.
Baer, L., Durell, J., Bunney, W. E., Levy, B. S., Murphy, D. L., Greenspan, K. and Cardon, P. V. (1970a). *Archs gen. Psychiat.* **22**, 40–44.
Baer, L., Kassir, S. and Fieve, R. R. (1970b). *Psychopharmacologia* **17**, 216–224.
Baer, L., Platman, S. R. and Fieve, R. R. (1970c). *Archs gen. Psychiat.* **22**, 108–113.
Baer, L., Platman, S. R., Kassir, S. and Fieve, R. R. (1971). *J. psychiat. Res.* **8**, 91–105.
Barnett, E. C. and Nordin, B. E. C. (1960). *Clin. Radiol.* **11**, 166–174.
Bartter, F. C. (1953). *Res. Publ. Assoc. nerv. ment. Dis.* **32**, 1–20.
Beaugé, L. A. and Ortiz, O. (1970). *Biochim. biophys. Acta.* **219**, 479–483.
Birch, N. J. (1970). *Brit. J. Psychiat.* **116**, 461.
Birch, N. J. and Hullin, R. P. (1972). *Life Sci.* **11**, 1095–1099.
Birch, N. J. and Jenner, F. A. (1973). *Brit. J. Pharmacol.* **47**, 586–594.
Bishop, C. C. and Gill, J. E. (1971). *Biochim. biophys. Acta.* **227**, 97–105.
Bjørum, N. (1972). *Acta psychiat. scand.* **48**, 59–68.
Bjørum, N., Mellerup, E. T. and Rafaelsen, O. J. (1972). *Acta psychiat. scand.* **48**, 337–349.
Brink, F. (1954). *Pharmacol.* **6**, 243–298.
Brooksbank, B. W. L. and Coppen, A. (1967). *Brit. J. Psychiat.* **113**, 395–404.
Brougher, J. C. (1927). *Amer. J. Physiol.* **80**, 411–415.

Brown, D. G., Hullin, R. P. and Roberts, J. M. (1963). *Brit. J. Psychiat.* **109**, 395–398.

Cade, J. F. J. (1964). *Med. J. Aust.* **1**, 195–196.

Christie–Brown, J. R. W. (1968). *Proc. R. Soc. Med.* **61**, 41–44.

Coppen, A. J. (1960). *J. Neurol. Neurosurg Psychiat.* **23**, 156–161.

Coppen, A. (1967). *Brit. J. Psychiat.* **113**, 1237–1264.

Coppen, A. and Shaw, D. M. (1963). *Brit. med. J.* **2**, 1439–1444.

Coppen, A. and Shaw, D. M. (1967). *Lancet,* **2**, 805–806.

Coppen, A., Malleson, A. and Shaw, D. M. (1965). *Lancet* **1**, 682–683.

Coppen, A., Shaw, D. M. and Mangoni, A. (1962). *Brit. med. J.* **2**, 295–298.

Coppen, A. Shaw, D. M. Malleson, A. and Costain, R. (1966). *Brit. med. J.* **1**, 71–75.

Cox, J. R., Pearson, R. E. and Speight, C. J. (1971). *Gerontol. Clinica.* **13**, 233–245.

Creek, R. D., Lund, P., Thomas, O. P. and Pollard, W. O. (1971) *Poultry Sci.* **50**, 577–580.

Davenport, V. D. (1950). *Amer. J. Physiol.* **163**, 633–641.

de Meis, L. (1969). *J. biol. Chem.* **244**, 3733–3739.

de Meis, L. (1971). *J. biol. Chem.* **246**, 4764–4773.

Ellman, G. L. and Gan, G. L. (1973) *Toxic. appl. Pharmacol.* **25**, 617–620.

Faragalla, F. F. and Flach, F. F. (1970). *J. nerv. ment. Dis.* **151**, 120–129.

Flach, F. F. (1964). *Brit. J. Psychiat.* **110**, 588–593.

Flach, F. F. and Faragalla, F. F. (1970). *Brit. J. Psychiat.* **116**, 437–438.

Flynn, F. and Maizels, M. (1949). *J. Physiol.* **110**, 301–318.

Fotherby, K., Ashcroft, G. W., Affleck, J. W. and Forrest, A. D. (1963). *J. Neurol. Neurosurg. Psychiat.* **26**, 71–73.

Foulks, J., Mudge, G. H. and Gilman, A. (1952). *Amer. J. Physiol.* **168**, 642–649.

Frankenhaeuser, B. and Hodgkin, A. L. (1957). *J. Physiol.* **138**, 218–244.

Frizel, D., Coppen, A. and Marks, V. (1969). *Brit. J. Psychiat.* **115**, 1375–1377.

Ghosh, M. and Straub, R. W. (1967). *Experientia,* **23**, 255–256.

Giacobini, E. and Stepita-Klauco, M. (1970). *Acta. physiol. Scand.* **80**, 519–527.

Gibbons, J. L. (1960). *Clin. Sci.* **19**, 133–138.

Gibbons, J. L. (1963). *Postgrad. med. J.* **39**, 19–25.

Gibbons, J. L. and McHugh, P. R. (1962) *J. psychiat. Res.* **1**, 162–171.

Glen, A. I. M., Ongley, G. C. and Robinson, K. (1968). *Lancet,* **2**, 241–242.

Gutman, Y., Benzakein, F. and Livneh, P. (1971). *Eur. J. Pharmacol.* **16**, 380–385.

Harris, E. J. (1954). *Symp. Soc. exp. Biol.* **8**, 228–241.

Harris, E. J. and Maizels, M. (1957). *J. Physiol.* **113**, 506–524.

Harrop, G. A. and Benedict, E. M. (1924). *J. biol. Chem.* **29**, 683-697.

Ho, A. K. S., Gershon, S. and Pinckney, L. (1970). *Archs int. Pharmacodyn. Ther.* **186**, 54–65.

Hullin, R. P., Bailey, A. D., McDonald, R., Dransfield, G. A. and Milne, H. B. (1967a). *Brit. J. Psychiat.* **113**, 573–583.

Hullin, R. P., Bailey, A. D., McDonald, R., Dransfield, G. A. and Milne, H. B. (1967b). *Brit. J. Psychiat.* **113**, 584–592.

Hullin, R. P., Bailey, A. D., McDonald, R., Dransfield, G. A. and Milne, H. B. (1967c). *Brit. J. Psychiat.* **113**, 593–600.

Hullin, R. P., Swinscoe, J. C., McDonald, R. and Dransfield, G. A. (1968). *Brit. J. Psychiat.* **114**, 1561–1573.

Hutter, O. F. and Kostial, K. (1954). *J. Physiol.* **124**, 234–241.

Inoue, A. and Iwata, H. (1971). *Biochim. biophys. Acta.* **242**, 459–469.

Katz, B. (1966). *In* "Nerve, Muscle and Synapse". McGraw-Hill, New York.

Kerry, R. J. and Owen, G. (1970). *Archs gen. Psychiat.* **22**, 301–303.

Keynes, R. D. and Swan, R. C. (1959). *J. Physiol.* **147**, 626–638.

Kjeldsen, C. S., Lund-Andersen, H. and Hertz, L. (1973). *Biochem. Soc. Trans.* **1**, 56–59.

Ljungberg, S. and Paalzow, L. (1969). *Acta psychiat. scand.* suppl. **207**, 68–82.

Maas, J. W. (1972). *J. psychiat. Res.* **9**, 227–241.

Maizels, M. (1954). *Symp. Soc. exp. Biol.* **8**, 202–227.

Malleson, A., Friezel, A. and Marks, V. (1968). *Brit. J. psychiat.* **114**, 631–633.

Malm, O. J. (1958). *Scand. J. clin. lab. Invest.* **10**, 528–536.

Mangoni, A., Andreoli, V., Cabibbe, F. and Mandelli, V. (1970). *Acta psychiat. scand.* **46**, 244–257.

McConaghey, P. D. and Maizels, M. (1962). *J. Physiol.* **162**, 485–509.

McKusick, V. A. J. (1954). *Clin. Invest.* **33**, 598–610.

Mellerup, E. T., Plenge, P., Ziegler, R. and Rafaelsen, O. J. (1970). *Int. Pharmacopsychiat.* **5**, 258–264.

Mellerup, E. T., Plenge, P. and Rafaelsen, O. J. (1973a). *Int. Pharmacopsychiat.* **8**, 178–183.

Mellerup, E. T., Plenge, P. and Rafaelsen, O. J. (1973b). *Biochem. Soc. Trans.* **1**, 54–56.

Mills, N., Helbacka, N. V. and Creek, R. D. (1969). *Poultry Sci.* **48**, 1766–1767.

Murphy, D. L. and Bunney, W. E. (1971). *J. nerv. ment. Dis.* **152**, 381–389.

Murphy, D. L., Goodwin, F. K. and Bunney, W. E. (1969). *Lancet* **2**, 458–461.

Naylor, G. J., Fleming, L. W. and Stewart, W. K. (1972). *Brit. J. Psychiat.* **120**, 683–684.

Naylor, G. J., McNamee, H. B. and Moody, J. P. (1970a). *J. Psychosom. Res.* **14**, 173–177.

Naylor, G. J., McNamee, H. B. and Moody, J. P. (1970b). *J. Psychosom. Res.* **14**, 179–186.

Naylor, G. J., McNamee, H. B. and Moody, J. P. (1971). *Brit. J. Psychiat.* **118**, 219–223.

Nielsen, J. (1964). *Acta psychiat. scand.* **40**, 190–196.

Nordin, B. E. C. (1971). *Brit. med. J.* **1**, 571–576.

Palmer, R. F. and Posey, V. A. (1967). *J. gen. Physiol.* **50**, 2085–2095.

Pappano, A. J. and Volle, R. L. (1966). *Science* **152**, 85–87.

Pappano, A. J. and Volle, R. L. (1967). *J. Pharmacol. exp. Ther.* **157**, 346–355.

Platman, S. R., Fieve, R. R. and Pierson, R. N. (1970). *Archs gen. Psychiat.* **22**, 297–300.

Plenge, P., Mellerup, E. T. and Rafaelsen, O. J. (1971). *Int. Pharmacopsychiat.* **6**, 52–59.

Ponder, E. (1950). *J. gen. Physiol.* **33**, 745–757.

Radomski, J. L., Fuyat, H. N., Nelson, A. A. and Smith, P. K. (1950). *J. Pharmacol. exp. Ther.* **100**, 429–444.

Rose, B. and Loewenstein, W. R. (1971). *J. membrane Biol.* **5**, 20–50.

Rubin, R. P. (1970). *Pharmacol. Rev.* **22**, 389–428.

Russell, G. F. M. (1967). *Clin. Sci.* **19**, 327–336.

Schottstaedt, W. W., Grace, W. J. and Wolff, H. G. (1956a). *J. psychosom. Res.* **1**, 147–159.

Schottstaedt, W. W., Grace, W. J. and Wolff, H. G. (1956b). *J. psychosom. Res.* **1**, 287–291.

Schou, M. (1957). *Pharmacol. Rev.* **9**, 17–58.

Schou, M. (1973). *Biochem. Soc. Trans.* **1,** 26–32.

Shaw, D. M. (1971). *Brit. J. Psychiat.* **119,** 114–115.

Shaw, D. M. and Coppen, A. (1966). *Brit. J. Psychiat.* **112,** 269–276.

Shopsin, B. Sathananthan, G. and Gershon, S. (1973). *Clin. Pharmacol. Ther.* **14,** 561–564.

Sjodin, R. A. and Beaugé, L. A. (1968). *J. gen. Physiol.* **52,** 389–407.

Skou, J. C. (1957). *Biochim. biophys. Acta* **23,** 394–401.

Solomon, A. K. (1952–53). *J. gen. Physiol.* **36,** 57–110.

Taggart, J. V., Silverman, L. and Trayner, E. M. (1953). *Amer. J. Physiol.* **173,** 345–350.

Trautner, E. M., Morris, R., Noack, C. H. and Gershon, S. (1955). *Med. J. Aust.* **42,** 280–291.

Tupin, J. P., Schlagenhauf, G. K. and Creson, D. L. (1968). *Amer. J. Psychiat.* **125,** 536–543.

Ueno, Y., Aoki, N., Yabuki, T. and Kuraishi, F. (1961). *Folia. psychiat. neurol. Jap.* **15,** 304–326.

Valencia, R. (1955). *C. R. Soc. Biol.* **241,** 244–246.

Weston, P. G. and Howard, M. O. (1922). *Neurol.* **8,** 179–182.

Wolff, J. Berens, S. C. and Jones, A. B. (1970). *Biochem. biophys. res. Commun.* **39,** 77–82.

23

LITHIUM AND CARBOHYDRATE METABOLISM

E. T. MELLERUP and O. J. RAFAELSEN

I. Introduction

Lithium may influence carbohydrate metabolism at various levels. Primarily, certain enzymes are affected by lithium, and secondary to these effects overall carbohydrate metabolism is influenced. In addition, the serum levels of both insulin and glucagon are changed after administration of lithium. These different effects, as well as their importance for the weight gain seen in some lithium treated patients, will be discussed. Changes in electrolyte metabolism, which are probably secondary to the lithium induced changes in carbohydrate metabolism, will also be mentioned.

II. Intermediary Metabolism

An increasing number of enzymes are being reported to be influenced by lithium. Most, if not all, of these enzymes are either activated or inhibited by sodium, potassium, magnesium or calcium. The effects of lithium may possibly depend upon the chemical similarity between lithium and these four cations (see

Chapter 21), because lithium may, under various conditions, substitute for one or another of the cations, thereby changing the properties of the enzyme. Furthermore, the effects of lithium may also be due to changes in the substrates; for example, many of the enzymes influenced by lithium have ATP as a substrate, and it has been suggested that lithium, by competitive replacement of magnesium, may form a lithium-ATP complex (Balan et al., 1970; Birch, 1973).

Among the enzymes affected by lithium are several belonging to, or related to, carbohydrate metabolism. The first step in intermediary glucose metabolism is the uptake of glucose into the cells; in experiments with 3-0-methyl-glucose it was found that replacement of sodium with lithium stimulated uptake of this sugar and probably also of glucose (Kohn and Clausen, 1971). After entering the cell, glucose is phosphorylated to glucose-6-phosphate by ATP, this reaction being catalysed by the magnesium-activated enzyme hexokinase, which in rat brain and erythrocytes has been claimed to be slightly activated by lithium (Balan et al., 1970). One of the steps in glycolysis is the formation of pyruvate and ATP from phosphoenol pyruvate and ADP, catalysed by pyruvate kinase. This enzyme, which is activated by potassium and magnesium, has been reported to be inhibited by lithium (Kachmar and Boyer, 1953; Balan et al., 1970). The inhibition of pyruvate kinase may explain the observation of decreased lactate production in muscles incubated in lithium-containing medium (Clausen, 1968).

Although the effect of lithium on glucose uptake, on activation of hexokinase and on inhibition of pyruvate kinase is probably slight, they may all lead to more glucose-6-phosphate being available for glycogen synthesis. However, enzymes which are directly involved in the metabolism of glycogen are also influenced by lithium. Glycogen is synthetized from UDPG (uridine diphosphate glucose), which in a reaction catalysed by a glycogen synthetase adds a glucose residue to a glycogen molecule and releases UDP (uridine diphosphate). The enzyme glycogen synthetase exists in two forms, the one being more active than the other. The active enzyme is converted to that of lesser activity by phosphorylation in a reaction with ATP catalysed by a protein kinase. This protein kinase is inhibited by lithium (Horn et al., 1973) so that a larger fraction of the glycogen synthetase will remain in the active form, giving rise to increased glycogen synthesis. The protein kinase (and hence the glycogen) is under control of the cyclic AMP system; activation of adenyl cyclase is followed, via cyclic AMP, by a stimulation of the protein kinase and thus an increased conversion of glycogen synthetase to the lesser active form, thereby decreasing glycogen synthesis. However, adenyl cyclase from several tissues is inhibited by lithium (Birnbaumer et al., 1969; Douša and Hechter, 1970; Forn and Valdecasas, 1971; Marcus and Aurbach, 1971), an effect which also may tend to increase glycogen synthesis. Thus in the literature are found reports of five different effects of lithium which would all give the same net result—an increased glycogen synthesis (see Fig. 1).

This effect of lithium was first observed by Bhattacharya (1959, 1961, 1964), who found increased amounts of glycogen in muscles incubated in a lithium containing medium, and in muscles and adipose tissue from animals treated with lithium. These results were confirmed by other authors (Clausen,

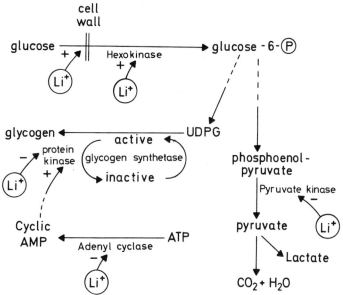

FIG. 1. Five different effects of lithium which may be of importance for the increased glycogen content in brain, muscle and adipose tissue seen after lithium administration. A stimulating effect is indicated by + and an inhibitory effect by —.

1968). It was also found that lithium increased glycogen synthesis in the brain after both intraperitoneal and intracisternal injection (Plenge et al., 1970).

Besides the above-mentioned examples where enzymatic and metabolic effects agree quite well, lithium has other effects, the importance of which are more difficult to evaluate. Fructose-1,6-diphosphatase, which catalyses the hydrolysis of fructose-1,6-diphosphate to fructose-1-phosphate and inorganic phosphate, is inhibited by lithium (Black et al., 1972), indicating that lithium inhibits the reversal of glycolysis, e.g., the gluconeogenesis from amino-acids. Also, brain pyrophosphates (Hadarag and Buruiana, 1972) and other phosphatases (Jaklinski et al., 1972) have been reported to be influenced by lithium, possibly giving rise to numerous, but perhaps minor, changes in carbohydrate metabolism. The recently reported alteration in urinary excretion of tricarboxylic acid cycle intermediary metabolites after lithium administration (Lee and Pollitt, 1973) is, on the other hand, not easily related to any enzyme effects of lithium known at the present time (see Chapter 30).

III. Insulin and Glucagon

In vitro experiments with pieces of rat pancreatic tissue have shown that insulin secretion is reduced when sodium is partially replaced by lithium (Malaisse *et al.*, 1971). This effect of lithium may be related to the function of calcium in the secretory process. In many secretory cells an influx of calcium (or, more generally, an increase in intracellular calcium concentration) is a necessary element in the secretion mechanism, and it has been found that calcium uptake into isolated islets of Langerhans is inhibited by lithium (Malaisse and Malaisse-Lagae, 1970). In agreement with these findings lithium administration to rats has been found to decrease serum insulin values shortly after lithium administration. At the same time, however, insulin secretion may possibly be stimulated due to an increase in the blood content of glucose, glucagon and calcium (see below), leading to an increase in serum insulin (Mellerup *et al.*, to be published). This biphasic effect of lithium with respect to serum insulin may explain the results obtained in a study of lithium-treated manic-depressive patients. No differences were found in fasting serum insulin levels when the patients were compared with normal controls, whereas drug-free manic-depressive patients had lower serum insulin compared with both the lithium-treated patients and the normal controls (both groups of patients were in neutral mood and had been so for several months) (Mellerup *et al.*, 1972).

In contrast to the decrease in rat serum insulin seen shortly after lithium administration, plasma glucagon has been found to increase, this effect lasting for 18 hours after a single injection (Mellerup *et al.*, 1970a). The increase might be due either to an increased secretion or to an inhibited degradation of glucagon.

IV. Glucose Homeostasis

The effect of lithium on carbohydrate metabolism in the whole organism is determined by the cellular as well as the hormonal effects. As these effects may vary both with time after administration and with the lithium dose used, and are probably also species dependent, it is difficult to extrapolate or make predictions from the basic biochemical effects to the physiological changes.

In the rat, shortly after injection of lithium, liver glycogen decreased and consequently blood glucose increased (Plenge *et al.*, 1970); as liver phosphorylase activity is also increased these effects were probably due to the observed increase in plasma glucagon. Later, blood glucose decreased below control values; this effect was probably secondary to the increased glucose uptake and glycogen synthesis in muscle, brain and adipose tissue. While the initial increase in blood glucose reached its maximum value two hours after the lithium administration the decrease in blood glucose persisted for almost 24 hours (see Fig. 2).

Following long-term lithium treatment of animals, the cellular effects of lithium might be more important than the effects on the hormonal systems, because it has been shown that rats which were treated chronically with lithium increased their liver glycogen content (Krulík and Zvolský, 1970). In *man* the cellular effect of lithium might likewise be more important, because after a

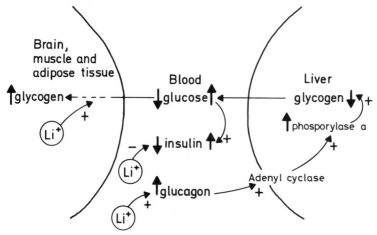

FIG. 2. Direct as well as indirect effects of lithium which may influence glucose homeostasis. A stimulating effect is indicated by + and an inhibitory effect by −.

single administration no changes in blood glucose were observed (Vendsborg *et al.*, 1973) when the patients were used as their own controls. In contrast to this observation (but in agreement with the animal studies) others have found an increase in blood glucose in man half an hour after administration of lithium capsules (Shopsin *et al.*, 1972). As no control experiments were performed in this study, and as the serum lithium concentration was barely measurable at the time of blood sugar increase, the effect might possibly be due to adrenaline mobilization.

Long-term lithium treatment of manic-depressive patients was in one study found to increase oral glucose tolerance (van der Velde and Gordon, 1969), whereas other workers, using the intravenous glucose tolerance test, found no significant effect after chronic administration of lithium to manic patients

(Heninger and Mueller, 1970). The acute effect of lithium was investigated in ten non-manic-depressive patients, using intravenous administration of glucose, and it was found that the glucose tolerance increased in all ten patients (Vendsborg and Rafaelsen, 1973). In relation to these studies it is of interest that in 1924 lithium was used in the treatment of 40 diabetic patients (Weiss, 1924) and it was claimed that the glucose tolerance increased. In the same study it was also reported that glucose and ketone bodies in the urine decreased, and that the body-weight increased. The untenable theoretical basis for using lithium salts and the fact that insulin treatment of diabetic patients was introduced at the same time, provoked rather sharp reactions (Depisch, 1924; Isaac, 1924). Recently the effect of lithium on alloxan and streptozotocin diabetic rats was tested, and it was found that acute administration of lithium increased glucose tolerance and decreased urinary glucose and ketone bodies (Männistö and Koivisto, 1972).

V. Weight Gain

The weight gain which often accompanies prolonged lithium administration, and which may be a severe side effect for many patients, may be secondary to the lithium effects on several enzymes, on the hormonal balance, on glycogen synthesis, and on glucose tolerance. Some authors have suggested that the weight gain is an adjustment to the weight which these patients might have reached had they not been ill (Kerry et al., 1970). However, other studies have shown that the body weight of healthy controls, drug-free manic-depressive patients, and lithium-treated patients without weight gain, was 7 to 9 kilograms above the desirable weight of each group as expressed in tables from a life insurance company (Metropolitan), whereas lithium-treated patients having a weight gain during treatment showed 16 kilogram overweight compared with the desirable body weight (Mellerup et al., 1972).

If the weight gain is based on cellular and enzymatic effects of lithium it is noteworthy that not all lithium-treated patients show this side effect. In lithium-treated rats a weight gain above the controls may be seen in each rat if some precautions are taken; firstly sodium chloride should be co-administered in order to avoid lithium toxicity; secondly lithium should not be given in the food as this procedure may decrease food intake; thirdly the cages should be kept dry during the lithium-induced polyuria; and finally the rats should be placed in relatively quiet and isolated rooms (Plenge et al., 1973).

If such precautions are not taken, lithium treatments may lead to weight decreases, as has been reported numerous times; even a moderate increase in the noise level, or an increase in the number of animals in each cage, may have the effect that only some of the rats show an increased weight (Plenge et al., 1973).

VI. Intestinal Glucose Absorption

The importance of oral lithium administration for the absorption of glucose is difficult to evaluate because in the *in vitro* studies which have been done in this field very high lithium concentrations have been used. It is generally accepted that glucose is absorbed from the small intestine by a sodium dependent process and that no other cation can replace sodium; however, lithium may stimulate sugar entry more effectively than potassium or choline (Bihler and Adamic, 1967). It has also been shown that in the rat lithium inhibits the absorption of glucose but not of xylose (Rosensweig *et al.*, 1965). Such an effect of lithium probably does not contribute significantly to changes in blood glucose, but might eventually play a role with respect to insulin response.

VII. Carbohydrates and Electrolytes

Lithium may influence electrolyte metabolism simply by substituting for the chemically similar sodium, potassium, magnesium or calcium. However, electrolyte metabolism may also be affected secondarily to changes in carbohydrate metabolism. Thus it has been shown that the effects of lithium on carbohydrate metabolism may be followed by an increased uptake of phosphate into muscle, liver and brain, leading to a decrease in serum phosphate and a decrease in uptake of phosphate in bone (Plenge *et al.*, 1971; Vendsborg *et al.*, 1973). This increased uptake of phosphate into certain tissues and the resultant decreases in others were not direct lithium effects, as *in vitro* experiments showed no lithium effect on phosphate uptake into muscles when glucose was omitted from the medium (Plenge *et al.*, 1971). Secondary to the changes in bone phosphate metabolism parallel changes occurred in magnesium and calcium metabolism; in particular a decrease occurred in calcium and magnesium uptake into bone, leading to increased serum concentration of calcium (Mellerup *et al.*, 1970b) and magnesium (Mellerup *et al.*, 1973). The possibility that these lithium induced changes in phosphate, calcium and magnesium metabolism were secondary to the effects of lithium on glucose uptake and glycogen synthesis, was supported by the findings of similar electrolyte changes after insuli⸱ administration (Mellerup, 1974).

VIII. Conclusion

Lithium influences carbohydrate metabolism in several ways; some effects may counteract and others reinforce each other. Whereas the qualitative aspects may to some degree be similar in different systems or species, the quantitative aspects seem to show great variations. It is difficult to determine the significance of these lithium effects with respect to treatment; they probably form the basis for the weight gain which is a severe side effect for many patients, but do they bear any relationship to the therapeutic and prophylactic action of lithium against mania and depression? Apart from a direct effect on nerve cell energy metabolism, the indirect effects of lithium, especially on calcium and magnesium metabolism, may be the way in which changes in carbohydrate metabolism can be related to changes in nervous function.

References

Balan, G., Cernatescu, D., Trandafirescu, M. and Ababei, L. (1970). 7th Congress CINP, Prague. (Abstracts **1**, 19).
Bhattacharya, G. (1959). *Nature* **183**, 324–325.
Bhattacharya, G. (1961). *Biochem. J.* **79**, 369–377.
Bhattacharya, G. (1964). *Biochim. biophys. Acta* **93**, 644–646.
Bihler, I. and Adamic, S. (1967). *Biochim. biophys. Acta* **135**, 466–474.
Birch, N. J. (1973). *Lancet* **2**, 46.
Birnbaumer, L., Pohl, S. L. and Rodbell, M. (1969). *J. biol. Chem.* **244**, 3468–3476.
Black, W. J., van Tol, A., Fernando, J. and Horecker, B. L. (1972). *Archs Biochem.* **151**, 576–590.
Clausen, T. (1967). *Biochim. biophys. Acta* **150**, 66–72.
Depisch, F. (1924). *Wien klin. Wschr.*, **37**, 1216.
Douša, T. and Hechter, O. (1970). *Life Sci.* **9**, 765–770.
Forn, J. and Valdecasas, F. G. (1971). *Biochem. Pharmacol.* **20**, 2773–2779.
Hadarag, E. and Buruiana, L. M. (1972). *Stud. Cercet. Biol.* **15**, 31–41.
Heninger, G. R. and Mueller, P. S. (1970). *Archs gen. Psychiat.* **23**, 310–319.
Horn, R. S., Walaas, O. and Walaas, E. (1973). *Biochim. biophys. Acta* **313**, 296–309.
Isaac, S. (1924). *Wien klin. Wschr.*, **37**, 1263
Jaklinski, A., Kleinrok, Z., Bryc, R., Wielosz, M. and Lukasiewicz, J. (1972). *Diss. pharm. pharmacol.* **24**, 165–175.
Kachmar, J. F. and Boyer, P. D. (1953). *J. biol. Chem.* **200**, 669–682.
Kerry, R. J., Liebling, L. I. and Owen, G. (1970). *Acta psychiat. scand.* **46**, 238–243.
Kohn, P. G. and Clausen, T. (1972). *Biochim. biophys. Acta* **255**, 798–814.
Krulík, R. and Zvolský, P. (1970). *Activ. nerv. sup. (Praha)* **12**, 279–283.
Lee, C. R. and Pollitt, R. J. (1973). *Biochem. Soc. Trans.* **1**, 53–54.
Malaisse, W. J. and Malaisse-Lagae, F. (1970). *Diabetes* **19**, 363.
Malaisse, W. J., Malaisse-Lagae, F. and Brisson, G. (1971). *Horm. Metab. Res.* **3**, 65–70.
Marcus, R. and Aurbach, G. D. (1971). *Biochim. biophys. Acta* **242**, 410–421.
Mellerup, E. T. (1974). *Acta endocr.* (Kbh) **75**, 748–755.
Mellerup, E. T., Thomsen, H. Grønlund, Plenge, P. and Rafaelsen, O. J. (1970a). *J. psychiat. Res.* **8**, 37–42.
Mellerup, E. T., Plenge, P., Ziegler, R. and Rafaelsen, O. J. (1970b). *Int. Pharmacopsychiat.* **5**, 258–264.
Mellerup, E. T., Thomsen, H. Grønlund, Bjørum, N. and Rafaelsen, O. J. (1972). *Acta psychiat. scand.* **48**, 332–336.
Mellerup, E. T., Plenge, P. and Rafaelsen, O. J. (1973). *Int. Pharmacopsychiat.* **8**, 178–183.
Männistö, P. and Koivisto, V. (1972). *Lancet* **2**, 1031.
Plenge, P., Mellerup, E. T. and Rafaelsen, O. J. (1970). *J. psychiat. Res.* **8**, 29–36.
Plenge, P., Mellerup, E. T. and Rafaelsen, O. J. (1971). *Int. Pharmacopsychiat.* **6**, 52–59.

Plenge, P., Mellerup, E. T. and Rafaelsen, O. J. (1973). *Int. Pharmacopsychiat.* **8,** 234–238.

Rosensweig, N. S., Cocco, A. E. and Hendrix, T. R. (1965). *Biochim. biophys. Acta* **109,** 312–313.

Shopsin, B., Stern, S. and Gershon, S. (1972). *Archs gen. Psychiat.* **26,** 566–571.

van der Velde, C. D. and Gordon, M. W. (1969). *Archs gen. Psychiat.* **21,** 478–485.

Vendsborg, P. B. and Rafaelsen, O. J. (1973). *Acta psychiat. scand.* **49,** 601–610.

Vendsborg, P. B., Mellerup, E. T. and Rafaelsen, O. J. (1973). *Acta psychiat. scand.* **49,** 97–103.

Weiss, H. (1924). *Wein klin. Wschr.,* p. **37,** 1142.

24

LITHIUM AND ACETYLCHOLINE METABOLISM

E. S. VIZI

I. Introduction

The similarities which exist between sodium and lithium in a wide range of physical, chemical and biological properties have made lithium a candidate for ionic replacement studies of many physiological processes. The successful introduction of lithium in the therapy of some psychiatric disorders, notably the recurrent affective disorders, has also led to increased interest in the biological effects of lithium in its own right. Whilst the effects of lithium on noradrenaline and serotonin release and metabolism have been extensively studied (see

o

Chapter 25) the acetylcholine system has been relatively neglected. Paton *et al.* (1971) first showed that lithium affects the release of acetylcholine from nerve terminals of the Auerbach plexus of guinea-pig ileum, and this work provided a stimulus for further studies on the effects produced by lithium on the acetylcholine system. Acetylcholine being a transmitter in the central and peripheral nervous system, any effect of lithium on acetylcholine release and metabolism might be important in the understanding of the clinical actions of lithium.

II. The Effect of Lithium on the Synthesis of Acetylcholine

A. Effects on enzyme activity and the uptake of choline and glucose

The acetyl-coenzyme-A which is involved in the synthesis of acetylcholine is itself originally formed in mitochondria under the influence of acetyl-coenzyme-A synthetase (Schuberth, 1965; Tucek, 1967, 1970). Choline-acetyl-transferase then catalyses the formation of acetylcholine from acetyl-coenzyme-A and choline. There is, as yet, no information about the action of lithium on choline-acetyl-transferase activity.

1. *Acetyl-coenzyme-A synthetase activity*

It has been shown (von Korff, 1953; Webster, 1966) that sodium and lithium can inhibit acetyl-coenzyme-A synthetase at concentrations in excess of 10 mM (Fig. 1): certain other monovalent cations (NH_4^+, K^+ and Rb^+), on the other

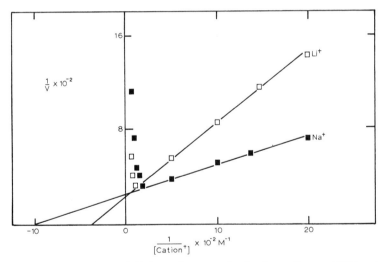

Fig. 1. The kinetics of acetyl-CoA-synthetase activation by sodium and lithium ions. Lineweaver-Burks plot. Note that Na^+ and Li^+ ions inhibited the activity of acetyl-CoA-synthetase in concentrations higher than 5 mM for Na^+ and 8 mM for Li^+. (Reproduced with permission from Webster (1966).)

hand, stimulate the enzyme's action at fairly low concentrations. The inhibition produced by sodium and potassium ions at concentrations in the region of six to ten-fold their respective apparent K_m concentrations (10 to 30 mM) may be overcome by the activator ions, NH_4^+, K^+ or Rb^+, but only when the latter are present in relatively high concentrations (of the order of 50 to 100 mM). The effect of potassium in overcoming the inhibition of acetyl-coenzyme-A synthetase by sodium ions is shown in Fig. 2. With concentrations of 15 mM sodium chloride, approximately 100 mM ammonium, 200 mM potassium, or 225 mM

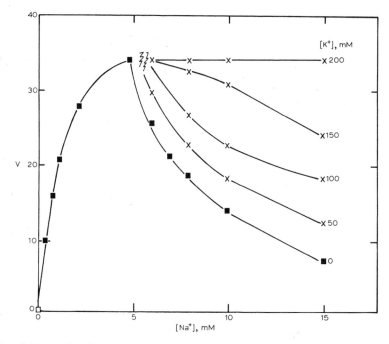

FIG. 2 Prevention by potassium ions of sodium-induced inhibition of acetyl-CoA-synthetase vs. rate of reaction. Note that the higher the concentration of sodium the lower is the enzyme activity. Also note that the inhibition by sodium of enzyme activity could be overcome by increasing the concentration of potassium. (Reproduced with permission from Webster (1966).)

rubidium chloride, were needed to restore the optimal reaction rate, and similar concentrations of these substances were required to overcome the inhibition produced by 16 mM of lithium chloride (Webster, 1966). Since the intracellular concentration of potassium ions in mammalian C fibres is as high as 98·0 mM, the corresponding value for sodium (42·0 mM) being less than half of this, it is possible that potassium ions may play an important role in maintaining the rate of synthesis of acetylcholine by virtue of their activating action on acetyl-coenzyme-A synthetase. Lithium ions enter the nerve fibre as readily as do sodium ions but since they are less efficiently transported out of the cell by the sodium pump mechanism (Keynes and Swan, 1959) their intracellular concentration can exceed the extracellular (Wespi, 1969): it is, therefore, possible for lithium ions to reach a sufficiently high intracellular concentration to compete with potassium ions and to produce a marked inhibition of acetyl-coenzyme-A synthetase, and hence of acetylcholine synthesis.

2. The transport of choline

Active processes have been shown to be involved in the uptake of both acetylcholine (Polak and Bertols-Meeuws, 1966; Bertols-Meeuws and Polak, 1968; Polak, 1969) and choline (Schuberth et al., 1966, 1967).

The uptake of choline is sensitive to the presence of sodium ions in the extracellular medium (Schuberth et al., 1966, 1967) and lithium ions cannot be substituted for sodium ions if choline accumulation by rat brain is to be maintained (Cooke and Robinson, 1971).

The addition to, or removal from, the incubation medium of 50 mM sodium chloride has been shown not to affect the uptake of labelled choline (^{3}H-choline) by rat brain slices, whereas the addition to the medium of 50 mM lithium chloride produced a significant reduction in the uptake rate (Cooke and Robinson, 1971). This finding suggests that lithium ions per se possess an inhibitory effect. Diamond and Kennedy (1969) also demonstrated an inhibitory action of lithium on the accumulation of choline by synaptosomes.

The inhibitory effect of lithium on choline uptake is not likely to play a significant role in its inhibitory action on acetylcholine synthesis (Vizi et al. 1972) since it has been shown that bound choline—e.g., as phosphatidylcholine (Ansell and Spanner, 1968)—can be released for acetylcholine synthesis (Collier et al., 1972), and choline is not, therefore, essential in the medium to maintain the release of acetylcholine (Quastel et al., 1936; Paton, 1963; Bhatnagar and McIntosh, 1967; Browning and Schulman, 1968; Dawes and Vizi, 1973).

3. Glucose transport and glycolysis

Several studies have shown that glucose is important in the synthesis of acetylcholine and any effect which lithium may have upon glucose transport and the subsequent course of glycolysis may be expected to be reflected in alterations in acetylcholine production.

Quastel et al. (1936) demonstrated that brain tissue incubated in the absence of glucose failed to synthesize acetylcholine. Similar conclusions have been reached by McIntosh (1938) and by Crossland et al. (1955). Confirmation was provided by Browning and Schulman (1968) using labelled substances.

Paton and Zar (1968) showed that in the Auerbach plexus of guinea-pig ileum, in the absence of glucose, the output of acetylcholine in response to stimulation declined sharply after the first 5 or 10 minutes, reaching a level of only 10% of normal after 50 to 60 minutes. Similar findings have been reported for the superior cervical ganglion (Kahlson and McIntosh, 1939).

Glucose is a pyruvate-yielding compound, and it has been demonstrated that pyruvate can give rise to acetyl-coenzyme-A (and hence, indirectly, to acetyl-choline) in the presence of NAD-lipase-linked pyruvate dehydrogenase (Tucek and Cheng, 1970). The role of glucose and pyruvate as acetylcholine precursors has been demonstrated by Mann et al. (1938) and verified by Browning and Schulman (1968) using labelled substances.

The intestinal absorption of sugar is inhibited by lithium and potassium when these substances are used to replace sodium (Bosacková and Crane, 1965): if it were to be shown that lithium ions produced a similar inhibition of glucose uptake into nerve terminals this would account for the observed inhibition of acetylcholine synthesis. However, when a comparison was made of the glucose uptake by the diaphragm in the presence of equivalent amounts of the alkali metal ions in the medium (Bhattacharya, 1959, 1961) it was found that the uptake was greatest in the presence of lithium ions and least with caesium ions, and followed the order: $Li^+ > Na^+ > K^+ = Rb^+ > Cs^+$.

In slices of rat cerebral cortex glycolysis is inhibited in a lithium medium (Pappius et al., 1958) and the course of glucose metabolism swings away from the production of pyruvate (and consequently from acetylcholine) and towards the enhanced synthesis of glycogen (see Chapter 23).

B. The effect of lithium on the rate of acetylcholine synthesis

It has been shown (Birks, 1963; Paton et al., 1971) that extracellular sodium ions are essential for the synthesis of acetylcholine. When the extracellular sodium was reduced there was a resultant decrease in the rate of acetylcholine synthesis in the cervical ganglia of the cat (Birks, 1963) and in the nerve terminals of the Auerbach plexus (Paton et al., 1971). When sodium chloride in Krebs' solution was replaced by lithium chloride, the lithium ions were not able to substitute effectively for the sodium ions in supporting the synthesis of acetylcholine (Vizi et al. 1972).

Usually, the synthesis of acetylcholine keeps pace with its release (Paton et al., 1971), but when lithium ions were present the rate of synthesis was inhibited even though the release, during resting conditions, was enhanced (Vizi et al., 1972). Table I shows that lithium in concentrations of 117·9 and 27·6 mM inhibited the synthesis of acetylcholine in isolated cortical slices. It is the

TABLE I. Effect of lithium on acetylcholine synthesis

$(Na^+)_o$ mM	Treatment	n	ACh content initial[a] (nmol/g)	final[b] (nmol/g)	Gain(+) or loss(−) (nmol/g)	Total ACh release (nmol/g. 2h)	Synthesis rate (nmol/g. 2h)
142·7	—	3	6·66 ± 1·35	6·04 ± 1·53	−0·58 ± 0·36	2·34 ± 0·25	1·72 ± 0·66
24·8	233·6 mM glucose	3	3·99 ± 0·99	2·34 ± 0·37	−1·65 ± 0·18	3·33 ± 0·62	1·68 ± 0·33
24·8	117·9 mM Li$^+$	6	4·79 ± 0·55	0·80 ± 0·15	−3·92 ± 0·69	3·15 ± 0·69	0
						(nmol/g. h)	(nmol/g. h)
138·0	—	3	4·24 ± 0·29	4·80 ± 0·29	+0·56	0·92 ± 0·11	1·55 ± 0·33
110·4	27·6 mM Li$^+$	3	8·59 ± 0·15	6·38 ± 0·70	−2·21	1·73 ± 0·41	0

[a] Initial refers to the ACh content of the contralateral cortex of the rat.
[b] Final refers to the ACh content of cortex slices at the end of the experiment.

accumulation of lithium ions, rather than the replacement of sodium ions *per se*, which is most likely to be responsible for the inhibitory effect, since when the extracellular sodium was lowered by 80% and replaced by glucose (Table I) synthesis rate of acetylcholine was still maintained.

Even when the rate of synthesis of acetycholine is enhanced by the presence of 31 mM of potassium chloride, the replacement of sodium by lithium ions in the medium results in this rate falling considerably (Grewaal and Quastel, 1973).

III. The Effect of Lithium on the Release of Acetylcholine

A. Neuromuscular junction

Kelly (1968) showed that substitution of sodium chloride by lithium chloride resulted in an increase of miniature excitatory end-plate potentials (MEEP) at frog neuro-muscular junctions: there was, however, a progressive decrease in the amplitude of the end-plate potential (EPP) itself and 10 to 20 minutes after all the sodium chloride had been replaced the EPP disappeared completely. The MEEP represents the resting release of acetylcholine at the neuromuscular junction whilst the EPP arises as a result of the acetycholine release which occurs as an evoked response to stimulation.

The lithium-induced failure of neuromuscular transmission as indicated by the loss of the EPP cannot be attributed to a reduction in the sensitivity of the post-synaptic membrane to acetylcholine since MEEPs could be recorded for at least two hours after the exchange of lithium for sodium. Moreover, Fatt (1950) showed that the depolarising response to acetylcholine recorded from the whole muscle was unaltered following the replacement of sodium by lithium.

Onodera and Yamakawa (1966), using frog muscle, noted that the ionic replacement resulted in the quantal content of acetylcholine being reduced by a factor of $1 \cdot 7$, thereby directly linking the lithium-induced impairment of the EPP to a pre-synaptic effect involving the acetylcholine releasing system subsequent to motor nerve stimulation. It would appear from these data that lithium ion accumulation inside the nerve terminals at neuromuscular junctions produces opposing effects—a decrease in the evoked release of acetylcholine but an increase in its release during the resting phase.

B. Ganglia

In the ganglia of the autonomic nervous system neuro-chemical transmission has been shown to be by means of acetylcholine, and any effects which lithium might have upon the metabolism or mechanisms of uptake and release of acetylcholine would be expected to be particularly evident in these regions of the nervous system.

1. *Electrophysiological evidence*

(a) Mammalian ganglia: The replacement of sodium by lithium has been shown to produce a depolarisation of ganglion cells in the cervical ganglion of the rabbit (Woodward and Wallis, unpublished data). This could mean that the ganglion cell membrane is very much more permeable to lithium than to sodium ions, but alternative explanations are possible, such as a lithium-induced inhibition of membrane ATP-ase which would also result in depolarisation.

Similar depolarisation resulting from lithium treatment was observed on the cell membrane of the crayfish stretch receptor neuron (Obara and Grundfest, 1968) and certain other types of cell (Böhm and Straub, 1962; Yonemura and Sato, 1967; Rose and Loewenstein, 1969). It has been observed that the replacement of sodium by lithium abolishes transmission in mammalian sympathetic ganglia (Klingman, 1966; Pappano and Volle, 1966, 1967). Pappano and Volle (1967) showed that in the cervical ganglion of the cat perfusion with lithium-Locke's solution resulted in an inhibition of impulse transmission (Fig. 3) and in a concomitant prevention of depolarisation by acetylcholine. However, ganglionic depolarisation by potassium chloride was not affected (Fig. 3). In contrast, Sanghvi *et al.* (1970) showed that serum lithium in concentration of $1\cdot81$ mEq/l had no significant effect on the cat nictitating membrane response to preganglionic nerve stimulation.

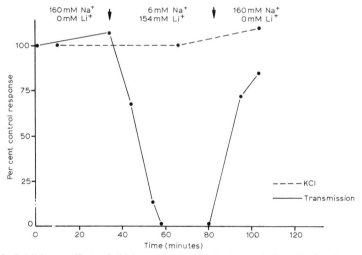

FIG. 3. Inhibitory effect of lithium on ganglionic transmission. Perfused superior cervical ganglion of the cat. The ordinate indicates amplitude of action potentials (transmission) and the depolarisation induced by potassium (1 mg). Note that perfusion with Li^+-Locke's solution completely blocked transmission whereas the depolarisation evoked by KCl was not affected. (Reproduced with permission from Pappano and Volle (1967).)

Lees and Wallis (personal communication) also observed that, in the presence of lithium, acetylcholine does not produce a detectable depolarisation of ganglion cells in the cervical ganglion of the rabbit, as measured by the sucrose gap technique. Further, replacement of sodium by lithium rapidly blocked synaptic transmission (Kosterlitz *et al.* 1970), whereas the conducted potential in the unmyelinated axons of the internal carotid nerve is much less affected by this procedure.

(b) Invertebrate ganglia: In the abdominal ganglion of *Aplysia californica* lithium, in concentrations of 10 to 20 mEq/l, reduced the neurochemical transmission and its effect proved to be presynaptic as evidenced by Waziri (1968) using electrophysiological techniques.

2. *Direct measurement of acetylcholine release*

On the replacement of the sodium chloride of Krebs' solution by lithium chloride the resting release of acetylcholine ($90 \cdot 0 \pm 31 \cdot 0$ pmol/g min) from the isolated superior cervical ganglion of the rabbit has been increased by about 300% (Dawes and Vizi, 1973). In the presence of lithium the stimulated release of acetylcholine at 10 Hz was reduced by 71% (Fig. 4), the output being

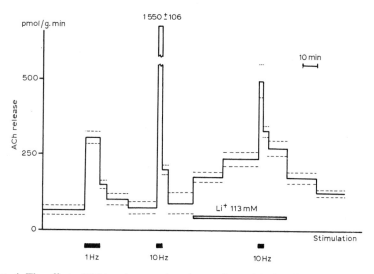

FIG. 4. The effect of lithium ions on the release of acetylcholine from isolated superior cervical ganglion of the rabbit. Eserinized Krebs' solution (Eserine sulphate, 2×10^{-6} g/ml). 95% O_2 + 5% CO_2. Stimulation ($0 \cdot 1$ msec; 2V) was applied via an isolation transformer. Note that the replacement of the NaCl by LiCl reduced the stimulated release at 10 Hz by about 71% but increased the resting release threefold. (Reproduced with permission from Dawes and Vizi (1973).)

1550 ± 106 pmol/g min in the absence of lithium and $450 \cdot 0 + 48 \cdot 0$ pmol/g min in its presence. This differential between the effects of lithium on resting and evoked release of acetylcholine parallels the findings with neuromuscular junctions as previously discussed.

C. Brain cortex

1. *Isolated brain cortical slices*

Lithium chloride in place of sodium chloride in Krebs' solution enhanced the resting release of acetylcholine from isolated cortical slices of rat brain (Vizi and Illés, 1970; Vizi *et al.*, 1972; Vizi, 1972). This effect of lithium proved to be concentration-dependent.

Experiments involving Krebs' solutions with differing sodium : lithium ratios, but with constant osmolarity, showed that maximal acetylcholine release was reached at a concentration of $117 \cdot 9$ mM (Fig. 5). The view that it is the presence of lithium ions, and not the concomitant reduction of sodium ions (at

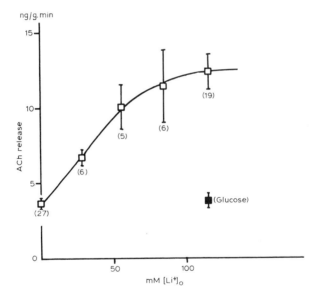

FIG. 5. The increase of resting acetylcholine release from cortical slice of the rat by different concentrations of lithium. Vertical lines indicate the standard error of the mean. In brackets are indicated the number of experiments. The highest release in 50 min was taken into account. 10 min collection periods. Li$^+$-Krebs' solution (NaCl was replaced by equimolar quantity of LiCl). 5% CO_2 in oxygen was used in the presence of eserine sulphate (2×10^{-6} g/ml). Closed symbols represent the release of acetylcholine when NaCl was replaced by an equiosmotic amount of glucose. (Reproduced with permission from Vizi *et al.* (1972).)

117·9 mM of lithium, 25 mM of sodium ions are still present) which was responsible for the enhanced acetylcholine release, is strengthened by the finding that when isoosmolarity was maintained by glucose, instead of by lithium ions, there was no significant increase in acetylcholine release.

The acetylcholine output induced by lithium was transient (Fig. 6). After

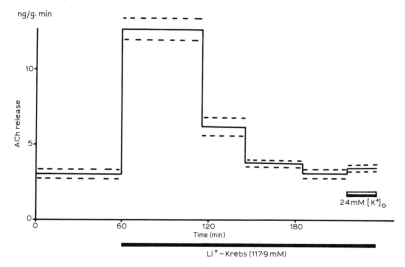

FIG. 6. Time course of the effect of lithium on the acetylcholine resting release from cortical slice of the rat. The data represent the mean of 3 experiments. the dotted lines indicate the standard errors of the means. Eserinized Krebs' solution (Eserine sulphate, 2×10^{-6} g/ml). 95% O_2 + 5% CO_2. When the LiCl (117·9 mM) was added, or KCl concentration was enhanced, the concentration of NaCl was concomitantly reduced to maintain isoosmolarity. Note the increase by lithium of acetylcholine resting release and the lack of potassium-excess (24 mM) induced increase of acetylcholine release. (Reproduced with permission from Vizi *et al.* (1972).)

150 minutes exposure to lithium (117·9 mM) potassium excess (24 mM) did not enhance the release of acetylcholine; in the absence of prior lithium exposure the release increased to 11·27 ± 1·15 ng/g. min.

A similar observation was made by Grewaal and Quastel (1973) in cortical slices when sodium was replaced by lithium in Locke-bicarbonate medium. Bowers and Rozitis (1970), on the other hand, did not find any differences in acetylcholine output in response to stimulation between the cortical slices taken from control or lithium-treated rats.

On omitting the extracellular calcium the acetylcholine releasing effect of lithium was prevented (Vizi *et al.* 1972). This fact indicates that an increased calcium influx may play a role in the acetylcholine release induced by lithium.

An increased calcium influx was, in fact, found in squid axon by Baker *et al.* (1969) and in guinea-pig cortical slices by Stahl and Swanson (1972).

2. *In vivo experiments*

Replacement of sodium chloride (137 mM) of Ringer-Locke solution by lithium chloride, inhibited the release of acetylcholine from the exposed surface of the contralateral sensory cortex of the cat in response to peripheral sensory nerve stimulation (Bjegovic and Randič, 1971). The release of acetylcholine during resting conditions, however, was unchanged.

D. Parasympathetic neuro-effector transmission

1. *Neurochemical transmission in the Auerbach plexus-longitudinal muscle strip of guinea-pig ileum preparations*

Vizi *et al.* (1972) reported that, under *in vitro* conditions when the sodium content of Krebs' solution was partly replaced by lithium chloride (11·9 mM), there was a transient contraction of the guinea-pig ileum preparation, followed by an insensitivity of the effector cells to different stimulants as indicated by a reduction in, or even complete inhibition of, the effects of acetylcholine, serotonin or potassium ions. This transient contraction of the smooth muscle preparation was blocked by atropine (10^{-7} g/ml) indicating that it was the release of acetylcholine which had caused the contraction to occur. Pfaffman *et al.* (1965) also observed in the taenia coli of the guinea pig that when sodium chloride was replaced by lithium chloride the tonic response to potassium-excess (40 mM) was abolished. Using the sucrose gap technique Bülbring and Tomita (1969) showed on the guinea-pig taenia coli preparation that when sodium is replaced by lithium the spike activity stops and the tissue becomes depolarised. The contractions of the longitudinal muscle in response to field stimulation (i.e., nerve stimulation) were reduced in a Krebs' solution in which the concentration of lithium ions was as low as 30 mM. Since the sensitivity of the smooth muscle itself was only slightly impaired at this lithium concentration, the progressive reduction of neurally-evoked contraction was possibly due to a decrease in acetylcholine output (Vizi, unpublished).

2. *The release of acetylcholine from the Auerbach plexus of the guinea-pig ileum*

(a) Resting release of acetylcholine: Paton *et al.* (1971) measured the resting acetylcholine release from the longitudinal muscle strip of guinea-pig ileum and showed that when the sodium ions of the Krebs' solution were replaced by lithium the output was enhanced by more than 250% (Fig. 7). The release of acetylcholine was much higher in lithium-Krebs than in media in which the sodium ions had been replaced by sucrose or trometamol (Paton *et al.*, 1971).

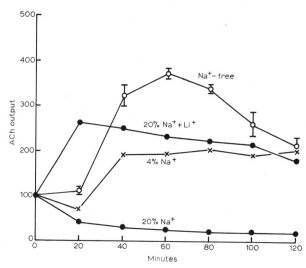

FiG. 7. Resting release of acetylcholine from the nerve terminals of Auerbach plexus. Longitudinal muscle strip of guinea-pig ileum. Krebs' solution. Sucrose substitution except when LiCl was used instead of NaCl. Initial rate of acetylcholine release in presence of normal Krebs solution taken as 100%. Each point represents the acetylcholine released during the preceding period. (Reproduced with permission from Paton *et al.* (1971).)

When 27·6 mM of sodium was still present in the medium, 110·4 mM of sodium chloride having been replaced by sucrose, the release of acetylcholine was lowered. However, when lithium was used in place of sucrose to maintain osmolarity the output of acetylcholine was increased by more than 280% (Paton *et al.* 1971). These facts indicate that lithium ion *per se*, accumulating intracellularly, is partly responsible for the acetylcholine release.

The acetylcholine release induced by 117·9 mM LiCl from the longitudinal muscle strip of guinea-pig ileum was not reduced by noradrenaline (10^{-6} g/ml) (Vizi and Illés, 1970), a substance able to inhibit the release of acetylcholine produced by low frequency of stimulation (Vizi, 1968; Paton and Vizi, 1969).

(b) Acetylcholine output in response to stimulation: The action of lithium on acetycholine output due to stimulation was examined by Vizi *et al.* (1972) in longitudinal muscle strip preparations of guinea pig ileum (Fig. 8). Lithium (117·9 mM) increased the resting acetylcholine release from the nerve terminals of the strip from 160·5 pmol/g min to 710·7 pmol/g min, but the volley output (i.e. output in response to neural stimulation) was reduced.

IV. The Effects of Lithium on Acetylcholine Content of the Brain

Birks (1963) showed that the superior cervical ganglion of the cat, when

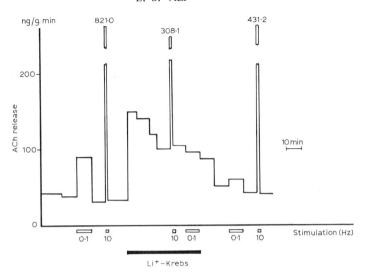

FIG. 8. The effect of lithium on the acetylcholine output during rest and stimulation conditions. Longitudinal muscle strip of guinea-pig ileum. Eserinized Krebs' solution (Eserine sulphate, 2×10^{-6} g/ml). 95% O_2 + 5% CO_2. Field stimulation, (10 V/cm, 1 msec, 0·1 and 10 Hz) was delivered as indicated. Li$^+$-Krebs (117·9 mM LiCl). Note that output induced by stimulation is reduced in Li$^+$-Krebs. However, the release during rest was enhanced. (Reproduced with permission from Vizi *et al.* (1972).)

perfused with choline-Locke's solution, is not able to maintain a high rate of acetylcholine release (produced by 40 mM potassium) when the extracellular sodium is low, and moreover that at least part of this effect is due to the exhaustion of the acetylcholine stores. Bhatnagar and McIntosh (1967) reported that brain tissue, incubated in the absence of sodium, loses about 85% of its stored acetylcholine, a finding subsequently confirmed by Paton *et al.* (1971) using the nerve terminals of the Auerbach plexus, and by Collier *et al.* (1972) using mouse brain. In cortical slices of rat brain the rate of acetylcholine synthesis was inhibited completely by lithium replacement of sodium (Vizi *et al.* 1972)—see Table I.

The final content of the cortex was as low as $0·8 \pm 0·15$ nmole/g, less than 20% of the initial content. However, when 233·6 mM glucose replaced sodium chloride, the content was not reduced to the same extent, being $2·34 \pm 0·37$ nmole/g.

However, this kind of *in vitro* experiment is very difficult to interpret as far as the clinical use of lithium is concerned. The lithium concentrations used have generally been much higher than those which occur in patients during lithium therapy, or in *vivo* experiments involving animals treated with lithium. To approximate more closely the therapeutic situation, studies have been commenced (Rónai and Vizi, unpublished) into the effects of low concentrations of lithium on acetylcholine synthesis of rat brain cortical slices *in vitro*, and also of the changes which occur in acetylcholine levels in different parts of the brain during sub-chronic *in vivo* lithium administration.

The lithium-treated animals typically exhibited diarrhoea, sweating and increased ingestion of water during the period of treatment. Immediately after lithium injection the rats behaved aggressively, an effect which is probably attributable to the local irritative effects of the lithium solution. There were no other behavioural changes observed during the experiment. These findings are in good agreement with those of King *et al.* (1969) in mice.

The acetylcholine content of different brain regions in both control and lithium-treated animals can be seen in Table II. There was a significant decrease in acetylcholine levels in the medulla oblongata-pons-mesencephalon complex ($p < 0.05$), but the values for the diencephalon, cerebellum and cortex levels in lithium-treated animals failed to differ significantly from those of control subjects.

TABLE II. Acetylcholine contents of different parts of rat's brain after subchronic LiCl treatment. 200 mg/kg was injected intraperitoneally in 0.1 ml/100 g aqueous solution, twice daily for five doses.

	Control nmole/g	Li$^+$-pretreated nmole/g	P
1. Cortex	4.82 ± 0.55 ($n=4$)	4.08 ± 0.6 ($n=4$)	$p > 0.3$
2. Diencephalon	9.39 ± 0.87 ($n=4$)	7.17 ± 0.50 ($n=4$)	$0.05 < p < 0.1$
3. Medulla oblongata	8.00 ± 0.48 ($n=4$)	6.10 ± 0.40 ($n=4$)	$p < 0.05$
4. Cerebellum	4.29 ± 0.30 ($n=4$)	3.16 ± 0.51 ($n=4$)	$p > 0.1$

Adult albino rats, 100–150 g. Means $\pm$ S.E.M.

One hour after the injection the rats were stunned and killed by decapitation; the brain was carefully removed, blotted and chilled. Four regions were separated and called by the following simplified names: (1) cortex, (2) diencephalon, (3) medulla oblongata, (4) cerebellum. The diencephalon corresponds to the thalamus and nucleus caudatus; the medulla oblongata corresponds to the medulla oblongata, pons and mesencephalon.

V. Summary and Review of Mechanisms

It has been shown that lithium in the extracellular fluid is able to affect the cholinergic neurochemical transmission, the effects being both pre- and post-synaptic and including:

1. An increase in the resting release of acetylcholine;
2. An inhibition of the synthesis of acetylcholine;

3. A reduction in the amount of acetylcholine released in response to stimulation;

4. A reduction in the acetylcholine content of tissues;

5. A reduction in the sensitivity of the post-synaptic membrane to stimulants.

A. Resting release

The transient increase in the release of acetylcholine during rest might be due to the combined effects of several mechanisms, including membrane depolarisation, increased calcium influx, and a partially reduced stimulation of Na^+-K^+-activated ATPase, all of which effects are produced by lithium accumulated inside the nerve terminals.

It is well-established that lithium, accumulating inside the nerve, produces depolarisation (Ritchie and Straub, 1957; Böhm and Straub, 1962; Giacobini and Stepita-Klauco, 1970).

Baker et al. (1969) showed that lithium enhances calcium influx; in view of the finding by Vizi et al. (1972) that calcium removal reduces the release of acetylcholine, lithium-induced calcium influx might be expected to produce an increase in acetylcholine release.

Gardner and Kerkut (1968) presented convincing evidence that lithium ions could mimic sodium ions carrying inward current, but that once inside the nerve lithium was not able to replace sodium inside the nerve terminals. Lithium was not able to stimulate the sodium pump ATPase system as sodium does. Skou (1957; 1960) showed that lithium is much less effective in stimulating the Na^+-K^+-activated ATPase of crab nerve than sodium. Baker (1965) and Baker and Shaw (1965a, b) found that under normal circumstances the internal inorganic phosphate level of crab nerve fibres increased during nerve transmission, but that if the sodium was replaced by lithium then this rise did not occur. This fact indicates that the inhibition of ionic pump mechanisms by lithium is probably a result of a failure to stimulate the membrane ATPase to break down ATP. Paton et al. (1971) and Vizi (1972) presented evidence that the reduction or inhibition of Na^+-K^+-activated ATPase is likely to result in the release of acetylcholine. Therefore it is likely that the lack of stimulation by lithium of membrane ATPase might also be responsible for the transient increase of acetylcholine.

B. Acetylcholine synthesis

Direct evidence (Vizi et al., 1972) has been provided that lithium inhibits the synthesis of acetylcholine and this may be directly responsible for the reduction by lithium of acetylcholine output in response to stimulation (Vizi and Illés, 1970; Vizi et al., 1972; Dawes and Vizi, 1973). The impairment by lithium

ions of acetylcholine synthesis (Fig. 9) might be attributed to the inhibitory effect of lithium on
1. The uptake of choline;
2. Acetyl-coenzyme-A synthetase;
3. Glucose—pyruvate transformation.

It is likely that the last two of these effects are most important; the inhibition of choline uptake seems not to be important in this respect since the tissues are able to synthesize acetylcholine in the absence of extracellular choline from choline of exogenous origin.

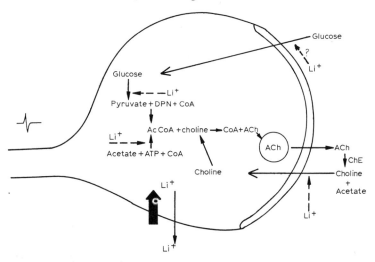

FIG. 9. A diagrammatic summary of the various actions of lithium ions on the metabolism of acetylcholine.

C. Acetylcholine output in response to nerve activity

Lithium reduces the amount of acetylcholine released by stimulation (Vizi *et al.*, 1972; Dawes and Vizi, 1973). The reduction of acetylcholine output in response to stimulation is partly due to the lithium-induced inhibition of acetyl choline synthesis and impairment of nerve conduction (Fig. 10). It has been shown that lithium carbonate reduces the frequency of seizures and may also be effective in some cases of temporal lobe epilepsy (see Chapter 6). These effects of lithium may also be related to its inhibitory effect on the release of acetylcholine induced by nerve activity.

Since lithium, even at low extracellular (plasma) concentrations, is capable of accumulating inside nerves, thereby reducing or inhibiting completely axonal conduction and/or impulse generation, this mechanism may also be involved in the inhibitory action of lithium on acetylcholine release.

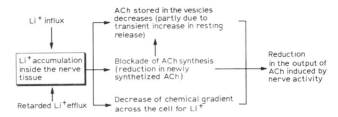

FIG. 10. The inhibitory effect of lithium on acetylcholine release.

D. Acetylcholine content of tissues

The brain content of acetylcholine is reduced by lithium ions as a direct result of the inhibitory action of lithium on acetylcholine synthesis.

E. Sensitivity of effector cells

Whilst the sensitivity of striated muscle to acetylcholine is not changed by acetylcholine (Fatt, 1950), lithium-treated smooth muscle cells have been found to have reduced sensitivity to a variety of stimulants (Pfaffman *et al.*, 1965; Vizi *et al.*, 1972), and the same has been observed in ganglion cells with respect to sensitivity to acetylcholine. Moreover, Bülbring and Tomita (1969) showed that when sodium was replaced by lithium, spike activity of guinea-pig taenia coli stopped and the tissue became depolarised and insensitive to stimulants.

VI. Concluding Remarks

It is clear that lithium treatment may lead to changes in those physiological and biochemical systems which involve acetylcholine, though several quite separate mechanisms may be involved in bringing about these changes. The understanding of the therapeutic action of lithium salts requires that both lithium effects on acetylcholine and the involvement of acetylcholine in determining the affective states should be elucidated.

References

Ansell, G. B. and Spanner, S. (1968). *Biochem. J.* **110**, 201–206.

Baker, P. F. (1965). *J. Physiol.* **180**, 383–423.

Baker, P. F. and Shaw, T. I. (1965a). *J. Physiol.* **180**, 383–423.

Baker, P. F. and Shaw, T. I. (1965b). *J. Physiol.* **180**, 424–438.

Baker, P. F., Blaustein, M. P., Hodgkin, A. L. and Steindhardt, R. A. (1969). *J. Physiol.* **200**, 431–458.

Bertols-Meeuws, M. M. and Polak, R. L. (1968). *Brit. J. Pharmacol* **33**, 368–380.

Bhatnagar, S. P. and MacIntosh, F. C. (1967). *Can. J. Physiol. Pharmacol.* **45**, 249–268.

Bhattacharya, G. (1959). *Nature* **183**, 324–325.

Bhattacharya, G. (1961). *Biochem. J.* **79**, 369–377.

Birks, R. I. (1963). *Can. J. Biochem. Physiol.* **41**, 2573–2577.

Bjegovic, M. and Randič, M. (1971). *Nature* **230**, 587–588.

Bosackova, J. and Crane, B. K. (1965). *Biochim. biophys. Acta* **102**, 423–435.

Bowers, M. B. and Rozitiz, A. (1970). *J. Pharm. Pharmacol.* **22**, 647.

Böhm, H. W. and Straub, R. W. (1962). *Pflügers Archs ges. Physiol.* **274**, 468–479.

Browning, E. T. and Schulman, M. P. (1968). *J. Neurochem.* **15**, 1391–1405.

Bülbring, E. and Tomita, T. (1969). *Proc. R. Soc. B.* **172**, 103–119.

Collier, B., Boon, P. and Salehmoghaddam, S. (1972). *J. Neurochem.* **19**, 51–60.

Cooke, W. J. and Robinson, J. D. (1971). *Amer. J. Physiol.* **22**, 218–225.

Crossland, J., Elliott, K. A. C. and Pappius, H. M. (1955). *Amer. J. Physiol.* **183**, 32–34.

Dawes, P. M. and Vizi, E. S. (1973). *Brit. J. Pharmacol.* **48**, 225–232.

Diamond, I. and Kennedy, E. P. (1969). *J. biol. Chem.* **244**, 3258–3263.

Fatt, P. (1950). *J. Physiol.* **111**, 408–422.

Giacobini, E. and Stepita-Klauco, M. (1970). *Acta physiol. scand.* **80**, 519–527.

Gardner, D. R. and Kerkut, G. A. (1968). *Comp. Biochem. Physiol.* **25**, 33–48.

Grewaal, D. S. and Quastel, J. H. (1973). *Biochem. J.* **132**, 1–14.

Kahlson, G. and MacIntosh, F. C. (1939). *J. Physiol.* **96**, 2555–2571.

Kelly, J. S. (1968). *Q. Jl. exp. Physiol.* **53**, 239–249.

Keynes, R. D. and Swan R. C. (1959). *J. Physiol.* **147**, 591–625.

King, L. J. Carl, J. L., Archer, E. G. and Castellanet, M. (1969). *J. Pharmacol.* **168**, 163–170.

Klingman, J. D. (1966). *Life. Sci.* **5**, 365–373.

Korff, R. W. Von. (1953). *J. Physiol.* **93**, 46–60.

Kosterlitz, H. W., Lees, G. M. and Wallis, D. J. (1970). *Brit. J. Pharmacol.* **40**, 275–293.

MacIntosh, F. C. (1938). *J. Physiol.* **93**, 46–60.

Mann, P. J. G., Tennenbaum, M. and Quastel, J. H. (1938). *Biochem J.* **32**, 243–253.

Obara, S. and Grundfest, H. (1968). *J. gen. Physiol.* **51**, 635–654.

Onodera, K. and Yamakawa, K. (1966). *Jap. J. Physiol.* **16**, 541–550.

Pappano, A. J. and Volle, R. L. (1966). *Science* **152**, 85–87.

Pappano, A. J. and Volle, R. L. (1967). *J. Pharmacol. exp. Ther.* **157**, 346–355.

Pappius, H. M., Rosenfeld, M. Johnson, D. M. and Elliot, K. (1958). *Can. J. Biochem.* **36**, 217–226.

Paton, W. D. M. (1963). *Can. J. Biochem. Physiol.* **41**, 2637–2653.

Paton, W. D. M. and Zar, A. M. (1968). *J. Physiol.* **194**, 13–33.

Paton, W. D. M. and Vizi, E. S. (1969). *Brit. J. Pharmacol.* **35**, 10–28.

Paton, W. D. M., Vizi, E. S. and Zar, A. M. (1971). *J. Physiol.* **215**, 819–848.

Pfaffman, M., Urakawa, N. and Holland, W. C. (1965). *Amer. J. Physiol.* **208**, 1203–1205.

Polak, R. L. (1969). *Brit. J. Pharmacol.* **36**, 144–152.

Polak, R. L. and Bertols-Meeuws, M. M. (1966). *Biochem. Pharmac.* **15**, 989–992.

Quastel, J. H., Tennenbaum, M. and Wheatley, A. H. M. (1936). *Biochem J.* **30**, 1668.

Ritchie, J. M. and Straub, R. W. (1957). *J. Physiol.* **136**, 80–97.

Rose, B. and Loewenstein, W. R. (1969). *Biochim. biophys. Acta* **173**, 146–148.

Sanghvi, I., Urquiaga, X. and Gershon, S. (1970). *Pharmacol. res. Commun.* **4**, 361–388.

Schuberth, J. (1965). *Biochem. biophys. Acta* **98**, 1–7.

Schuberth, J., Sundwall, A., Sorbo, B. and Lindel, J. O. (1966). *J. Neurochem.* **13**, 347–352.

Schuberth, J., Sundwall, A. and Sorbo, B. (1967). *Life Sci.* **6**, 291–295.

Skou, J. C. (1957). *Biochim. biophys. Acta* **23**, 394–401.

Skou, J. C. (1960). *Biochim. biophys. Acta* **42**, 6–23.

Stahl, W. L. and Swanson, P. D. (1972). *J. Neurochem.* **19**, 2395–2407.

Tucek, S. (1967). *J. Neurochem.* **14**, 531–545.

Tueck, S. (1970). *In* "Drugs and Cholinergic Mechanism in the CNS" (E. Heilbron and A. Winter, eds), pp. 117–131. Research Institute of National Science, Stockholm.

Tueck, S. and Cheng, S. C. (1970). *Biochim. biophys. Acta* **208**, 538–540.

Vizi, E. S. (1968). *Archs exp. Path. Pharmacol.* **259**, 199–200.

Vizi, E. S. (1972). *J. Physiol.* **226**, 95–117.

Vizi, E. S. and Illés, P. (1970). CINP VII. Congress. Abstracts. p. 459.

Vizi, E. S., Illés, P., Rónai, A. and Knoll, J. (1972). *Neuropharmacol* **11**, 521–530.

Waziri, R. (1968). *Life Sci.* **7**, 865–873.

Webster, L. T. (1966). *J. biol. Chem.* **561**, 5504–5510.

Wespi, H. H. (1969). *Pflügers Archs ges. Physiol.* **306**, 262–280.

Yonemura, K. and Sato, M. (1967). *Jap. J. Physiol.* **17**, 678–697.

25

LITHIUM AND AMINE METABOLISM

D. M. Shaw

I. Introduction

Of the hypotheses which attempt to explain the biochemical basis of the affective disorders the ones implicating the amines, particularly noradrenaline and 5-hydroxytryptamine (5HT), have received the most continuous support (Schildkraut, 1965; Coppen et al., 1963). Interest arose initially from the finding that depression may be precipitated by reserpine in susceptible individuals and that the illness may persist after withdrawal of the drug (Muller et al., 1955; Lemieux, 1956). Reserpine also depletes the body of amines by preventing their storage and the two observations were linked together in the now well-known 'catecholamine hypothesis' (Schildkraut and Kety, 1967). Subsequently it has been suggested that 5-hydroxytryptamine (5HT) or both 5HT and noradrenaline, or possibly dopamine, might be important. To date there is only a small amount of direct evidence supporting the amine hypothesis and indeed several studies have suggested that the original views were oversimplified (Shaw et al., 1972, 1973; Shaw, 1973a). Nevertheless, the fact remains that indirect and circumstantial evidence continues to point to some involvement of amines in the pathological processes underlying affective illness, perhaps in a more complex way than was originally envisaged. The exact nature and degree of their implication in the syndromes has yet to be defined.

As has been discussed in detail elsewhere in this book, lithium has clinical interest because of two main therapeutic actions in patients suffering from affective disorder. In patients with bipolar illness, where there are attacks of both mania and depression, the symptoms of the manic phase may be alleviated by the use of lithium salts—an effect which appears within the first week of treatment (Chapter 3). The second therapeutic action of lithium is its ability to prevent or attenuate episodes in individuals with either bipolar or unipolar (depression only) forms, turning a periodic form of illness into either a less troublesome form or suppressing its manifestations altogether (Chapter 5).

II. Difficulties in Interpreting the Experimental Data

It is hardly surprising that the empirical finding of lithium's therapeutic properties has led to a search for the particular biological actions responsible, and considerable attention has been paid to effects on amine metabolism. There are, however, particular reasons why this search and the interpretation of the resultant data, particularly in this area, have run into some difficulties.

The main problem is in the dosage given and the time allowed to elapse before assays are made. In man the therapeutic range lies at dosages which give serum concentrations in the region of $0.7–1.2$ mM/l (these vary considerably about an approximate average of, say, 0.5 mM/kg body weight) and toxic dosages when serum concentration rises to 2.0 mM/l or higher. This means that therapeutic and toxic dosages are not widely separated from each other and therefore that one cannot be certain whether the effects on amine metabolism, particularly in the animal experiments, are related to the therapeutic or to the toxic action. In addition, many systems show biphasic or perhaps even more complex reactions to lithium in relationship to time, so that what is happening during the first few days of administration may have little similarity to results 2, 3 or more weeks later. Many of the biochemical processes change in opposite directions at different times.

It seems probable that the studies least likely to give relevant information are "early" *in vitro* studies where tissues or organs are exposed to quite high concentrations of lithium *for the first time. In vivo* the tissue has been subject to the secondary effects of modification of endocrine and other systems, but perhaps most important of all, usually sufficient time has elapsed for the lithium ion to have reacted on intracellular as well as extracellular compartments. Results obtained in such circumstances cannot be compared easily with a virginal cell or tissue suddenly presented with a significant amount of lithium in the extracellular compartment only. The data from "intermediate" times should not be neglected, however, because it should be remembered that we do not know if the biological actions of lithium are the same when it is acting in a relatively acute way as an antimanic agent as those which are at work when it is operating in its "prophylactic" capacity, in the setting of a longer exposure to lithium.

There is uncertainty also about whether effects at the "therapeutic concentration" in animals can be extrapolated back to man when general and organ tolerances to lithium vary between the species. For instance, the central nervous system is the organ most vulnerable to toxicity in man, whereas the kidney is the most susceptible organ in the rat, so that considerable caution is needed in comparing results in different species.

A further and very important complication is that we do not know if the "important" action of lithium, i.e. its therapeutic effects, are central or peripheral.

It is unfortunate, therefore, that so much work has not taken account of these problems and difficulties. Many studies have been made *in vivo* and *in vitro* at dose levels which were quite obviously toxic or would have been toxic had they been prolonged for any length of time, and even some of the chronic studies have been completed with animals in moderate or even advanced stages of lithium poisoning. Clearly the effects observed in these studies may be those of lithium's toxic actions rather than analogous to its prophylactic functions in man. With many of the studies these limitations need to be kept in mind.

Finally it should be pointed out that Donaldson *et al.* (1973) have highlighted an important possible artifact of studies of lithium. They demonstrated changes in amine metabolism in the brain of mice induced by the injection of lithium carbonate. However, the changes proved to be not an effect of the lithium ion *per se* but a feature of the high alkalinity of the salt used. When the lithium carbonate was neutralized prior to injection the initial findings could not be confirmed.

III. Experimental Studies

It is convenient to discuss the effects of lithium on amine metabolism in terms of three periods: viz., the first, or 'acute', phase when the individual is initially exposed to lithium and covering the time during which lithium is accumulating rapidly in the body; a second, 'subacute' stage when presumably readjustments to the appearance of the cation are being made; and thirdly, the time after this, the 'chronic' phase, when biochemical effects are remaining on a long-term basis.

If the actions of lithium as an antimanic agent are the same as those determining its prophylactic properties, some effect which is present in the initial phase of treatment will presumably have to remain unaltered into the phase of long-term effects, whilst if the actions are different obviously we shall need to identify quite separate processes and mechanisms.

A. Acute effects of lithium on amine metabolism

The acute effects of lithium have been taken arbitrarily, for the purposes of the present discussion, as those occurring immediately after exposure to lithium and for up to 4 days thereafter and as including *in vitro* experiments where the tissues used were derived from animals who had not been treated with lithium or had received it for four days or less (Shaw, 1973b).

1. *5-hydroxytryptamine metabolism*

One of the earliest studies in this area was carried out by Corrodi *et al.* (1967) who failed to find any effects of doses of up to 15 mEq/kg of lithium chloride on 5HT turnover in rat brain; neither brain concentrations, nor rate of depletion following administration of tryptophan hydroxylase inhibitor (which reduces the synthesis of 5HT), were affected. Katz *et al.* (1968, 1969), and Katz and Kopin (1969) studied the release of labelled amine from brain slices which had previously been allowed to accumulate either tritiated noradrenaline or 5HT. Addition of lithium to the incubation medium at 2·4 mM/l did not change the rate of spontaneous release, but decreased the amount liberated by electrical stimulation. In *in vivo* experiments, Schildraut *et al.* (1969b) used the technique of injecting ^{14}C-labelled 5HT intracisternally into rats which subsequently received lithium intraperitoneally (50 mg/kg × 2 or 200 mg/kg × 2, administered as the chloride). Disappearance of radioactive amine was slowed by lithium, suggesting decreased turnover, but this did not seem compatible with the presence in the animals' brains of increased amounts of the labelled deaminated metabolite, 5-hydroxyindoleacetic acid (5HIAA).

The finding of a possible decreased turnover of 5HT by Schildkraut and his colleagues has not been confirmed by other studies. Lapin and Oxenkrug (1969) and Kiseleva and Lapin (1969), for example, investigating the head-twitches produced in mice by the injection of 5-hydroxytryptophan (5HTP), noted that the effect was antagonised by lithium, suggesting a selective central antiserotonin effect. Lithium did not change the level of 5HT in the brain but prevented the 5HTP-induced increase in this amine. These and other data led the authors to conclude that lithium accelerates the destruction of 5HT in the brain. Sheard and Aghajanian (1970) measured the amounts of 5HT and 5HIAA in the forebrain of rats in which they had stimulated the median forebrain bundle. This procedure resulted in an increase in the amounts of both 5HT and 5HIAA in the forebrain, indicating enhancement of a neuronally activated metabolism of 5HT. In animals treated with lithium (2·5 to 5 mM/kg for 2 or 4 days, or 7·5 mM/kg for 2 days) the increments in 5HT and 5HIAA were greater than in the controls, suggesting that lithium accelerated the turnover of 5HT. The authors felt that the change in turnover was probably in intracellular metabolism rather than in extraneuronal release because there was no change in the firing rates of the neurones.

In acute experiments, and using the thrombocyte as the "test system" Genefke (1972a) showed that in man the uptake of 5HT was inhibited by only 5% at a concentration which is well into the toxic range. In rats treated for 2 days or longer with lithium to give serum levels in the range of 0·4 to 0·7 mM/l there were no changes either in the content or in the uptake rates of 5HT by the platelets.

Recently, Knapp and Mandell (1973) have studied the effects of lithium on tryptophan hydroxylase activity and on the transport of tryptophan into striate synaptosomes. In the acute phase of treatment, 3 to 5 days in this case, there was a significant decrease in soluble tryptophan hydroxylase activity but nevertheless increased synthesis of serotonin in the nerve endings.

2. Noradrenaline metabolism

The data on the acute effects of lithium on noradrenaline metabolism provide a more coherent pattern than the studies on 5HT. Corrodi et al. (1967) treated rats intraperitoneally with doses of lithium of 2·5–15 mM/kg body weight, and assayed noradrenaline in the brain from several minutes up to 48 hours later. They gave a tyrosine hydroxylase inhibitor to block synthesis of noradrenaline and used the "fall-off" in concentration of noradrenaline as a measure of turnover. Under these conditions the noradrenaline turnover was greater in lithium-treated animals. Dopamine levels were unchanged, as were concentrations of 5HT after inhibition of tryptophan hydroxylase.

A number of experiments have been done on the acute effects of lithium using the technique of the intracisternal injection of labelled noradrenaline (Schildkraut et al., 1966; 1969a; Schanbert et al., 1967). The treatment schedules involved giving two or three injections of lithium salts over several hours at doses in the range of 1·2–2·4 mM/kg—somewhat above that of the equivalent maintenance therapy in man. Control and lithium-treated animals were killed at various times after the intracisternal injection of tritiated noradrenaline, and the main findings with lithium were an increase in the production of labelled deaminated catecholamines and a decrease in formation of tritiated normetanephrine.

Sterne et al. (1969) studied rats given lithium at doses of 2·5 or 3·75 mM/kg body weight for 2 days, which gave plasma levels within the toxic range for these animals. Noradrenaline turnover was followed by blocking tyrosine hydroxylase with α-methyltyrosine and observing the decline of the amine with time. There was a 95% increase in turnover of noradrenaline in the brain and a similar but much smaller change in the heart.

The data from the acute studies thus suggest a lithium-induced increase in the intracellular (presynaptic) degradation of noradrenaline, retention of the amine presynaptically and a generally enhanced rate of turnover.

More recently, Frazer et al. (1972) have investigated the effect of lithium at concentrations of 10 mM/l on the response of the perfused heart of the guinea pig to catecholamines. The results are important in that they suggest that lithium's action may be post-synaptic, a view based on the fact that lithium decreased the effect of isoproterenol, a sympathomimetic amine which is not taken up by adrenergic nerve terminals.

B. Subacute effects of lithium on amine metabolism

The subacute studies have been taken arbitrarily as those in which lithium has been given for 5–10 days inclusively and also include the *in vitro* studies where the tissues were from similarly treated animals. Schildkraut *et al.* (1969a) included in their experiments involving intracisternal injection of tritiated noradrenaline, rats treated on the subacute time schedule (2·4 mM/kg × 2/day for 7 days). The results were similar to those of the acute studies in that lithium caused a significant reduction in the amount of labelled noradrenaline and metabolites present (and this was not due to reduced uptake), while the deaminated and free deaminated O-methylated metabolites represented a larger fraction of the total brain radioactivity. There was also a small but significant reduction in labelled normetanephrine.

Several groups have done *in vitro* studies using synaptosomes from lithium-treated animals (Colburn *et al.*, 1967; Baldessarini and Yorke, 1970; Kuriyama and Speken, 1970). The experiments of Colburn *et al.* and Baldessarini and Yorke were on rats given 2 mM/kg of lithium in food for 5–7 days and for 3–5 days respectively, sufficient to give serum levels of 1 mM/l. Lithium produced a significant increase in the uptake of noradrenaline by synaptosomes in both experiments and the former group also showed that adding lithium *in vitro* to synaptosomes of untreated animals was without effect. Kuriyama and Speken made similar observations on synaptosomes from the brains of mice treated with lithium chloride 3·75 mM/kg every 12 hours for 5 days. Brain concentrations were quoted as 2·84 mM/g (which seems unlikely) and serum concentrations as 0·83 mM/l. The concentrations of both noradrenaline and 5HT were reduced in the synaptosomes. Synaptosomes from the lithium-treated animals showed an increased uptake of labelled noradrenaline, whereas addition of lithium in considerable concentrations *in vitro* (between 2 and 10 mM/l) had no effect on content and uptake of either noradrenaline or 5HT by synaptosomes and mitochondria. Whole brain concentrations of 5HT and noradrenaline were reported by Kuriyama and Speken to remain unchanged, whereas another group, working with rats, found an increase of both 5HT and 5HIAA in brain (Perez-Cruet *et al.*, 1971) and suggested that at the dose levels used (1·6–2·0 mM/kg twice a day for 5 days), the turnover of 5HT was accelerated.

The discordant findings in these two studies on mice and rats may indicate valid differences in the effects of lithium on these two species. The findings of

Perez–Cruet et al., might have been predicted by their parallel study (Tagliamonte et al., 1971) where they showed that doses of lithium of 3·3 mM/kg for 5 days resulted in increased concentrations of tryptophan in plasma and brain of rats, and the concentration of tryptophan in brain may be the rate-limiting step in the synthesis of 5HT.

Opitz et al. (1971) studied the influence of lithium on the oxygen uptake and the calorigenic actions of noradrenaline, isoprenaline, amphetamine and 2,4-dinitrophenol. The reduced calorigenic response to noradrenaline and other sympathomimetic amines in the presence of lithium did not appear to be due to hypothyroidism but could have been caused by altered uptake and release of monoamines.

In a different type of experiment, Greenspan et al. (1970a) felt that lithium may change storage and metabolism of noradrenaline. They showed that 10 days' administration of lithium at 3 mM/kg body weight produced overactivity, mydriasis and exophthalmos in rats given a monoamine oxidase inhibitor (MAOI). In other animals (without MAOI) efflux of ^{3}H-noradrenaline from the brain was more than doubled. There was a raised proportion of total radioactivity in ^{3}H-O-methylated metabolites at the expense of ^{3}H-noradrenaline. The increase of endogenous noradrenaline produced by MAOI was less than in control animals.

After a 7-day span of treatment with lithium at 100 mg/kg body weight Oxenkrug and Kiseleva (1971) were unable to find any change in the concentration of 5HT in the brain of mice, but it prevented the rise seen after the administration of 5HTP. The activity of 5HTP was unaffected by lithium. The authors felt that lithium probably activated the catabolism of 5-HT.

Schubert (1973) also used the 7-day period of treatment with lithium in two dose levels which gave concentrations in the serum in the region of 0·4 and 0·7 mM/l respectively. The smaller dose of lithium was without effect on amine metabolism in the brain but with the higher there was an increase in the accumulation of labelled 5HT and 5HIAA in the brain during venous infusion of ^{3}H-tryptophan. Disappearance of labelled 5HT was reduced also, suggesting reduction in the release of the amine from storage sites. The concentration of tryptophan in brain rose. Similar experiments on labelled dopamine and noradrenaline from ^{14}C-tyrosine demonstrated no effects and the experiments as a whole suggested effects of lithium on indolamines but not on catecholamines.

The paper by Knapp and Mandell (1973) was mentioned in the section on acute effects of lithium. In the experiments conducted over the subacute-chronic time span, that is rats treated for 10–21 days, the biosynthesis of 5-hydroxytryptamine returned to normal but cell body tryptophan hydroxylase remained significantly below control levels.

Shaw et al. (1972) attempted a somewhat different type of experiment. They gave lithium in drinking water to rabbits in doses which resulted in a mean serum concentration of 1·3 mM/l by the seventh day. They injected ^{14}C-l-tryptophan intravenously and the curve of changes in plasma radioactivity was subjected to multiple compartmental analysis. The preliminary analysis suggested that lithium altered the partitition of the amino acid in the body in favour of the extracellular space and at the expense of the intracellular compartment.

C. Chronic effects of lithium on amine metabolism

Relatively few chronic experiments have been completed successfully and in those that have been published there were often signs of incipient toxicity in the animals treated with lithium.

Corrodi *et al.* (1969) gave rats lithium at doses of about 2 mM/kg at which dosage some animals were experiencing polyuria and diarrhoea. Under these conditions concentrations of noradrenaline, dopamine and 5HT in the brain did not change. Blocking the appropriate hydroxylating enzyme did not give evidence of change in turnover of noradrenaline, but there was an increased turnover of dopamine in the infundibular area and a decrease in the mesotelencephalic region, and the turnover of 5-hydroxytryptamine was reduced.

An even longer-term experiment was completed by Ho *et al.* (1970) who gave 2 mM/kg of lithium for 28 days to rats and also ended up with animals which had signs of toxicity, as shown by polyuria, diarrhoea, weight loss and the death of a few animals. Estimating turnover from rate of accumulation of amine after monoamine oxidase inhibition, they found a decreased rate for dopamine in brainstem and for noradrenaline in hypothalamus. The concention of noradrenaline, again failed to reveal differences between the lithium-rate of turnover was decreased in hypothalamus, diencephalon and brainstem.

Bliss and Ailion (1970) fed lithium carbonate to rats in their diet over a 14-day period and then examined the animals' brains for changes in noradrenaline, 5-hydroxytryptamine and dopamine. Brain concentrations of noradrenaline did not differ from those of control subjects; blocking noradrenaline synthesis for one hour by α-methyl-*p*-tyrosine, and following the ensuing rates of degradation of noradrenaline, again failed to reveal differences between the lithium-treated and control animals. The only difference which was observed was a slight decrease in the percentage recovery of deaminated metabolites following the intracisternal injection of tritiated noradrenaline into lithium treated rats. The authors concluded that lithium probably did not affect the level or rate of metabolism of noradrenaline in rat brain. The metabolism of 5-hydroxytryptamine also appeared to be relatively unaffected by lithium treatment; brain levels did not change, though slight increases were observed in 5-HIAA levels. Blockage of 5HT degradation by the administration of pheniprazine also revealed no difference in 5HT degradation or synthesis rates in lithium-treated animals as compared with control subjects. Dopamine metabolism, too, was not changed by the lithium treatment. Commenting on the differences between their negative results and the effects of lithium on amine metabolism reported by other investigators, Bliss and Ailion suggested that the discrepancy might relate either to the length of time for which the lithium had been administered, or to the final concentration of lithium in the serum (0·5 to 1·0 mEq Li$^+$/l) achieved by the treatment. They concluded that it may not be the case that the therapeutic actions of lithium are mediated by changes in cerebral amine metabolism, though they conceded that specific regional effects might be involved. In this respect, it is interesting to compare the results of Bliss and Ailion with those of Ho et al. (1970) mentioned above.

Genefke (1972b) also used rats in experiments where lithium was given for 1–7 weeks. Polyuria was present after three weeks and although the animals gained weight this was less than in controls. No changes in concentration of 5HT in grey or white matter were observed but, after more than four weeks on lithium, concentrations of 5HT rose by 19% in the hypothalamus.

Murphy et al. (1969) showed that in platelets taken from manic-depressive patients being treated chronically with lithium, the uptake of 5HT during the first 10 minutes of incubation was accelerated as compared to rates before treatment.

D. Experiments on dopamine

Friedman and Gershon (1973) carried out one of the few experiments which have involved dopamine. Acute treatment by injection of lithium at a dose level of 2–4 mM/kg body weight had no effect on endogenous dopamine nor on its synthesis in striatal slices. However, doses of 1 and 2 mM/kg body weight for 14 days inhibited the synthesis of dopamine in the striatum by 34% and 62% respectively. In vitro replacement of 4–18 mMol/l of sodium by lithium ion in the media incubating striatal slices did not affect synthesis of dopamine.

These data agree in part with the earlier observations of Corrodi et al. (1969) who showed no change in levels of whole brain dopamine and slightly decreased turnover in rats treated for three weeks with lithium, but a localized increase in turnover in the tubero-infundibula region and increase in the mesotelencephalic region.

After a longer period of treatment (4 weeks) Ho et al. (1970) could demonstrate no changes in dopamine turnover in several regions of the brain, so it may be that alterations do not extend into the chronic period of treatment.

IV. Changes in Amine Metabolism during Lithium Therapy

Despite the great interest which clearly attaches to information about changes in amine metabolism brought about by lithium, there have been relatively few studies specifically designed to examine this aspect of the actions of lithium within the clinical context. The early findings were, in any case, not particularly clear-cut and this may have led to the feeling that no information of any great value was likely to emerge from investigations in this area.

Bowers *et al.* (1969), reporting on four manic patients, noted only a slight decrease in homovanillic acid (HVA) in cerebrospinal fluid and even this was statistically non-significant. No change was found in 5HIAA levels in the cerebrospinal fluid of the same patients. Haskovec and Rysanek (1969) were also unable to find changes in 5HIAA excretion following lithium; however, these investigators examined non-psychiatric patients and their results may not be directly comparable to those obtained from investigations of manic patients. Haskovec and Rysanek administered lithium carbonate to their subjects over a 5-day period and monitored excretory rates of various products of amine metabolism over this time: they reported that 3-methoxy-4-hydroxyvanillyl-mandelic acid (VMA) excretory rates were elevated during the first two days of treatment, but that thereafter there was no significant increase, whilst a significant decrease in normetanephrine and metanephrine excretion occurred on days five and six.

In the following year, Greenspan *et al.* (1970b) reported a statistically significant decrease in normetanephrine and metanephrine excretion following lithium treatment in manic-depressive patients, and Messiha *et al.* (1970) noted that lithium treatment reduced dopamine excretion (which was elevated during the manic state) but had no effect on the excretion of VMA.

Mendels (1971) showed that 5HIAA levels in cerebrospinal fluid were decreased during manic episodes and elevated again as a result of lithium therapy, but since only two patients were involved in these investigations their generality is uncertain. However, Wilk *et al.* (1972) have confirmed the finding of a rise in 5HIAA in cerebrospinal fluid; they also reported that 3-methoxy-4-hydroxyphenylglycol (MHPG) levels, which were increased during mania, were reduced by lithium, whilst HVA levels were increased (the latter finding being contrary to that reported by Bowers, *et al.*, 1969).

V. Conclusions

Although patterns can be discerned in the various experiments it is most difficult to say which are the most significant or even which are the valid observations. As stated above, many of the effects may be secondary to toxic processes or to the stress of being in a toxic state. If we ignore these provisos, then the main demonstrated acute effect of lithium seems to be an enhancement of the intraneuronal retention and turnover of noradrenaline, but it is not at all clear what happens to 5HT in the brain or whether the platelet experiments are strictly relevant.

In the subacute experiments, the most clear-cut data were once again on noradrenaline, suggesting increased synaptosomal uptake, increased intraneuronal degradation and limitation of release. The picture for 5HT was much less clear.

Chronic treatment with lithium seems to affect turnover of both 5HT and dopamine, the most consistent finding being decreased turnover of 5HT in several areas of the brain.

It is manifestly not possible, at this point in time, to make any definite statements about the mechanisms whereby lithium brings about its effects on amine metabolism. In the first place, the experimental and clinical investigations which have been carried out have revealed such a variety of effects that it must be suspected that more than one mechanism is involved. Secondly, it is not always possible to tell from the clinical studies which of the changes in amine metabolism are direct results of lithium administration and which are secondary effects consequent upon clinical improvement. The differences noted previously in this chapter between the effects of lithium administered for varying periods of time have also to be encompassed in any satisfactory model of lithium involvement in amine metabolism: the interpretation of this aspect of lithium's effects is of crucial importance in developing our understanding of the relationship between therapeutic regimes of an acute nature (as in the treatment of mania) or of more extended duration (as in lithium prophylaxis of recurrent disorders).

There are several possible points at which lithium may have a more or less direct effect on amine function in neurones. In theory the effects may be upon the availability and transport of substrates, upon synthesis or upon the concentration, storage and release of amine neurotransmitters from synaptic vesicles, upon the reuptake mechanism from the synaptic cleft, upon postsynaptic processes, especially the receptors, and finally upon the catabolic processes. It is known that lithium interacts with the various monovalent and divalent cations (see Chapter 22) and enzyme systems (see Chapter 33) which are associated with the integrity of vesicles. Schildkraut (1973) has suggested recently that lithium may affect transmitter release from vesicles, the release being intra-, rather than extra-neuronal, and leading to catabolism of the biogenic amines within the neurone. Once released from the neurone into the synaptic space, the amines may have their reuptake rates modified as a result of lithium (see the earlier comments on the work of Colburn *et al.*, 1967; Baldessarini and Yorke, 1970; and Kuriyama and Speken, 1970), or their extra-neuronal catabolism may be changed. Postsynaptic receptor sites may respond to lithium by becoming less sensitive to neurotransmitter substances. The work of Fann *et al.* (1972) has led to the suggestion that this may be an important aspect of lithium's effects, and this is supported by the *in vitro* studies of Frazer *et al.* (1972) mentioned previously. Receptor processes are now known to be dependent upon adenyl cyclase activity and in Chapter 29 it is demonstrated that lithium may have important effects here which could determine some of its actions on amine metabolism.

The most important question, of course, centres on whether the effects of lithium on amines have any therapeutic significance. If at this point in time we could say in what ways amines are involved in the aetiology of affective illness, we would be in a much better position to assess the importance of the effects of lithium on amines. We might be able to decide whether or not these actions are connected with either of lithium's two main therapeutic roles. Unfortunately we can say only that amines are likely to play some part in causing the illness, a part which may be in a less central position than was conceived in the original versions of the amine hypothesis.

If we were to speculate, however, that lithium does act therapeutically via aminergic pathways, then clearly considerable interest would focus on the acute effects of lithium on noradrenaline (for its antimanic actions) and on the chronic effects of this cation on 5HT turnover (for its preventative activity). It may be that the suggested post-synaptic actions could be the most significant of all.

References

Baldessarini, R. J. and Yorke, C. (1970). *Nature* **228**, 1301–1303.

Bliss, E. L. and Ailion, J. (1970). *Brain Res.* **24**, 305–310.

Bowers, M. B., Heninger, G. R. and Gerbode, F. (1969). *Int. J. Neuropharmacol.* **8**, 255–259.

Colburn, R. W., Goodwin, F. K., Bunney, W. E. and Davis, J. M. (1967). *Nature* **215**, 1395–1397.

Coppen, A., Shaw, D. M. and Farrell, J. P. (1963). *Lancet* **1**, 79–81.

Corrodi, H., Fuxe, K., Hökfelt, T. and Schou, M. (1967). *Psychopharmacologia* **11**, 345–353.

Corrodi, H., Fuxe, K. and Schou, M. (1969). *Life Sci.* **8**, 643–651.

Donaldson, J., Minnich, J. L. and Barbeau, A. (1973). *Un. méd. Can.* **102**, 907–911.

Fann, W. E., Davis, J. M., Janowsky, D. S., Cavanaugh, J. H., Kaufmann, J. S., Griffith, J. D. and Oates, J. A. (1972). *Clin. pharmacol. Ther.* **13**, 71–77.

Frazer, A., Hancock, A., Mendels, J. and MacIntire, R. (1972). *Biol. Psychiat.* **5**, 79–87.

Friedman, E. and Gershon, S. (1973). *Nature* **243**, 520–521.

Genefke, I. K. (1972a). *Acta psychiat. scand.* **48**, 394–399.

Genefke, I. K. (1972b). *Acta psychiat. scand.* **48**, 400–404.

Greenspan, K., Aronoff, M. S. and Bogdanski, D. F. (1970a). *Pharmacology* **3**, 129–136.

Greenspan, K., Schildkraut, J. J., Gordon, E. K., Baer, L., Aronoff, M. S. and Durrell, J. (1970b). *J. psychiat. Res.* **7**, 171–183.

Haskovec, L. and Rysanek, K. (1969). *Arzneimittel-Forsch.* **19**, 426–427.

Ho, A. K. S., Loh, H. H., Craves, F., Hitzemann, R. J. and Gershon, S. (1970). *Eur. J. Pharmacol.* **10**, 72–78.

Katz, R. I., Chase, T. N. and Kopin, I. J. (1968). *Science* **162**, 466–467.

Katz, R. I., Chase, T. N. and Kopin, I. J. (1969). *J. Neurochem.* **16**, 961–967.

Katz, R. I. and Kopin, I. J. (1969). *Biochem. Pharmacol.* **18**, 1935–1939.

Kiseleva, I. P. and Lapin, I. P. (1969). *Pharmacol. res. Commun.* **1**, 108–114.

Knapp, S. and Mandell, A. J., (1973). *Science* **180**, 645–647.

Kuriyama, K. and Speken, R. (1970). *Life Sci.* **9**, 1213–1220.

Lapin, I. P. and Oxenkrug, G. F. (1969). *New Eng. J. Med.* **281**, 218.

Lemieux, G., Davignon, A. and Genest, J. (1956). *Can. med. Ass. J.* **74**, 522–526.

Mendels, J. (1971). *Lancet* **1**, 342.

Messiha, F. S., Agallianos, D. and Clower, C. (1970). *Nature* **225**, 868–869.

Muller, J. C., Pryor, W. W., Gibbons, J. E. and Orgain, E. S. (1955). *J. Amer. med. Ass.* **159**, 836-839.

Murphy, D. L., Colburn, R. W., Davis, J. M. and Bunney, W. E. (1969). *Life Sci.* **8**, 1187–1193.

Opitz, K., Chu, H. and Grüter, H. (1971). *Naunyn-Schmiedebergs Archs exp. Pathol. Pharmakol.* **268**, 379–391.

Oxenkrug, G. F. and Kiseleva, I. P. (1971). *Farmakol. Toksikol.* **34**, 405–408.

Perez-Cruet, J., Tagliamonte, A., Tagliamonte, P. and Gessa, G. L. (1971). *J. Pharmacol. exp. Ther.* **178**, 325–330.

Schanberg, S. M., Schildkraut, J. J. and Kopin, I. J. (1967). *Biochem. Pharmacol.* **16**, 393–399.

Schildkraut, J. J. (1965). *Am. J. Psychiat.* **122**, 509–522.

Schildkraut, J. J. (1973). *In* "Lithium: Its Role in Psychiatric Research and Treatment" (S. Gershon and B. Shopsin, eds), pp. 51–73. Plenum Press, New York.

Schildkraut, J. J. and Kety, S. S. (1967). *Science* **156**, 21–37.

Schildkraut, J. J., Logue, M. A. and Dodge, G. A. (1969a). *Psychopharmacologia* **14**, 135–141.

Schildkraut, J. J., Schanberg, S. M., Breese, G. R. and Kopin, I. J. (1969b). *Biochem. Pharmacol.* **18**, 1971–1978.

Schildkraut, J. J., Schanberg, S. M. and Kopin, I. J. (1966). *Life Sci.* **5**, 1479–1483.

Schubert, J. (1973). *Psychopharmacologia* **32**, 301–311.

Shaw, D. M. (1973a). *Brit. J. hosp. Med.* **10**, 609–616.

Shaw, D. M. (1973b). *Trans. Biochem. Soc.* **1**, 78–81.

Shaw, D. M. Johnson, A. J. and Short, R. (1972). *Math. Biosci.* **15**, 137–151.

Shaw, D. M., O'Keeffe, R., MacSweeney, D. A., Brooksbank, B. W. L., Noguera, R. and Coppen, A. (1973). *Psychol. Med.* **3**, 333–336.

Sheard, M. H. and Aghajanian, G. K. (1970). *Life Sci.* **9**, 285–290.

Sterne, D. N., Fieve, R. R., Neff, N. H. and Costa, E. (1969). *Psychopharmacologia* **14**, 315–322.

Tagliamonte, A., Tagliamonte, P., Perez-Cruet, J. and Gessa, G. L. (1971). *Nature New Biology* **229**, 125–126.

Wilk, S., Shopsin, B., Gershon, S. and Suhl, M. (1972). *Nature* **235**, 440–441.

P

26

LITHIUM AND AMINO ACID METABOLISM

S. Berl and D. D. Clarke

I. Introduction

The efficacy of lithium therapy in the treatment of mania has been attributed in part to its effect on the metabolism of monoamine neurotransmitters (Schou, 1971; Schildkraut and Gershon, 1971); this is amply demonstrated in this book (Chapter 25). It has been found, however, that drugs such as reserpine (Berl and Frigyesi, 1969), 6-hydroxydopamine (Nicklas and Berl, 1973) and L-DOPA (Nicklas et al., 1974), which also affect catecholamine metabolism, alter as well the metabolism in brain of glutamine, glutamic acid, aspartic acid and γ-aminobutyric acid (GABA), the latter three of which have also been described as neurotransmitters or neuromodulators and, increasingly, studies on the metabolic relationships between catecholamine and amino acid metabolism have added proof that they are interdependent. The question posed by these investigations is whether unbalancing one set of transmitters, such as the catecholamines, will result in the metabolism of other related transmitter substances, such as the amino acids, also being unbalanced.

Support for an anticipated effect of lithium on the metabolism of glutamic acid and GABA derives from the dependence which the high affinity uptake of these amino acids into nerve endings has on the concentrations of Na⁺ (Bennett *et al.*, 1973); Li⁺ would be expected to compete with Na⁺ in such an active uptake process, although attempts to demonstrate such an effect on GABA uptake by slices from various regions of rat brain were not successful (Bond, 1973).

II. Amino Acids as Transmitters

The concept that amino acids may function as neurotransmitters arose largely from the discoveries in the late 1950's that GABA is present in brain in relatively high concentrations (Roberts, 1960), and that it is inhibitory in the stretch receptor of the cray fish (Florey, 1960) as well as in the central nervous system. Soon afterwards it was shown that glutamic acid, the precursor of GABA, was excitatory when iontophoretically applied in the CNS (Curtis and Watkins, 1965). In similar experiments aspartate was also found to be excitatory. On the other hand, their amides, glutamine and asparagine, were pharmacologically inactive. While glutamic acid is present in all tissues, its concentration in brain is two to ten times higher than in other tissues (Tallan, 1962). If one were to assume that the difference in levels between brain and other tissues are related to a special function such as neurotransmission, then it might be expected that glutaminergic nerve endings would be found to predominate in the CNS. Following the same argument, GABA is generally not detectable in other tissues (Roberts, 1960) and its major function appears to be that of an inhibitory transmitter (Curtis and Johnston, 1970). These ideas are bolstered by the estimates of Snyder and others (Snyder *et al.*, 1973) that cholinergic and catecholaminergic endings make up no more than about 15% of the nerve endings.

Clearly, a major use of amino acids in all tissues is for protein synthesis: in view of the above discussion it might be anticipated that in brain only a small portion of glutamic acid and its associated metabolites would be utilized for this purpose. Thus it is not surprising that the metabolism of glutamic acid shows a distinct compartmentation in the brain, existing in several metabolically discrete pools (Berl and Clarke, 1969). Consequently, studies of amino acid metabolism in brain which have not been cognizant of this fact often require re-evaluation. In addition, studies designed to demonstrate the metabolism of transmitter pools of glutamic acid are rendered much more difficult than metabolic studies in other tissue. Studies based exclusively on changes in levels of amino acids after various types of treatment, including Li⁺, offer only a limited view which is easily subject to ambiguous interpretation. The use of tracer amounts of radioactive precursors (Reiner, 1953) gives additional information about fluxes of materials which aids in the interpretation of the

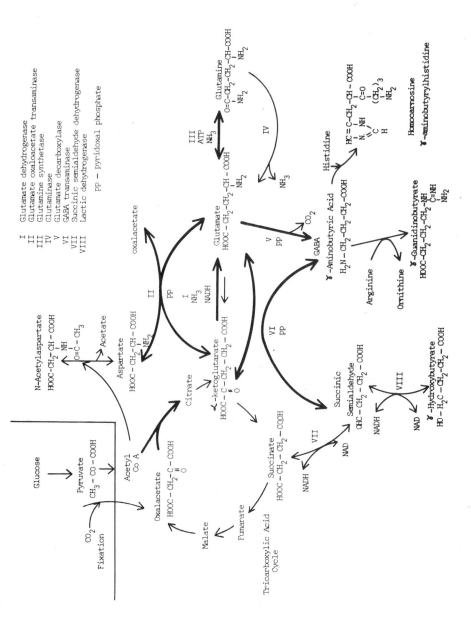

FIG. 1. Metabolic relationships between glucose oxidation, the tricarboxylic acid cycle and glutamic acid as well as related amino acids.

metabolic studies by removing some of the ambiguities and allowing sharper focus on the effects of the drug treatment.

III. Metabolism of Glutamic Acid

A flow chart depicting the metabolic relationships between glucose oxidation, the operation of the tricarboxylic acid cycle and the biosynthesis of glutamate and related amino acids is shown in Fig. 1. In early studies of the nature of the blood–brain barrier to glutamic acid, utilizing ^{14}C-labelled glutamic acid (Lajtha *et al.*, 1959), it was observed that the metabolic transformation of this amino acid to glutamine showed unusual product-precursor relationships. These suggested that either metabolic pathways existed in brain which had not been previously demonstrated in other organs,or that glutamate metabolism in brain was heterogenous to a degree not previously noticed in studies with this tissue (Berl *et al.*, 1961). Further studies indicated that not only were there at least two pools of glutamate, but that the tricarboxylic acid cycle intermediates associated with these pools of glutamate were also compartmented (Waelsch *et al.*, 1964; Gaitonde, 1965; Van den Berg *et al.*, 1966). These tracer studies were followed by attempts to develop quantitative models for these compartments using the computer simulation methods of Garfinkel (1966).

Figure 2 presents a description of such a model developed by Van den Berg and Garfinkel (1971). A key assumption in this model is that GABA is metabolized at a site different from that at which it is synthesized. The kinetics of the data required that part of the glutamate formed in a relatively small pool

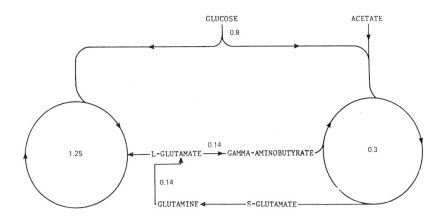

FIG. 2. Relationship of "small" (S) and "large (L) pools of glutamic acid in mouse brain. The numbers represent the flux of glucose in μ mol/min/g wet weight of tissue. (From Van den Berg and Garfinkel (1971), with permission.)

must flow back to a relatively large pool, presumably as glutamine, which in part is then recycled to glutamate and GABA. This kinetic model is supported by recent studies of the enzymes required for the formation and degradation of GABA which indicate differential localization of glutamic acid decarboxylase (E.C.4.1.1.15) and GABA transaminase (E.C.2.6.1.19), (Baxter, 1970). From developmental studies of the compartmentation of glutamate, it has been suggested by Balázs (Balázs et al., 1973) that the small pool of glutamate and its related tricarboxylic acid cycle is associated with the glia, and the large pools with the neurons (see Watkins, 1973 for a review). In view of what has been previously said about the probable role of GABA and glutamate as neurotransmitters, it would seem likely that this flow of amino acids is occurring at nerve endings and probably in response to nerve stimulation.

IV. Effects of Li⁺ on Amino Acid Metabolism

Recently it has been suggested that lithium carbonate may be of aid in the treatment of Huntington's chorea (Dalén, 1973; Manyam and Bravo-Fernandez, 1973); preliminary trials appear to support this suggestion. The rationale for this form of therapy derives from (1) the findings that GABA (Perry et al., 1973) as well as glutamic acid decarboxylase (GAD) Bird et al., 1973; McGeer et al., 1973), the enzyme responsible for GABA formation from

TABLE I. Effect of OHP (oxygen high pressure) on brain GABA in rats pretreated with various cations. (From Radomski and Watson (1973) with permission.)

Group	Dose (mmol/kg)	Injection time prior to OHP	Brain GABA (μmol/g wet wt)	% Decrease from control
Non-exposed	—	—	$1\cdot60 \pm 0\cdot03$	—
Water	—	15 min	$1\cdot29 \pm 0\cdot04$**	-19
Li	4·7	15 min	$1\cdot39 \pm 0\cdot04$**	-13
	4·7	1 hr	$1\cdot46 \pm 0\cdot05$*	-9
	4·7	24 hr	$1\cdot34 \pm 0\cdot02$**	-16
Li	9·4	15 min	$1\cdot55 \pm 0\cdot04$	-3
	9·4	1 hr	$1\cdot60 \pm 0\cdot04$	0
	9·4	24 hr	$1\cdot34 \pm 0\cdot02$**	-16
Mg	1·0	15 min	$1\cdot39 \pm 0\cdot02$**	-13
Zn	0·5	15 min	$1\cdot34 \pm 0\cdot06$**	-16
Mn	0·1	15 min	$1\cdot37 \pm 0\cdot02$**	-14

Data for brain GABA represent the mean $\pm$ SEM for at least 8 brains.
Values significantly different from the non-exposed group:
 * $p < 0\cdot05$
 ** $p < 0\cdot001$

glutamic acid, are decreased in Huntington's chorea; (2) a decrease of brain GABA precedes convulsions and lung edema due to breathing oxygen at high pressures (5·5 atm.) in rats (Fig. 3, Table I; Radomski and Watson, 1973); (3) lithium at 9·4 mmol/kg proved to be highly effective in inhibiting the development of the convulsions and lung edema and to prevent as well the

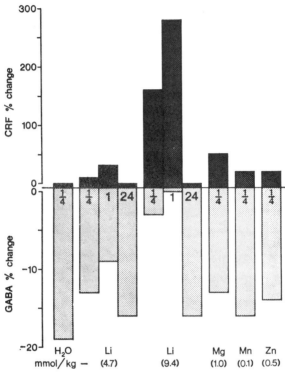

FIG. 3. Comparison of the decrease in brain GABA to the convulsion reduction factor (CRF) for various cation treatments. The figures shown in the bars represent the time of injection of lithium prior to exposure. (From Radomski and Watson (1973) with permission.)

decrease in brain GABA (Fig. 4, Table I; Radomski and Watson, 1973). This protective effect of lithium was evident at 15–60 minutes after injection corresponding to the time of peak serum levels of lithium. It was absent 24 hours after injection at which time brain lithium levels were maximal while serum levels had returned to near pre-drug values. This suggests that either the action of lithium in the CNS is secondary to a peripheral effect (possibly on the metabolism of norepinephrine in the adrenal medulla), or that lithium under-

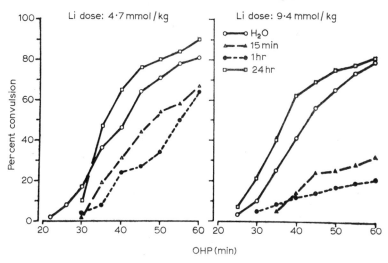

FIG. 4. The effect of two doses of lithium at various times of injection on convulsions induced by OHP. Doses are shown in the Figure. The times indicated for each curve represent the time that lithium was injected prior to exposure to OHP (Oxygen high pressure). (From Radomski and Watson (1973) with permission.)

goes redistribution in the brain, becoming concentrated in non-synaptic sites where it is sequestered and no longer effective. In support of the former explanation, it has been reported that administered Li^+ decreases the sensitivity of man to infused noradrenaline (Fann *et al.*, 1972). It has been suggested (Radomski and Watson, 1973) that Li^+ may counteract the release of sympathoadrenal hormones induced by oxygen high pressure, by decreasing the sensitivity of receptor sites normally responsive to these hormones. On the other hand, or in addition, lithium may counteract any oxygen high pressure-induced acceleration of membrane transport of GABA (Radomski and Watson, 1973) in the brain. Li^+ produces a decrease in brain Na^+ (Davenport, 1950; King *et al.*, 1969), an effect which may inhibit the binding and transport of free GABA from the synaptic cleft into metabolic sites (Radomski and Watson, 1973); thus the concentration of GABA in synaptic clefts would be prolonged. Na^+ is required for the binding and transport of GABA into intracellular neuronal sites (Kuriyama *et al.*, 1969): it is also required for the high affinity uptake of glutamate and aspartate by synaptosomal preparations (Bennett *et al.*, 1973).

Although Li^+ does not alter the levels of GABA in the whole brain of animals not subjected to high oxygen pressure (De Feudis and Delgado, 1970; Gottesfeld *et al.*, 1971; Radomski and Watson, 1973) (Table II), it has been

TABLE II. Effect of cations on brain GABA levels in rats not exposed to OHP (oxygen high pressure). (From Radomski and Watson (1973) with permission.)

Group	Dose (mmol/kg)	Time after[a] injection	Brain GABA (μmol/g wet wt)
Water	—	45 min	1.60 ± 0.03
Li	4.7	24 hr	1.61 ± 0.02
	9.4	1.5 hr	1.56 ± 0.04
	9.4	24 hr	1.55 ± 0.03
Mg	1.0	45 min	1.52 ± 0.03
Zn	0.5	45 min	1.53 ± 0.05
Mn	0.1	45 min	1.64 ± 0.03
	0.3	45 min	1.57 ± 0.04

Values for brain GABA represent the mean $\pm$ SEM of at least eight brains.

[a]The time of sacrifice after injection in the non-exposed animals corresponds in exposed animals (Table I), to the time of injection prior to exposure plus 30 min of exposure to OHP.

reported that a significant increase in glutamate and GABA does occur in the hypothalamus of the rat one hour after a single dose of 20 mEq/g (Gottesfeld *et al.*, 1971). Chronic treatment for five days with a twice daily injection of 2 mEq/g had similar effects. Li^+ treatment also lowered the Na^+ and K^+ levels in the hypothalamus (Ho *et al.*, 1970). Gottesfeld *et al.* (1971) suggested that these changes may be the responsible mode of action.

The finding that Li^+ does not alter the overall level of GABA in the brain is not subject to simple interpretation for a number of reasons. If, as indicated in Fig. 2, the formation of GABA (in neurons) is linked to a large extent to the flux of S-glutamate (small pool; from glia), Li^+ could slow the net flux of these two amino acids without any change in their levels; GABA levels depend on the flow of transmitter glutamate from neurons to glia. A further complicating feature is that GABA metabolism is also compartmented (Clarke and Garfinkel, unpublished observations). The ratio of pool sizes and flux rates are, no doubt, different in different brain areas and therefore it is possible to see changes in levels in one area even though this is not apparent in the whole brain. Such differences in compartmentation in brain areas have been demonstrated in previous studies where leucine and acetate (both preferential precursors of the small pool of glutamate) labelled amino acids differently in caudate nucleus and cortex (Berl and Frigyesi, 1968).

The picture is confused by possible species differences, since a decrease in mouse whole brain glutamate has been found one hour following intraperitoneal administration of 0·25–0·5 mmol of Li⁺ (De Feudis and Delgado, 1970). Alternately, this may not be a species problem since, as discussed above, whole brain may not be adequately compared with specific areas because of differences in compartmentation between areas. Similarly, the lack of an effect of Li⁺ on the activities of glutamic acid decarboxylase (E.C.4.1.1.15) and γ-aminobutyrate aminotransferase (E.C.2.6.1.19) of whole brain (Rees, 1972) does not justify the conclusion that the glutamate $-\gamma-$ aminobutyrate enzyme system is not concerned in the mechanism of action of therapeutic lithium. The flow of radioactivity from [6-^{14}C]–D–glucose into the total amino acid pool was also decreased by about 10–20% (De Feudis and Delgado, 1970), although the flow of radioactivity from [U^{14}C]–D–glucose into brain and liver was increased (De Feudis, 1971).

The two studies taken together suggest that Li⁺ causes a decrease in the accumulation of radioactivity from glucose into amino acids even though more glucose enters the brain and possibly accumulates in glycolytic or Krebs cycle intermediates. This suggests that a greater proportion of glucose is being used for ATP production rather than for amino acid "transmitter" formation. This would follow the dissipation of energy needed for the pumping of Li⁺ which has leaked into nerve cells. This would be consistent with the computer simulation model (Fig. 2), if it is assumed that the increased flux of glucose is predominantly toward that Krebs cycle which contains the large pools of intermediates and is more intimately associated with energy metabolism (Berl and Clarke, 1969).

The emotional state of mice apparently also determines the action of administered lithium on amino acids (De Feudis, 1972a, b; De Feudis and Paolino, 1972). In mice made aggressive by isolation the subcellular distribution of the lithium is altered in favour of a greater synaptosomal distribution of the cation and an enhanced effect is observed on the incorporation of carbon atoms of [1–^{14}C–] pyruvate into brain. Such environmental manipulation also enhances the effect of Li⁺ on the binding of GABA to crude synaptosomal preparations. Li⁺ affects the binding of GABA to such nerve ending preparations and less GABA is bound by preparations from "isolated" mice as compared with "aggregated" mice.

Other *in vitro* studies also support an effect of Li⁺ on the binding, uptake and metabolism of GABA and glutamate. Thus Li⁺ causes release of GABA from brain slices and from the exposed cerebral cortex of the rat (De Feudis and Mitchell, 1970), as well as from isolated synaptic vesicles (Kuriyama *et al.*, 1968). Replacement of Na⁺ by Li⁺ also progressively inhibits L-glutamate transport into rat cerebral cortex slices (Brechtlová and Laššánová, 1971).

In our studies (Berl and Clark, 1972) with rat brain cortex slices it was found that substitution of Li⁺ for Na⁺ enhanced the leakage from the tissue into the incubation medium of glutamate, glutamine, aspartic acid and GABA, with the

TABLE III. Levels of amino acids in guinea pig brain slices, incubation and preincubation media (μmoles/g tissue wet weight ± S.E.M.) Guinea pig brain slices (approximately 75 mg) were preincubated for 10 min at 37°C in 2·5 ml Krebs-Ringer phosphate medium containing 55 mM glucose and 1·55 mM Ca^{2+}. They were then transferred to fresh medium, 2 μCi of [1-^{14}C]acetate (58 μCi/μmole) added and incubated for 20 min at 37°C. Preincubation and incubation were carried out either in air or 100% O_2. Where Li^+ was added, an equivalent amount of NaCl was replaced by LiCl except in the last set of experiments where 0·1 M LiCl was added without reduction of Na^+ (0·1 M $Li^+ + Na^+$). N = 4 for all samples except for controls with 100% O_2 (N = 17) and 0·1 M Li^+ in 100% O_2 (N = 7). (From Berl and Clarke (1972) with permission.)

	In air				In 100% oxygen			
	Slices	Incubation medium	Preincubation medium	Total	Slices	Incubation medium	Preincubation medium	Total
Glutamic acid								
Control	8·68±0·38	0·28±0·05	1·65±0·15	10·61±0·29	7·85±0·16	0·24±0·03	0·74±0·09	8·87±0·15
0·04 M Li^+	8·18±0·18	0·82±0·04**	2·42±0·12**	11·23±0·21	8·36±0·41	0·26±0·03	1·15±0·23	9·77±0·50*
0·10 M Li^+	6·19±0·07**	1·67±0·11**	2·87±0·10**	10·73±0·23	6·76±0·24**	0·31±0·04	2·01±0·15**	9·08±0·38
0·1 M $Li^+ + Na^+$					6·75±0·34**	0·35±0·13	1·77±0·14**	8·86±0·41
Glutamine								
Control	2·65±0·13	0·96±0·07	1·41±0·16	5·01±0·27	1·85±0·12	1·18±0·08	1·82±0·10	4·85±0·25
0·04 M Li^+	2·54±0·22	1·18±0·04*	1·63±0·14	5·34±0·22	1·79±0·15	1·56±0·08*	2·21±0·52	5·55±0·46
0·10 M Li^+	1·80±0·33*	1·45±0·07**	2·27±0·20*	5·52±0·35	1·71±0·17	1·64±0·08**	2·73±0·32**	6·07±0·43*
0·1 M $Li^+ + Na^+$					1·64±0·17	1·47±0·20	3·20±0·18**	6·11±0·35*
Aspartic acid								
Control	2·00±0·18	0·09±0·06	0·28±0·06	2·37±0·12	2·41±0·05	0·12±0·01	0·18±0·02	2·70±0·06
0·04 M Li^+	1·51±0·12*	0·11±0·06	0·41±0·09	2·02±0·08	1·93±0·11**	0·05±0·01*	0·26±0·06	2·24±0·07**
0·10 M Li^+	1·13±0·18**	0·20±0·08	0·46±0·12	1·79±0·19*	1·19±0·05**	0·23±0·04**	0·52±0·06**	1·93±0·09**
0·1 M $Li^+ + Na^+$					1·51±0·05**	0·21±0·01**	0·21±0·06	1·93±0·07**
GABA								
Control	4·01±0·35	0·40±0·05	0·42±0·06	4·82±0·33	2·42±0·17	0·39±0·03	0·66±0·06	3·47±0·86
0·04 M Li^+	3·60±0·27	0·46±0·05	0·55±0·08	4·61±0·32	2·80±0·14	0·53±0·08	0·76±0·15	4·08±0·27
0·10 M Li^+	3·09±0·15*	0·87±0·09**	0·94±0·05**	4·89±0·19	1·85±0·34	0·54±0·06*	1·08±0·19**	3·47±0·45
0·1 M $Li^+ + Na^+$					3·48±0·27**	0·66±0·05**	1·25±0·19**	5·40±0·43**
Sum of the amino acids								
Control	17·34±1·04	1·73±0·23	3·76±0·43	22·81±1·01	14·53±0·50	1·93±0·15	3·40±0·27	19·89±1·32
0·04 M Li^+	15·83±0·73	2·57±0·19*	5·01±0·43*	23·20±0·83	14·88±0·81	2·40±0·20	4·38±0·96	21·64±1·30
0·10 M Li^+	12·13±0·73**	4·19±0·35**	6·54±0·47**	22·93±0·96	11·51±0·80	2·72±0·22	6·34±0·73**	20·55±1·35
0·1 M $Li^+ + Na^+$					13·38±0·83	2·69±0·39	6·34±0·57**	22·30±1·26

* $p<0.05$ by Student 't' test.
** $p<0.01$ by Student 't' test.

most marked effect on glutamate (Table III). The use of 100% oxygen rather than air as the gas phase counteracted in part the leakage of glutamate, indicating that the leakage is dependent upon the energy state of the tissue (see above). The sum of the levels of the amino acids in the slices plus media were relatively constant and approximated the values observed in fresh tissue (except for GABA). The addition of Li^+ rather than the replacement of NaCl (the condition which would prevail *in vivo*) greatly elevated the level of GABA in the slices. This may have some relevance to the protective effect of Li^+ on the GABA brain level under conditions of high oxygen pressure discussed previously.

Since [1-^{14}C]–acetate preferentially labels a pool or pools of glutamate active in glutamine formation (Berl and Clarke, 1969), this tracer was used in the study of the effect of Li^+ on glutamate metabolism. The distribution of radioactivity from this precursor in the individual amino acids showed specific effects of Li^+ (Table IV). The cation decreased the percentage of radioactivity in the sum of the four amino acids. Particularly evident was a decrease in the amount of radioactivity in glutamine while that in glutamic acid tended to increase. Thus the flux of glutamic acid to glutamine was apparently decreased. Although it is not very likely, this inhibition of glutamine labeling could be due to inhibition of glutamine synthetase (E.C.6.3.1.2). A second hypothesis is that the pool of ATP required for the operation of the Na^+– K^+ pump is either the same as, or closely related to, the pool of ATP required for glutamine synthesis. The assumption would be that this pool of ATP is depleted by replacement of Na^+ by Li^+ as suggested above.

A third hypothesis which would not necessarily exclude the second is that a small pool of glutamate (transmitter glutamate at nerve endings?) formed at one site, must be transported to another site for conversion to glutamine. Such an effect on the active transport of glutamate would be similar to that of ouabain. The presence of ouabain (an inhibitor of the Na^+–K^+ pump) in the incubation medium has been found to depress the formation of labeled glutamine (Berl *et al.,* 1970). In addition, the presence of Ca^{2+}, (a cation essential for release of transmitter substance at nerve endings) is also required for glutamine formation in brain tissue. This supports the idea that release of "transmitter" glutamate determines the rate of glutamine synthesis rather than predominantly the activity of glutamine synthetase (6.3.1.2). Metabolic inactivation of "transmitter" glutamate may also be postulated. If glutamate released by synaptic stimulation entered the post synaptic site with the influx of Na^+, glutamine synthetase concentrated in the endoplasmic reticulum (Salganicoff and De Robertis, 1965) would convert it to glutamine which is pharmacologically inactive (Bradford and McIlwain, 1966). A relationship between cellular influx of glutamate and Na^+ has been amply demonstrated. Another very likely site for inactivation of released glutamate would be the glia. It has been suggested that

TABLE IV. Per cent distribution of radioactivity in amino acids[a]. (From Berl and Clarke (1972) with permission.)

| | Slices | | | | Medium | | | |
| | In air | | In 100% O_2 | | In air | | In 100% O_2 | |
	%	N	%	N	%	N	%	N
Glutamic acid								
Control	26.2 ± 1.3	4	25.4 ± 1.2	17	16.0 ± 3.7	4	3.6 ± 0.3	17
0.04 M Li⁺	28.3 ± 2.0	4	33.0 ± 2.6*	4	32.5 ± 2.4**	4	4.5 ± 0.5	4
0.10 M Li⁺	33.5 ± 2.0*	2	39.0 ± 0.9***	7	54.5 ± 3.0***	4	11.6 ± 1.4**	7
0.10 M Li⁺ + Na⁺	—		30.7 ± 3.7	4	—		13.5 ± 3.1*	4
Glutamine								
Control	30.1 ± 2.1	4	45.7 ± 2.1	17	83.4 ± 3.9	4	95.5 ± 0.3	17
0.04 M Li⁺	14.3 ± 0.8***	4	37.2 ± 3.8	4	67.4 ± 2.4*	4	94.5 ± 0.5	4
0.10 M Li⁺	3.5 ± 0.4***	4	21.9 ± 2.1***	7	40.9 ± 3.0***	4	86.2 ± 1.7***	7
0.10 M Li⁺ + Na⁺	—		15.7 ± 0.8**	4	—		84.5 ± 3.3**	4

TABLE IV—*continued*

Aspartic acid								
Control	3·4±0·2	4	3·7±0·2	17	0·4±0·07	2	0·4±0·05	17
0·04 M Li⁺	3·3±0·1	4	4·5±0·3*	4	1·7±0·04**	2	0·7±0·19	4
0·10 M Li⁺	3·0±0·5	4	6·3±0·5**	7	4·7±0·32**	3	1·6±0·26**	7
0·10 M Li⁺ + Na⁺	—		5·6±0·8**	4	—		1·5±0·22**	4
GABA								
Control	1·4±0·3	4	1·1±0·1	15	0·4±0·11	4	0·5±0·11	17
0·04 M Li⁺	1·0±0·1	4	0·9±0·3	2	0·6±0·08	4	0·6±0·15	4
0·10 M Li⁺	0·5±0·1*	4	0·9±0·1	5	1·1±0·27	4	0·5±0·08	4
0·10 M Li⁺ + Na⁺	—		1·4±0·1*	4	—		0·5±0·05	4
Total								
Control	61·1±3·9		75·9±3·6					
0·04 M Li⁺	46·9±3·0*		75·6±7·0					
0·10 M Li⁺	40·5±3·0*		68·1±4·6					
0·10 M Li⁺ + Na⁺	—		53·4±5·4*					

^{a}Calculations for the slices are based on the total radioactivity in the trichloroacetic acid extract of the slices; for the media the percentages are based on the total radioactivity in the amino acids.

 * $p < 0.005$ by Student 't' test.
 ** $p < 0.001$ by Student 't' test.

the glia of the immediate extraneural space at areas of synaptic contact act as a buffer against increases in external K^+ concentration that accompany synaptic activity (Trachtenberg and Pollen, 1970). Increasing the concentration of K^+ in the medium does stimulate the labeling of glutamine from $[1-^{14}C]$–acetate as well as from other radioactive precursors (Berl et al., 1968). It has also been reported that the substitution of Li^+ for Na^+ in the incubation medium causes the loss of K^+ to the same extent as that found in brain slices under anaerobic conditions (Pappius et al., 1958). Li^+ also inhibits the uptake of K^+ by brain slices previously depleted of K^+ by anaerobiosis (Israel et al., 1966). It is now generally accepted that glia constitute a compartment in which glutamate is rapidly converted to glutamine (Balázs et al., 1973). If Li^+ were to inhibit the reuptake of glutamate it would presumably be free to diffuse out into the medium in vitro or out into the spinal fluid in vivo. This might also be true for GABA although this compound is ordinarily not detected in the cerebrospinal fluid. Whether GABA and glutamate levels are elevated in the CSF during Li^+ therapy appears to be worth investigating.

V. Points of Interaction Between Amino Acid and Catecholamine Metabolism

Evidence is coming to light (Nicklas and Berl, 1973; Nicklas et al., 1974) that drugs which alter catecholamine metabolism, or their uptake or storage mechanisms, also affect the metabolism of those amino acids proposed as neurotransmitters and associated with the tricarboxylic acid cycle, i.e. glutamate, aspartate and GABA. Reserpine administered to cats at low doses caused a threefold increase in the rate of turnover of these amino acids in cortex, caudate and thalamus (Berl and Frigyesi, 1969). At larger doses of reserpine the levels of these amino acids were decreased both in the brain and other neuronal structures of the cat supplied by noradrenergic terminals (Santini and Berl, 1972). Pargyline also significantly decreased the levels of glutamate, glutamine, aspartate and alanine plus glycine in dorsal root ganglia, but not in sympathetic ganglia (Santini and Berl, 1972).

The exact mechanisim of the interaction between catecholamine metabolism and that of amino acids related to the tricarboxylic acid cycle remains to be clarified. However, there are several points at which they could affect each other: (1) The availability of tyrosine for catecholamine formation may be partially regulated by tyrosine aminotransferase which transfers the amino group of tyrosine to α-oxoglutarate (E.C.2.6.1.5.) to form glutamate. The competition for the co-factor, pyridoxal-5-phosphate by norepinephrine has been suggested as a controlling factor for this enzyme (Black and Axelrod, 1969). Since this enzyme appears to be localized in brain mitochondria (Mark et al., 1970) the pools of glutamate and oxoglutarate associated with the tricarboxylic acid cycle are involved as co-substrates. (2) Dicarboxylic acids such as fumarate (which is an intermediate in the trycarboxylic acid cycle) enhance the activity of dopamine-β-hydroxylase (Goldstein et al., 1968) apparently decreasing the Km of the enzyme for oxygen. Oxygen consumption might therefore play a regulatory role in bridging the relationships between these different types of neurotransmitters.

The question therefore arises as to whether Li^+ affects one of these neurotransmitters primarily and then acts secondarily upon the other type, or whether it acts on each type independently. Insofar as the high affinity uptake system for amino acids has an absolute dependence on Na^+ it would seem possible that competition between Li^+ and Na^+ at the synaptic junction would provide a plausible basis for the inhibition of the excitatory effects of glutamic and aspartic acids, or for the prolongation of the inhibitory effects of GABA. This, however, does not rule out a direct effect for Li^+ on the inhibitory action of catecholaminergic neurons.

VI. Therapeutic Action—Possible Explanations

In *in vitro* studies the levels of Li^+ used are usually considerably higher than the levels used in treatment or which can be tolerated by the living animal. This does not necessarily mean that similar phenomena are not involved. Rather it would seem to be an indication that the biochemical techniques available are not sufficiently sensitive to detect the subtle changes involved at specific areas in the brain. The larger doses may be looked at as producing an amplification of effects occurring at the lower doses. Determination of the levels of Li^+ in relatively large areas of brain may not truly reflect its concentration at subcellular active sites. However, it must be borne in mind that extrapolation from *in vitro* studies may be at times misleading in attempting to evaluate therapeutic action of the drug. The metabolic effects of Li^+ reported in the literature often appear to be contradictory but this may be more apparent than real since the conditions in different experiments are often not directly comparable.

In considering the therapeutic action of Li^+ it may be suggested that its primary effect is in the interaction between excitary and inhibitory synapses. From a theoretical point of view it would seem that excitation and inhibition must be in balance for normal brain function (Roberts and Matthysse, 1970). This would lead us to propose that the mood cycles evident in the manic-depressive psychosis may be the result of a metabolic imbalance in the flow of excitatory and inhibitory transmitters in mood-controlling areas of the brain. It appears from the experiments cited that Li^+ can effect the metabolism of the putative excitatory transmitter glutamic acid as well as the putative inhibitory transmitters GABA and norepinephrine. Can it be that Li^+ acting on both systems has a leveling effect on mood?

Acknowledgements

This work was supported in part by Grants NS-07890 and NS-10670 (D.D.C.) and Grants NS-04064 and the Clinical Center for Research in Parkinson's and Allied Diseases, NS-05184 (S.B.).

References

Balázs, R.. Patel, A. J. and Richter, D. (1973). *In* "Metabolic Compartmentation in Brain" (R. Balazs and J. Cremer, eds), pp. 167–184. Macmillan, London.

Baxter, C. F. (1970). *In* "Handbook of Neurochemistry" (A. Lajtha, ed.), Vol. 3, pp. 289–353, Plenum Press, New York.

Bennett, Jr. J. P., Logan, W. J. and Snyder, S. H. (1973). *J. Neurochem.* **21**, 1533–1550.

Berl, S. and Clarke, D. D. (1969). *In* ..Handbook of Neurochemistry". (A. Lajtha, ed.), Vol. 2 pp. 447–442. Plenum Press, New York.

Berl, S. and Clarke, D. D. (1972). *Brain Res.* **36**, 203–213.

Berl, S. and Frigyesi, T. L. (1968). *J. Neurochem.* **15**, 965–970.

Berl, S. and Frigyesi, T. L. (1969). *Brain Res.* **14**, 683–695.

Berl, S., Lajtha, A. and Waelsch, H. (1961). *J. Neurochem.* **7**, 186–197.

Berl, S., Nicklas, W. J. and Clarke, D. D. (1968). *J. Neurochem.* **15**, 131–140.

Berl, S., Clarke, D. D. and Nicklas, W. J. (1970). *J. Neurochem.* **17**, 999–1007.

Bird, E. D., Mackay, A. V. P., Rayner, C. N. and Iversen, L. L. (1973). *Lancet* **1**, 1090–1092.

Black, I. B., and Axelrod, J. (1969). *J. biol. Chem.* **244**, 6124–6129.

Bond, P. A. (1973). *J. Neurochem.* **20**, 511–517.

Bradford, H. F. and McIlwain, H. (1966). *J. Neurochem.* **13**, 1163–1177.

Brechtlová, M. and Laššánová, M. (1971). *Physiol Bohemoslov*, **20**, 241–248.

Curtis, D. R. and Johnston, G. A. R. (1970). *In* "Handbook of Neurochemistry" (A. Lajtha, ed.), Vol. 4, pp. 115–134. Plenum Press, New York.

Curtis, D. R. and Watkins, J. C. (1965). *Pharmacol. Rev.* **17**, 347–392.

Dalen, P. (1973). *Lancet* **1**, 107.

Davenport, V. D. (1950). *Am. J. Physiol.* **163**, 633–641.

De Feudis, F. V. (1971). *Archs int. Pharmacodyn. Ther.* **193**, 322–329.

De Feudis, F. V. (1972a). *Neuropharmacology* **11**, 879–888.

De Feudis, F. V. (1972b). *Brain Res.* **43**, 686–689.

De Feudis, F. V., and Delgado, J. M. R. (1970). *Nature.* **225**, 749–750.

De Feudis, F. V. and Mitchell, F. F. (1970). *J. Physiol.* **210**, 83P.

De Feudis, F. V. and Paolino, R. M. (1972). *Experientia* **28**, 309.

Fann, W. E., Davis, J. M., Janowsky, D. S., Cavanaugh, J. H., Kaufmann, J. S., Griffith, J. D. and Oates, J. A. (1972). *Clin. Pharmacol. Therap.* **13**, 71–77.

Florey, E. (1960). *In* "Inhibition in the Nervous System and γ-Aminobutynic acid" (E. Roberts, ed.), pp. 72–84. Pergamon Press, New York.

Gaitonde, M. K. (1965). *Biochem. J.* **95**, 803–810.

Garfinkel, D. (1966). *J. biol . Chem.* **241**, 3918–3929.

Goldstein, M., Joh, T. H. and Garvey, T. Q. (1968). *Biochem.* **7**, 2724–2730.

Gottesfeld, Z., Ebstein, B. S. and Samuel, D. (1971). *Nature New Biology* **234**, 124–125.

Ho, A. K. S., Gershon, S. and Pinckney, L. (1970). *Archs Intern. Pharmacodyn. Therap.* **186**, 54–65.

Israel, Y., Kalant, H. and Le Blanc, A. E. (1966). *Biochem. J.* **100**, 27–33.

King, L. J., Carl, J. L., Archer, E. G. and Castallanet, M. (1969). *J. Pharmac. exp. Therap.* **168**, 163–170.

Kuriyama, K., Roberts, E. and Vos, J. (1968). *Brain Res.* **9**, 231–252.

Kuriyama, K. Winstein, H. and Roberts, E. (1969). *Brain Res.* **16**, 479–492.

Lajtha, A., Berl, S. and Waelsch, H. (1959). *J. Neurochem.* **3**, 322–332.

Manyam, N. V. B. and Bravo-Fernandez, E. (1973). *Lancet,* **1**, 1010.

Mark, J., Pugge, H. and Mandel, P. (1970). *J. Neurochem.* **17,** 1393–1401.

McGeer, P., McGeer, E. G. and Fibiger, H. C. (1973). *Lancet.* **2,** 623–624.

Nicklas, W. J. and Berl, S. (1973) *Brain Res.* **61,** 343–356.

Nicklas, W. J., Berl, S. and Clarke, D. D. (1974). *J. Neurochem.* **23,** 149–157.

Pappius, H. M., Rosenfeld, M., Johnson, D. M. and Elliot, K. A. C. (1958). *Canad. J. Biochem. Physiol.* **36,** 217–226.

Perry, T. L., Hansen, S. and Kloster, M. (1973). *New Engl. and J. Med.* **288,** 337–342.

Radomski, M. W. and Watson, W. J. (1973). *Aerospace Med.* **44,** 387–392.

Rees, J. R. (1972). *Life Sci* **11,** 925–928.

Reiner, J. M. (1953). *Archs Biochem. Biophys.* **46,** 53–99.

Roberts, E. (1960). *In* "Inhibition in the Nervous System and γ-Aminobutyric Acid" (E. Roberts, ed.), pp. 144–158. Pergamon Press, New York.

Roberts, E. and Matthysse, S. (1970). *A. Rev. Biochem.* **39,** 77–820.

Salganicoff, L. and De Robertis, E. (1965). *J. Neurochem.* **12,** 287–309.

Santini, M. and Berl, S. (1972). *Brain Res.* **47,** 167–176.

Schildkraut, J. J. and Gershon, E. S. (1971). *In* "Handbook of Neurochemistry" (A. Lajtha, ed.), Vol. 6, pp. 135–141. Plenum press, New York.

Schou, M. (1971). In "Handbook of Neurochemistry" (A. Lajtha, ed.), Vol. 6, pp. 387–393. Plenum Press, New York.

Snyder, S. H., Young, A. B., Bennett, J. P. and Mulder, A. H. (1973). *Fed. Proc.* **32,** 2039–2047.

Tallan, H. H. (1962). *In* "Amino Acid Pools" (J. T. Holden, ed.), pp. 471-485. Elsevier, Amsterdam.

Trachtenberg, M. C. and Pollen, D. A. (1970). *Science* **167,** 1248–1252.

Van den Berg, C. J. and Garfinkel, D. (1971). *Biochem. J.* **123,** 211–218.

Van den Berg, C. J., Mela, P. and Waelsch, H. (1966). *Biochem. biophys. Res. Comm.* **23,** 479–484.

Waelsch, H., Berl, S., Rossi, C. A., Clarke, D. D. and Purpura, D. P. (1964). *J. Neurochem.* **11,** 717–728.

Watkins, J. C. (1973). *Biochem Soc. Symp.* **36,** 33–47.

27

THE ENDOCRINE EFFECTS OF LITHIUM

S. C. BERENS and J. WOLFF

I. Introduction

Of the many side reactions observed during the course of Li^+ therapy, those involving the endocrine glands, and especially the thyroid, have received particular attention because of the great ease with which changes in endocrine function are measured and because simple tests are available to shed light on possible mechanisms for the effects produced by Li^+. Nevertheless, since the primary concern of Li^+ therapy is not with the endocrine glands, documentation of the side effects has often been inadequate. We have attempted, in this chapter, to summarize clinical and laboratory findings of Li^+ effects on the adrenal cortex, thyroid and posterior pituitary gland and to point out the many gaps in our knowledge. Data on anterior pituitary or gonadal function are so fragmentary as not to permit even a summary, whereas certain other endocrine effects are discussed in Chapters 28 and 29.

II. Adrenal Cortex

Numerous studies have been carried out in an effort to define possible roles for adrenal steriods in the Li^+ response of manic-depressive patients. At the outset it should be recalled that this illness can, in the absence of drug therapy, alter the output of steroids from the adrenal cortex (see Noyes *et al.*, 1971). Hence differentiation between a direct effect of Li⁺ and a change in the status of the disease will be difficult. Nevertheless, Li⁺ treatment does appear to cause changes in cortisol metabolism, and despite conflicting results the following summary appears to be consonant with studies published to date. As is the case with the thyroid, there are acute and chronic effects which are often in opposite directions. The possibility of significant interaction between the thyroid and adrenal in the Li⁺ response should also be kept in mind, although direct studies bearing on this are wanting in the case of Li⁺ therapy.

Platman and Fieve (1968) found that Li⁺ therapy led to a small but significant rise in the 8 a.m. plasma cortisol levels (from 18 to 25 μg/100 mg) early after the start of Li⁺, and again when toxic serum Li⁺ levels were reached. If Li⁺ therapy was continued for more than one week, the drug tended to depress plasma 17-hydroxycorticoids (Platman *et al.*, 1971). On the other hand Sachar *et al.* (1970) were unable to detect such changes in patients who had gone into clinical remission. Moreover, a strict relation between cortisol response and blood lithium levels has not been established, although toxic levels of lithium are associated initially with increased plasma levels and excretion of steroids (Männistö, 1973).

The cortisol production rates were not consistently altered by Li⁺ (Sachar *et al.*, 1970; Platman *et al.*, 1971) nor was the excretion of urinary cortisol metabolites (tetrahydrocortisol, allotetrahydrocortisol and tetrahydrocortisone) (Sachar *et al.*, 1970). However, in an extensive study, Noyes *et al.* (1971) showed that Li⁺ increased urinary 17-hydroxycorticoid secretion transiently in four out of seven manic patients and all of five depressed subjects; the change was not sustained. Moreover, excretion fell rapidly with cessation of Li⁺ therapy and rose promptly again when it was reinstituted. Sodium excretion fluctuated in parallel with steroid secretion. Since this is also a period of considerable diuresis, it seems unlikely that the electrolyte changes were caused by the steroid changes. The reverse cannot be ruled out.

Murphy and coworkers (1969) have documented a 50% increase in aldosterone excretion during the period of sodium retention that follows the initial diuresis caused by Li⁺. On the other hand, Demers *et al.* (1972) found no such changes. When changes do occur, they may be related to sodium retention and poor urine output although the sodium retention is in excess of that lost during diuresis. In rats, substantial doses of Li⁺ lead to a doubling of aldosterone production from labeled progesterone, as well as a significant increase in adrenal weight (Krulik, 1971).

Because of the difficulty in separating direct from indirect Li⁺ effects in manic depressive patients, Halmi *et al.* (1972) studied adrenal function in normal volunteers. The diurnal variation in serum cortisol was slightly diminished by Li⁺ therapy (due to somewhat lower morning values) whereas the

TABLE I. The effect of lithium ion on steroid secretion by Y-1 mouse adrenal tumor cells.

Activator	Lithium concentration mM	Steroid output[a] μg/mg/h
Control	—	0·61
Control	10	0·51
ACTH (15 mU/ml)	—	2·07
ACTH (15 mU/ml)	2	1·84
ACTH (15 mU/ml)	10	1·61
ACTH (15 mU/ml)	20	1·30

[a]Measured fluorometrically and expressed as 20α-dihydroprogesterone as previously described (Temple and Wolff, 1973).

response to exogenous ACTH (after dexamethasone suppression) was not.

The possibility that diminished steroid levels are due to an inhibition of the ability of adrenal tissue to respond to ACTH with increased steroid secretion has been investigated in adrenal tumor cells in culture. As seen in Table I, Li$^+$ concentrations from 2 to 20 mM in the incubation medium caused a progressive inhibition of the output of steroids from these cells. Since such cells store very little steroid the effect is primarily on the synthesis of steroid. Halmi *et al.* (1974) have shown that ACTH-stimulated adenylate cyclase of rat adrenal homogenates is inhibited by 25 mM Li$^+$. However, the Li$^+$ effect on steroid output is not necessarily on the ACTH receptor since cAMP-mediated steroid secretion is equally inhibited (Wolff and Cook, unpublished observation). Nevertheless, in animals at least, the lithium concentrations required are so much higher than those encountered clinically that it is unlikely that such observations explain the clinical findings.

In conclusion, it seems unlikely that the sustained therapeutic effect of Li$^+$ is mediated by changes in corticosteroid metabolism, although no knowledge yet exists about changes in the size of the cortisol pool. More probably the changes which are seen are the result of stress or electrolyte changes early in therapy and a later suppression of secretion.

III. Thyroid Gland

Clinical evidence for a lithium effect on thyroid function stems mainly from goiter and hypothyroidism seen in a number of manic patients undergoing lithium therapy. This has led to extensive laboratory testing and has revealed frequent abnormal test results. Investigators should not be led to the erroneous conclusion that the hypothyroid state is an intrinsic and important component of the beneficial effect of Li^+ in mania. There is no support for such a mechanism since the majority of favourable responses occur without any evidence of hypothyroidism.

A. Incidence of goiter and hypothyroidism

There have been 97 patients reported in whom hypothyroidism and/or goiter have been ascribed to lithium therapy. In addition, many more patients have been noted to have only abnormal thyroid function tests with Li^+ administration. The effects on the thyroid seen in patients receiving Li^+ can be classed into the following three groups: 1) goiter without overt hypothyroidism (37 cases); 2) hypothyroidism with or without goiter (60 cases); 3) laboratory abnormalities only.

1. *Goiter*

To date there have been 45 cases of goiter or thyroid enlargement observed during Li^+ therapy (Table II). Eight of these patients had thyroid enlargement detectable by scanning techniques only (Lazarus and Bennie, 1972). Goiters have been limited in size and have been diffuse rather than nodular (Schou *et al.*, 1968; Emerson *et al.*, 1973). However, four patients had thyroids large enough to produce difficulties with swallowing (Schou *et al.*, 1968). In nine studies attempts have been made to estimate the incidence of goiter in the Li^+-treated populations with the following results: 1/69 (Gonzales and Lauter, 1969); 12/330 (Schou *et al.*, 1968); 3/16 (Sedvall, *et al.*, 1968); 0/13 (Sedvall *et al.*, 1969); 2/13 (Burrow *et al.*, 1971); 1/60 (Bennie and Lazarus, 1972); 8/13 (Lazarus and Bennie, 1972); 6/255 (Emerson *et al.*, 1973); 1/334 (Lindstedt *et al.*, 1973); the mean incidence for these studies being $34/1103 \simeq 3 \cdot 1\%$. This is essentially the same incidence as the single series originally reported by Schou *et al.* (1968).

Of the 12 cases with goiter reported by Schou *et al.* (1968), three may have shown signs of the goiter before lithium was started, but the glands increased in size during the treatment. In the remaining nine, goiter developed after lithium had been administered from 5 months to 2 years. In three patients, lithium therapy was interrupted and the goiters decreased in size within 2 to 3 months. Burrow *et al.* (1971) reported the development of goiter in 2 patients out of a group of 13 treated with Li^+. One developed after only 5 weeks of therapy and subsided when thyroid replacement was given. In another case a thyrotoxic gland increased significantly in size after only three weeks of lithium therapy (Gerdes *et al.*, 1973). Since the incidence of goiter in a comparable normal population (of the same geographic and dietary distribution) is not generally reported, the significance of such numbers is obscure (Fieve and Platman, 1968, 1969; Cooper and Simpson, 1969). Despite the fact that small goiters are often missed, when one considers the widespread use of Li^+ and the small

TABLE II. Clinical hypothyroidism and/or goiter developing during lithium administration[a]

Author	Number of Case	Age	Sex	Time on Li$^+$ (months)	PBI or T$_4$[b] on Li$^+$ (µg%)	131I Uptake (24 hrs.)	TSH (µU/ml)	Thyroid Anti-bodies	Comments: clinical and laboratory data
I. GOITER WITHOUT HYPOTHYROIDISM									
Gonzales and Lauter (1968)	1/69	—[c]	—	—	—	—	—	—	—
Halberg et al. (1968)	2	35 37	M M	— —	— —	83% 82%	— —	— —	Non-toxic goiter Non-toxic goiter
Schou et al. (1968)	12/330	18–51	5F 7M	5–24	2·3–7·4	↑[d] in 6/10 at 2½ hrs.	—	none in 10/10	↑ thy[e] iodine clearance
Sedvall et al. (1968)	3/16	—	—	—	—	—	—	—	—
Wiggers (1968)	2	55 54	F M	— —	Normal Normal	↑ ↑	— —	— —	— —
Burrow et al. (1971)	2/13	— —	— —	5 weeks —	— —	47%	— —	— —	RAIU[f] ↓[g] to 22% four weeks after Li$^+$ stopped, and goiter size ↓
Bennie and Lazarus (1972)	1/60	45	M	12	—	—	—	—	Large goiter, 60–70 gms.
Lazarus and Bennie (1972)	8/13	—	—	—	—	—	—	—	Quantitative scan used to diagnose enlarged thyroid

TABLE II.—continued

Author	Number of Cases	Age	Sex	Time on Li+ (months)	PBI or T4(b) on Li+ (µg%)	131I Uptake (24 hrs.)	TSH (µU/ml)	Thyroid Anti bodies	Comments: clinical and laboratory data
Emerson et al. (1973)	6/255	— —	— —	9 14 4 cases no data	— — —	— — —	Normal Normal (b)	None None (b)	All goiters palpable but not visible. 4/6 had ATA[i]. 2 of these 4 had ↑ TSH
II. GOITER WITH HYPOTHYROIDISM									
Shopsin et al. (1969)	1	41	F	24	1·2	9·3%	—	1:512	[131]I uptake ↑ to 25% off Li+ for 5 days
Lauter (1971)	1	52	F	6	—	—	—	—	Goiter ↓ when thy. hormone given and Li+ continued
Candy (1972)	1	48	F	2	0·8	—	—	—	Pre Li+ PBI = 5·8
Crowe et al. (1973)	1	36	F	36	1·0	2%	—	1:20,480	After 24 mos. of Li+, PBI = 3·7. 12 mos. later, PBI = 1·0 with myxedema
Edhag et al. (1973)	1	34	F	(b)	(b)	(b)	—	1:500	Goiter present prior to Li+. Myxedema symptoms 1 week after Li started. Tenderness in neck on Li+. When off Li+ for ~9 mos., PBI ≅ 4·0 and normal RAIU. Biopsy consistent with DeQuervain's thyroiditis

TABLE II.—*continued*

Author	Number of Cases	Age	Sex	Time on Li+ (months)	PBI or $T_4^{(b)}$ on Li+ (μg%)	131_I Uptake (24 hrs.)	TSH (μU/ml)	Thyroid Anti-bodies	Comments: clinical and laboratory data
Lindstedt et al. (1973)	1/334	27	F	48	$131^{(b,j)}$ nmoles/l	—	$41^{(k)}$	None	Rapid development of goiter when Li+ initiated. Clinically hypothy, despite normal T_4. FHx of thy. disorders
Pousset et al. (1973)	2	48	F	~12	2·0 $2·2^{(b)}$	41%	82	1:100	8 weeks after Li+ stopped, PBI ↑ to 3·2, T_4 6·8
		39	F	(h)	3·9 $2·3^{(b)}$	12%	—	1:30	Progressive hypothy. symptoms from start of Li+. No TSH or Li+. 4 weeks after Li+ stopped, PBI ↑ to 6·5, T_4 = 6·0, TSH = 59

III. HYPOTHYROID WITHOUT GOITER

Author	Number of Cases	Age	Sex	Time on Li+ (months)	PBI or $T_4^{(b)}$ on Li+ (μg%)	131_I Uptake (24 hrs.)	TSH (μU/ml)	Thyroid Anti-bodies	Comments: clinical and laboratory data
Sedvall et al. (1968)	1/16	—	—	—	—	—	—	—	—
Wiggers (1968)	1	64	F	5	3·7	—	—	—	—
Halberg et al. (1968)	1	43	M	4	1·4	Low	—	High	Thy. biopsy: Hashimoto's thyroiditis
Luby et al. (1971)	1	45	M	6	1·1	—	—	—	Pre Li+ PBI = 6·8

TABLE II.—*continued*

Author	Number of Cases	Age	Sex	Time on Li+ (months)	PBI or T₄(b) on Li+ (µg%)	¹³¹I Uptake (24 hrs.)	TSH (µU/ml)	Thyroid Anti-bodies	Comments: clinical and labatory data
O'Connell (1971)	2/44	—	F	—	1·5	Low	—	—	—
		—	F	—	2·0	Low	—	—	—
Rogers and Whybrow (1971)	2	59	F	20	1·2	—	—	—	Pre Li+ PBI = 3·0
		37	F	3	1·8	—	—	—	
Bennie and Lazarus (1972)	1/60	55	F	20	—	—	—	—	—
Birch et al. (1972)	1	29	M	22	1·5	4%	—	—	—
Hanna et al. (1972)	1	61	M	36	3·9	12%	—	None	—
Myers (1972)	2	21	F	—	0·8	—	—	—	—
		36	F	—	2·1	—	—	—	—
Vestergaard and Poulson (1972)	5	47	F	7	0·08⁽¹⁾	—	—	—	—
		63	F	8	0·07	11·4%	—	—	—
		50	F	14	0·18	25·3%	—	—	—
		43	F	10	0·05	9·1%	—	—	—
		43	F	11	0·18	—	—	—	Pre Li+ PBI = 0·46 µmol/l
Whybrow (1972)	1	—	—	—	—	—	—	—	—
Crowe et al. (1973)	1	26	F	72	1·9	57%	—	None	—

TABLE II.—*continued*

Author	Number of Cases	Age	Sex	Time on Li+ (months)	PBI or T$_4$ (b) on Li+ (µg %)	^{131}I Uptake (24 hrs.)	TSH (µU/ml)	Thyroid Anti-bodies	Comments: clinical and laboratory data
Edhag et al. (1972)	2	63	F	7	(h)	1%	—	None	Li+ stopped 2 mos. prior to lab tests. **PBI** = 0·3 mg%. Cholesterol 465. **BMR** −19%. No evidence of panhypopituitarism
		57	F	4	1·4 0·6(b, h)	—	340(h)	None	4 mos. after Li+ started, PBI = 1·4. At 5 mos., PBI = 4·8, BMR −31%, cholesterol 415 mg%. RAIU 40% at 24 hours, normal thy. scan. TSH sampled at 7 mos. (very high). Thy. biopsy = diffuse lymphomatous thyroiditis
Emerson et al. (1973)	6(h)	—	—	13	1·0(b)	—	50	—	Data given for only 1 of these 6 patients. 3 had pre-existing thy. disease, but not hypothy.
Lindstedt et al.	11	56	F	—	1·5	—	>100	1:250	Normal thy. biopsy
		57	F	—	2·1	—	44	—	—
		44	F	—	3·8	—	43	—	—
		69	F	—	3·0	—	(h)	1:250,000	TSH = 39 after 13 days of thyroxine therapy
		47	F	—	30(b)(j)	—	>100	None	Thy. biopsy = chronic thyroiditis
		52	F	—	52(b)	—	80	—	Thy. biopsy = chronic thyroiditis
		58	F	—	14(b)	—	55	None	—
		67	M	—	61(b)	—	50	None	—
		47	F	—	28(b)	—	37	None	—
		47	F	—	34(b)	—	29	1:2500	—
		47	F	—	57(b)	—	23	1:250,000	—

TABLE II.—*continued*

Author	Number of Cases	Age	Sex	Time on Li$^+$ (months)	PBI or T$_4$ (b) on Li$^+$ (μg%)	131$_I$ Uptake (24 hrs.)	TSH (μU/ml)	Thyroid Anti-bodies	Comments: clinical and laboratory data
Segal et al. (1973)	12/100	—	—	—	<3·5	—	—	—	—
Shopsin et al. (1973)	1	46	M	28	2·0$^{(b)}$	7%	100	Only at 1:16 = not signi-ficant	Pre Li$^+$ thy. function tests all normal. 12 weeks after Li$^+$ stopped, patient euthyroid, T$_4$ ↑ to 3·9, TSH ↓ to 30, RAIU 18%. Became hypothy. when SSKI given without Li$^+$

(a) There are no double entries for patients in this table. However, one study may be cited in more than one section. When hypothyroidism or goiter were not specifically mentioned in a paper, they were assumed to be absent.

(b) T$_4$

(c) — means no data given

(d) ↑ = increased

(e) Thy. = thyroid

(f) RAIU = radioactive iodine uptake

(g) ↓ = decreased

(h) See comments

(i) ATA = antithyroid antibodies

(j) T$_4$ normal range for this study = 58–167 nmoles/l

(k) Normal TSH for this study <8 mU/l

(l) PBI normal range for this study = 0·32–0·58 μmoles/l

number of goiters reported to develop under Li⁺ therapy, it seems probable that the incidence is truly low. Nevertheless, the response of thyroid size to manipulations of Li⁺ administration and withdrawal make it appear likely that goiter is a significant side effect.

A single case of neonatal goiter in a child whose mother was on lithium therapy (Amdisen, 1969) serves as warning of the considerable danger of a respiratory obstruction during delivery. This is also seen after iodides (Wolff, 1969), and must be anticipated when cessation of therapy in the mother is not feasible.

Four patients with Li⁺-induced goiter were continued on Li⁺ and received thyroid therapy. Three of these goiters decreased (Schou et al., 1968; Lauter, 1971), providing evidence for the role of pituitary TSH in goitrogenesis produced by lithium.

Of the total group of 45 goitrous patients, 37 occurred without overt hypothyroidism (Table II). These cases presumably reflect adequate compensation for hormone deficiency. Although data were not always available, these goiters were generally accompanied by a tendency for the serum PBI[1] or T_4 to fall somewhat and for the TSH to show a small, and frequently transient, increase (Lindstedt et al., 1973). Some patients show increased TSH without detectable decreases in serum PBI (Lazarus and Bennie, 1972); however information about T_3 levels will be required before it is possible to interpret such discrepancies.

2. Hypothyroidism

As seen in Table II, there are 60 reported cases of myxedema clearly related to initiation of lithium therapy (eight cases, all female, of hypothyroidism with goiter; 52 cases, 26 female, six male and 20 of unspecified sex, of hypothyroidism without goiter). Villeneuve et al. (1973) reported another 22 cases of "hypothyroidism" out of a series of 149 patients, but they only reported a fall in PBI from $4 \cdot 9$ to $3 \cdot 3 \, \mu g/100$ ml and in T_4 $6 \cdot 7$ to $4 \cdot 7 \, \mu g/100$ ml in this group. There was no mention of symptoms of clinical hypothyroidism, and we doubt that they would be very noticeable with serum thyroxine levels in this range. Therefore, these cases are not included in the summary table. Hypothyroidism, when induced by Li⁺, resembles primary hypothyroidism in many respects, both in clinical manifestation and laboratory tests. It may occur in the absence of goiter (Vestergaard and Poulsen, 1972; Shopsin et al., 1973) but is *probably* more often accompanied by goiter, although only eight patients have been clearly identified with both (Table II) (Shopsin et al., 1969; Lauter, 1971; Candy, 1972; Crowe et al., 1973; Edhag et al., 1973; Lindstedt et al., 1973). In most reports the presence or absence of goiter is unfortunately not

---

[1] Abbreviations used are: T_4 for thyroxine, T_3 for triiodothyronine, PBI for serum protein-bound iodine and cAMP for cyclic adenosine-3,5-monophosphate.

mentioned. Full-blown myxedema has been seen not infrequently. The earliest symptoms of clinical hypothyroidism have been detected one week after institution of Li⁺ therapy (Edhag *et al.*, 1973; Pousset *et al.*, 1973) and a new goiter has been documented as early as 5 weeks after the start of Li⁺ administration (Burrow *et al.*, 1971). However, signs or symptoms of myxedema may appear many years after Li⁺ administration has been started without any obvious precipitating event (Table II). Attempts to relate the incidence or severity to blood Li⁺ levels have not been successful since essentially all cases have had serum Li⁺ levels in the therapeutic range. On the other hand, in three patients reported by Lindstedt *et al.* (1973), reduction of lithium intake by as little as one third resulted in the partial normalization of the laboratory findings over a period of weeks. It had been known earlier that cessation of Li⁺ therapy led to reduction of the goiter and the depressed PBI (Schou *et al.*, 1968; Shopsin *et al.*, 1969; Burrow *et al.*, 1971).

Segal *et al.* (1973) have reported a surprisingly high incidence of unilateral or bilateral proptosis without signs of malignant exophthalmos in patients treated over periods of 4 to 30 months. The proptosis did not correlate with hypothyroidism. Although this finding has not been reported in other studies, exophthalmometry should probably be part of the workup for Li⁺-treatment.

An outstanding difference from primary hypothyroidism is the normal or elevated ¹³¹I uptake observed in some patients who have become hypothyroid under Li⁺ therapy (Sedvall *et al.*, 1968; Hanna *et al.*, 1972; Vestergaard and Poulsen, 1972; Crowe *et al.*, 1973; Pousset *et al.*, 1973). Radioiodine uptakes that were either abnormally high or significantly above pre-lithium levels were also seen in some clinically euthyroid patients (Schou *et al.*, 1968; Sedvall *et al.*, 1969; Cooper and Simpson, 1969; Fyrö *et al.*, 1973). Sedvall *et al.* (1968) first suggested that this might be the result of decreased thyroidal iodine turnover (see also Pousset *et al.*, 1973). The importance of this in explaining the mechanism of lithium action will become apparent below. Many other patients, however, show low 24-hour ¹³¹I uptakes, and it appears probable that some of these patients constitute a separate group, unable to compensate for decreased hormone release by enhanced iodine metabolism. Crowe *et al.* (1973) have similarly concluded that there are two groups of patients that develop hypothyroidism on Li⁺: 1) those without preexisting thyroid disease or family history, and 2) those in whom the additional insult to thyroid function superimposed on preexisting thyroiditis or parenchymal damage leads to myxedema. As in the case of iodide goiter (Wolff, 1969), preexisting thyroid damage prevents adequate compensation of thyroid function and contributes to overt signs of hypothyroidism with chronic use of excess iodide (Braverman *et al.*, 1969). The evidence suggests that similar under-lying factors may be responsible in those patients who develop myxedema or sizeable goiters as a result of Li⁺ therapy. Evidence of low thyroid reserve or of preexisting thyroid disease appears in a substantial fraction of the published reports of clinical hypothyroidism in Li$^+$-treated patients.

Preexisting thyroid dysfunction has, for example, been noted by Halberg *et al.* (1968); Wiggers (1968); and Luby *et al.* (1972); none of five patients developing myxedema developed goiters (Vestergaard and Poulsen, 1972; Rogers and Whybrow, 1971; Whybrow, 1972). One case of thyroiditis developed on Li$^+$ therapy (Halberg *et al.*, 1968).

A poor response to TSH was noted by Shopsin *et al.* (1969) and Vestergaard and Poulsen, 1972.

High antithyroid antibody titers have been reported by Shopsin *et al.* (1969), Sedvall *et al.* (1968), Lazarus and Bennie (1972), Lauter (1971), Lindstedt *et al.* (1973), Crowe *et al.* (1973), Edhag *et al.* (1973), and Pousset *et al.* (1973), but not necessarily in all cases of goiter (Halberg *et al.*, 1968). Of the eight cases with both goiter and hypothyroidism (Table II), six had antibody titers measured and five of these had elevated titers. All eight patients were females. There is a high incidence of positive antibody titers (29%) in patients with elevated TSH, whereas titers were significantly elevated in only 9% of other patients (Emerson *et al.*, 1973).

Positive iodide-perchlorate tests (Anderson, 1973) may signal a preexisting limitation of the capacity to oxidize iodide.

These findings raise enough suspicion that all patients who must receive Li$^+$ and who are known to have, or have had, thyroiditis, subtotal thyroidectomy or ^{131}I therapy, should be considered high risks for the development of hypothyroidism.

The possibility that some patients with low iodine uptakes have undamaged thyroid parenchyma cannot be ruled out.

3. *Euthyroid patients with laboratory test abnormalities only*

Many patients who receive lithium never develop either goiter or hypothyroidism, yet they can be shown to have transient changes in thyroid function tests. This probably represents the overwhelming majority of lithium-treated patients. In prospective studies of 27 patients, Emerson *et al.* (1973) were able to demonstrate a rise in serum TSH in the first 3 months of treatment, although serum thyroxine levels did not change significantly. In a similar study, Lindstedt *et al.* (1973) found a large group of euthyroid Li$^+$-treated patients with a slightly increased range of serum TSH levels (9–13 μU/ml) and a 20% decrease in serum T_4 levels. In one case chemical evidence of interference with thyroid hormone secretion occurred after three weeks of Li$^+$ therapy (Shopsin *et al.*, 1973). Moreover, Cooper and Simpson (1969) found a drop in serum PBI and free thyroxine which was maximal at 10–14 days after Li$^+$ was started and which showed a variable return toward the baseline after one to three months of continued therapy. A significant decrease in serum thyroxine in normal volunteers given Li^+ for 13 days was noted by Halmi and Noyes (1972), and transient or persistent minor decreases in PBI were noted by Hullin et al. (1972). Isolated cases of transient upward TSH and/or downward T_4 changes have been observed by us and others. The critical need for T_3 determinations in such patients is obvious.

The large increases in serum creatine phosphokinase that have been reported to occur in Li^+ treatment of manic patients (Gosling et al., 1972) may be due to hypothyroidism, although such a cause was not considered by these authors.

B. Experimental studies

1, Acute effects

The foregoing clinical findings (Table II) have made it abundantly clear that Li^+ ion, at therapeutic levels, can, in some patients, produce hypothyroidism, enhance TSH secretion and eventually cause goiter. The locus of this interference with iodine metabolism has not been established in these clinical studies, although Sedvall et al. (1968) postulated an impaired release of iodine from the thyroid to explain the elevated uptakes of ^{131}I.

The mechanisms of the antithyroid effect has been studied in animals by several groups of investigators. The nature of the effects obtained is dose-dependent, and clear differentiation between acute, toxic effects and effects of a chronic nature occuring at lower dosage has not been made in many studies. As a result, a great deal of confusion has arisen by ascribing mechanistic significance to toxic effects. It is also important to note that, except for bone, the thyroid gland appears to concentrate more Li^+ than any other organ. This amounts to between 2·5 and 5 times the concentration present in serum (Schou et al., 1968; Shopsin et al., 1969; Berens et al., 1970b; Burrow et al., 1971; Männistö, 1973). Whether this fact accounts for the more frequent reports of interference of function in the thyroid as compared to other endocrine glands is a matter for speculation. Although the thyroid Li^+ is in rapid equilibrium with that of serum, it is possible that a substantial fraction of thyroid Li^+ is distributed extracellularly, i.e. in the follicular lumen, hence the cellular concentration of Li^+ is a matter of considerable uncertainty in this tissue (Berens et al., 1970b). Berens et al. (1970a) showed in the rat that large concentrations of Li^+ (3–4 mEq/l) depressed all parameters of iodine metabolism that were measured; namely, iodide transport, ^{131}I uptake and ^{131}I release rates from the thyroid. Similarly, generalized antithyroid effects with large Li^+ dosage have been obtained by Männistö (1973) and Männistö et al. (1971). These inhibitions occurred at the level of the thyroid gland and were not primarily mediated via the pituitary. Similar toxic effects on iodine uptake and turnover of the rat thyroid were also reported by Hullin and Johnson (1970), Cooper et al. (1970) and Ljunggren et al. (1971). Toxic serum levels of Li^+ may also be

.associated with diminished levels of serum PBI (Sedvall *et al.*, 1968; Ljunggren *et al.*, 1971).

The mechanism of the acute, toxic inhibition of thyroid function that occurs at high ambient levels of Li⁺ ion is unknown. It does not appear to be mediated via the pituitary gland since similar results can be obtained in hypophysectomized rats maintained on exogenous TSH (Berens *et al.*, 1970a). Birnbaumer *et al.* (1969) were the first to show that Li⁺ inhibited adenylate cyclase in the fat cell, but this occurred at concentrations where ionic strength effect seemed likely. However, Li⁺ ion has been shown to inhibit beef thyroid membrane adenylate cyclase activity with a half-maximal effect occurring at 4 mM Li⁺. The sensitivity to Li⁺ can be increased by reduction of Mg^{++}, an effect that may have its origin in the similarity of the crystal radii of the two cations (Wolff *et al.*, 1970). These results have been confirmed (Burke, 1970), and occur also in intact mouse thyroids when cyclase activity is measured by the formation of cAMP from [³H]adenine (Kendall-Taylor, 1972). While the Li⁺ concentrations used in some studies (thyroid and brain) were sufficiently low to be clinically significant (Wolff *et al.*, 1970; Forn and Valdecasas, 1971), the difficulty of simulating cytosol condition *in vitro,* and the argument presented below for the thyroid gland, suggests that considerable caution is warranted in using such cyclase inhibitions to formulate mechanisms for the Li⁺ effect. There was no effect on cyclic AMP phosphodiesterase activity. Preliminary results suggested that Li⁺ interfered with Mg^{++} binding to plasma membrane preparations (Wolff *et al.*, 1970). It is of interest, therefore, that the Na⁺–K⁺ ATPase was *not* inhibited at Li⁺ concentrations that clearly inhibit the cyclase (Wolff *et al.*, 1970; Burrow *et al.*, 1971).

2. *Chronic effects*

A much higher degree of specificity of action on iodine metabolism is observed with chronic, low concentration Li⁺ treatment. The minimum serum levels necessary to obtain effects have not been measured, but in rats the effective range is from 0·35 to 0·70 mEq/l and in man is from 0·5 to 1·0 mEq/l, i.e. somewhat lower than the serum level aimed for in the treatment of mania.

(a) *Iodide uptake:* Under normal conditions the rate-limiting step for thyroid hormone biosynthesis is the rate of transport of iodide into the gland. Entry of iodide into the thyroid depends on the ratio of renal clearance to thyroid clearance (normally this ratio is about 2 : 1). Renal clearance of I⁻ has been stated to be normal in the presence of therapeutic concentrations of Li⁺ (Hullin and Johnson, 1970; Lazarus and Bennie, 1972) but few data have been supplied.

The iodide concentrating mechanism is not inhibited during chronic Li⁺ treatment and may even be hyperactive in some animals showing a goitrous response (Berens *et al.*, 1970a; Burrow *et al.*, 1971). Nevertheless, the saliva/plasma ratio showed significant decreases after Li^+ therapy (more seriously at 3 than 20 months) (Lazarus and Bennie, 1972). Because of the similarity of the salivary iodide transport mechanism to that of the thyroid (Wolff, 1964), it had been concluded that the inhibitory effects of Li^+ could be explained on the basis of an inhibition of the iodide concentrating mechanism (Lazarus and Bennie, 1972). However, the above data in rats, and the kinetic data in thyrotoxic patients to be presented below, make it unlikely that this contributes more than a small fraction to the total antithyroid effect of lithium.

As noted in many patients (see above), total iodine uptake is increased in rats (Berens et al., 1970a), though there are exceptions (Shopsin et al., 1969). In general the increment over control values is greater at later intervals (greater than 4 h after ^{131}I). Similar findings have been obtained in the Li^+-treated ewe (Abuzzahab, 1972). While iodine uptakes are increased, the clearance is not (Lazarus and Bennie, 1972), and it is apparent that increased uptakes are likely to be due to changes in the outflow of iodine from the gland.

The iodide taken up by the thyroid gland in the presence of Li^+ is apparently converted normally to the iodoamino acids. The distribution of label may show a depression in the fraction present as iodothyronines (T_3 and T_4) (Berens et al., 1970a; Burrow et al., 1971; Männistö et al., 1971, 1973), but the drop may be small, and was not found at all in another study (Cooper et al., 1970). Determination of a true "coupling" effect would require a study under equilibrium, rather than pulse-label, conditions. Furthermore, the sucrose-gradient sedimentation pattern of thyroglobulin was not significantly altered by Li^+ treatment (Ljunggren et al., 1971). Additional evidence for grossly normal rates of organic iodine formation comes from the common findings of negative perchlorate discharge tests in Li^+-treated patients (Halberg et al., 1968; Jensen et al., 1968, Shopsin et al., 1969). However, when an iodide load was imposed during the discharge test (iodide-perchlorate test) four out of 15 patients showed significant loss of label from the thyroid (Andersen, 1973). Two of these four patients had known thyroid dysfunction and it may be that these tests are positive only in glands with preexisting limited thyroid reserve.

(b) *Secretion:* The "uptake" of ^{131}I by the thyroid gland at any time is a function (algebraic sum) of the unidirectional clearance of ^{131}I and the exit rate. In attempting to explain the increased uptake of ^{131}I seen in Li^+-treated patients, Sedvall and coworkers (1968, 1969) were the first to propose, on the basis of a prolonged thyroidal ^{131}I half-life, that Li^+ might act by inhibiting release of iodine from the gland. Berens et al. (1970a) provided direct evidence in rats that the release of ^{131}I from prelabeled thyroids could be depressed by as much as 90% by lithium feeding.

The secretion of thyroid hormone is a complex process that is initiated by apical pseudopod formation, engulfment of follicular colloid by these pseudopods, endocytosis of the engulfed colloid droplets, migration of droplets and lysosomes leading to fusion of these organelles, proteolysis, release of iodoa-mino acids from the lysosomes and eventual movement of T_3 and T_4 out of the cell[2]. The process is very responsive to TSH stimulation. Several aspects of the secretory process can be directly measured *in vitro*, namely endocytosis and overall release of iodine into the medium. Lithium ion, administered either *in vivo* or *in vitro*, inhibits both of these processes in concert. The inhibition of endocytosis suggests that an early step in secretion is inhibited (Williams *et al.*, 1971; Kendall-Taylor, 1972).

Since secretion is normally under direct control of TSH, and since it has been shown that TSH-stimulated adenylate cyclase could be inhibited by Li^+ (Wolff *et al.*, 1970), the possibility existed that Li^+ interfered at this locus with TSH stimulation of secretion. That this was *not* the case in chronically Li^+-treated animals is shown by the following:

1. Li^+ inhibits secretion stimulated by dibutyryl cyclic AMP, i.e., it can act at a step beyond the adenylate cyclase (Williams *et al.*, 1971; Kendall-Taylor, 1972).

2. Li^+ does not inhibit, and may even enhance, the stimulation of various metabolic indices by TSH in some thyroid tissues, such as $^{14}CO_2$ production from [1-^{14}C]glucose or [1-^{14}C]pyruvate, and ^{32}P incorporation into lipid (Berens *et al.*, 1971).

3. Cyclic AMP accumulation in mouse thyroid lobes following TSH stimulation is not altered even by large concentrations of Li^+ (Williams and Wolff, 1972).

4. The production of goiter would seem to be incompatible with an inhibition of the ability to respond to TSH.

5. Binding of [^{125}I]TSH to beef thyroid membranes is not significantly affected by Li^+ concentrations that inhibit secretion (Moore and Wolff, in press).

In addition it has been shown that 12 mM Li^+ had no effect on three separate cyclic AMP-dependent protein kinase activities of the thyroid (Spaulding *et al.*, 1972).

(c) *Circulating hormone:* The obvious sequel to be expected from an interference with hormone secretion is a decreased level of circulating T_4 and T_3. This has been amply demonstrated in man, although decreases are usually small (see above), less striking in experimental animals (Sedvall *et al.*, 1968; Ljunggren *et*

[2] It has recently been shown that one component of the secretory system for thyroid hormone may be the cytoplasmic microtubules. Agents which disrupt microtubules of the mitotic spindle or the neurotubules, such as colchicine or vinblastine, interfere with endocytosis of colloid and iodine secretion at very low concentrations (Williams and Wolff, 1970, 1972). The striking resemblance of these effects to those of Li^+ prompted us to investigate the effect of Li^+ on microtubules in neuroblastoma axons (Wolff and Williams, 1973). Although Li^+ has been reported to increase colchicine binding to tubulin (Harris and Teller, 1973), it produced none of the morphological changes that result from colchicine-induced microtubular disaggregation, and it seems probable that the antisecretory effect of Li^+ does not operate through disruption of microtubules. The ultrastructural or molecular locus for Li^+ action has thus yet to be identified.

al., 1971), and were not observed in two other studies (Berens *et al.*, 1970a; Männistö *et al.*, 1971). However, now that the critical role of T_3 is better understood, these studies need to be repeated with serum T_3 measurements, especially where changes in T_4 seem to be paradoxically small. In one patient studied by us the T_3 values fell 35% within 24 hours of the onset of Li^+ therapy.

(d) *TSH levels:* A necessary consequence of these reductions in circulating thyroid hormone levels is an elevation of serum TSH. The clinical data have permitted the conclusion that prolonged high levels of TSH after Li^+ therapy are indicative of hypothyroidism probably resulting from low thyroid reserve, whereas smaller and transient rises are to be expected in patients with otherwise normal thyroid glands (Burrow *et al.*, 1971; Lazarus and Bennie, 1972; Emerson *et al.*, 1972; Lindstedt *et al.*, 1973). High circulating TSH levels in patients with fully reversible hypothyroidism and with no evidence of paren-chymal damage have also been reported (Pousset *et al.*, 1973). Transient increases in circulating TSH were also seen in Li^+-treated rats (Berens *et al.*, 1970a) even though T_4 levels were not changed. T_3 values would be likely to give better correlations. Interpretation of TSH levels is complicated, however, by the fact that toxic doses of Li^+ cause depression of serum TSH levels in rats (Männistö *et al.*, 1973).

It is of interest that the diurnal variation of iodine secretion from the thyroid is blunted in some patients receiving lithium (Carlson *et al.*, 1974). It is uncertain, however, whether this effect is directly on the thyroid or operates at higher levels, since similar changes occur in the cortisol pattern (Halmi *et al.*, 1972).

(e) *Goiter:* A further effect to be expected from the decreased secretion → decreased circulating hormone → increased TSH sequence is the formation of goiter. The clinical experience has been tabulated (Table II). Small goiters have been observed in rats fed lithium salts (Cooper *et al.*, 1970; Berens *et al.*, 1970; Ljunggren *et al.*, 1971; Heltne and Ollerich, 1973). In one study the goitro-genic effect of submaximal doses of carbimazole was markedly enhanced by concomitant administration of LiCl (Männistö *et al.*, 1971). The histological appearance of these goiters did not differ markedly from the controls (Berens *et al.*, 1970a; Ljunggren *et al.*, 1971). However, in another study, chronic lithium feeding led to enlargement of the colloid goiter type with enlarged Golgi apparatuses (Heltne and Ollerich, 1973). This is of some interest in view of the fact that a certain type of colloid goiter is seen after treatment of rats with iodide, another antisecretory agent.

If, in fact, most of the biosynthetic steps are unimpaired during chronic lithium treatment, then a reduced output from the gland should lead to an increased thyroidal iodine content. This has been found to be the case in Li^+-fed rats (Berens *et al.*, 1970a) and could be computed in thyrotoxic patients treated with Li^+ (see below). As a consequence, if all other factors (and especially the change in secretion rate) remain constant, one would predict that the Li$^+$ effect would be transient. The *amount* of hormone secreted (as opposed to the fractional rate) would be expected to return to pretreatment levels when the thyroidal iodine pool is increased by the reciprocal of the fraction to which the secretory rate is reduced. This is indeed the case in the rat (as judged by goiter size) (Berens *et al.*, 1970a), and probably explains the circulating T$_4$ of thyrotoxic patients treated with Li$^+$ to be described below. Increase in the iodine pool of the gland may also contribute to the transience of the serum T$_4$ and TSH changes reported in many patients (Berens *et al.*, 1970a; Lazarus and Bennie, 1972). A particularly clear example has been shown in the PBI and free T$_4$ responses of the patients studied by Cooper and Simpson (1969). It may well be that when such reversal in hormone output fails to occur, other (toxic?) effects of Li$^+$ may be present or the thyroid reserve may be so low as to prevent a sizeable increase in the thyroidal iodine pool.

3. *Thyrotoxic patients*

The thionamides block organic iodine formation and reduce circulating hormone levels only when the bulk of the thyroidal iodine stores are depleted[3]. If the major antithyroid effect of Li$^+$ is to inhibit the secretion of hormone, it resembles the antisecretory effect of iodide or Lugol's solution and may thus be useful in the *rapid* treatment of hyperthyroidism without, at the same time, obscuring certain of the diagnostic tests as does iodide. For this reason, the usefulness of Li$^+$ in the treatment of thyrotoxicosis was investigated in two laboratories (Temple *et al.*, 1972a,b; Burrow *et al.*, 1971; Spaulding *et al.*, 1972). The high turnover of thyroidal ^{131}I permits more accurate kinetic analysis of ^{131}I metabolism in such patients. Spaulding *et al.* (1972) determined a significant decrease in secretion from the thyroid gland and a more modest reduction (18%) of the PBI in 5 days after the onset of Li therapy. Li$^+$ levels varied from 0·39–1·45 mEq/l but did not correlate with the antithyroid effectiveness.

Temple *et al.* (1972b), used the least squares fit of thyroid serum and urine ^{131}I data in a 20-compartment model. The strategy was to adjust a single kinetic parameter during lithium administration to test whether this was sufficient to fit the data. In eight studies the data-fitting process required that the Li$^+$ inhibited total iodine secretion (hormonal and non-hormonal) from the thyroid by 30 to 80% when serum Li$^+$ levels ranged from 0·5 to 1·0 mEq/l. Adjustment of a number of other parameters of intrathyroidal iodine metabolism was not required to obtain good fits (within an estimated error of about 20%), thus various aspects of iodine entry into the gland were not altered from the pre-lithium thyrotoxic levels. The 20-min. ^{99m}TcO$_4^-$ uptake of twelve other thyro-

[3] However, the inhibition of the peripheral conversion of T$_4$ to T$_3$ may be an important additional factor in speeding the response to, e.g., propylthiouracil.

toxic patients was unaffected by Li⁺ therapy (Gerdes *et al.*, 1973). The serum T_4 fell between 21–30% in 6 to 8 days and tended to level off or rise again after two weeks. The reason for this discrepancy with secretion is explained below.

Gerdes *et al.* (1973) treated eight patients with "thyrotoxic crisis" and twelve other severely hyperthyroid patients with lithium. Changes in ^{131}I kinetics resembled those obtained by Temple *et al.* (1972b). There was a 30% reduction in serum T_4 within 7 days, and a gratifying early improvement in patients with thyroid storm.

When methimazole was used together with Li⁺, T_4 values continued to decline (Temple *et al.*, 1972b). The apparent escape of the serum T_4 values when Li⁺ was used alone may be ascribed to increasing thyroidal iodine pools, as in the rat (Berens *et al.*, 1970a). For prolonged therapy, therefore, a thionamide must be used together with Li⁺, the cation serving largely to accelerate the reduction in circulating hormone levels.

Recovery toward the original secretion rate upon cessation of Li⁺ administration was often incomplete both in our series and in other studies (Shopsin *et al.*, 1969; Spaulding *et al.*, 1972; Temple *et al.*, 1972a; Carlson *et al.*, 1973). Since the thyroid concentrates Li⁺ (Schou *et al.*, 1968; Berens *et al.*, 1971; Burrow *et al.*, 1971), it was possible that it would retain significant quantities of the cation. However, the thyroid Li⁺ concentration appears to be in rapid equilibrium with the serum (Berens *et al.*, 1971), and it seems more likely that bone Li⁺ (Birch and Hullin, 1972; Birch and Jenner, 1973) will be the major reservoir for continued Li⁺ release. In one case Li⁺ excretion continued for months after cessation of lithium treatment (Hullin *et al.*, 1968). Whether or not sufficient amounts can be released from bone to explain the persistent antithyroid effect is not known and requires further study.

4. *Extrathyroidal effect of Li⁺ on iodine metabolism*

In a number of cases the kinetic analysis of Temple *et al.* (1972b) required a second Li⁺ effect in order to obtain satisfactory fits of the model with the data. This second action was an inhibition of T_4 disappearance from the blood[4], and amounted to a reduction of 0–70% of the pre-lithium rate. Its net effect is to reduce the apparent Li⁺ effect on secretion as measured by serum T_4. Such an effect was first proposed by Ohlin and Söderberg (1970), but no data were supplied. Direct measurement of the effect of Li⁺ on the disappearance of labeled T_4 from the circulation have confirmed this computer prediction (Spaulding *et al.*, 1972; Temple *et al.*, 1972b; Carlson *et al.*, 1973). In thyrotoxic patients, the mean decreases were 33% and 36% of the pre-lithium rate.

---

[4] T_3 is a small quantity not readily separately analyzed under the current model restrictions. A Li⁺ effect on its disappearance rate has yet to be investigated. The major mechanism for increased disappearance appears to be deiodination and not fecal excretion (Temple *et al.*, 1972a; Carlson *et al.*, 1973).

However, in euthyroid patients Spaulding *et al.* (1972) found a 30% decrease whereas Carlson *et al.* (1973) failed to see any change. It is, nevertheless, important to keep this site of Li^+ action in mind when evaluating Li^+ effects in manic patients. Thus, because of her high iodine turnover, the thyrotoxic patient is an excellent model for the study of the antithyroid actions of Li^+. The findings so obtained confirm and extend findings obtained from the rat and from some manic patients, that the major component of the effect is the inhibition of secretion of iodine from the thyroid gland. Other effects are likely to be of small magnitude or should be ascribed to large, toxic doses. A second action, on peripheral degradation of thyroid hormone may not always accompany the intrathyroidal effect, but tends to diminish its effect on blood hormone levels when present. Whether or not the reduced release rate of ^{131}I due to Li^+ will prove to be useful in the reduction of ^{131}I doses for radiation therapy remains to be determined.

5. *Synergism with iodide*

Finally, the similarity of Li^+ and I^- effects on secretion by the thyroid gland suggests that these two agents may act synergistically. While no direct evidence has, so far, been obtained, the possibility has been raised repeatedly (Luby *et al.,* 1971; Wiener, 1972; Vesterdal-Jorgensen *et al.,* 1973). In two patients recently described (Shopsin *et al.,* 1973) previous Li^+ treatment sensitized the patients to subsequent iodide myxedema. Synergism may have occurred but this could not be proved since duration of treatment with each drug alone and together was not controlled. Interestingly, neither patient showed evidence of preexisting thyroid damage. The question of synergism could be most satisfactorily answered by a detailed kinetic study in thyrotoxic patients as carried out for Li^+ alone (Temple *et al.,* 1972a, b). The problem of synergism of Li^+ with other drugs to which manic patients are so often exposed (Rogers and Whybrow, 1971) requires further attention.

6. *Summary*

If we assume that the effect of Li^+ seen at the lowest concentration is likely to be the most specific one, then we can summarize the foregoing as follows: Li^+ ion, which is concentrated to some extent in the thyroid, leads to decrease in the secretion of all forms of iodine (I^-, T_3, T_4) from the normal and thyrotoxic gland. This leads to a lowering of the circulating hormone, which, if sufficient, stimulates TSH secretion, which, if sufficient, leads to goiter. In the absence of thyroid damage, goiter and the decrease of serum hormone levels are transient, since hormone stores build up in the gland and compensate for the decreased fractional release rate.

An additional effect at these lithium levels is to reduce peripheral T_4 deiodination which tends to blunt the fall in serum T_4 but may exacerbate T_3 deficiency.

Depending on the extent of inhibition of secretion and compensation, the clinical picture may be limited to laboratory findings, may include goiter (usually diffuse), or may progress to clinical hypothyroidism and classical myxedema. When compensation is limited by preexisting thyroiditis or other thyroid damage (as shown by biopsy or antibody titers), effects are less likely to be transient and hypothyroidism is more likely.

It is obvious that a thorough clinical and laboratory investigation, and particularly antibody studies, should precede initiation of lithium therapy and should be pursued throughout the course of such therapy.

IV. The Effects of Lithium on Antidiuretic Hormone

The development of a vasopressin-resistant diabetes insipidus-like syndrome was one of the earliest side effects recognized in patients and animals receiving Li^+. As early as 1950, Radomski et al., described polyuria in dogs fed LiCl. Schou (1958) and Thomsen (1970) characterized the polyuria and polydipsia observed in rats fed Li^+ as vasopressin resistant. It was completely reversible and urine flow decreased to pretreatment levels within 5 to 8 days after cessation of Li^+ administration. Harris and Jenner (1969a) further characterized the time-course of Li^+ interference with vasopressin (or antidiuretic hormone, ADH) action. They demonstrated a 40 to 70% decrease in the response to vasopressin in rats within 10 minutes of starting intravenous Li^+. The effect was reversible, and large doses of exogenous vasopressin would produce some antidiuretic action in Li^+-fed rats with polyuria (Schreiber and Roháčová, 1971). Harris and Jenner (1969b) also showed that the effect was specific for Li^+ and was not seen with potassium, rubidium, calcium, magnesium, or strontium. The effect was not dependent upon total body or serum Li^+ levels (Harris and Jenner, 1971a). Harris and Dirks (1973) further described a decrease in sodium concentration in the inner medulla of the kidney. They showed that the concentrating defects caused by therapeutic levels of Li^+ are due to distal rather than proximal tubule effects.

The *clinical* observation of a diabetes insipidus-like syndrome associated with Li^+ treatment was made by Trautner et al. (1955), who described a short diuretic phase after a single dose of oral Li^+ in man. They also described a rise in urinary pH by 1 to 1·5 units; strongly acidic urine became less acid; neutral urine reached pH values up to between 7·5 to 7·8. Defective urinary acidification after Li^+ treatment was also noted by Viol and Smith (1971), and the effect has been demonstrated in dogs (Orloff and Kennedy, 1952).

Although there have been only 11 reported cases of Li^+-induced polyuria-polydipsia (see Table III), Forrest et al. (1971) have stated that "about $\frac{1}{3}$ of patients given Li^+ . . . complain of polydipsia and polyuria" (p. 32A), although no data were supplied. O'Connell (1971) also stated that "many patients reported increased thirst and polydipsia," (p. 226) but no incidence was given. While there are no exact statistics published, the syndrome is probably more common than one would guess from the number of case reports, since patients, especially those either manic or depressed, may not notice the thirst or increased urine volume. Ramsey *et al.* (1972) reported one patient who did not notice a urine volume of 6 liters per day.

As seen in Table III, the onset of polyuria/polydipsia was from 2 weeks to 18 months after onset of Li^+ treatment. The cases were approximately equally divided between sexes, and there was no predisposing renal disease reported. In the case reported by Levy *et al.* (1973), polyuria began several days after Li^+-induced electroencephalographic changes were noted. In the nine cases in which there are data, five patients were essentially resistant to exogenous vasopressin, while four showed a partial response.

Whereas those cases with total resistance to ADH have been cited as evidence for a pure nephrogenic effect of Li^+, partial responses could be interpreted as showing either some lack of circulating ADH (Brightwell *et al.*, 1973) or a partial defect at the renal level overcome by high exogenous ADH levels. In support of the former concept, Sörensen *et al.* (1973) have stated that "intranasal 1-deamino-8-d-arginine-vasopressin may effectively counteract the lithium-induced polyuria/polydipsia" (p. 39) in man. The case described by Brightwell *et al.* (1973) would also support this view. Torp-Pedersen and Thorn (1973) showed that pre-incubation of isolated hemilobes of rat neuro-hypophyses with lithium caused a greater release of ADH into the *in vitro* medium than controls. When rats were fed LiCl to subtoxic serum levels of Li^+, histologic examination of the hypophysis revealed profound depletion of the neurosecretory material and there was swelling of the cells of the supraoptic nucleus; these were similar to findings in rats given excessive NaCl (Ellman and Gan, 1973). These two studies suggest greater than normal hypophyseal ADH secretion with Li^+ in the environment. Thus, while the case of Brightwell *et al.* (1973) and the animal data of Schreiber and Roháčová (1971) might be construed to support the view that some cases of Li^+-induced polyuria/polydipsia may be partly due to a defect in the hypothalamo-neurophypophyseal system, the overwhelming majority of the *in vivo* data support the view of a nephrogenic type of diabetes insipidus.

The mechanisms by which Li^+ inhibits the action of ADH may be through interference with hormone-activated adenylate cyclase. Dousa and Hechter (1970) demonstrated inhibition of ADH interaction with rabbit kidney adeny-late cyclase at Li^+ concentrations of 25 and 50 mM. Beck *et al.* (1971) showed that 10 mM Li^+ significantly inhibited cAMP production in dog kidney slices. This inhibition applied to both ADH- and isoproterenol-stimulated production of cAMP. The log-dose response relationship between Li^+ and inhibition of vasopressin effect was linear and significant over the range of 0–100 mM Li^+. Parathormone-induced cAMP production in kidney cortex was not inhibited

TABLE III. Clinical Case Reports: Lithium Induced Diabetes Insipidus

Author	Age	Sex	Time on Li to Onset of P/P[a]	Vasopressin Resistance	Comments
Trautner et al. (1955)	—	—	—	"Reacts"	No data given
Angrist et al. (1970)	24	F	2 weeks	Resistant	Normal urine concentrating ability 28 days after Li discontinued
	54	F	7 months	Resistant	No P/P 18 days after Li stopped
Lee et al. (1971)	54	F	P/P after 2 months. When Li stopped and restarted, P/P within 7 days	Resistant	On Li for 2 years, but P/P started after 2 months of treatment. Diabetic.
O'Connell (1971)	—	F	—	—	—
Viol and Smith (1971)	54	F	On Li $2\frac{1}{2}$ yrs. when studied. P/P marked during that time	Partial resistance	Urinary acidification defect demonstrated; normalized off Li
Ramsey et al.[a] (1972)	27	M	2 weeks	Resistant	
	43	M	2 months	Partial resistance	
	53	M	6 weeks or less	Resistant	

TABLE III.—*continued*

Author	Age	Sex	Time on Li to Onset of P/P[a]	Vasopressin Resistance	Comments
Brightwell *et al.* (1973)	27	M	2 months	Responded to vasopressin normally after H₂O deprivation	Normal water deprivation test. Possible mild decrease in hypothalamo-neurohypophysial system. Urine volume normal after 1 week on placebo
Levy *et al.* (1973)	54	F	18 months	Almost complete resistance	Treatment with chlorothiazide reduced polyuria and permitted patient to continue Li therapy but at lower dose due to toxicity

[a] P/P = polyuria/polydipsia
[b] Singer (1972) also reported these 3 cases of Ramsey *et al.* (1972) in more detail.

Note added in proof: Recently, Forrest *et al.* (1974) reported a 40% incidence of polydipsia and 12% incidence of polyuria (>3 litres/day) in 96 patients receiving lithium. The patients were unable to concentrate urine and were resistant to vasopressin. This high sensitivity to Li⁺ may be due to the high concentration of this cation in the renal medulla and papillae. (*J. clin. Invest.* **53**, 1115–1123, 1974).

by Li^+. These data are strongly supported by the work of Singer and colleagues (1972, 1973). Using the toad urinary bladder *in vitro* model, they showed that Li^+ blocked the ADH-induced short circuit current and water flow at concentrations which did not affect cAMP-induced changes in these parameters. This suggests that Li^+ interferes with ADH-activation of adenylate cyclase to produce cAMP. The crystal radius of Li^+ resembles that of both Mg^{++} and Ca^{++}. Since both of the divalent cations have marked effects on vasopressin binding and the subsequent activation of the cyclase (Campbell *et al.*, 1972), ion competition may be partly responsible for the Li^+ effect. Increased urinary potassium or hydrogen ion prevented Li^+-inhibition of ADH-induced responses, suggesting that urine composition may be important in both production and prevention of lithium-induced nephrogenic diabetes insipidus. Since a urinary acidification defect has been demonstrated in two patients (Trautner, 1955; Viol and Smith, 1971) receiving Li^+ therapy, an acidification defect may contribute to the subsequent development of impaired concentrating ability.

Lithium may also act at a step beyond cAMP. Harris and Jenner (1971b) demonstrated *in vitro* in the toad bladder preparation that Li^+ inhibits the effect of cAMP on water transport. They later showed (Harris and Jenner, 1972) that the effect was cation-specific; similar concentration of potassium, rubidium, strontium, magnesium, calcium and choline had no effect. This was a similar specificity as that seen in the intact animal (Harris and Jenner, 1969b). Forrest *et al.* (1971) showed that Li^+-induced polyuria in rats is *not* interrupted by intravenous dibutyryl-cAMP, whereas water diuresis in normal rats is.

In summary, Li^+ has been demonstrated to produce a reversible nephrogenic diabetes insipidus-like syndrome. While the syndrome occurs regularly in rats fed Li^+, it is only occasionally a significant problem in the clinical situation. However, the signs and symptoms of mildly increased thirst and mild polyuria-polydipsia are relatively common if patients are questioned closely. The mechanism of this syndrome may involve inhibition of the adenylate cyclase response to ADH and the function of cAMP itself in the distal tubular system of the kidney (see Chapters 28 and 29).

Finally, it must be pointed out that lithium has numerous other effects on the kidney that may influence its overall response to ADH. These include changes in adrenal steroid output; stimulation of the Na^+-K^+-ouabain-sensitive ATPase (Willis and Fang, 1970; Gutman *et al.*, 1973a); pathological tissue changes (Salomon *et al.*, 1972); and increases in plasma renin activity (Gutman *et al.*, 1971; Demers *et al*, 1972). Such increases may be toxic effects since in the rat, at least, low doses of Li^+ produced decreases in plasma renin activity (Gutman *et al.*, 1973b). It is, therefore, hazardous to draw mechanistic conclusions from the present evidence.

V. Concluding Remarks

In conclusion, the effects of Li$^+$ on the adrenal cortex, thyroid gland, or the kidney—ADH system resemble each other in that all three tissues possess an adenylate cyclase whose hormonal stimulation can be interfered with by the addition of Li$^+$, albeit at rather different concentrations. They are also alike in that each system has at least one other locus for lithium action beyond the cyclase in the "stimulus-secretion" sequence, and this site may be the more sensitive one, at least in the thyroid and adrenal glands. Because of the multiplicity of lithium effects, careful attention must be paid to the *lowest* lithium concentration that can elicit pharmacologic effects so that embarrassing mechanistic interpretations are avoided.

References

Abuzzahab, F. S. (1972). *Archs int. Pharmacodyn. Ther.* **198**, 5–8.

Amdisen, A. (1969). *Acta psychiat. Scand. Suppl.* **207**, 67.

Andersen, B. F. (1973). *Acta Endocrinol.* **73**, 35–42.

Angrist, B. M., Gershon, S., Levitan, S. J. and Blumberg, A. G. (1970). *Compreh. Psychiat.* **11**, 141–146.

Beck, N. P., Reed, S. W. and Davis, B. B. (1971). *Clin. Res.* **19**, 684 (abstract).

Bennie, E. H. and Lazarus, H. J. (1972). *Lancet* **2**, 44–45.

Berens, S. C., Bernstein, R. S., Robbins, J. and Wolff, J. (1970a) *J. clin. Invest.* **49**, 1357–1367.

Berens, S. C., Wolff, J. and Murphy, D. L. (1970b) *Endocrinol.* **87**, 1085–1087.

Berens, S. C., Williams, J. A. and Wolff, J. (1971). *Biochem. biophys. Acta* **252**, 314–323.

Birch, N. J. and Hullin, R. P. (1973). *Life Sci.* **11**, 1095–1099.

Birch, N. J. and Jenner, F. A. (1973). *Brit. J. Pharmacol.* **47**, 586–594.

Birch, C. R., Jolley, D. J., Hay, G. G. and Dymock, I. W. (1972). *Brit. med. J.* **4**, 233.

Birnbaumer, L, Pohl, S. L. and Rodbell, M. (1969). *J. biol. Chem.* **244**, 3468–3476.

Braverman, L. E., Woeber, K. A. and Ingbar, S. M. (1969). *New Engl. J. Med.* **281**, 816–821.

Brightwell, D. R., Halmi, K. A. and Finn, R. (1973). *Biol. Psychiat.* **7**, 167–172.

Burke, G. (1970). *Biochim. biophys. Acta* **220**, 30–41.

Burrow, G. N., Burke, W. R., Himmelhoch, J. M., Spencer, R. P. and Hersham, J. M. (1971). *J. clin. Endocrinol. Metab.* **32**, 647–652.

Campbell, B. J., Woodward, G. and Borberg, V. (1972). *J. biol. Chem.* **247**, 6167–6175

Candy, J. (1972). *Brit. med. J.* **3**, 277.

Carlson, H. E., Robbins, J. and Murphy, D. L. (1974). *Psychopharmacologia* **35**, 249–256.

Carlson, H. E., Temple, R. and Robbins, J. (1973). *J. clin. Endocrinol. Metab.* **36**, 1251–1254.

Cooper, T. B. and Simpson, G. M. (1969). *Curr. ther. Res.* **11**, 603–608.

Cooper, T. B., Wagner, B. M. and Kline, N. S. (1970). *Biol. Psychiat.* **2**, 273–278.

Crowe, M. J., Lloyd, G. G., Bloch, S. and Rosser, R. M. (1973). *Psychol. Med.* **3**, 337–342.

470   S. C. BERENS and J. WOLFF

Demers, R. G., Hendler, R., Allen, R. P. and Boyd, J. (1972). *Behav. Neuropsych.* **3**, 20–24.

Dousa, T. and Hechter, O. (1970). *Life Sci.* **9**, 765–770.

Edhag, O., Swahn, A. and Wester, P. O. (1973). *Acta med. Scand.* **193**, 553–555.

Ellman, G. L. and Gan, G. L. (1973). *Toxicol. appl. Pharmacol.* **25**, 617–620.

Emerson, G. H., Dyson, W. L. and Utiger, R. D. (1973). *J. clin. Endocrinol. Metab.* **36**, 338–346.

Fieve, R. R. and Platman, S. (1968). *Amer. J. Psychiat.* **125**, 527–530.

Fieve, R. R. and Platman (1969). *Amer. J. Psychiat.* **125**, 1443–1445.

Forrest, J. N., Cohen, A. D. and Torretti, J., unpublished results.

Forrest, J. N., Jr., Cohen, A. D., Torretti, J. and Epstein, F. H. (1971). *J. clin. Invest.* **50**, 32A (abstract).

Forn, J. and Valdecasas, F. B. (1971). *Biochem. Pharmacol.* **20**, 2773–2779.

Fyrö, B., Petterson, U. and Sedvall, G. (1973). *Acta psychiat. Scand.* **49**, 230–236.

Gerdes, H., Littmann, K. P., Joseph, K. and Mohlstedt, J. (1973). *Deut. med. Worchenschr.* **98**, 1551–1554.

Gonzales, R. and Lauter, H. (1968). *Der Nervenarzt* **39**, 11–16.

Gosling, R., Kerry, R. J. and Owen, G. (1972). *Brit. med. J.* **2**, 327–329.

Gutman, Y., Benzakein, F. and Livneh, P. (1971). *Eur. J. Pharmacol.* **16**, 380–384.

Gutman, Y., Hochman, S. and Wald, H. (1973a). *Biochim. biophys. Acta* **298**, 284–290.

Gutman, Y., Tamir, N. and Benzakein, F. (1973b). *Eur. J. Pharmacol.* **24**, 347–351.

Halberg, P., Dige-Petersen, H., Werdelin, O., Simornsen, J. and Rafaelsen, O. J. (1968). *Ugeskr. Laeg.* **130**, 1521.

Halmi, K. A., Halmi, N. S. and Anderson, D. J. (1974). *Proc. Soc. exp. Biol.* (in press).

Halmi, K. A. and Noyes, R. (1972). *Biol. Psychiat.* **5**, 211–215.

Halmi, K. A., Noyes, R. and Millard, S. A. (1972). *Clin. pharmacol. Therap.* **13**, 699–703.

Hanna, S. M., Jenner, F. A., Pearson, I. B., Sampson, G. A. and Thompson, E. A. (1972). *Brit. J. Psychiat.* **121**, 271–280.

Harris, C. A. and Dirks, J. H. (1973). *Fed. Proc.* **32**, 381.

Harris, C. A. and Jenner, F. A. (1969a). *J. Physiol.* **200**, 59P.

Harris, C. A. and Jenner, F. A. (1969b). *J. Physiol.* **203**, 73P–74P.

Harris, C. A. and Jenner, F. A. (1971a). *J. Physiol.* **214**, 43P–44P.

Harris, C. A. and Jenner, F. A. (1971b). *J. Pharmacologie* **2**, 215–216.

Harris, C. A. and Jenner, F. A. (1972). *Brit. J. Pharmacol.* **44**, 223–232.

Harris, C. E. and Teller, D. C. (1973). *Fed. Proc.* **32**, 1809A.

Heltne, C. E. and Ollerich, D. A. (1973). *Amer. J. Anat.* **136**, 297–303.

Hullin, R. P. and Johnson, A. W. (1970). *Life Sci.,* **9**, 9–20.

Hullin, R. P., McDonald, R. and Allsopp, M. N. E. (1972). *Lancet* **1**, 1044–1046.

Hullin, R. P., Swincoe, J. C., McDonald, R. and Dransfield, C. A. (1968). *Brit. J. Psychiat.* **114**, 1561–1573.

Jensen, S. E., Amdisen, A., Olsen, T. and Schou, M. (1968). *Ugeskr. Laeg.* **130**, 1518.

Kendall-Taylor, P. (1972). *J. Endocrinol.* **54**, 137–145.

Krulik, R. (1971). *Arzneimittel Forsch.* **21**, 889–890.

Lauter, H. (1971). *Deut. med. Wchschr.* **96**, 805.

Lazarus, J. H. and Bennie, E. H. (1972). *Acta Endocrinol.* **70**, 266–272.

Lee, R. V., Jampol, L. M. and Brown, W. V. (1971). *New Engl. J. Med.* **284**, 93–94.

Levy, S. T., Forrest, J. N. and Heniger, G. R. (1973). *Amer. J. Psychiat.* **130**, 1014–1017.

Lindstedt, G., Lundberg, P. A., Tofft, M., Akesson, H. O. and Öhman, R. (1973). *Clinica chim. Acta* **48**, 127–133.

Ljunggren, J. C., Sedvall, G., Levin, K. and Fyrö, B. (1971). *Acta Endocrinol.* **67**, 784–792.

Lloyd, G. G. (1973). *Lancet* **2**, 619.

Luby, E. D., Schwartz, D. and Rosenbaum, H. (1971). *J. Amer. med. Assoc.* **218**, 1298–1299.

Männistö, P. T. (1973). *Ann. Med. exp. Biol. Fenniae* **51**, 42–45.

Männistö, P. T., Leppäluoto, J. and Virkkunen, P. (1973). *Acta Endrocrinol.* **74**, 492–500.

Männistö, P., Linnoila, M. and Leppäluoto, J. (1971). *Life Sci.* **10**, 9–19.

Murphy, D. L., Goodwin, F. K. and Bunney, W. E. (1969). *Lancet* **2**, 458.

Myers, E. D. (1972). *Lancet* **1**, 1287.

Noyes, R., Ringdahl, I. C. and Andreasen, N. J. C. (1971). *Compreh. Psychiat.* **12**, 337–347.

O'Connell, R. A. (1971). *Compreh. Psychiat.* **12**, 224–229.

Ohlin, G. and Söderberg, U. (1970). *Acta physiol. Scand.* **79**, 24A–25A.

Orloff, J. and Kennedy, T. (1952). *Fed. Proc.* **11**, 115.

Platman, S. R. and Fieve, R. R. (1968). *Archs gen. Psychiat.* **18**, 591–594.

Platman, S. R., Hilton, J. G., Koss, M. C. and Kelly, W. G. (1971). *Dis. nerv. Syst.* **32**, 542–544.

Pousset, G., Briere, J., Berthezene, F., Tourniaire, J. and Devic, M. (1973). *Ann. Endocrinologie* **34**, 454–456.

Radomski, J. L., Fuyat, H. N., Nelson, A. A. and Smith, P. A. (1950). *J. Pharmacol. exp. Ther.* **100**, 429–444.

Ramsey, T. A., Mendels, J., Stokes, J. W. and Fitzgerald, R. G. (1972). *J. Amer. med. Assoc.* **219**, 1446–1449.

Rogers, M. P. and Whybrow, P. C. (1971). *Amer. J. Psychiat.* **128**, 158–163.

Sachar, E. J., Hellman, L., Kream, J., Fukushima, D. K. and Gallagher, T. F. (1970). *Arch. gen. Psych.* **22**, 304–307.

Salomon, M. I., King, E. J. and Gallo, G. (1972). *Dis. nerv. Syst.* **32**, 483–485.

Schou, M. (1958). *Acta Pharmacol. Toxicol.* **15**, 70–84.

Schou, M., Amdisen, A., Jensen, S. E. and Olsen, T. (1968). *Brit. med. J.* **3**, 710–713.

Schreiber, V. and Roháčová, J. (1971). *Acta Endocrinol.* **68**, 686–695.

Sedvall, G., Jönsson, B. and Pettersson, U. (1969). *Acta psychiat. Scand.* Suppl. **207**, 59–66.

Sedvall, G., Jönsson, B., Pettersson, U. and Levin, K. (1968) *Life Sci.,* **7**, 1257–1264.

Segal, R. L., Rosenblatt, S. and Eliasoph, I. (1973). *New Engl. J. Med.* **289**, 136–138.

Shopsin, B., Blum, M. and Gershon, S. (1969). *Comprehens. Psychiat.* **10**, 215–223.

Shopsin, B., Shenkman, L., Blum, M. and Hollander, S. C. (1973). *Amer. J. Med.* **55**, 695–699.

Singer, I. and Franko, E. A. (1973). *Kidney Internat.* **3**, 151–159.

Singer, I., Rotenberg, D. and Puschett, J. B. (1972). *J. clin. Invest.* **51**, 1081–1091.

Sörensen, R., Jensen, J., Mulder, J. and Schou, M. (1973). *Acta psychiat. Scand. Suppl.* **243**, 39.

Spaulding, S. W., Burrow, G. N., Bermudez, F. G. and Himmelhoch, J. M. (1972). *J. clin. Endocrinol. Metab.* **35**, 905–911.

Temple, R., Berman, M., Carlson, H. E., Robbins, J. and Wolff, J. (1972a). *Mayo Clin. Proc.* **47**, 872–878.

Temple, R., Berman, M., Robbins, J. and Wolff, J. (1972b). *J. clin. Invest.* **51,** 2746–2756.

Temple, R. and Wolff, J. (1973). *J. biol. Chem.* **248,** 2691–2698.

Thomsen, K. (1970). *Int. Pharmacopsychiat.* **4,** 233–241.

Torp-Pedersen, C. and Thorn, N. A. (1973). *Acta Endocrinol.* **73,** 665–671.

Trautner, E. M., Morris, R., Noack, C. H. and Gershon, S. (1955). *Med. J. Austr.* **2,** 280–291.

Vesterdal-Jorgensen, J., Brandrup, F. and Schroll, M. (1973). *J. Amer. med. Assoc.* **223,** 192–193.

Vestergaard, P. A. and Poulsen, J. C. (1972). *Lancet* **2,** 427–428.

Villeneuve, A., Gautier, J., Jus, A. and Perron, D. (1973). *Lancet* **2,** 502.

Viol, G. W. and Smith, E. K. M. (1971). *New Engl. J. Med.* **284,** 674.

Whybrow, P. C. (1972). *J. Amer. med. Assoc.* **221,** 506.

Wiener, J. D. (1972). *J. Amer. med. Assoc.* **220,** 587.

Wiggers, A. S. (1968). *Ugeskr. Laeg.* **130,** 1523.

Williams, J. A., Berens, S. C. and Wolff, J. (1971). *Endocrinol.* **88,** 1385-1388.

Williams, J. A. and Wolff (1970). *Proc. nat. Acad. Sci.* **67,** 1901–1908.

Williams, J. A. and Wolff, J. (1972). *J. cell Biol.* **54,** 157–165.

Willis, J. S. and Fang, L. S. T. (1970). *Biochim. biophys. Acta* **219,** 486–489.

Wolff, J. (1964). *Physiol. Rev.* **44,** 45–90.

Wolff, J. (1969). *Amer. J. Med.* **47,** 101–129.

Wolff, J., Berens, S. C. and Jones, A. B. (1970). *Biochem. biophys. Res. Commun.* **39,** 77–82.

Wolff, J. and Williams, J. (1973). *Rec. Prog. Horm. Res.* **29,** 229–285.

28

LITHIUM AND POLYURIA

Sheila MacNeil and F. A. Jenner

I. Introduction

Lithium ions induce polyuria and polydipsia which can vary from a negligible side effect in clinical practice to a major problem of a full blown nephrogenic vasopressin resistant syndrome of diabetes insipidus (cf. eg. Schou, 1968). The degree to which the problems will arise in an individual and the factors which make some and not other persons react in this way are unknown. Similar responses in rats, however, occur in all animals as a dose dependent effect. Forrest (1974) in a very comprehensive article, suggests that reversible concentrating defects in the kidney are probably present in the majority of patients and rats treated with lithium.

The evidence indicates that the increased intake and excretion of water are very significantly, but not completely, explained by inhibition of vasopressin-sensitive adenyl cyclase in the kidney.

There is little evidence that these striking effects are helpful in explaining the therapeutic activity of lithium, but in the absence of any clear understanding of the clinical response they have justified, and received, considerable attention.

II. Clinical Presentation

Angrist *et al.* (1970) reported two patients with "pitressin resistant (apparent) diabetes insipidus due to lithium carbonate treatment". This confirmed Schou's (1968) earlier reports. As is quite characteristic, the enormous increase in urine volume in the two patients followed periods of two weeks and of seven months respectively of only minimal increase of polydipsia and polyuria. Both patients had shown good therapeutic responses, but there is little reason to believe that any correlation between successful treatment and the diabetes insipidus syndrome exists. Clearly, however, persons with good responses to lithium are likely to be those who continue to receive the treatment, and hence they have more time to present the, as yet, unpredictable polyuria. Angrist *et al.* postulated that a potassium deficient state occurred in the kidney, but they themselves showed in their own patients that there was no hypokalemia. Despite the work of Smith and Lasater (1950), which Angrist *et al.* quote and which showed how dogs can be given a diabetes insipidus-like syndrome by administering a severely potassium-deficient diet, it does not seem likely that low intracellular potassium explains this particular lithium effect in manic depressive patients.

Brightwell *et al.* (1973) review some of the more recent literature and report on a 27 year old male who developed a gross polyuria after two months of lithium therapy. The serum lithium levels varied from 0·64–0·78 mEq/l and no other significant toxic effects were noted, but his urine volume increased to 4·7 l and the diuresis was unaffected by vasopressin. The patient was very unusual in excreting a hyperosmolar urine of large volume. One wonders what he was eating. When he was given a placebo his urine output became about 1·6 l. This patient, however, probably did not secrete vasopressin maximally when water was withheld as he was able to further concentrate his urine. He also showed a borderline abnormal responsiveness of adrenocorticotrophic hormone and growth hormone secretion. On this limited, but interesting, evidence the authors postulated a hypothalamo-neurohypohyseal defect, itself an imprecise concept, which either preceded the patient's treatment or was due to lithium. Further examples of such responses would be extremely interesting to consider. As will become apparent, however, most of the evidence suggests that a renal action of lithium explains most of the volume changes which occur, but certainly other actions are also involved.

Two sets of workers report abnormalities of glucose metabolism in patients showing the lithium-induced diabetes insipidus syndrome. In the patient reported by Lee *et al.* (1971), frank diabetes mellitus with a blood sugar up to 972 mg per hundred millilitres of blood was present, and insulin treatment was required. Nevertheless, in addition to any osmotic diuresis due to glucose, a clear lithium effect was present with low serum values (0·41–0·77 mEq/l). When lithium was withdrawn, the urine volume was reduced from 6 to 2·5 l per 24h. The polyuria did not respond to 5 Units of pitressin, and this response was still limited three weeks after stopping lithium. After eight weeks, a normal response occurred. Lithium was, for various clinical reasons, started and stopped on two occasions, and with about a week's delay the urine volume respectively increased or decreased.

The other report of a lithium-induced diabetes insipidus-like state associated with abnormal glucose tolerance came from Viol and Smith (1971). In this case, abnormal urine acidification was noted as well as a defective response to vasopressin. It would naturally be of interest to have more information on glucose tolerance in other patients with lithium-induced diabetes insipidus-like syndromes, as at present one can only suspect that these particular patients show a fortuitous association of diabetes insipidus and mellitus. Indeed, Ramsey *et al.* (1972), while attempting to characterise the common features of the patients they were able to study, were forced to point out the lack of evidence of discernible factors leading to any useful prediction of this complication. The patients were without previous renal disease, their serum lithium levels were not particularly high, and indeed the degree of polyuria was quite independent of the serum lithium levels within the therapeutic range, and the time of onset of grossly increased diuresis seemed an iodiosyncrasy of each of the individuals.

Brightwell *et al.* (1973) also emphasise that of the cases designated lithium-induced nephrogenic vasopressin resistant diabetes insipidus, there is a considerable variability in the degree to which they are unable to concentrate their urine following 12 hours without water on 5 units of vasopressin. This is well shown in the study of three patients by Singer *et al.* (1972) and the patients already mentioned with frank or borderline diabetes mellitus, where each showed some concentrating ability following withdrawal of water and vasopressin administration.

The patient reported by Trautner *et al.* (1955) very interestingly showed increased lithium excretion before the polyuria and polydipsia, despite a constant dose of lithium. This patient responded with an antidiuresis to vasopressin administration but not to water deprivation, hence there may have been inadequate formation or release of vasopressin, either independently of, or in part due to, a reduced renal sensitivity.

Despite these complicating possibilities in some patients, it is clear that an idiosyncratic polyuria is a moderately common side effect of lithium therapy, and the major factor inducing this state arises from the inhibition by lithium of the antidiuretic activity of vasopressin.

Among others, the following papers refer to further examples of diabetes insipidus-like states induced by lithium therapy: Rotenberg *et al.* (1971); Rybakowski and Daszynska (1972); Schrub *et al.* (1972); Sober and Gorden (1972).

III. Treatment of the Diabetes Insipidus-Like State

Until recently, little could be done for patients beset by gross urine loss, and it was often necessary to stop treatment however successfully their mental state had been controlled (see e.g. Dostal, 1971). Levy *et al.* (1973), however, reported that chlorothiazide reduced the lithium-induced polyuria and permitted their patient to continue receiving lithium treatment. A fourfold increase of sodium intake, however, had no effect.

It has, of course, long been recognised that chlorothiazide and related drugs produce a paradoxical antidiuresis in naturally occurring diabetes insipidus. These drugs are themselves diuretics in normal persons. Earley and Orloff (1962) induced antidiuresis in nephrogenic or vasopressin-resistant diabetes insipidus using hydrochlorothiazide. They suggest that this is due to an effect of the drug increasing sodium depletion and they conclude that a potassium rich and sodium depleted diet would be of value with hydrochlorothiazide in these patients. In view of the finding by Levy *at al.* (1973) of the ineffectiveness of sodium loading in lithium-induced nephrogenic diabetes insipidus, further studies of the effects of sodium and potassium intake with chlorothiazides in lithium-induced polyuria seem warranted.

Sorensen *et al.* (1973) raise the further possibility of using l-deamino-8-d-arginine vasopressin (DDAVP), a synthetic analogue of the antidiuretic hormone. They claim in a preliminary report that intranasal application as a snuff effectively controls the polyuria and polydipsia caused by lithium. DDAVP is interesting in being a powerful antidiuretic and not having the same magnitude of pressor activity as vasopressin. It can therefore be used in much larger doses than can vasopressin (see e.g. Andersson and Arner, 1972 and Edwards *et al.*, 1973).

IV. Structural Renal Changes Due to Lithium

There is no evidence that the diabetes insipidus like state is irreversible. In both animals and man, complete recovery follows stopping lithium administration. Very large doses of lithium leading to serum levels above 4 mEq/l lead to clear damage to proximal tubules, and to a lesser extent to the glomeruli and intertubular arteries (Lavender *et al.*, 1973). Evans (1973) has demonstrated a change in the mitochondria in the kidney which is dose-dependent and which leads to renal degeneration in the course of time. It seems unlikely that significant risk is involved with serum lithium levels below 2 mEq/l. Reports of renal failure in patients with moderate serum levels of lithium are characteristically accompanied by reports of other pathology, as for example in the patient reported by Dias and Hocken (1973). In fact the very wide-scale use of lithium and the limited reports of toxic effects make it most likely that reports of associated renal failure are fortuitous. This must be so until a statistically higher incidence of renal failure can be shown to have occurred in lithium treated patients compared to control subjects. Naturally, considerable caution is required if iatrogenic illness is to be avoided.

V. The Mode of Action of Vasopressin

The inhibition by lithium of the antidiuretic activity of vasopressin in the kidney must, of course, be explored in relationship to current concepts of the mode of action of the antidiuretic hormone, vasopressin, itself. The lithium effect also gives another approach to the problems involved in understanding the action of the hormones. These questions are only broached here.

The "current view" strongly implies that vasopressin, only facilitates passive movement of water by diffusion and down the osmotic and electrochemical gradients across cells and membranes. This can be visualised as though membrane pore size is increased and resistance to flow is thereby reduced. The concomitant movement of urea and electrolytes is due to a "wash through" effect of going along with the tide. Perhaps a separate barrier of "pores" is affected which selectively limits passive transport of sodium and water. Schwartz and Schwartz (1967) have edited a very helpful collection of papers in this field in the American Journal of Medicine.

Vasopressin, like many other hormones, is thought to act on a specific adenyl cyclase which converts adenosine triphosphate to cyclic adenosine monosphate (cAMP). This latter affects the membrane permeability but is itself converted to 5'adenosine monophosphate by cyclic nucleotide phosphodiesterase. Theophylline as well as other drugs inhibits the diesterase and increases sodium and water transport in many biological preparations (Orloff and Handler, 1967).

cAMP in very large doses will cause water retention even in hypophysectomised patients with diabetes insipidus (Levine, 1968). cAMP, of course, has innumerable effects in the body but this result is consistent with the view that its release by vasopressin is a stage in the action of the antidiuretic hormone (see also Dousa et al., 1972).

The effects of vasopressin on water and sodium movements can be separated by increased calcium or magnesium concentrations, and it is possible that the water facilitating effect only is mediated by cyclic AMP. To preserve the view that vasopressin does not affect the active pumping of sodium, but that it can affect sodium and water separately, the double diffusion barrier in the mucosal border of the tubular cells is postulated. One barrier is freely permeable to water but not to sodium, the other to sodium but not to water. Relative effects on the two barriers could explain the available results (see Singer et al., 1969).

For early but helpful general accounts of the membrane effects of lithium, the reader is referred to Leaf (1967) and Pitts (1968).

VI. Animal and *In Vitro* Studies of the Inhibition of the Effect of Vasopressin by Lithium

The rat in particular is a suitable laboratory animal in which to study the renal effects of lithium. Rats can be kept in metabolic cages without too much expense, and they have been widely used for assay of vasopressin (see e.g. Bisset, 1962).

The toad bladder and frog skin also offer useful biological preparations on which the effect of vasopressin seems analogous to its action on the renal tubule. These almost one cell thick poikilothermic tissues allow one to study mucosal and serosal changes as well as investigating the intracellular, or at least tissue, content alterations in a variety of experimental situations.

The anuran's bladder and skin do seem to act like the mammalian tubule in the animal's economy, but despite the apparent elegance of the experimental preparations which can be made, results recorded in the literature tend to be contradictory. The tissues are not as easy to handle as may appear to be so at first sight. Nevertheless, a good deal has been done using lithium and vasopressin on such tissues.

Naturally, slices of rabbit, cat, dog and other kidneys have been studied, and some of the results to be reported come from these animals as well as from mice and hamsters, etc.

VII. The Production of Nephrogenic Diabetes Insipidus in The Rat by Lithium

Feeding lithium to rats always induces a marked polyuria and polydipsia if the dose is high enough, water is available, and the experiment is continued long enough. The rat is more predictable and does not show the characteristic idiosyncratic response of the individual so striking in man. There is no known explanation for this. Because of this, and for other reasons to be highlighted, the extrapolation from one to another species is, as always, somewhat suspect but unavoidable. However, there are many different features in common between the polyuria in man and the rat. The increased urine volume only occurs after a delay of up to 20 days in the rat, so it is not an immediate response in man or rat despite a wide range of doses. In both, the effect is reversible in 5–6 days. In rat and man the excess intake and excretion of water remains stable over an indefinite period if the lithium continues to be administered. In both, there is an inadequate and often negligible response to large doses of pitressin (15 Units per kilogram body weight in the rat). Though the rat is more sensitive in terms of serum levels of lithium, in both rat and man the polyuria can occur without significant defect to the animal and in the absence of any indication of other renal defect. In both, the urine volume remains elevated even when lithium levels in serum and tissues must be very low. Thomsen (1970a, b) in particular brings out most of the above points, which are also in keeping with the studies of Smith *et al.* (1970), Gutman *et al.* (1971), Schreiber *et al.* (1971), Geisler *et al.* (1972) and Rafaelsen (1972).

As has been pointed out, in man the inhibition of the action of vasopressin alone cannot totally explain the findings. Smith *et al.* (1970) also produce evidence for a direct effect of lithium on the lateral hypothalamus in the rat. Lesions in this area stop the immediate drinking which classically follows intragastric administration of lithium to the rat.

VIII. The Inhibition of Vasopressin Activity in Rat by Lithium Ions

Harris and Jenner (1972), using alcohol anaesthetized and water-loaded rats, were able to show a very clear acute inhibition of the antidiuretic activity of intravenous pitressin. Alcohol is used as an anaesthetic which does not itself cause the posterior pituitary and hypothalmus to secrete vasopressin, but as one which is fairly unique in stopping the release of vasopressin. The experimental design involved water loading by intravenous infusion, which could be changed in its contents to and from equivalent amounts of sodium and lithium. The inhibitory effect produced is quick and apparent in 10 minutes (using 13 mmol/l of lithium chloride at 0·2 ml per minute). It is maximal in 30 minutes when serum levels of lithium are still fairly low. Harris and Jenner (1972) claim that the inhibition is reversible at a rate much in excess of that which might be predicted by the slowly dropping plasma, tissue or whole body lithium levels, and no inhibition can be demonstrated when these levels are still higher than was initially required to produce profound effects. The latter point of the apparent irrelevance of plasma levels of lithium might imply that the effect depends on the direction of movement of the lithium ion or on its relative distribution. This would argue against a simple inhibition of vasopressin sensitive adenyl cyclase as the explanation of the major effect on the kidney.

Torp-Pederson and Thorn (1973), while confirming much of Harris and Jenner's (1972) study, and indeed essentially using their procedures, cast considerable doubt on one point. Studying animals for up to 120 minutes after lithium, they found negligible return of sensitivity to vasopressin. Harris and Jenner (1972) report a complete return to normal sensitivity in about half an hour. The authors of this chapter, however, still feel from further, as yet unpublished, studies that inhibition can be reversed in the presence of fairly high persisting plasma levels of lithium. The two sets of authors should of course, resolve this difference in due course.

Harris and Jenner's (1972) study also clearly showed that in their preparation lithium was different from rubidium, potassium, strontium, magnesium, choline and calcium.

The body's handling of these different ions administered intravenously or orally is quite different and it takes different periods of infusion to produce similar renal levels (see e.g. Bond and Jenner, 1974). Hence, while it is likely that inhibition of vasopressin is characteristic of lithium rather than other group I and II ions, the evidence is not totally adequate.

The rapid inhibition of the antidiuretic effect of vasopressin by lithium shown by Harris and Jenner (1972) and Torp-Pederson and Thorn (1973) could be due to inhibition of adenyl cyclase. If, however, what occurs in ten minutes is to be seen as analogous to the clinical situation, or indeed the chronic rat preparation which, with similar serum levels, takes three weeks to show this effect, some compensatory mechanisms must be postulated. Perhaps increased amounts of vasopressin are produced to compensate for its relative lack of effect. Recent unpublished studies by the present authors have, indeed, shown that, in the rat at least, vasopressin is produced, and excreted, in increased amounts following lithium treatment. Although it is possible that the acute and chronic effects of lithium on vasopressin sensitivity are due to a similar mechanism (e.g. the inhibition of vasopressin sensitive adenyl cyclase) it is also possible that the two effects are due to different actions of lithium in the kidney.

IX. The Inhibition of Adenyl Cyclase by Lithium

Using large doses of lithium, Dousa and Hechter (1970a, b) clearly demonstrated inhibition of vasopressin sensitive adenyl cyclase in rabbit kidney preparations. Less lithium chloride, but still more than 25 mmol/l, was required when 15 mmol/l of sodium were present. Geisler *et al.* (1972), at much more relevant plasma levels, compared the adenyl cyclase activity of rats made polyuric by adding lithium to their food. They found less stimulation by vasopressin in these as compared to control animals. This assay was performed on kidneys extracted in such a way that neither group had significant lithium levels in the extracts when the assays were performed. This implies that lithium causes an alteration of some intermediary which itself affects adenyl cyclase. The results are of clear interest but they require confirmation and their detailed interpretation remains complex.

Lithium does undoubtedly inhibit a number of adenyl cyclases other than the renal vasopressin sensitive enzyme: inhibition of rabbit brain adrenaline stimulated adenyl cyclase (Dousa and Hechter, 1970a); stimulation of rat glial adrenaline stimulated adenyl cyclase (Schimmer, 1971); inhibition of rabbit renal cortex parathyroid sensitive adenyl cyclase (Dousa and Hechter, 1970a); inhibition of rat renal cortex parathyroid sensitive adenyl cyclase (Marcus and Aurbach, 1971); inhibition of bovine thyroid stimulating hormone sensitive adenyl cyclase (Wolff and Jones, 1971); inhibition of mouse thyroid stimulating hormone sensitive adenyl cyclase (Kendall-Taylor, 1972); inhibition of rabbit liver glucagon sensitive adenyl cyclase (Dousa and Hechter, 1970a). Presumably many other adenyl cyclases are affected and this factor alone would give lithium almost as many effects as cAMP itself.

The pituitary response, however, to antidiuretic hormone in patients with lithium-induced diabetes insipidus is reported to be normal by Sober and Gorden (1972) who measured the steroid rise mediated by adrenocorticotrophic hormone release induced by administered vasopressin.

Because lithium inhibits adenyl cyclase this does not exclude the possibility that it also inhibits the effects of cAMP as well. Toad bladder results do seem to show this (Harris and Jenner, 1972), and Bentley and Wasserman (1972) and Singer and Franko (1973) suggest this might well be the case particularly at high levels of lithium concentration.

Confirmatory evidence of lithium effects on vasopressin sensitive adenyl cyclase comes from direct studies of cAMP production. Beck *et al.* (1971) studied dog kidney slices. Lithium alone did nothing to cAMP concentrations, but it did reduce the degree to which vasopressin can increase the slice cAMP. In this particular preparation, parathormone increased cAMP levels and this effect was not inhibited by lithium. The authors argue that this indicates the specificity of the lithium effect despite the studies of Marcus and Aurbach (1971) and Dousa and Hechter (1970a), of which the authors would not be aware at their time of writing.

The general interest in the physiological significance of prostaglandins and their known modulating effect on the stimulation of adenyl cyclase by vasopressin must lead to studies on the degree to which lithium might also act on these mechanisms (see e.g. Hinman, 1972). The adenyl cyclase studies must also be considered in relation to changes due to lithium of renin activity reported by Gutman *et al.* (1973) and on renal microsomal ATPases in the rat kidney (Gutman *et al.*, 1973) and of course on aldosterone (see Murphy *et al.*, 1969).

X. Studies in Toad Bladder and Frog Skin Preparations

The effects of lithium on biological transport systems have been widely studied using simple pieces of toad bladder or frog skin as the membranes across which transport occurs.

The lithium ion itself is actively transported in these tissues (Zerahn, 1955 and Herrera *et al.*, 1971). In the toad bladder, ouabain inhibits this process in the same way as it inhibits sodium transport. Hence it would seem that as in muscle (Keynes and Swan, 1959) lithium is actively pumped by the cellular sodium pump. This seems to be confirmed by the inhibition by amiloride of the transport of both sodium and lithium (Herrera, 1972).

The transport of lithium is assumed, especially in muscle, to be low compared to that of sodium, but Herrera *et al.* (1971) show that in the toad bladder with lithium on the mucosal surface, its transport and the short circuit current (a measure of net cation movement) can be almost identical. The transport of lithium across these amphibian tissues is itself stimulated by vasopressin

(Natochin and Leont'ev, 1964).

It seems that lithium itself limits the vasopressin facilitated passage of water and sodium across these isolated tissues (Zerahn, 1955; Natochin and Leont-'ev, 1964; Herrera et al., 1971; Herrera, 1972; Singer and Franko, 1973; Bentley and Wasserman, 1972; and Harris and Jenner, 1972; etc.), but studying details of these processes reveals contradictory findings in the literature.

Harris and Jenner (1972) find inhibition of the facilitated water transport due to vasopressin or due to cAMP, with 2 mmol/l of lithium on the serosal surface. Bentley and Wasserman (1972) found no effect of 11 to 111 mmol/l on either side. Singer and Franko (1973) using the same technique as other authors found no inhibition unless the lithium was on the mucosal side when it inhibited vasopressin induced water movement. As Harris and Jenner (1972) found no effect with lithium on the mucosal side, the simultaneous interpretation of the results of these three groups is really impossible.

Currently available studies of lithium's effect on vasopressin stimulated sodium transport are less discrepant (see Bentley and Wasserman, 1972; Singer and Franko, 1973; Singer et al., 1972). They are, however, probably less relevant to the clinical problem posed and which is among the excuses for studying the lowly anuran's isolated tissues.

XI. Conclusions

Lithium ions probably inhibit the increased activity of the specific adenyl cyclase responsive to vasopressin in the kidney. It is likely that lithium interferes with several other processes.

It is quite clear that, from time to time, clinical use of lithium is limited by the enormous water loss which can be induced in some unfortunate subjects.

It is possible that new analogues of vasopressin or chlorothiazide may be helpful for this iatrogenic state though Olesen (1974) has recently hinted that potassium loading may prove to be a useful way of ameliorating the condition.

There is certainly a need for a clearer scientific understanding of the situation, but no obvious reason to believe this will explain much about the centrally interesting question: how does lithium help in the treatment of affective psychoses?

References

Andersson, K. E. and Arner, B. (1972). Acta med. Scand. 192, 21–27.
Angrist, B. M., Gershon, S., Levitan, S. J. and Blumberg, A. G. (1970). Compreh. Psychiat. 11, 141–146.
Beck, N. P., Reed, S. W. and Davis, B. B. (1971). Clin. Res. 19, 684.
Bentley, P. J. and Wasserman, A. (1972). Biochem. biophys. Acta 266, 285–292.
Bisset, G. W. (1962). Brit. J. Pharmacol. 18, 405–420.
Bond, P. A. and Jenner, F. A. (1974). Brit. J. Pharmacol. 50, (in Press).
Brightwell, D. R., Halmi, K. A. and Finn, R. (1973) Biol. Psychiat. 7, 167–171.
Dias, N. and Hocken, A. G. (1973). Nephron 10, 264–249.

Dostal, T. (1971). *In* "Proc. 4th U.E.P. Congr., Stockholm", 491–498.

Dousa, T. and Hechter, O. (1970a). *Lancet* 1, 834.

Dousa, T. and Hechter, O. (1970b). *Life Sci.* 9, 765–770.

Dousa, T. P., Walter, R., Schwartz, I. L., Sands, H. and Hechter, O. (1972). *In* "Advances in Cyclic Nucleotide Research" (P. Greengard, ed.), Vol. 1, pp. 121–135. Raven Press, New York.

Earley, L. E. and Orloff, J. (1962). *J. clin. Invest.* 41, 1988–1997.

Edwards, C. R. W., Kitau, M. J., Chard, T. and Besser, G. M. (1973). *Brit. Med. J.* 3, 375–378.

Evans, A. P. (1973). *Toxic. appl. Pharmacol.* 24, 413–422.

Forrest, J. N. (1974). *J. clin. Invest.* 53, 1115–1123.

Geisler, A., Wraae, O. and Olesen, O. V. (1972). *Acta Pharmacol. Toxic.* 31, 203–208.

Gutman, Y., Benzakein, F. and Livneh, P. (1971). *Eur. J. Pharmacol.* 16, 380–384.

Gutman, Y., Hockman, S. and Wald, H. (1973). *Biochim. Biophys. Acta* 298, 284–290.

Gutman, Y., Tamir, N. and Benzakein, F. (1973). *Eur. J. Pharmacol.* 24, 347–351.

Harris, C. A. and Jenner, F. A. (1972). *Brit. J. Pharmacol.* 44, 223–232.

Herrera, F. C. (1972). *Amer. J. Physiol.* 222, 499–502.

Herrera, F. C., Egea, R. and Herrera, A. M. (1971). *Amer. J. Physiol.* 220, 1501–1508.

Hinman, J. W. (1972). *Ann. Rev. Biochem.* 41, 161–178.

Kendall–Taylor, P. (1972). *J. Endocrinol.* 54, 137–145.

Keynes, R. D. and Swan, R. C. (1959). *J. Physiol.* 147, 591–625.

Lavender, S., Brown, J. N. and Berrill, W. T. (1973). *Postgrad. med. J.* 49, 277–279.

Leaf, A. (1967). *Am. J. Med.* 42, 745–756.

Lee, R. B., Jampol, L. M. and Braun, W. B. (1971). *New Engl. J. Med.* 284, 93.

Levine, R. A. (1968). *Clin. Sci.* 34, 253–260.

Levy, S. T., Forrest, J. N. and Heninger, G. R. (1973). *Am. J. Psychiat.* 130, 1014–1018.

Marcus, R. and Aurbach, G. D. (1971). *Biochim. biophys. Acta* 242, 410–421.

Murphy, D. L., Goodwin, F. K. and Bunney, W. E. (1969). *Lancet* 2, 458–461.

Natochin, Y. V. and Leont'ev, V. G. (1964). *Fiziol. Zh. SSSR im. I. M. Sechenova* 50, 618–625.

Olesen, O. V. Paper presented at IX C.I.N.P., Paris.

Orloff, J. and Handler, J. (1967). *Am. J. Med.* 42, 757–768.

Pitts, R. F. (1968). *In* "Physiology of the Kidney and Body Fluids", 2nd Ed., p. 213. Year Book Medical Publishers, Inc.

Rafaelsen, O. J. (1972). Report for the Year 1972. Psychochemistry Institute, Rigshospitalet, Copenhagen.

Ramsey, T. A., Mendels, J., Stokes, J. W. and Fitzgerald, R. G. (1972). *J. Am. Med. Assoc.* 219, 1446–1449.

Rotenberg, D., Puschett, J. B., Ramsey, P., Stokes, J. Mendels, J. and Singer, I. (1971). *Clin. Res.* 19, 546.

Rybakowski, J. and Daszynska, M. (1972). *Pol. Tyg. Lek.* 27, 1527–1528.

Schimmer, B. P. (1971). *Biochim. biophys. Acta* 252, 567–573.

Schou, M. (1968). *J. psychiat. Res.* 6, 67–95.

Schreiber, V., Rohacova, J. and Pribyl, T. (1971). *Physiol. Bohemoslov.* 20, 249–254.

Schrub, J. C., Wolf, L. M., Courtois, M., Vuillermet, P. and Marel, U. (1972). *La Nouvelle Presse Medicale* 1, 2109–2110.

Schwartz, I. L. and Schwartz, W. B. (1967). *Am. J. Med.* 42, 651–827.

Singer, I. and Franko, E. A. (1973). *Kidney International* **3**, 151–159.

Singer, I., Civan, M. M., Baddour, R. F. and Leaf, A. (1969). *Amer. J. Physiol.* **217**, 938–945.

Singer, I., Rotenberg, D. and Puschett, J. B. (1972). *J. clin. Invest.* **51**, 1081–1091.

Smith. D. F.. Balagura. S. and Lubran. M. (1970). *Science* **167**, 297–298.

Smith, S. G. and Lasater, T. E. (1950). *Proc. Soc. exp. Biol. Med.* **74**, 427–431.

Sober, A. J. and Gorden, P. (1972). *J. clin. Endocrin. Metab.* **35**, 924.

Sorensen, R., Jensen, J., Mulder, J. and Schou, M. (1973). *Acta psychiat scand. Suppl.* **243**, 39.

Thomsen, K. (1970a). Paper read at Symposium VII C.I.N.P. Meeting in Prague.

Thomsen, K. (1970b). *Int. Pharmacopsychiat.* **5**, 233–241.

Torp–Pedersen, C. and Thorn, N. A. (1973). *Acta Endocrinol.* **73**, 665–671.

Trautner, E. M., Morris, R., Noack, C. H. and Gershon, S. (1955). *Med. J. Aust.* **2**, 280–291.

Viol, G. W. and Smith, E. K. M. (1971). *New Engl. J. Med.* **284**, 674–675.

Wolff, J. and Jones, A. B. (1971). *J. biol. Chem.* **246**, 3939–3947.

Zerahn, K. (1955). *Acta physiol. Scand.* **33**, 347–358.

29

LITHIUM AND CYCLIC AMP

J. Forn

I. Introduction

Adenosine 3′,5′-monophosphate (cyclic AMP) was discovered by Sutherland and his co-workers as the intracellular mediator of the glycogenolytic effect of norepinephrine and glucagon in the liver (Sutherland and Rall, 1958). Since then, the role of cyclic AMP as intracellular mediator or "second messenger" of the action of many hormones in their corresponding target cells has been clearly established. Most of this evidence has been recently summarized (Robison *et al.*, 1971; Sutherland, 1972; Greengard and Robison, 1973).

The conversion of ATP to cyclic AMP is catalyzed by adenylate cyclase, a membrane-bound enzyme that requires a divalent cation, usually magnesium. The concentration of cyclic AMP is also regulated by phosphodiesterase, an enzyme that opens the cyclic phosphate bond and converts the cyclic nucleotide into an inactive derivative.

In recent years it has been observed that lithium inhibits adenylate cyclase activity in homogenates of several tissues, as well as the hormone-induced accumulation of cyclic AMP in some *in vitro* tissue preparations containing intact cells. Due to the key role of cyclic AMP as the intracellular mediator of many hormones, these effects of lithium might explain some of its therapeutic and toxicological properties. In this chapter, the effects of lithium on the cyclic AMP system of several tissues, and the possible relationship between these effects and some pharmacological properties of lithium, will be discussed.

II. Brain

A. Characteristics of the brain cyclic AMP system

The importance of cyclic AMP in the central nervous system is suggested by the finding that the activity of adenylate cyclase and phosphodiesterase is higher in the brain than in other tissues (Sutherland *et al.*, 1962).

The sensitivity of brain adenylate cyclase to different neurohormones is lost or greatly reduced when broken cell preparations are used. However, fluoride, by an as yet unknown mechanism, is able to stimulate adenylate cyclase activity of cell free systems of many issues, including the brain (Perkins, 1973). Kakiuchi and Rall (1968a, b) demonstrated that several agents affected the cyclic AMP levels of slices of either cerebellum or cerebrum of rabbit brain. Some biogenic amines, direct electrical stimulation, and several agents that depolarize electrically excitable tissues have been shown by several groups to increase the cyclic AMP content of brain slices incubated *in vitro* (Kakiuchi *et al.*, 1969; Shimizu *et al.*, 1970; Shimizu *et al.*, 1972). The effect of any given neurohormone depends on the region of the brain and also on the animal species (Forn and Krishna, 1970); However, the complexity of these preparations severely limits the conclusions that can be drawn from these observations. Brain slices, even of a well defined region, are composed of neurons, glia cells and cells of connective tissue. It has not yet been possible in most cases to determine which cell types are responsible for the observed changes in cyclic AMP concentration in response to norepinephrine and to other neurotransmitters, and any extrapolation from these preparations to the function of an intact brain has to be made with great caution. It has been shown that in cells derived from neuronal tumors (neuroblastomas) prostaglandin E_1 causes an increase in cyclic AMP accumulation (Gilman and Nirenburg, 1971a), whereas in cells from glial tumors cyclic AMP levels were unaffected by prostaglandins but were greatly increased by norepinephrine or isoproterenol (Gilman and Nirenberg, 1971b). The functional significance of these alterations on cyclic AMP content is, however, unknown.

The possibility that cyclic AMP functions in brain as a second messenger for one or more neurotransmitters is supported by studies in which the cyclic nucleotide was directly injected into specific brain regions. Injection of dibutyryl cyclic AMP, a lipid-soluble derivative of cyclic AMP, into the lateral ventricles of rats, produced increased motor activity, catatonia and convulsions. Injection in more definite areas of the cat brain with permanently implanted cannulae produced more specific vegetative and behavioral effects. Opposite effects, like sedation or excitation, adrenergic or cholinergic stimulation, could be obtained depending on the area in which the nucleotide was injected. The presence of the cyclic AMP moiety was essential for these effects (Gessa *et al.,* 1970).

There is some evidence to implicate cyclic AMP in the physiology of synaptic transmission. For example, adenylate cyclase and phosphodiesterase have highest specific activity in preparations of synaptic membranes (De Robertis *et al.,* 1967). With a histochemical method, phosphodiesterase has been localized in post-synaptic nerve endings in the cortex of the rat brain (Florendo *et al.,* 1971). It has been shown (Hoffer *et al.,* 1972) that the hyperpolarization produced by norepinephrine in cerebeller Purkinje cells is mediated by cyclic AMP. Dopamine produces a hyperpolarization of the post-ganglionic neurons of the superior cervical ganglion, and it has been demonstrated that these effects are also mediated by an increase in cyclic AMP levels (McAfee and Greengard, 1972). These cyclic AMP-mediated effects take place at a post-synaptic level. Moreover, some experimental results suggest that cyclic AMP may also regulate the excitation-coupled release of neurotransmitters at the nerve ending (Peach, 1972; Wooten *et al.,* 1973).

B. Cyclic AMP and the affective disorders

On the basis of an increased urinary excretion of cyclic AMP in manic patients, and of opposite changes in depressed patients, Abdulla and Hamadah (1970) have put forward the hypothesis that depressive illness is due to a fall in cyclic AMP concentrations in the cells of all tissues, including the brain. Paul *et al.* (1970a) had reported similar results in a group of manic patients. However, in further studies (Paul *et al.,* 1970b, 1970c) it was reported that in the manic group the urinary volume was consistently higher than in normal or depressed groups, and that if the cyclic AMP excretion was expressed in concentration values the difference between the manic and the control groups was not significant.

It has been suggested that the variations in urinary cyclic AMP output during different phases of affective illness may be due to changes in motor activity. Eccleston *et al.,* (1970), in a study with three normal volunteers, found that exercise increases the 24-hour excretion of cyclic AMP. They found that this increase was not related to changes in the volume of urine. However, Murad and Park (1972) did not see an increase in cyclic AMP urinary output in normals due to exercise, and Paul *et al.* (1971) did not observe any elevation in daily cyclic AMP excretion in agitated psychotically depressed patients. They also found no difference between the amount of cyclic AMP excreted by ten hyperkinetic children and by an age-matched group of normal controls. Furthermore, after physical activity in seven normal subjects they saw no significant difference between the pre- and post-excercise output of urinary cyclic AMP.

It has been also reported that in patients with manic-depressive illness there is a marked elevation of urinary cyclic AMP excretion on the same day of switch from a depressed into a manic state (Paul et al., 1971). The increase in cyclic AMP output was not accompanied by a similar increase in urinary volume, and consequently there was a significant increase in urinary concentration of the cyclic nucleotide. In this study they observed that in five out of seven episodes the cyclic AMP output decreased after the initial increase on the switch day. Only in a subgroup of patients did the post-switch values remain elevated during all the manic episode, although in a previous study Paul et al. (1970c) had reported higher urinary output of cyclic AMP in all manic patients studied. It is interesting, although it may require further confirmation, that a significant reduction has been observed in urinary excretion of cyclic AMP in manic patients who improved under lithium therapy (Paul et al., 1970b).

In order to determine if urinary cyclic AMP excretion may reflect changes in cyclic AMP metabolism in the central nervous system, Robison et al. (1970) measured the concentrations of cyclic AMP in the cerebrospinal fluid of several patients with affective disorders. No differences were observed between manic and depressive patients. This study does not offer any support for the idea of a correlation between urinary cyclic AMP excretion and central nervous system activity.

C. Lithium effects on brain cyclic AMP

An interaction of lithium with the brain adenylate cyclase system has been observed by several authors. Dousa and Hechter (1970b) reported that concentrations of lithium between 25 and 50 mM inhibited fluoride-stimulated adenylate cyclase activity in rabbit brain. They did not report the effect of lower concentrations of lithium. Forn and Valdecasas (1971) observed that concentrations of lithium as low as 2 mM produced a small but significant inhibition of NaF-activated adenylate cyclase of rabbit and rat cerebral homogenates.

Norepinephrine is the neurotransmitter that induces the greatest formation of cyclic AMP in incubated slices of rat cerebral cortex, while histamine is the most potent inducer in slices of rabbit cerebral cortex. Forn and Valdecasas (1971) also observed that low concentrations of lithium inhibited significantly the norepinephrine and histamine induced accumulation of cyclic AMP in rat and rabbit cerebral cortex slices. Uzunoff and Weiss (1972) later reported similar results in rat brain stem slices. They observed that concentrations of lithium of 5 mM completely abolished the accumulation of cyclic AMP induced by norepinephrine. This result indicates that brain stem adenylate cyclase may be more sensitive to the inhibitory effect of lithium than cerebral cortex adenylate cyclase. Uzunoff and Weiss (1972) have also made studies *in vivo*, and they have found that a dose of lithium of 4 mmol/kg administered intraperitoneally in rats 15 and 2 hours before decapitation completely blocks the rise of cyclic AMP in cerebellum that occurs immediately after decapitation.

Schimmer (1971) obtained completely different results in cultured glial tumor cells. He observed that lithium increases epinephrine-sensitive adenylate cyclase activity. The different functions of neuronal and glial cells may account for these discrepancies.

III. Thyroid

The interference of lithium with human thyroid physiology is well known (see Chapter 27). Chronic lithium administration produces a reversible goiter in a small percentage of patients (Schou *et al.*, 1968). Significantly elevated levels of TSH have been observed in about 30% of the lithium-treated patients (Emerson *et al.*, 1973). Lower serum protein-bound iodine and free thyroxine in the lithium treated patients were also observed (Cooper and Simpson, 1969), and with less frequency there is clinical evidence of hypothyroidism (Shopson, 1970). The reduced serum thyroxine and the elevated serum TSH levels suggest that lithium blocks the TSH-induced release of thyroxine from the thyroid gland.

A. Cyclic AMP and thyroid function

It has been demonstrated that the release of thyroid hormone induced by TSH is mediated by cyclic AMP. TSH stimulates adenylate cyclase in thyroid membrane preparations (Klainer *et al.*, 1962; Pastan and Katzen, 1962) and also increases the levels of cyclic AMP in thyroid gland slices (Gilman and Rall, 1968). In this study it was also observed that theophylline, a phosphodiesterase inhibitor, potentiates the TSH effect on cyclic AMP formation. Moreover, cyclic AMP and its dibutyryl derivative, when added to thyroid slices incubated *in vitro*, promote the formation of coloid droplets and an increase in thyroid hormone release (Dumont *et al.*, 1971).

B. Lithium effects on thyroid cyclic AMP

Lithium strongly inhibits the TSH-stimulated adenylate cyclase activity. With beef thyroid membrane preparations, Wolff *et al.* (1970) obtained a 50% reduction in the TSH effects with lithium concentrations from 4 to 8 mM. A competition between lithium and magnesium was observed. When 5 mM magnesium was present, a 30 mM concentration of lithium was required to obtain a 50% inhibition. The inhibitory effect was quite specific for lithium, other monovalent ions having much weaker inhibitory effects. Lithium did not modify the basal adenylate cyclase activity, and much higher lithium concentrations were required to inhibit the fluoride-stimulated adenylate cyclase activity.

Considering that lithium concentrations in the thyroid gland may be 2 to 3 times higher than in plasma (Berens *et al.*, 1970a), these results might explain the inhibitory effects of lithium on thyroid function. However, some other TSH-dependent functions of the thyroid gland, like glucose oxidation (Berens *et al.*, 1971) and iodine uptake (Berens *et al.*, 1970b) were stimulated by chronic lithium treatment. This indicates that lithium may also affect iodine metabolism at some points that are not dependent on cyclic AMP formation.

IV. Kidney

A. Lithium effects on the kidney

It has been frequently reported, since the first observation by Schou (1958), that polydipsia and polyuria may appear during treatment with lithium. Some effects of lithium on electrolyte metabolism may be explained by partial substitution of lithium for sodium or potassium in renal transport mechanisms. However, the polyuria that has been observed in patients and animals treated with lithium is most probably related to an inhibition of the effect of ADH on the kidney (Singer *et al.*, 1972; Ramsey *et al.*, 1972; Lee, 1971). ADH controls the osmolarity of the plasma by increasing the permeability of the collecting ducts to water. In the absence of ADH the collecting ducts are impermeable to water. In this situation, water cannot flow to the hyperosmolar region of the kidney medulla and a polyuria appears. The ADH-induced water flow can be observed also in the toad urinary bladder. While in the mammalian kidney ADH controls only water transport, in the toad bladder it also stimulates sodium transport.

The intravenous infusion of lithium inhibits the antidiuretic action of ADH in rats (Harris and Jenner, 1972). Also, an acute infusion of lithium in rats causes an inhibition of the effect of ADH on urine osmolality (Torp-Pedersen and Thorn, 1973). This effect is very specific for the lithium ion, since similar concentrations of potassium, rubidium, strontium, magnesium and calcium had no effect.

The polyuria induced by lithium in patients is refractory to doses of ADH that are effective for the treatment of diabetes insipidus (Ramsey *et al.*, 1972). Studies in lithium-treated polyuric patients have shown that these patients have no abnormalities of sodium transport, although they have an impaired capacity to reabsorb solute-free water and do not respond to exogenous ADH (Singer *et al.*, 1972).

At very low concentrations (0·7 mM), lithium inhibits the basal short-circuit current in toad urinary bladder; at higher concentrations (11 mM) lithium inhibits also the short-circuit current responses to ADH (Singer *et al.*, 1972). These concentrations are in the range of those found in the urine of lithium-treated patients (Trautner *et al.*, 1955). Lithium effects are greater when lithium is applied to the mucosal surface of the toad bladder, which may indicate that in man the urinary levels of lithium may be more important than the blood levels in the production of nephrogenic diabetes insipidus. (See also Chapter 28.)

B. Cyclic AMP and kidney function

Experimental evidence supports the view that cyclic AMP serves as a mediator of the action of ADH (Orloff and Handler, 1967). It has been observed that cyclic AMP and theophylline, similarly to ADH, increase water flow in the isolated perfused rabbit collecting tubules (Grantham and Burg, 1966). More recently it has been shown that in the mammalian kidney there are two different hormone-sensitive adenylate cyclases. One is located in the kidney cortex, and is stimulated by parathyroid hormone, and the other is located in the kidney medulla and is specifically stimulated by ADH (Chase and Aurbach, 1968).

Strong evidence for cyclic AMP as a mediator of ADH effect has been obtained in the toad bladder. Cyclic AMP levels increase in this tissue following incubation with ADH (Handler et al., 1965). Furthermore, the effects of ADH on water flow and sodium transport can be mimicked when cyclic AMP or theophylline are applied to the serosal surface of the toad bladder (Orloff and Handler, 1967).

C. Lithium effects on kidney cyclic AMP

Lithium does not modify the cyclic AMP-induced water flow in the toad bladder (Singer et al., 1972). This suggests that lithium prevents in some way the formation of cyclic AMP. This is supported by the finding that lithium, at a 25 mM concentration, and in the presence of 150 mM sodium chloride, exerts a significant inhibitory influence on ADH-stimulated adenylate cyclase on the kidney medulla (Dousa and Hechter, 1970a). Since lithium accumulates in the kidney medulla, these results might have physiological significance.

It has also been reported that in kidneys of rats made polyuric by chronic administration of lithium chloride there is a diminished ADH-sensitive adenylate cyclase activity (Geisler et al., 1972). In these experiments, there was no detectable lithium during the assay of the adenylate cyclase activity of kidney homogenates, and the results observed must be the consequence of some interaction of lithium with the kidney during the pretreatment of the animals.

Although these data support an effect of lithium at the level of the formation of cyclic AMP in the kidney, the possibility has been raised that lithium-induced polyuria might be due to some other factor. For instance, Forrest et al (1971) have reported that lithium blocks the cyclic AMP effect on urine osmolarity in rats. This would indicate that lithium interacts with the action of ADH at a site beyond the production of cyclic AMP. Different results have been obtained in experiments using toad bladder, in which the cyclic AMP effect was not blocked by lithium (Singer et al., 1972).

V. Other Tissues

Lithium has some effects on the cyclic AMP system of other tissues. These effects are in most cases of small intensity, and it has not been demonstrated that they have any physiological of pharmacological implication, as far as the therapeutic effects of lithium are concerned.

For example, Birnbaumer et al. (1969) found that lithium, at 100 mM, inhibits fluoride- and ACTH-stimulated adenylate cyclase activity in fat cell ghosts by 35% and 52%, respectively, while it stimulated basal activity by 36%.

It has been reported that in the isolated perfused guinea pig heart, lithium, at a concentration 10 mM, significantly decreases the positive inotropic effect induced by norepinephrine and isoproterenol (Frazer et al., 1972). Since a great deal of experimental evidence suggests that the positive inotropic response to catecholamines is mediated by an increase in the intracellular level of cyclic AMP (Murad et al., 1962; Robison et al., 1967), it is possible that the above described effect of lithium on the heart is mediated by interference with cyclic AMP formation.

Prostaglandins stimulate adenylate cyclase activity in platelets, both in intact and in broken cell preparations (Wolfe and Shulman, 1969). It has been reported that in platelets obtained from patients under chronic lithium treatment, with serum lithium levels between $0 \cdot 9$ mM and $1 \cdot 5$ mM, there was a 50% reduction of the prostaglandin E_1-induced formation of cyclic AMP when compared to controls (Murphy et al., 1973). The norepinephrine-induced reversal of the prostaglandin stimulation was also inhibited significantly in the platelets from the lithium treated group of patients. In acute experiments in vitro, greater concentrations of lithium were required to produce a similar inhibition of prostaglandin-induced cyclic AMP formation. This study is interesting because it suggests that the effects of chronic lithium administration on other systems may be greater than the results of experiments in vitro might indicate.

Katz et al. (1968) have shown that lithium, at concentrations as low as $1 \cdot 2$ and $2 \cdot 4$ mM, decreases the amount of norepinephrine and serotonin released from brain slices in response to electrical stimulation. It has been found also that lithium, at a dose of $1 \cdot 2$ m mole/kg, modifies the metabolism of intracisternally injected norepinephrine (Schildkraut et al., 1966). A decrease in 0-methylated metabolites and a simultaneous increase in deaminated metabolites suggests that less norepinephrine is released in active form. The norepinephrine release in response to nerve stimulation of isolated spleens is also significantly reduced by the addition of 4 mM lithium to the perfusion medium (Bindler et al., 1971). The mechanism by which lithium inhibits the release of biogenic amines is unknown. However, it has recently been shown that cyclic AMP is involved in the mechanism of release of norepinephrine in several sympathetic nerve endings (Peach, 1972. Wooten *et al.*, 1973). We might therefore speculate that lithium interferes with transmitter release through an inhibition of cyclic AMP formation. This is at this point merely an hypothesis that will require further studies.

VI. Discussion

The finding that lithium inhibits the hormone-induced formation of cyclic AMP in several tissues seems to provide a unique mechanism of action for some therapeutic and toxic effects of lithium. However, two important points must be kept in mind. First, lithium, as a partial substitute for sodium and potassium, alters the normal electrolyte balance and may modify the ionic environment necessary for some metabolic or enzymatic activities and interfere with functions of the cell that are not cyclic AMP-mediated. Second, concentrations of lithium similar to the ones that can be reached during lithium treatment of patients, produce, in the most favorable cases, only a small inhibition of adenylate cyclase activity in broken cells and of cyclic AMP accumulation in intact cells; we do not know with certainty if this small impairment of cyclic AMP formation is of physiological significance.

Lithium has many physical and chemical properties similar to sodium and potassium (see Chapter 21). Lithium may cross all cell boundaries, but since it cannot substitute completely for sodium or potassium, one potential mechanism of action for lithium in intact cells may be its interference with the fine regulation of intracellular and extracellular ionic concentrations. However, lithium modifies cyclic AMP formation not only in intact cells, but also in homogenates. Due to its special physicochemical characteristics, such as high water solubility and high ionization potential, lithium might affect the properties of complex organic molecules, changing their conformation and biological properties. In this way lithium might modify the intimate structure of cell membranes, and alter subsequently the activity of the membrane-bound adenylate cyclase.

It is commonly accepted that adenylate cyclase has at least two components: a regulatory or receptor sub-unit, with tissue specificity for different hormones, and a catalytic sub-unit activated through the regulatory sub-unit (Perkins, 1973). The fact that lithium blocks the adenylate cyclase activity of different tissues, as well as the fluoride-stimulated adenylate cyclase activity in broken cells preparations, suggests that lithium acts at the level of the catalytic sub-unit.

Adenylate cyclase activity requires the presence of magnesium and, due to some chemical similarities between lithium and magnesium, a possible competitive action between the two might be considered. This possibility has not been well investigated, although it has been found that lithium competes with magnesium in the activation of thyroid membranes by TSH.

Much speculation about the mode of action of lithium in mania has involved its effects on catecholamine metabolism in the brain. The so-called "catechol-amine hypothesis" of affective disorders (Schildkraut, 1965. Schildkraut *et al.*, 1967) predicts that drugs such as imipramine and monoamine oxidase inhi-bitors, which increase functional free norepinephrine in the brain, will be effective in the treatment of depressed patients, while drugs like reserpine, which decrease brain norepinephrine, will cause sedation and even clinical depression. It has already been mentioned that lithium increases the intraneuronal inactiva-tion of norepinephrine and decreases the levels of functionally active norepinephrine available to adrenergic receptors; it also decreases the amount of norepinephrine released by electrical stimulation of brain slices and by nerve stimulation of the spleen. It has been postulated that norepinephrine release is cyclic AMP-mediated, and although it has not been proved, there is a possibi-lity that lithium inhibits norepinephrine release by interfering with cyclic AMP formation at presynaptic level. At the postsynaptic level it has been shown that lithium blocks the norepinephrine-induced accumulation of cyclic AMP in rat brain slices. Although the mechanism of action of lithium in mania cannot be determined at the present moment, all these various effects tend to decrease the noradrenergic tone in the brain and may very well account for the efficacy of lithium in manic states.

Several publications have tried to relate changes in cyclic AMP excretion with mania. These studies are controversial, since it is doubtful that urinary cyclic AMP concentration may reflect any change in the cyclic nucleotide metabolism in the brain. First of all, cyclic AMP is not lipid soluble and does not easily cross cell membranes or the blood-brain barrier. It has been shown that there is no difference in cerebrospinal fluid cyclic AMP concentration between depressed and manic patients. Also, in several of the published papers, although there is an increased output of urinary cyclic AMP in mania, this is accompanied by an increase in volume without any change in the urinary concentration of the cyclic nucleotide. In normal subjects, only 15% of the total plasma cyclic AMP is eliminated by the kidney, and about one third of the total urinary cyclic AMP is formed by the kidney itself (Broadus *et al.*, 1969). The relatively minor role played by renal excretion makes it less likely that changes in urinary cyclic AMP reflect changes in brain cyclic AMP metabolism. Furthermore, the urinary excretion of cyclic AMP is influenced by several hormones. The parenteral administration of parathyroid hormone causes a marked increase in urinary cyclic AMP excretion in rats and humans (Chase and Aurbach, 1967). Glucagon also increases urinary cyclic AMP excretion in man (Broadus *et al.*, 1969). Even physical exercise may increase urinary cyclic AMP excretion, and this might be an important factor in the variations observed in manic patients, although such an increase after exercise has been observed by other authors.

Lithium affects the adenylate cyclase system of several other tissues. Its effects on the thyroid and on the kidney have been more extensively studied. In both cases a significant inhibition of cyclic AMP formation has been observed at lithium concentrations that can be reached in patients under lithium treatment. However, some effects of lithium on the thyroid are not cyclic AMP-dependent, suggesting that lithium may interfere with the thyroid gland at more than one site. The possibility has been discussed that lithium affects the ADH effect on the kidney at a point beyond the formation of cyclic AMP, although the evidence is stronger in support of an effect by inhibition of the kidney adenylate cyclase.

References

Abdulla, Y. H. and Hamadah, K. (1970). *Lancet* 1, 378–381.

Berens, S. C., Wolff, J. and Murphy, D. L. (1970a). *Endocrinology* 87, 1085–1087.

Berens, S. C., Bernstein, R. S., Robbins, J. and Wolff, J. (1970b). *J. clin. Invest.* 49, 1357–1367.

Berens, S. C., Williams, J. A. and Wolff, J. (1971). *Biochim. biophys. Acta* 252, 314–323.

Bindler, E. H., Wallach, M. B. and Gershon, S. (1971). *Archs Int. Pharmacodyn.* 190, 150–154.

Birnbaumer, J., Pohl, S. L. and Rodbell, M. (1969) *J. biol. Chem.* 224, 3468–3476.

Broadus, A. E., Northcutt, R. C., Hardman, J. G., Kaminsky, N. I., Sutherland, E. W. and Liddle, G. W. (1969). *Clin. Res.* 17, 65–72.

Chase, L. R. and Aurbach, G. D. (1967). *Proc. natn. Acad. Sci. U.S.A.* 58, 518–522.

Chase, L. R. and Aurbach, G. D. (1968). *Science* 159, 545–547.

Cooper, T. B. and Simpson, G. M. (1969). *Curr. ther. Res.* 11, 603–608.

De Robertis, E., De Lores Arnaiz, G. R., Alberici, M., Butcher, R. W. and Sutherland, E. W. (1967). *J. biol. Chem.* 242, 3487–3493.

Dousa, T. and Hechter, O. (1970a). *Life Sci.* 9, 765–770.

Dousa, T. and Hechter, O. (1970b). *Lancet* 1, 834–835.

Dumont, J. E., Willems, C., Van Sande, J., Neve, P. (1971). *Ann. N. Y. Acad. Sci.* 185, 291–316.

Eccleston, D., Loose, R., Pullar, I. A. and Sugden, R. F. (1970). *Lancet* 2, 1028–1029.

Emerson, C. H., Dyson, W. L. and Utiger, R. D. (1973). *J. clin. Endocrinol. Metab.* 36, 338–346.

Florendo, N. T., Barnett, R. J. and Grengard, P. (1971). *Science,* 173, 745–748.

Forn, J. and Krishna, G. (1970). *Pharmacology* 5, 193–204.

Forn, J. and Valdecasas, F. G. (1971). *Biochem. Pharmacol.* 20, 2773–2779.

Forrest, J. N. Jr., Cohen, A. D., Torreti, J. and Epstein, F. H. (1971). *J. clin. Invest.* 50, 32a–33a.

Frazer, A., Hancock, A., Mendels, J. and MacIntire, R. (1972). *Biol. Psychiat.* 5, 79–86.

Geisler, A., Wraae, O. and Olesen, O. V. (1972). *Acta Pharmacol. Toxicol.* 31, 203–208.

Gessa, G. L., Krishna, G., Forn, J., Tagliamonte, A. and Brodie, B. B. (1970). *In* "Advances in Biochemical Psychopharmacology" (P. Greengard and E. Costa, eds.), Vol. 3. pp. 371–381, Raven press, New York.

Gilman, A. G. and Nirenberg, M. (1971a) *Nature* 234, 356–358.

Gilman, A. G. and Nirenberg, M. (1971b). *Proc. natn. Acad. Sci. U.S.A.* 68, 2165–2168.

Gilman, A. G. and Rall, T. W. (1968). *J. biol. Chem.* **243,** 5867–5871.

Grantham, J. J. and Burg, M. B. (1966). *Amer. J. Physiol.* **211,** 255–259.

Greengard, P. and Robison, G. A. (eds.), (1973). *In* "Advances in Cyclic Nucleotide Research). Vol 3. Raven Press, New York.

Handler, J. S., Butcher, R. W., Sutherland, E. W. and Orloff, J. (1965). *J. biol. Chem.* **240,** 4524–4526.

Harris, C. A. and Jenner, F. A. (1972) *Brit. J. Pharmacol.* **44,** 223–232.

Hoffer, B. J., Siggins, G. R., Oliver, A. P. and Bloom, F. E. (1972). *In* "Advances in Cyclic Nucleotide Research". (P. Greengard, R. Paoletti and G. A. Robison, eds.), Vol. 1, pp. 411–423, Raven Press, New York.

Kakiuchi, S. and Rall, T. W. (1968a). *Mol. Pharmacol.* **4,** 367–378.

Kakiuchi, S. and Rall, T. W. (1968b). *Mol. Pharmacol.* **4,** 379–388.

Kakiuchi, S., Rall, T. W. and McIlwain, H. (1969). *J. Neurochem.* **16,** 485-491.

Katz, R. I., Chase, T. N. and Kopin, I. J. (1968). *Science* **162,** 466–467.

Klainer, L. M., Chi, Y. M., Freidberg, S. L., Rall, T. W. and Sutherland, E. W. (1962). *J. biol. Chem.* **237,** 1239–1243.

Lee, R. V., Jampol, L. M. and Brown, W. V. (1971) *New Engl. J. Med.* **284,** 93–94.

McAfee, O. A. and Greengard, P. (1972). *Science* **178,** 310–312.

Murad, F. and Park, C.Y.C. (1972). *New Engl. J. Med.* **286,** 1382–1387.

Murad, F., Chi, Y. M., Rall, T. W. and Sutherland, E. W. (1962). *J. biol. Chem.* **237,** 1233–1238.

Murphy, D. L., Donnelly, C. and Moskowitz, J. (1963). *Clin. Pharmac. Therapeut.* **14,** 810–814.

Orloff, J. and Handler, J. S. (1967). *Amer. J. Med.* **42,** 757–768.

Pastan, I. and Katzen, R. (1962). *Biochem. biophys. Res. Comm.* **29,** 792–798.

Paul, M. I., Ditzion, B. R. and Janowski, D. S. (1970a). *Lancet* **1,** 88.

Paul, M. I., Cramer, H. and Goodwin, F. K. (1970b) *Lancet* **1,** 996.

Paul, M. I., Ditzion, B. R., Pauk, G. L., and Janowski, D. S. (1970c). *Amer. J. Psychiat.* **126,** 1493–1497.

Paul, M. I., Cramer, H. and Bunney, W. E. (1971). *Science* **171,** 300–303.

Peach, M. J. (1972). *Proc. natn. Acad. Sci. U.S.A.* **69,** 834–836.

Perkins, J. P. (1973). *In* "Advances in Cyclic Nucleotide Research". (P. Greengard and J. A. Robison, eds.). Vol. 3. pp. 1–64, Raven Press, New York.

Ramsey, T. A., Mendels, J., Stokes, J. W. and Fitzgerald, R. G. (1972). *J. Amer. med. Ass.* **219,** 1446–1449.

Robison, G. A., Butcher, R. W. and Sutherland, E. W. (1967). *Ann. N.Y. Acad. Sci.* **139,** 703–723.

Robison, G. A., Coppen, A. J., Whybrow, P. C. and Prange, A. J. (1970). *Lancet* **2,** 1028–1029.

Robison, G. A., Butcher, R. W. and Sutherland, E. W. (1971). *In* "Cyclic AMP", Academic Press, New York and London.

Schildkraut, J. J. (1965). *Amer. J. Psychiat.* **122,** 509–522.

Schildkraut, J. J., Schanberg, S. M. and Kopin, I. J. (1966). *Life Sci.* **5,** 1479–1483.

Schildkraut, J. J., Schanberg, S. M., Breese, G. R. and Kopin, I. J. (1967). *Amer. J. Psychiat.* **124,** 600–608.

Schimmer, B. P. (1971). *Biochim. biophys. Acta* **252,** 567–573.

Schou, M. (1958). *Acta Pharmacol. Toxicol* **15,** 70–84.

Schou, M., Amdisen, A., Jensen, S. E. and Olsen, T. (1968). *Brit. med. J.* **3,** 710–713.

Shimizu, H., Creveling, C. R. and Daly, J. W. (1970). *J. Neurochem.* **17,** 441–444.

Shimizu, H., Creveling, C. R. and Daly, J. W. (1972). *Mol. Pharmacol.* **6,** 184–188.

Shopsin, B. (1970). *Dis. nerv. Syst.* **31**, 237–244.

Singer, I., Rotenberg, D. and Puschett, J. B. (1972). *J. clin. Invest.* **51**, 1081–1091.

Sutherland, E. W. (1972). *Science* **177**, 401–408.

Sutherland, E. W. and Rall, T. W. (1958). *J. biol. Chem.* **232**, 1077–1091.

Sutherland, E. W., Rall, T. W. and Menon, P. (1962). *J. biol. Chem.* **237**, 1220–1227.

Torp-Pedersen, C. and Thorn, N. A. (1973). *Acta Endocrinol.* **73**, 665–671.

Trautner, E. M., Morris, R., Noack, C. H. and Gershon, S. (1955). *Med. J. Aust.* **42**, 280–291.

Uzunoff, P. and Weiss, B. (1972). *In* "Advances in Cyclic Nucleotide Research", (P. Greengard, R. Paoletti and G. A. Robison, eds.) vol. 1, pp. 435–453, Raven Press, New York.

Wolfe, S. M. and Shulman, N. R. (1969). *Biochem. biophys. Res. Commun.* **35**, 265–272.

Wolff, J., Berens, S. C. and Jones, A. B. (1970). *Biochem. biophys. Res. Commun.* **39**, 77–82.

Wooten, G. F., Thos, N. B., Kopin, I. J. and Axelrod, J. (1973). *Mol. Pharmacol.* **9**, 178–183.

30

THE EFFECTS OF LITHIUM ON ORGANIC ACID EXCRETION

P. A. BOND and F. A. JENNER

I. Introduction

As there is, as yet, no clear and unequivocal explanation of how lithium ions achieve their therapeutic effects, studies of their influence on almost all aspects of metabolism have stimulated interest. One very clear effect which lithium ions have is to increase the renal excretion of 2-oxoglutarate and other dicarboxylic acids with a chain length of C_4 to C_6. As some of these metabolites are involved in the Krebs' tricarboxylic acid cycle of the final aerobic metabolism of carbohydrates and other metabolites, a possible action of lithium ions through this aspect of cellular energy metabolism has been sought.

The studies which have been carried out to date on this subject have tended to emphasize renal rather than cerebral effects, although, as will be discussed later, there is some suggestion that the renal studies may turn out to be analogues of investigations involving the nervous system (Jenner, 1973; Bailey et al., 1974).

II. The Range of Organic Acids Affected

In both normal and manic-depressive persons it has been shown (Bond et al., 1972) that following the establishment of measurable blood levels of lithium there is an acute (within minutes) increase in the urinary levels of 2-oxoglutarate and glutarate, but not of citrate, pyruvate nor lactate. Lee and Pollitt (1973) subsequently undertook an investigation of the effects of lithium administration on excretion rates of a range of dicarboxylic acids to provide a better basis for interpreting the phenomenon. They obtained complete urine collections from four patients undergoing lithium therapy and obtained metabolic profiles of the urinary acids by gas–liquid chromatography. The profiles were very complex and in the region of 70 distinct peaks were observed on the records. In their study, Lee and Pollitt concentrated on methylmalonate, succinate, glutarate, adipate, pimelate and suberate. Comparisons of urine collected on three days prior to lithium treatment with that collected on three days during treatment revealed increases in excretory rates of succinate, glutarate and adipate which were statistically highly significant. An increase in malate excretion was also noted. A modification in the analytic procedure showed that lithium treatment led to a four-fold increase in excreted fumarate; discontinuation of lithium treatment was followed by a return of the fumarate excretion levels to pretreatment values.

III. Lithium-Induced Alkalosis: A Contributory Factor?

The initial period of lithium administration in therapeutic doses leads to the production of alkaline urine due to an increased excretion of bicarbonate ions; this lasts for 24 hours and is associated with a natriuresis and increased urine volume. Alkalosis alone is known to increase organic acid excretion in man and animals (Jenner, 1973) but the observed lithium-induced elevation of 2-oxoglutarate excretion is not a simple response to the changing alkalinity since under conditions of alkalosis there is usually a much greater rise of citrate than of 2-oxoglutarate excretion (Crawford *et al.*, 1959), the reverse of the situation noted following lithium administration.

In this respect it is also of some interest to note that there is little evidence in studies with snail giant neurones and in studies of red blood cells with 5,5-dimethyl-2,4,oxazolidinedione that lithium affects intracellular pH (S. MacNeil personal communication). Hence, neither urinary nor intracellular changes of acid-base equilibrium explain the changes of organic acid excretion.

Bond *et al.* (1972) demonstrated a dissociation between 2-oxoglutarate excretion rates and the urinary levels of bicarbonate ions which also argues against an explanation of changes in organic acid excretion in terms of a response to alkalosis. They noted that the amount of 2-oxoglutarate excreted showed a gradual increase over several months of lithium treatment, although it bore a close relationship to the amount of lithium also excreted, and on cessation of treatment both lithium and 2-oxoglutarate excretion rates fell together with similar timing. In contrast, the bicarbonate excretion rate was raised only on the first day of treatment, thereafter returning to control values and maintaining an equilibrium state (as indicated by a compensatory fall in bicarbonate excretion on the day after cessation of lithium treatment).

Recent work by Bond and Hill (personal communication) on the effect of chronic administration of lithium in food on levels of 2-oxoglutarate and citrate in kidney clearly distinguishes the effect of this ion from that due to alkalosis. In chronic alkalosis citrate levels are elevated in both kidney and liver, while in acidosis there is a fall (Adler *et al.*, 1971) and levels of 2-oxoglutarate in kidney have been shown to fall in chronic metabolic acidosis (Alleyne, 1968), though no levels in alkalosis were given. In contrast, chronic lithium administration (for 2 days, 2, 4 and 6 weeks) consistently produces lowered levels of both 2-oxoglutarate and citrate in kidney.

The effect of lithium on organic acid excretion is not, therefore, easily explained in terms of hydrogen ion changes.

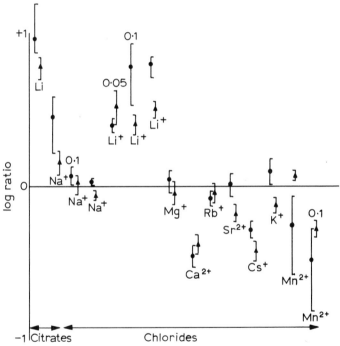

FIG. 1. *Acute effects of intraperitoneal injections on 2-oxoglutarate excretion.* 2-Oxoglutarate was measured in rat urine during the 3h preceding intraperitoneal injection of the salts and for 3h after the injection. Animals received 0·2 mEq of the cation unless another value is quoted. The lines represent the log of the mean ratio ±S.E.M. of the 2-oxoglutarate excretions before and after the injection, presented in terms of grams excreted (●) and of concentration (▲). (Reproduced from Jenner (1973), with permission.)

IV. Comparisons with the Effects of Other Cations

There is evidence that the increase in organic acid excretion which follows lithium administration is not a response to the presence of metallic cations in general, but that it is an effect which is specific to lithium ions as such.

Bond and Jenner (1974) have reported a study in which rats were injected with 0·2 mmol of the chloride or citrate of lithium or other ions, the injections being given intraperitoneally. Urine levels of 2-oxoglutarate and citrate were measured in the 3-hour period before injection and compared with the levels in the 3-hour post-injection period. It was found that whilst, like humans, the rats showed clear increases in the excretion of 2-oxoglutarate (both in absolute amounts and as measured as concentrations) after lithium treatment, they did not show comparable increases after the administration of the chlorides of sodium, rubidium, caesium, manganese, magnesium, potassium or strontium. Small diurnal increases were noted as well as an increase caused by sodium citrate, but this latter probably arose as a result of alkalosis. Manganese ions were generally toxic to the animals but the animals' behaviour and general condition seemed relatively unaffected by the other ions. Caesium, calcium and (though to a lesser extent) rubidium decreased 2-oxoglutarate excretion, an effect in the opposite direction to that observed with lithium. Figure 1 summarises the findings. Under the conditions of this study only lithium and magnesium ions were found in the urine as a significant proportion of the injected dose, but any suggestion that the effects of these ions might have been due to their presence in the kidney or urine can be discounted in view of subsequent studies in which rubidium and caesium were administered chronically in the food until they attained similar urinary excretion levels to those in rats on a lithium diet—the 2-oxoglutarate excretion levels were still suppressed by the rubidium and caesium (see Table I). Caesium and rubidium also reduce the renal excretion of citrate, as does calcium.

The rat is somewhat different from man in relying more strikingly on organic acids than on bicarbonate to control the urine pH, and this, together with a greater tendency for rats to show increases in citrate excretion following lithium administration, may to some extent limit the suitability of the rat as a model for understanding lithium affects in humans. Bond and Jenner (1974) do, however, demonstrate that even in the rat the effects on 2-oxoglutarate are more striking than are those on citrate.

V. Changes in Tissue Levels of Organic Acids

In addition to modifications in excretion rates, there have been reports of changes in the level of certain organic acids and associated enzymes in various body tissues. Krulík and Zvolsky (1970) reported significant increases of tissue levels of 2-oxoglutarate and pyruvate in rats after 7 days of lithium chloride administration. Other studies (Bond and Hill, personal communication), in

TABLE I. Urinary Excretion of 2-Oxoglutarate and Citrate and Titratable Acidity in Rats Given Lithium, Sodium, Rubidium or Caesium in the Diet.

Ion	Urine levels of administered ion (mEq/24 h)	Mean pH	Mean titratable acidity (mEq)	2-Oxoglutarate		Citrate		
				Conc. (mg/ml)	Amount (mg/sample)	Conc. (mg/ml)	Amount (mg/sample)	Urine vol. (ml)
Li	0·390 ± 0·021(48)	6·78 ± 0·049(24)	0·097 ± 0·011	1·63 ± 0·12	6·14 ± 0·68	2·05 ± 0·10	8·80 ± 0·46	4·5 ± 0·3
Na		6·88 ± 0·063(24)	0·069 ± 0·008	0·73 ± 0·063	2·60 ± 0·17	1·89 ± 0·10	7·08 ± 0·27	4·3 ± 0·2
Cs	0·272 ± 0·012(40)	6·84 ± 0·047(20)	0·100 ± 0·013	0·09 ± 0·011	0·34 ± 0·031	0·24 ± 0·03	0·95 ± 0·14	4·7 ± 0·4
Rb	0·500 ± 0·017(40)	6·72 ± 0·032(20)	0·136 ± 0·013	0·096 ± 0·009	0·37 ± 0·034	0·27 ± 0·04	1·11 ± 0·14	4·7 ± 0·20

Sodium chloride was administered at 0·33 mEq/day for 17 days to six animals. Lithium chloride at 0·35 mEq/day for 24 days to six animals. Rubidium chloride at 0·41 mEq/day for 31 days to five animals. Caesium chloride at 0·46 mEq/day for 45 days to five animals. Values are given with their s.e. mean. At this stage the excretion of the administered ion appeared constant and each animal was studied for six consecutive days. Where appropriate results are per 3 hours. (Reproduced from Bond and Jenner (1974) with permission.)

which lithium chloride was administered in the diet over varying periods from 2 days to 6 weeks, have shown marked effects on the levels of citrate and 2-oxoglutarate in kidney. Citrate levels were lowered by 45% after two days, thereafter increasing steadily to be only 14% below the controls after 6 weeks. 2-Oxoglutarate showed a maximum drop (45–53%) after two weeks, thereafter increasing to 12% (not significantly different) below control values. No consistent changes were seen in lactate, pyruvate or malate. In the liver there were no significant effects of lithium on levels of 2-oxoglutarate or citrate. It seems that while the urinary excretion of 2-oxoglutarate (and citrate in the rat) remains elevated for an indefinite period during lithium treatment, tissue levels revert gradually towards normal levels, suggesting the existence of some homeostatic mechanism.

Administration (for 2 weeks) of rubidium, the salts of which have been reported to have opposite behavioural effects to lithium (Carroll and Sharp, 1971), also produced opposite effects on levels of 2-oxoglutarate and citrate in kidney. 2-oxogluturate was elevated by 89% in the kidneys of rubidium-fed animals, as opposed to the 45% drop caused by lithium. In the liver also, rubidium produced a marked increase in levels of 2-oxoglutarate (76%) and citrate (89%) while lithium produced a small but insignificant decrease in levels of 2-oxoglutarate.

It has been claimed (King *et al.*, 1969) that lithium causes increased accumulation of lactate by mouse brains, and in other studies organic acid levels in brain tissue have been reported to change; thus increases in glutamate and γ-aminobutyric acid have been noted in the amygdaloid nucleus of rats (Gottesfeld *et al.*, 1971). On the other hand, glutamate decarboxylase levels of these limbic system structures have been reported not to change following lithium administration (Gottesfeld *et al.*, 1973) and when the lithium doses were large and acute the mouse brain glutamate levels may even show some decrease (DeFeudis and Delgado, 1970).

VI. Mechanisms

In view of the fact that no discernible changes occur in plasma 2-oxoglutarate concentrations after lithium administration, the increased excretion rates seem consistent with an inhibition of net renal tubular reabsorption. The increased excretion of glutarate and of succinate, adipate, fumarate, α-hydroxy-glutarate and 2-hydroxy-4-oxoglutarate more recently demonstrated by Lee and Pollitt (1973) after lithium administration may be seen as in accord with this view. Lee and Pollitt (1973) point out that the organic acids which show increased excretory rates following the administration of lithium are linked more by their chemical structures than by their metabolic relationships. This might therefore imply that the lithium action is upon an active transport mechanism which they share, rather than upon a metabolic process *per se* as they share no metabolic pathway. However, metabolic accumulation of some of the acids could over-load the common transport pathway for all of them. In this respect, however, it is interesting that the increased accumulation of lactate by mouse brain, which was noted by King *et al.* (1969), can be abolished by ouabain which is itself a classical inhibitor of ion transport mechanisms. In considering where ion transport mechanism might be clinically relevant attention is necessarily drawn to ion concentration by mitochondria but no clear information is as yet available to us concerning lithium effects on this system (see Chapter 33).

The fact that fumarate, succinate and 2-oxoglutarate, all sequential steps in the tricarboxylic acid cycle, are each excreted in increased amounts, but not citrate, pyruvate or lactate, means a direct effect of lithium ions on enzymic processes in the tricarboxylic acid cycle cannot be ruled out

There is also some other evidence for a lithium-induced interference with a stage in the tricarboxylic acid cycle. Berl and Clarke (1972) have reported differences in incorporation of ^{14}C-acetate and the distribution of the label among amino acids derived from tricarboxylic acid cycle. These results could be explained by assuming an inhibition of some stages of the Krebs cycle, but they too could equally well be explained by effects on transport mechanisms. A report by Abreu and Abreu (1972) of an increase in brain succinate dehydro-genase after 80 days treatment by adding lithium to drinking water has not proved possible to repeat in our laboratories; Abreu and Abreu used mouse brains, however, and our replicatory studies involved rat brains.

VII. Conclusion

At this stage the finding that changes in organic acid excretion rates follow lithium administration can only be looked upon as a possible clue, the signifi-cance to something of clinical relevance of which remains uncertain. The relationship between the renal excretory studies and other work, involving glutamate changes in the brain is still to be decided. The earlier findings by Berl and Clarke (1972) and by DeFeudis and Delgado (1970) that lithium ions tend to lead to a decrease in brain glutamate raise the possibility that the renal studies may be analogues of changes induced in the nervous system.

This is clearly an area of investigation which requires much more work, but reports such as that of Wiechert and Knaape (1972) on the cerebral activity of glutamate derivatives lead one to hope that future findings may possibly advance our knowledge of the way in which lithium affects brain and behaviour.

References

Abreu, L. A. and Abreu, R. R. (1972). *Nature New Biology* **236**, 254–255.
Adler, S., Anderson, B. and Zemotel, L. (1971). *Amer. J. Physiol.* **220**, 986–992.
Alleyne, G. A. O. (1968). *Nature* **217**, 847–848.
Bailey, E., Bond, P. A., Brooks, B. A., Dimitrakoudi, M., Jenner, F. A., Judd, A., Lee,

C. R., Lenton, E. A., MacNeil, S., Pollitt, R. J., Sampson, G. A. and Thompson, E. A. (1974). *Progress in Medicinal Chemistry* **2** (in press).

Berl, S. and Clarke, D. D. (1972). *Brain Res.* **36**, 203–213.

Bond, P. A., Jenner, F. A., Lee, C. R., Lenton, E., Pollitt, R. J. and Sampson, G. A. (1972). *Brit. J. Pharmacol.* **46**, 116–123.

Bond, P. A. and Jenner, F. A. (1974). *Brit. J. Pharmacol.* **50** (in press).

Carroll, B. J. and Sharp, P. T. (1971). *Science* **172**, 1355–1357.

Crawford, M. A., Milne, M. D. and Scribner, B. H. (1959). *J. Physiol.* **149**, 413–423.

DeFeudis, F. V. and Delgado, J. M. R. (1970). *Nature* **225**, 749–750.

Gottesfeld, Z., Ebstein, B. S. and Samuel, D. (1971). *Nature New Biology* **234**, 124–125.

Gottesfeld, Z., Samuel, D. and Icekson, U. (1973). *Experientia* **29**, 68–69.

Jenner, F. A. (1973). *Biochem. Soc. Trans.* **1**, 88–93.

King, L. J., Carl, J. L., Archer, E. G. and Castellanet, M. (1969). *J. Pharmacol. exp. Ther.* **168**, 163–170.

Krulík, R. and Zvolsky, P. (1970). *Activ. nerv. super.* **12**, 279–283.

Lee, C. R. and Pollitt, R. J. (1973). *Biochem. Soc. Trans.* **1**, 108–109.

Wiechert, P. and Knaape, H. H. (1972). *Acta biol. med. Ger.* **28**, 145–155.

31

ELECTROENCEPHALOGRAPHIC EFFECTS OF LITHIUM

Maria Dimitrakoudi and F. A. Jenner

I. Introduction

Human electroencephalography remains an important, but very disappointing, field of enquiry. In the field of psychopharmacology the studies of Fink, Itil and others (see, for example, Fink, 1965 and Fink *et al.*, 1968) have possibly added a new dimension. They claim that the results of frequency analysis applied to EEG changes due to drugs are often more characteristic of the psychopharmacological activity of those drugs than of the particular chemical group to which they belong. This, it is claimed, led to the discovery of the antidepressive action of GB-94 (Itil *et al.*, 1972). Establishing that a substance is a valid antidepressant in clinical usage is, however, by no means easy, and combining the vagaries of EEGs with those of clinical trials often leaves open questions. The saga of demonstrating that lithium is active in affective psychoses itself shows the weak links in the chain of that sort of reasoning. The central nervous system is incredibly complex and different chemicals have more than one activity upon it: the scalp EEG is an integrated measure of all the various changes which reach the surface. These changes are not identical between different persons, nor within the same person from time to time.

II. The EEG of the Awake Subject

Studies of encephalographic traces must be severely empirical. At that level,

S

dimensions of arousal, susceptibility to convulsion, sleep or coma, can be measured with a degree of confidence.

Lithium, not surprisingly, has a profound effect on cerebral electrical activity, but it is not always easy, in the studies so far reported, to distinguish its direct effects from changes that might be secondary to the clinical response achieved. The changes are fairly dose dependent, but can lag behind dropping serum lithium levels when lithium treatment is discontinued. The best early study on these points was made by Mayfield and Brown (1966). They showed that controls and patients alike demonstrated profound changes in their EEG records as a result of lithium administration. These changes were characterized by a wider frequency spectrum, diffuse slowing or general amplitude increases with disorganization of the background rhythms. Thirty per cent of the subjects showed bilaterally synchronous paroxysms of delta activity. Changes in the straight resting EEGs became apparent with serum levels of 1·2 mmol/l of lithium, whilst all subjects showed some changes with lithium levels of 1·96 mmol/l. The changes always progressed if the serum values were further elevated. Hyperventilation produced clear changes at lower levels of serum lithium (down, in fact, to 0·76 mmol/l). While hyperventilation was reported to elicit more readily the EEG changes which arise anyway with higher lithium levels, these authors noted no increased sensitivity or response to intermittent photic stimulation. The authors commented on a slight lag in the return of the EEG to normal after lithium administration, but the delay was nothing like as long as that reported in some subsequent studies, such as that by Jenner (1973), though this latter may have been an idiosyncratic finding. Small *et al.* (1971a), however, report EEG anomalies persisting for five days after lithium withdrawal. Despite the small number of patients studied (five manic-depressive patients) Mayfield and Brown (1966) claimed dose-serum level-EEG-behavioural correlations of significance.

Platman and Fieve (1969), in a much larger double-blind study, denied any characteristic EEG pattern in manic-depressive illness which could give a baseline for improvement with lithium. While not describing a characteristic EEG pattern in affective psychoses, Harding *et al.* (1966) and Gjessing *et al.* (1967) discussed the problem and clearly demonstrated intraindividual correlations which varied concomitantly with mood. As a follow-up to these studies, Hanna *et al.* (1972) showed how these sequential changes in alpha amplitude and frequency disappeared when the mood became stabilized on lithium carbonate treatment. The changes were, of course, at least partially masked by the generalized EEG slowing with increased amplitude due to lithium which has, in fact, been reported by most investigators. The EEG of arousal, often found in mania, is usually one showing increased frequency, decreased amplitude and desynchronization.

The report by Hanna *et al.* (1972) shows, in an extensively studied individual, the close relationship which can be found between generalized slowing, increased amplitude, and lithium dose. Taking this into account makes many of the findings noted in the literature less contradictory than can often appear at first sight. Platman and Fieve (1969), for example, could find no simple correlations of significance between age, sex, serum lithium, duration of treatment, and the EEG findings, except for the fact that half of the patients treated showed deterioration of their EEG tracings as compared to controls. The levels of serum lithium in this study were, however, lower than those in the work of Mayfield and Brown (1966), a fact to which Platman and Fieve themselves drew attention and which might, in view of the findings of Hanna *et al.* (1972), have accounted for the failure of clear relationships to emerge.

Zakowska-Dabrowska and Rybakowski (1973) studied 30 persons, some with affective disorders, and some as controls. They determined lithium levels in plasma and in red cells. Generalized, focal and paroxysmal changes were seen after single doses and more reliably after two weeks of chronic treatment. No relationship was found between clinical outcome and serum lithium level, nor between clinical state and the form of the EEG, and this led the investigators to regard intracellular measurements as the relevant indices of lithium concentration in the body (see Chapter 4).

Paroxysmal slowing of the EEG trace following lithium administration was noted by Small *et al.* (1972), though this seemed to occur more commonly in control subjects than in patients given lithium salts. Slowing of the EEGs of normal individuals was reported by this group to persist for at least five days after stopping lithium administration, but paroxysmal slowing was less frequently noted in the post-lithium records.

The effects of lithium, both on the induction of epileptic fits and of epileptic EEG records, remain obscure, though it is not, perhaps, surprising that lithium intoxication can be accompanied by seizures (see Chapters 13 and 32). In an early study of lithium poisoning Corcoran *et al.* (1949) showed generalized slow activity of 4–6 Hz with an amplitude of $150\mu V$. Passouant *et al.* (1953) reported the production of EEG abnormalities resembling temporal epilepsy. Andreani *et al.* (1958), on the other hand, emphasized a tendency of lithium treatment to normalize desynchronized traces. Roberts (1950), Glesinger (1954), Schou *et al.* (1968), Lauter and Middelhoff (1969), Wharton (1969), Baldessarini and Stephens (1970), Demers *et al.* (1970) and Helmchen and Kanowski (1970, 1971) all claimed to have noted fits due to therapeutic doses of lithium while the serum lithium was still in the therapeutic range. On the other hand, Erwin *et al.* (1971) reported that lithium reduced the incidence of fits in epileptics with affective disorders, the affective component being successfully eliminated by the lithium. Under these conditions the EEG became normalized. More recently, Jus *et al.* (1973) have examined the effects of lithium carbonate on the EEG records of 18 female patients with temporal epilepsy. In all cases the EEG records were initially abnormal. Single doses of 600 to 900 mg of lithium carbonate, leading to serum levels of lithium within the range 0·68 to 1·15 mmol/l, left the EEG patterns virtually unchanged. Subsequently, eight of the patients were treated with 600 mg lithium carbonate daily for an extended period, in an attempt to assess the effects of chronic administration on the EEG recordings. Even though serum lithium levels did not exceed 0·58 mmol/l it was found that EEG abnormalities intensified in five out of the eight patients and this, coupled with increased seizure frequency and other behaviour impairments, led to the trial being terminated.

Differences between acute and chronic administration regimes have been noted in several studies. Acute administration of 750 mg of lithium carbonate (Johnson, 1969; Johnson et al., 1970) produced negligible EEG changes, despite some fluctuations of normal serum electrolytes. Chronic administration of lithium in the same studies led to the usual finding of generalized slowing and increased amplitude, but the authors also referred to an accentuation of focal abnormalities and a correlation between changes in the EEG with neurotoxicity (more details of neurotoxic effects of lithium are given in Chapters 13 and 32). These investigators attempted to correlate the EEG changes with variations in serum electrolytes, but found that the latter revealed no consistent pattern of changes. They emphasized that, although a correlation with lithium dose emerged, more important factors were patient specific, including the presence of organic disease, and that overall sodium balance might possibly be important. Most authors, however, consider sodium balance changes to be transient.

It is probably correct to conclude that, in general, lithium causes an increased amplitude and decreased frequency of the EEG. In the acute situation, however, different effects may occur, lithium either being without influence on the EEG or sometimes causing increases in both frequency and amplitude. Other ways of expressing EEG data may, of course, alter the interpretation to be placed upon lithium-induced changes: thus, Pfeiffer et al. (1969) used a measure of the mean energy content of the EEG as the dependent variable in a study of lithium effects. Lithium generally led to a dose-related increase in this value. The full implications of this work have yet to be assessed.

The effects of lithium on the EEG are usually found to be partially dose-dependent, but various individual factors alter sensitivity, persistence, and the tendency to display paroxysmal and epileptic type records. Helmchen and Kanowski (1971) summarize very helpfully the variety of effects produced by lithium and the methodological problems involved in their adequate interpretation.

III. The EEG of the Sleeping Subject

Clinical state has, of course, a profound effect on patterns of sleeping, times of waking, insomnia, etc. Lithium treatment, if successful, alters these measures and hence would be expected to change the nature of the sleeping EEG. Early studies, however, provided little evidence that lithium had any direct effect on rapid eye movement (REM) sleep or on the non-paradoxical stages of sleep. This was clearly shown in the studies of Mayfield and Brown (1966) and those of Brebbia et al. (1969).

In the work reported by Mayfield and Brown (1966) the sleep rhythms were generally less affected by lithium than were the waking EEGs. The investigators commented that it was often difficult to distinguish between lithium effects and those of sleep. Brebbia and his co-workers (Brebbia et al., 1969) took up this point, and in a study involving manic-depressive patients and control patients they recorded both EEGs and electromyograms both before and during lithium treatment whilst the subjects were sleeping. They were unable to report any systematic drug effects in either group of subjects.

Kupfer et al. (1970) noted that in the investigations undertaken by Brebbia and his associates the serum lithium levels failed to exceed 0·49 mmol/l in any subject, a value normally considered to be below the therapeutic range. They therefore undertook further investigations of lithium effects on sleeping EEGs using higher lithium dose levels (0·7 to 1·3 mmol/l), and this time marked effects were noted. In particular, there was a reduction in the percentage of Stage I REM sleep and a prolongation of the latency to first REM period. Delta sleep time (sleep Stages III and IV) was increased in a manner which was roughly dose-related.

More recently, Mendels and Chernik (1973) have looked at the effect produced by lithium carbonate in sleep patterns in five depressed patients. The study covered a period of 113 drug-free nights and 150 nights during lithium therapy. EOG and EMG recordings were made simultaneously with the EEGs. Lithium treatment resulted in a significant decrease in mean REM percentage (which had been elevated during depression) and an increased latency to first REM period. These findings clearly paralleled those of Kupfer et al. (1970). In addition, mean delta sleep time also increased significantly as a result of lithium treatment, again in accordance with the results reported by Kupfer and his colleagues. These effects were reversed on withdrawal of lithium. The EEG changes occurred within a day of the initiation of lithium treatment, and lithium withdrawal was followed within the same period by reversal of the Stage I REM and delta wave sleep changes, though the sleep changes were not necessarily accompanied by any concomitant deterioration in the clinical status of the patients.

Kupfer et al. (1970) noted that in some patients in whom delta wave sleep was totally absent before lithium administration there was no appearance of this type of sleep resulting from lithium therapy. A similar finding was reported by Mendels and Chernik (1973). In two non-depressed psychiatric patients a pre-drug absence of delta wave sleep was not modified by lithium. Mendels and

Chernik hypothesized that there might be some metabolic difference between those patients showing some delta wave sleep and those showing none, possibly based on 5-hydroxytryptamine and noradrenaline, both of which substances are known to be involved in the mediation of REM and delta wave sleep.

IV. Cortical Evoked Potentials: Contingent Negative Variation

Perhaps one of the most promising developments in electroencephalography of recent years has been the development of averaging techniques for the EEG, which allow one to study evoked potentials. The patient is repeatedly stimulated in some way (visually, electrically, auditorily, etc.), and from the immediate onset of each stimulus the EEG is recorded and the traces are averaged in terms of the amplitude against time from the stimulus. The resulting average curve has therefore filtered out influences not due to the stimuli being studied. The problems presented by the method are primarily those of describing the curves produced, and of obtaining from the descriptions adequate quantitative statements to allow meaningful and accurate comparisons to be made between different records.

The use of individuals as their own controls often helps to resolve this type of problem. Gartside *et al.* (1966), using this principle to some extent, showed in 17 normal subjects that lithium may affect cortical recovery following somatosensory stimulation. They noticed that lithium (1 g lithium carbonate daily for seven days) caused a reduction in the amplitude of the response to the second stimulus when paired stimuli sufficiently close together were used. This delayed recovery is similar to findings noted in psychotic depression which is not caused by lithium: the response is not, therefore, easy to interpret.

The amplitude of the EEG in general is, as has been mentioned previously, much increased following lithium administration. It is not, therefore, surprising that Mayfield and Brown (1966) found a generalized increase in the visual evoked potential response. Heninger (1969) investigating auditory, somatosensory and visually evoked potentials in 18 patients before and after lithium intervention, also noted increased amplitude of response, especially of the early primary positive component of the somatosensory response. The later components of all the responses showed only variable increases in amplitude and there were slight latency changes. There was negligible alteration in the recoveries of the somatosensory and auditory evoked responses. The changes which did occur began after three to five days of treatment and at levels above 1 mmol/l of lithium ions in the serum. The changes persisted despite negligible serum levels for up to four days. The magnitudes of the changes were related to dose.

Postulating that lithium might control the impulsiveness of manic patients by altering the evoked potentials between the amygdaloid nucleus and the orbito-frontal cortex, Creson *et al.* (1967) tried to study these potentials in cats. Following intravenous lithium administration only the cortical evoked potentials changed. There was an increased amplitude, a greater latency of the second peak, and a decrease in the average latency of the beginning of secondary activity. The limbic system did not show changes, although the experimenters used very large doses of lithium. The investigators felt that this might explain the discrepancy between their study and that of Gartside *et al.* (1966). Essentially similar results to those of Creson *et al.* (1967), however, were achieved when the same team repeated their work, again using cats, at a later date (Barratt *et al.*, 1968). The cortical, but not subcortical, responses were influenced by lithium. Lithium chloride differentially affected the behavioural and electrophysiological responses to auditory stimuli. Head-turning responses (orientation reactions) which normally occurred to a repeated tone stimulus were suppressed by lithium, but the evoked cortical potentials still occurred: moreover, the evoked cortical response was reported not to show habituation to repeated administration of the tone (see Chapter 20).

The development of toxic reactions to lithium is known to be related in part to the state of sodium balance in the individual (see Chapter 13) and it may be supposed that a similar relationship exists between sodium metabolism and sensitivity to lithium effects at subtoxic lithium levels. Heninger and Demers (1971) took this possibility into account in a study of lithium effects on somatosensory evoked potentials. They reported that the clinical improvement produced by lithium was accompanied by increased amplitudes in the primary positive components of the somatosensory evoked response. High-sodium diets occasionally offset this effect on the evoked response, suggesting to the authors that there was a close relationship between lithium effects, sodium metabolism, and clinical response.

Particular interest attaches to attempts to provide tests which will differentiate between lithium responders and lithium non-responders, as well as detecting changes associated with clinical improvement. Some progress in this direction was made in relation to EEG tests by Borge *et al.* (1971) and Buchsbaum *et al.* (1972) who showed that in patients suffering from bipolar affective disorders and likely to respond to lithium treatment, the average visual evoked potentials which were exhibited increased in magnitude as the eliciting stimuli became more intense. Clinical improvement following lithium was accompanied by a reduction in this so-called augmenting response. Unipolar patients, on the other hand, who were generally poor responders to lithium, showed the opposite effect—some reduction in average evoked potentials with increasing stimulus intensity, a relationship generally unaffected by lithium. Small *et al.* (1971a) reported that lithium produced negligible changes in average visual evoked responses when all patients' records were considered together. However, when the records of those patients who did not show mood changes with lithium were eliminated, it could be seen that certain changes in the form of the average visual and auditory evoked potentials did occur. In the case of the auditory evoked potentials, lithium produced increased amplitudes of response both in patients showing lithium-induced mood changes and in those showing no mood response.

Shagass *et al.* (1973) also found that lithium increased the amplitude of evoked responses (in this case somatosensory responses) in 14 patients. The somatosensory response recovery was enhanced by lithium treatment, a finding apparently contrary to those of Gartside *et al.* (1966); Shagass and his associates resolved the discrepancy, however, by pointing to differences in the way in which recovery characteristics were expressed in the two studies.

In normal subjects, Small *et al.* (1971b; 1972) reported that lithium sometimes shortened visual evoked response latencies, a finding which was not paralleled in studies with patients. Normal subjects, however, did not exhibit the variations in evoked potential amplitudes which were found in lithium-treated patients. The variations in the patients, though, seemed to be mood-dependent.

Studies illustrating the difficulties involved in interpreting EEG effects of lithium have followed work on the so-called contingent negative variation (CNV) in slow potential data (i.e., the variation found in d–c measures of amplitude when the subject has been conditioned to expect a second stimulus, the measures being taken before the onset of the expected stimulus). Walter (1971) noted that the d–c CNV response was increased in its negativity as a result of lithium therapy. Similar findings were reported by Small *et al.* (1971a): the slow potential variations were altered by lithium carbonate and negativity was significantly increased, though it was not possible to determine from the data whether or not this increase was maintained while the subject was on lithium. No information was available to indicate the reversibility of the effect following lithium withdrawal. The changes which occurred, however, were unrelated to the clinical status of the patients or to the nature of the clinical response shown to treatment. The subsequent studies of Small *et al.* (1971b; 1972) using normal volunteer subjects showed a variability in both pre- and post-lithium d–c amplitudes which makes comparisons with patients with mood disorders very difficult. Significant d–c amplitude changes occurred in different volunteers in both directions and even included reversal of the polarity after treatment with lithium, the nature of the change apparently depending in part upon the precise experimental circumstances. The d–c changes were still in evidence to some extent some five days after the cessation of lithium treatment. Small *et al.* (1971b; 1972) have suggested that the variability in the d–c responses amongst normal subjects may reflect the wide range of different attitudes towards the experiment which these subjects expressed, as contrasted with the more uniformly hopeful attitudes of the patients. If this is indeed the case, it is a factor which must be carefully monitored in future EEG studies of this kind before definitive conclusions can be drawn from any results obtained.

V. Modes of Action of Lithium on the EEG

It is probably premature to attempt to relate the EEG changes noted as a result of lithium treatment to the effects which lithium ions are known to have at the level of excitable cell membranes. Many of the *in vitro* studies upon which this knowledge is based have, in any case, involved lithium concentrations far in excess of those attained during lithium therapy and generalization of the information to the clinical situation is therefore undertaken only with extreme caution. Despite all these cautionary comments, however, it seems clear that the eventual description of the mechanisms underlying lithium-induced EEG changes will almost certainly involve references to the ability of lithium to substitute for other cations (see Chapters 21 and 22) particularly in those processes associated with nerve cell functioning.

The ease with which lithium can replace sodium in nerve action potential mechanisms is now well-documented (e.g., Ritchie and Straub, 1957; Keynes and Swan, 1959). This is due mainly to the fact that the nerve cell membrane is more or less equally permeable to sodium and lithium ions (Armett and Ritchie, 1963), a characteristic shown by other membranes, such as that of the erythrocyte. Several investigators, working with erythrocyte preparations, have made the point that, when lithium is inside the cell, it acts like sodium, stimulating sodium pump mechanisms (see Chapter 33). The situation is, however, complicated and it is possible that the nature of the lithium effect on neuronal functioning is to some extent related to the concentration of lithium in the tissues: thus, Giacobini and Stepita-Klauco (1970) have shown that the sodium-potassium pump mechanism in stretch-receptor neurones of the crayfish is inhibited by relatively high concentrations of lithium in the nutrient medium. Attention is drawn in Chapter 33 to further possible complications in the picture of lithium involvement in energetic processes similar to those associated with the nerve resting potential and with the production and subsequent recovery of the action potential.

Lithium concentrates intracellularly, suggesting that the active transport outwards across the cell membrane is inefficient as compared with the transport of sodium: the efflux rate for lithium has been put at about 12% that of sodium (see Giabocini, 1969). This may explain some of the persisting effects which lithium has on the EEG following withdrawal of lithium treatment, even when serum lithium can no longer be measured.

In addition to the marked effects which lithium produces on the mechanisms related to nerve impulse propagation as a result of its substitution for sodium, there are actions at the level of the synapse, probably more related to lithium substitution for calcium or magnesium, which may also be partly responsible for the gross EEG changes observed during lithium therapy. Neurotransmitter synthesis, vesicular concentration, intra- and extra-neuronal release, and re-uptake through the pre-synaptic membrane, are all processes potentially subject to the influences of lithium. Biogenic amine effects are discussed in Chapter 25, and in Chapter 24 the involvement of lithium with acetylcholine metabolism is outlined. Post-synaptic processes, too, may be altered, and Chapter 29 deals with the lithium-induced changes in cyclic-AMP metabolism which may affect post-synaptic receptor sensitivities. Although one might feel that the profound effects of lithium on the EEG are profitably to be considered as aspects of the therapeutic effect, one must take note of such findings as those produced by Platman and Fieve (1969). These authors failed to see EEG changes in patients who seemed to have responded therapeutically. This must argue in favour of the EEG changes largely measuring toxic or side effects of lithium, though it could be that the available scalp recording techniques are able to register EEG changes of clinical significance only when these are produced by sufficiently large doses (i.e., outside the normal range of doses used therapeutically) and are therefore very marked.

Another possible interpretation of lithium-induced EEG effects has been put forward by Reilly et al. (1973), who suggested that lithium serves merely to accentuate previously existing underlying EEG abnormalities. Their conclusions were based upon studies of normal volunteer subjects given lithium carbonate over a two-week period; six subjects developed EEG abnormalities, but four of these showed the same abnormalities in both control and lithium treatment periods. In support of the view that lithium may be acting to make pre-existing abnormalities more obvious, is the observation that the incidence of EEG abnormalities amongst manic-depressive patients is greater than amongst other patient populations (Hurst et al., 1954; Assael and Winnik, 1970).

The lack of clear evidence of limbic system changes makes it difficult to fit current findings in with available hypotheses of psychoses. Assistance may, however, come from another direction. As the behavioural effects of lithium on animals are more fully documented (see Chapters 19 and 20) it may be possible to relate EEG changes and evoked potential characteristics to these effects and so indirectly arrive at new hypotheses about the interrelationships between lithium, behaviour and neurophysiological response.

It is, of course, possible that refinements of electroencephalographic recording techniques will eventually make it possible to detect the neurophysiological concomitants of those aspects of the action of lithium which are important in determining its therapeutic effectiveness. Small and Small (1973), for example, have recently drawn attention to the increasingly sophisticated application of computer analyses to the examination of EEG records, which may increase both the sensitivity and precision of neurophysiological recordings.

References

Andreani, G., Casselli, G. and Martelli, G. (1958). *G. Psichiat. Neuropat.* **86**, 273–328.

Armett, C. J. and Ritchie, J. M. (1963). *J. Physiol.* **165**, 130–140.

Assael, M. and Winnik, H. Z. (1970). *Dis. nerv. Syst.* **31**, 695-701.

Baldessarini, R. and Stephens, J. (1970). *Archs gen. Psychiat.* **22**, 72–77.

Barratt, E. S., Creson, D. L. and Russell, G. (1968). *Amer. J. Psychiat.* **125**, 530–536.

Borge, G., Buchsbaum, M., Goodwin, F., Murphy, D. and Silverman, J. (1971). *Archs gen. Psychiat.* **24**, 501–504.

Brebbia, D. R., Altshuler, K. Z. and Kline, N. S. (1969). *Dis. nerv. Syst.* **30**, 541–546.

Buchsbaum, M., Goodwin, F., Murphy, D. and Borge, G. (1971). *Amer. J. Psychiat.* **128**, 19–22.

Corcoran, A., Taylor, C. and Page, L. H. (1949). *J. Amer. med. Assoc.* **139**, 685–688.

Creson, D. L., Barratt, E. S., Russell, G. V. and Schlagenhauf, G. K. (1967). *Texas Rep. Biol. Med.* **25**, 374–379.

Demers, R., Lukesh, R. and Prichard, J. (1970). *Lancet* **2**, 315–316.

Erwin, C. W., Gerber, C. J., Morrison, S. D. and James, F. (1971). Paper read at 5th World Congr. Psychiat. Mexico City.

Fink, M. (1965). *In* "Applications of Electroencephalography in Psychiatry" (W. P. Wilson, ed), pp. 226–240. Duke University Press, North Carolina.

Fink, M., Shapiro, D. M., Hickman, C. and Itil, T. (1968). *In* "Computers and Electronic Devices in Psychiatry" (W. S. Kline and E. Laska, eds), pp. 109–123. Grune and Stratton, New York.

Gartside, J. B., Lippold, O. C. J. and Meldrum, B. S. (1966). *Electroencephalog. clin. Neurophysiol.* **20**, 382–390.

Giacobini, E. (1969). *Acta psychiat. scand.* Suppl. **207**, 85–87.

Giacobini, E. and Stepita-Klauco, M. (1970). *Acta psychiat. scand.* **80**, 519–527.

Gjessing, L. R., Harding, G. F. A., Jenner, F. A. and Johannessen, N. (1967). *Brit. J. Psychiat.* **113**, 1271–1282.

Glesinger, B. (1954). *Med. J. Aust.* **41**, 277–283.

Hanna, S. M., Jenner, F. A., Pearson, I. B., Sampson, G. A. and Thompson, E. A. (1972). *Brit. J. Psychiat.* **121**, 271–280.

Harding, G., Jeavons, P. M., Jenner, F. A., Drummond, P., Sheridan, M. and Howells, G. W. (1966). *Electroencephalog. clin. Neurophysiol.* **21**, 59–66.

Helmchen, H. and Kanowski, S. (1970). *Int. Pharmacopsychiat.* **5**, 149–161.

Helmchen, H. and Kanowski, S. (1971). *Nervenartz.* **42**, 144–148.

Heninger, G. R. (1969). *Electroencephalog. clin. Neurophysiol.* **27**, 656.

Heninger, G. R. and Demers, R. (1971). *Electroencephalog. clin. Neurophysiol.* **31**, 287–298.

Hurst, L. A., Mundy-Castle, A. C. and Beerstecher, D. M. (1954). *J. ment. Sci.* **100**, 220–240.

Itil, T. M., Polvan, N. and Hsu, W. (1972). *Curr. ther. Res.* **14**, 395–413.

Jenner, F. A. (1973). *Biochem. Soc. Trans.* **1**, 88–93.

Johnson, G. (1969). *Electroencephalog. clin. Neurophysiol.* **27**, 656–657.

Johnson, G., Maccario, M., Gershon, S. and Korein, J. (1970). *J. nerv. ment. Dis.* **151**, 273–289.

Jus, A., Villeneuve, A., Gautier, J., Pires, A., Côté, J. M., Jus, K., Villeneuve, R. and Perron, D. (1973). *Int. J. clin. Pharmacol. Ther. Toxicol.* **7**, 67–74.

Keynes, R. D. and Swan, R. C. (1959). *J. Physiol.* **147**, 626–638.

Kupfer, D. J., Wyatt, R. J., Greenspan, K. and Snyder, F. (1970). *Archs gen. Psychiat.* **23,** 35–40.

Lauter, H. and Middelhoff, H. D. (1969). *Nervenartz.* **40,** 549–551.

Mayfield, D. and Brown, R. G. (1966). *J. psychiat. Res.* **4,** 207–219.

Mendels, J. and Chernik, D. A. (1973). *Int. Pharmacopsychiat.* **8,** 184–192.

Passouant, P., Duc, N. and Maurel, H. (1953). *Montpellier Méd.* **A96,** 38.

Pfeiffer, C. C., Singh, M. and Goldstein, L. (1969). *J. clin. Pharmacol.* **9,** 298–307.

Platman, S. R. and Fieve, R. R. (1969). *Brit. J. Psychiat.* **115,** 1185–1188.

Reilly, E., Halmi, K. A. and Noyes, R. Jr. (1973). *Int. Pharmacopsychiat.* **8,** 208–213.

Ritchie, J. M. and Straub, R. W. (1957). *J. Physiol.* **136,** 80–97.

Roberts, E. L. (1950). *Med. J. Aust.* **37,** 261–262.

Schou, M. (1968). *J. psychiat. Res.* **6,** 67–95.

Schou, M., Amdisen, A. and Trap-Jensen, J. (1968). *Amer. J. Psychiat.* **125,** 520–527.

Shagass, C., Straumanis, J. J. and Overton, D. A. (1973). *Psychopharmacologia* **29,** 185–196.

Small, J. G. and Small, I. F. (1973). *In* "Lithium: Its Role in Psychiatric Research and Treatment" (Gershon, S. and Shopsin, B. eds.) pp. 83–106. Plenum, New York.

Small, J. G., Milstein, V. and Small, I. F. (1971a). *Dis. nerv. Syst.* **32,** 818–821.

Small, J. G., Small, I. F. and Perez, H. C. (1971b). *Biol. Psychiat.* **3,** 47–58.

Small, J. G., Milstein, V., Perez, H. C., Small, I. F. and Moore, D. F. (1972). *Biol. Psychiat.* **5,** 65–77.

Walter, W. G. (1971). *Biol. Psychiat.* **3,** 59–68.

Wharton, R. N. (1969). *Amer. J. Psychiat.* **125,** 1446.

Zakowska-Dabrowska, T. and Rybakowski, J. (1973). *Acta psychiat. scand.* **49,** 457–465.

32

LITHIUM SIDE-EFFECTS AND TOXICITY: MECHANISMS

F. N. Johnson and L. Vacaflor

I. Introduction

For most practical purposes it is sufficient for the clinician merely to be aware of the symptomatic nature of the side-effects of lithium, their severity, and their frequency of occurrence, so that upon their appearance he may decide what action, if any, need be taken to alleviate them. Possibly for this reason the majority of reports of lithium side-effects, and in particular the early reports, tend to be purely descriptive: such suggestions as are put forward concerning their pathophysiological bases are made briefly and tentatively. It is, however, essential for the development of rational supplementary treatment procedures aimed at reducing or eliminating the more serious and lasting of these reactions, that the underlying mechanisms should be elucidated in as detailed a manner as possible.

The side-effects and other toxic manifestations of any drug may stem from two different sources. They may either be associated with physiological mechanisms which are also important in determining the drug's therapeutic efficacy, or they may involve quite separate and distinct processes. The implications for treatment are, of course, entirely different in the two cases if the drug therapy is to be continued. In the former instance, one would be inclined to adopt treatment procedures of a generally supportive kind which would minimize the consequences of the side-effects; alternatively, if active intervention seemed essential, the additional medication or other anti-side-effect procedure chosen would have to be one which did not counteract the drug's main action. In the event of the side-effects and the main therapeutic action being produced by separate biochemical or physiological mechanisms, the restrictions upon the choice of supportive medication will, of course, be fewer.

At the present time, the information relating to both the main effects and the side-effects of lithium is markedly insufficient for any clear differentiation, of the kind noted above, to be made, and the effectiveness of treatment procedures for side-effects vis-à-vis the continued efficacy of lithium treatment, must be assessed empirically.

There is a clear need for some measure of systematization of our knowledge about side-effect physiology so that we may begin to locate which of the physiological actions of lithium are necessary, and which are unnecessary, for the drug's therapeutic action; as a first step towards this an attempt will be made in this chapter to review the suggestions which have been made to account for the various types of side-effects and toxic reactions which are associated with lithium therapy. The task is not any easy one, for the information is scattered in the literature and frequently lacks cohesiveness or precision of statement.

II. Side-Effects and Toxic Reactions Related to Specific Organ Systems

A. Central nervous and neuromuscular systems

The neural effects of lithium which give rise to side-effects would appear to be of a subtle, rather than a gross, kind. In those cases of fatality directly linked to lithium ingestion in which post mortem brain examinations were carried out, no evidence of brain damage was reported (Roberts, 1950; Duc and Maurel, 1953; Trautner et al., 1955). However, Glessinger (1954) suggested that in these cases and in others (Corcoran et al., 1949; Hanlon et al., 1949; Stern, 1949) brain damage might well have occurred but of a type which would not normally be detected without microscopic histological analysis. Glessinger proposed that small, lithium-induced haemorrhages, possibly situated in the cortical grey matter close to the meninges, could be responsible for all the symptoms of encephalopathy. Such a condition might, he suggested, account for many of the observed features of lithium poisoning, including the occasional convulsion. No evidence is available to confirm or refute the notion of microscopic brain damage.

Other writers differ on the question of whether lithium produces its toxic effects on the nervous system directly, by modifying the brain tissues and their associated physiological processes, or indirectly as a result of metabolic disturbances induced elsewhere in the body.

Shopsin *et al.* (1970) suggested that a direct modification of brain tissue might be involved in view of the ability of lithium to reduce the threshold tolerance of the brain to other, previously tolerated, drugs. They noted that Moracci (1931) had shown that lithium salts, applied topically to the exposed motor cortex of dogs, could produce clonic seizures, and that Delgado and De Feudis (1969) had produced limbic system effects by direct injection of lithium salts into the amygdala and hippocampus of monkeys: such studies as these clearly suggest that lithium ions might act on the brain substance without the mediation of other, non-neural, physiological events. That this *could* happen is, however, far from a demonstration that, under normal administration procedures, it *does* happen, and some authors have preferred the view that central nervous effects are secondary to other events, such as an abnormally low serum potassium level (Corcoran *et al.*, 1949) or hypoglycaemia (Van der Velde, 1971).

The fact that central nervous and neuromuscular effects are not seen in all patients, coupled with the extreme variability noted in the severity of such symptoms when they do appear, has suggested to some authors that a predisposing intolerance or hypersensitivity to lithium effects may be present in some patients (Schou, 1969; Shopsin *et al.*, 1970). Johnson *et al.* (1970) and Reilly *et al.* (1973) provide some support for this view by observing that the presence of baseline abnormalities in the EEG is an indicator of extreme EEG changes following lithium administration. Shopsin *et al.* (1970) comment that the predisposing factor may either be itself neural, in the form of a baseline neuropathy, or non-neural, such as a renal handling insufficiency.

Changing serum levels of lithium may also predispose to the appearance of EEG abnormalities, these abnormalities disappearing as soon as the serum levels reach a constant value (James and Reilly, 1971). Homeostatic control mechanisms, it might be supposed, would be particularly sensitive to changes rather than constancies in the internal environment, and the appearance of various kinds of abnormalities associated with rapidly rising or falling lithium levels could reflect some changes (perhaps over-reactions) of the homeostatic processes.

B. Gastrointestinal system

Schou (1957) noted that the side-effects of lithium associated with the gut were unlikely to be caused by the absorption of lithium into the gut wall in view of the fact that the same, or similar, symptoms appeared even when other routes of administration were employed.

Rask-Madsen *et al.* (1972) tentatively proposed that the initial diarrhoea following lithium ingestion might be in some way related to an increase in transmucosal potential difference in the lower gut, indicative of a general disturbance of electrolyte balance, but the precise way in which this might produce the clinical symptoms was not elaborated upon.

Several writers have expressed the opinion that in some way the rate of change of lithium concentration in the tissues may be instrumental in producing gastrointestinal side-effects. Talso and Clarke (1951) recorded vomiting in dogs following intravenous lithium chloride injections, at a time when the serum lithium concentration would have been rising rapidly. Gattozzi (1970) similarly suggested that the occurrence of nausea, vomiting, diarrhoea and stomach pain might be related both to the peak serum levels and to the rate of rising blood concentration, whilst Prien *et al.* (1971) noted that the gastric symptoms generally subside once the patient has become adapted to the transient concentration changes which follow each administration of the drug.

C. Renal system

As with the central nervous system effects, there have been two possibilities expressed with regard to the renal symptoms associated with lithium treatment: they may be due either to a direct action of lithium on the kidney tubules or to an indirect renal response to some other, possibly more generalized, lithium toxicity operating at a different primary site.

Microscopic changes, of a degenerative nature, were recorded in the tubular epithelium by Radomski *et al.* (1955), Sivadon and Chanoit (1955) and Schou (1957, 1959) in the early days of lithium therapy. Glessinger (1954) noted the occurrence of albuminuria, again suggesting primary renal damage.

More recently, two reports have appeared which seem to confirm that renal structural changes may be consequent upon lithium treatment (though this in itself does not, of course, necessarily imply their involvement in producing side-effects). Lavender *et al.* (1973) found many minor changes in the glomeruli which were indicative of some degree of sclerosis: this finding was in accord with an earlier report by Schou *et al.* (1968b) of extensive renal vascular sclerosis in two patients. Evan (1973) described dose-related ultrastructural transformations which occurred in renal mitochondria following lithium treatment and suggested that there was some evidence (Gritzka and Trump, 1968; Goyer and Krall, 1969; Evan and Ollerich, 1972) to link certain of these changes (notably mitochondrial swelling) to an impaired phosphorylative ability which might, in its turn, be related to a general renal inadequacy.

One or two authors have briefly entertained the possibility of non-renal primary effects before finally coming down in favour of lithium-induced renal damage as the primary effect. Radomski *et al.* (1950) felt that the biochemical effects observed might equally well be a result of adrenal cortical insufficiency, but administration of large doses of desoxycorticosterone acetate or adrenal cortical extract did not alleviate the toxic symptoms and so Radomski and his colleagues were forced to the conclusion that a primary renal effect was involved. Similarly, Dias and Hocken (1972), whilst noting that the protracted hypotension and peripheral vascular failure shown by one of their patients were probably sufficient in themselves to account for the renal failure brought on by lithium, nevertheless felt that the evidence from other studies was probably strong enough to suggest that a primary nephrotoxic effect was indicated by the symptoms.

Theories of indirect lithium action on the kidneys have emphasized changes of either an electrolytic or hormonal nature, or a combination of the two. Radomski *et al.* (1950) noted an increase in the excretion of aldosterone in the urine in the first seven days after lithium administration, and Demers and Heninger (1970a) and Demers *et al.* (1971) suggested that the oedema sometimes associated with lithium therapy might be related to the impairment of aldosterone-stimulated reabsorption of sodium in the renal tubules. Stancer and Kivi (1971), whilst agreeing that sodium reabsorption effects might be involved in the oedematous reaction, could not rule out the alternative possibility that lithium potentiated the effects of other drugs which were being used concurrently. The importance of sodium excretion on renal functioning during lithium therapy was elegantly demonstrated by Gutman *et al.* (1971) who showed that lithium-induced polydipsia could be eliminated by nephrectomy or by ligaturing the ureters: this suggested that the polydipsia was maintained by the excretion of some component of the urine, and sodium ions appeared to be the most likely candidate for such a role. The initial natriuresis induced by lithium was proposed by Gutman and his colleagues as leading to increased plasma renin activity, and hence to elevated urine output.

Angrist *et al.* (1970) speculated that lithium produced a hypokalaemic nephropathy, leading to a diabetes insipidus-like syndrome by affecting the intra- to extra-cellular ratio of potassium ions. They noted, in support of this view, that Smith and Lasater (1950) had been able to induce a similar syndrome in dogs by providing the animals with a potassium-deficient diet, and also that Wolff *et al.* (1968) recorded defects in renal concentrating ability of psychiatric patients showing potassium depletion.

The renal concentrating failure following lithium treatment was considered by Ramsey *et al.* (1972) as possibly related to the inhibition by lithium of adenyl cyclase (Dousa and Hechter, 1970a, b; Wolff *et al.*, 1970). Both adenyl cyclase and cyclic-AMP are important in initiating the action of vasopressin, and in this respect it is interesting that Harris and Jenner (1969a, b) have reported a lithium-induced inhibition of vasopressin action in the kidney of the rat. See Chapters 27, 28 and 29 for elaboration of this point.

O'Connell (1971), whilst noting the possibility of a direct hypokalaemic nephropathy, has suggested that the major effect of lithium may be as remote as the posterior pituitary gland or even the hypothalamus where the release of pitressin might be affected.

As with the central nervous system side-effects, the possibility is sometimes suggested that there exists a predisposing kidney weakness in those patients who eventually succumb to renal complications whilst undergoing lithium therapy (Schou *et al.*, 1968b).

D. Cardiovascular system

The cardiovascular side-effects of lithium have not usually been linked to a direct toxic action, leading to actual tissue damage, on the heart muscle itself. The majority of writers favour the idea that electrolyte imbalance, particularly involving sodium, which results from lithium administration, leads to electrophysiological abnormalities of heart muscle (e.g., McKusick, 1954; Larson *et al.*, 1972). Some difference of opinion occasionally seems to exist, however, as to whether hyper- or hypo-kalaemic effects are involved. Thus, whilst Corcoran *et al.* (1949) noted that in a case of lithium-induced heart failure the serum potassium concentration was abnormally low, McKusick (1954) subsequently related amplitude increases in the T-wave component of the EKG to an increase in plasma potassium (with a concomitant intracellular decrease). Tangedahl and Gau (1972) noted that McKusick's work was carried out using high lithium dose levels, and that with the therapeutic doses given to patients hypokalaemia is the usual result since the depletion of intracellular potassium is accompanied by the renal elimination of this ion and is not, therefore, reflected in any elevation of serum potassium levels. Tangedahl and Gau suggest that the hypokalaemia may be expected to result in prolongation of repolarization and hence to lead to myocardial irritability by facilitating ectopic beats and arrhythmias of ventricular and supraventricular types (Surawicz, 1964).

Demers and Heninger (1970b) refer to one patient, showing persistent P and QRS amplitude alterations, in whom they could not rule out direct toxic effects of lithium on the myocardium, and Schou (1957) also suggests that, in moderate doses, such a direct action may occur, though in more severe states of intoxication the picture would be complicated by hypokalaemic effects consequent upon renal failure.

E. Endocrine system (thyroid gland)

The effects which lithium exerts on the endocrine system have been considered in more detail in Chapter 27 by Berens and Wolff, and therefore in the present chapter attention will be limited to those mechanisms which have been directly implicated in the goitrogenic and hypothyroidal properties of lithium by those investigators who have been primarily concerned with the study of lithium side-effects.

There is no doubt about the fact that lithium interferes with the functioning of the thyroid gland, but there is some disagreement about the precise nature of this interference. Schou *et al.* (1968a) reported that in patients exhibiting goitres as lithium side-effects the uptake of radioactive iodine into the thyroid was either increased or remained at a normal level, thereby suggesting that lithium did not affect iodine trapping. The administration of perchlorate did not produce elevated iodine release and this was held to show that lithium was not affecting the incorporation of iodine into tyrosine. Schou and his colleagues proposed a lithium-induced alteration in intrathyroidal metabolism which impaired thyroxine production: for example, hormone synthesis might, they suggested, be impaired by an inhibition of dehalogenation or of the coupling of iodotyrosines—hypotheses which Cooper *et al.* (1970) referred to as attractive but remote.

Cooper and his colleagues espoused the view that intrathyroidal processing of iodine was in fact normal in lithium-treated patients, the effect on iodine metabolism occurring prior to iodine trapping. They quoted the work of Sedvall *et al.* (1968) and Abuzzahab *et al.* (1969) in support of this contention. Cooper *et al.* (1970) also proposed that, in addition to impairing iodine uptake by the thyroid, lithium might also reduce the eventual release of hormone from the gland, possibly via an inhibition of TSH action or release. Rogers and Whybrow (1971) point out that the reduced hormone release would be expected to lead to increased TSH levels and consequent elevation in iodine uptake rates.

Fieve and Platman (1968), however, finding that iodine intakes in half of their patient sample were down to 15% or less, suggested that the incorporation of iodine into the thyroid was, in fact, reduced by lithium, and they advanced the idea that plasma corticosteroids, elevated as a result of lithium administration (Platman and Fieve, 1968) were directly responsible for the reduced iodine uptake. The concensus view, however, is that lithium treatment usually elevates iodine uptake.

Lazarus and Bennie (1972) demonstrated a clear tendency for lithium to stimulate iodine uptake into the thyroid, but they found that iodide concentration mechanisms were thereafter impaired, in agreement with similar findings by Sedvall *et al.* (1969), Cooper *et al.* (1970), Hullin and Johnson (1970) and Ljunggren *et al.* (1971). A decreased release of thyroidal iodine was also noted by Lazarus and Bennie (1972), as it had been previously by Berens *et al.* (1970) and Burrow *et al.* (1971), and this, in its turn, led to a slight, but significant, rise in TSH levels and to thyroid enlargement. Wolff *et al.* (1970) and Williams *et al.* (1971) drew attention to the lithium-induced inhibition of thyroidal adenyl cyclase and of the action of cyclic-AMP on the thyroid, and it may be that such effects are of fundamental importance in determining lithium's side-effects on thyroidal functioning. Halmi and Noyes (1972) agreed that this might lie behind the observed reduction in serum thyroxine levels following lithium administration, but they added that it was still difficult to interpret the hormone reduction which occurred within 24 hours of lithium being given, in view of the six-day half-life of thyroxine. It might, they suggested, simply be that the hormone level falls as a result of shifts in body fluids.

Villeneuve et al. (1973) suggested that lithium might act to trigger a latent hypothyroidism and that this would occur only in those patients so predisposed. Crowe et al. (1973) proposed that two types of hypothyroidism might be discerned in lithium-treated individuals, the one in patients in whom an underlying thyroiditis existed, and the other in patients in whom no thyroid abnormality could be detected. Crowe and his co-workers elaborated on their views by suggesting that in the second type of patients (i.e., the basically normal, in terms of thyroid function) a compensatory mechanism existed, whereby a rise in TSH secretion would lead to an increased iodine uptake in order to overcome the defect in iodine trapping: such a compensation would not occur in patients with a prior thyroid defect and in these latter an increased iodine uptake would not, therefore, be expected.

The thyroidal side-effects of lithium are clearly the result of a whole complex of mechanisms and it is unlikely that they will be susceptible to a single explanation: the reader is referred to Chapter 27 for further details of the hormonal effects produced by lithium.

F. Skin

The skin disorders which arise as a result of lithium treatment often subside spontaneously and Kusumi (1971) notes that, because of this, they may be missed by the clinician. It is possible that the disappearance of the lesions is associated with the establishment of a relatively stable level of lithium in the blood serum, and that it is the rapidly changing electrolyte environment which is responsible for the skin eruptions.

Kusumi (1971) feels that the abrupt appearance of the skin lesions in early treatment, followed by their eventual spontaneous subsidence and failure to reappear on resumed or continued lithium treatment, are indicative of an allergic hypersensitivity reaction, and five patients reported by Callaway et al. (1968) as showing lithium-induced pruritic maculo-papular rashes, did indeed respond to the administration of antihistamines or steroids.

Carter (1972) points out that methotrexate, an effective medication for psoriasis, is believed to act by inhibiting folate reductase, an effect which results in the prevention of tetrahydrofolate formation: this latter substance is a necessary coenzyme for thymidine synthesis and is thus necessary for the formation of DNA. Epithelial cell division involves DNA and is consequently reduced by methotrexate. In psoriasis the rate of cell division in the epithelium is abnormally high. Lithium induces psoriasis when it is administered shortly after methotrexate medication and Carter suggests that it may do so by reversing, or inhibiting, one of the steps which have been implicated in methotrexate action.

The question of a predisposition to skin disorders is raised by Carter (1972) who notes that most of the patients reported by O'Connell (1970) as showing lithium-induced skin lesions, had histories of such conditions in adolescence.

G. Blood

O'Connell (1970) dismissed the possibility of a direct toxic effect of lithium on the leukocyte-forming tissues on the grounds that the leukocytosis observed during lithium treatment is sporadic, whereas there is no reason to believe that the irritant effect of lithium would be anything but continuous. A similar view was expressed by Shopsin et al. (1971) who also rejected a secondary pathological leukocytosis resulting from acidosis, eclampsia or gout. Sternal punctures carried out by Shopsin and his co-workers also provided no further information about the origins of the leukocytosis, despite an early report of toxic bone-marrow changes by Bille and Plum (1955). Both O'Connell (1970) and Shopsin et al. (1971) put forward the view that the leukocytosis was stimulated by a change in steroid metabolism: it had already been established (Nelson et al., 1952) that corticosteroids elevated the leukocyte count and that neutro-philia in particular followed steroid administration (Mayfield and Brown, 1969). Moreover, lithium had been shown to produce a rise in plasma cortisol levels, particularly in those patients who showed a susceptibility to lithium toxicity (Platman and Fieve, 1968) and medullary and cortical adrenal hor-mones were found by Samuels (1951) to lead to leukocytosis and lymphocyto-paenia.

Alternative explanations have been aired, albeit more tentatively. Murphy et al. (1971), for example, note that the lithium-induced leukocytosis proceeds in the general direction of mature granulocytes and they suggest that the role of thyroid hormones (themselves known to be affected by lithium) on granulocyto-poiesis should be examined. Shopsin et al. (1971) refer briefly to the "alluring possibility" that the leukocytosis may be secondary to a central effect of lithium, possibly on neuroendocrine mechanisms.

H. Other systems (body weight)

Kerry et al. (1970) and O'Connell (1971) make the point that the weight gain reported in many lithium-treated patients is not due to water retention, but is a result of an increase in fat and other "solid" tissue. O'Connell suggested that this may reflect a decrease in metabolic rate secondarily to reduced thyroid functioning and that a hypothalamic mechanism might also be involved.

Kerry and his colleagues voiced the opinion that weight gain is not so much a side-effect as an indicator of therapeutic benefit. Lithium-treated patients may, upon an improvement in their clinical status, develop better appetites and pay more attention to their diet. This, coupled with an improved general health, may restore the patients to the weight they would have attained had they not been ill. If this is indeed the case, it may be that the frequent decision to put lithium patients on to reducing diets is misguided, and Furlong (1973) has in fact reported that unless such reducing diets are supplemented with sodium chloride tablets, the resultant drop in sodium intake may precipitate severe toxic reactions.

The process of weight gain has also been investigated by Mellerup *et al.* (1972) and Plenge *et al.* (1973). Plenge and his co-workers pointed out that in view of the known effects of lithium on various aspects of intermediary metabolism, reports by some investigators of a loss of weight amongst experimental animals treated with lithium are rather difficult to understand; accordingly, Plenge *et al.* (1973) examined lithium effects on weight gain in rats. They noted that their animals actually gained weight as a result of lithium treatment, but that the extent of the gain was a function of the conditions under which the animals were kept. Overcrowding reduced the size of average weight gain. The authors concluded that a gain of weight was to be expected as a normal accompaniment of lithium treatment, a failure for this to occur possibly indicating that the environmental conditions were stressful; mild stress, they point out, elevates blood corticosteroid levels and this results in decreased peripheral uptake of glucose. Results such as these argue against the view of Kerry and his co-workers that the weight gain is an indirect effect of lithium.

III. Proposals for Single Mechanisms Producing a Variety of Side-Effects

As early as 1954, Glessinger put forward the suggestion that many of the more commonly observed side-effects of lithium could be traced to an action of the drug on the central nervous system. Taking a patient described by Stern (1949) as a case in point, Glessinger supported his contention by a variety of arguments. He claimed that the swallowing difficulties which were reported were most appropriately related to bulbar, rather than peripheral muscular, actions since the muscles were, if anything, hyper-responsive; dorsiflexion of the big toes is a sign of cerebral interference, not of general poisoning; nystagmus is a well-known symptom of encephalopathy which can be traced to central lesions of the cerebellum or cerebrum; ataxia suggests cerebellar, spinal or brain stem defects.

Schou *et al.* (1968b) agree that the central nervous system is of major importance in determining the symptoms of lithium toxicity. An early tendency to regard the kidneys as the primarily affected organs may have been due to the reports of toxicity studies with animals in which relatively large doses of lithium were studied in comparison with the doses employed therapeutically.

O'Connell (1971) has, more recently, suggested that, in accordance with the principle of parsimony, lithium side-effects may all be related to a non-specific effect of the ion on the neuroendocrine axis, resulting in an inhibition of hypothalamic or other subcortical processes.

Other general principles, not specifically elaborated by any particular author but found running throughout the literature, relate to the rate of change of tissue concentrations of lithium, and to the presence of predisposing conditions of either an overtly pathological or subclinical nature.

IV. Conclusions

The picture which emerges when one surveys the ideas which have been advanced regarding the mechanisms of lithium side-effects and toxic reactions, is far from clear. The major research effort as far as lithium is concerned has manifestly been directed towards the elucidation of the biochemical and physiological mechanisms involved in the therapeutic actions of lithium, but if it is to find a lasting place in regular treatment it is essential that more attention should be given to its side-effects. It may, in any case, be a mistake to regard the two kinds of endeavour as entirely separable: just as much of our knowledge of the mechanisms of lithium toxicity stems from studies of its therapeutic action, so a closer study of individual side-effects may provide us with valuable clues to the way in which lithium produces its beneficial effects in alleviating affective disorders, and it may even shed light upon the biochemical and physiological bases of the affective disorders themselves.

References

Abuzzahab, F. S., Schrader, R. J. and Borgen, L. A. (1969). *Fed. Proc.* **28**, 260.

Angrist, B. M., Gershon, S., Levitan, S. J. and Blumberg, A. G. (1970). *Compreh. Psychiat.* **11,** 141–146.

Berens, S. C., Bernstein, R. S., Robbins, J. and Wolff, J. (1970). *J. clin. Invest.* **49,** 1357–1367.

Bille, M. and Plum, C. M. (1955). *Ugeskr. Laeg.* **117**, 293–297.

Burrow, G. N., Burke, W. R., Himmelhoch, J. M., Spencer, R. P. and Hersham, J. M. (1971). *J. clin. Endocrinol.* **32**, 647–652.

Callaway, C. L., Hendric, H. C. and Luby, E. D. (1968). *Amer. J. Psychiat.* **124**, 1124–1125.

Carter, T. N. (1972). *Psychosomatics* **13**, 325–327.

Cooper, T. B., Wagner, B. M. and Kline, N. S. (1970). *Biol. Psychiat.* **2**, 273–278.

Corcoran, A. C., Taylor, R. D. and Page, I. (1949). *J. Amer. med. Assoc.* **139**, 685–688.

Crowe, M. J., Lloyd, G. G., Bloch, S. and Rosser, R. M. (1973). *Psychol. Med.* **3**, 337–342.

Delgado, J. M. R. and De Feudis, F. V. (1969). *Expl. Neurol.* **25**, 255–267.

Demers, R. G., Hendler, R., Allen, R. P. and Boyd, J. (1969). *Expl. Neurol.* **25**, 255–267.

Demers, R. and Heninger, G. (1970a). *J. Amer. med. Assoc.* **214**, 1845–1848.

Demers, R. and Heninger, G. (1970b). *J. Amer. med. Assoc.* **218**, 381–386.

Demers, R. G., Hendler, R., Allen, R. P. and Boyd, J. (1971). *Physician's Drug Manual* **3**, 2–24.

Dias, N. and Hocken, A. G. (1972). *Nephron* **10**, 246–249.

Dousa, T. and Hechter, O. (1970a). *Life Sci.* **9**, 765–770.

Dousa, T. and Hechter, O. (1970b). *Lancet* **1**, 834–835.

Duc, N. and Maurel, H. (1953). *Concours méd.* **75**, 1817–1820.

Evan, A. P. (1973). *Toxic. appl. Pharmacol.* **24**, 413–422.

Evan, A. P. and Ollerich, D. A. (1972). *Amer. J. Anat.* **134**, 97–106.

Fieve, R. R. and Platman, S. (1968). *Amer. J. Psychiat.* **125**, 527–530.

Furlong, F. W. (1973). *Canad. psychiat. Assoc. J.* **18**, 75–76.

Gattozzi, A. A. (1970). "Lithium in the Treatment of Mood Disorders". National Clearinghouse for Mental Health Information, NIMH Publication Number 5033.

Glessinger, B. (1954). *Med. J. Aust.* **41**, 277–283.

Goyer, R. A. and Krall, R. (1969). *J. cell. Biol.* **41**, 393–400.

Gritzka, T. L. and Trump, B. F. (1968). *Amer. J. Pathol.* **52**, 1225–1227.

Gutman, Y., Benzakein, F. and Livneh, P. (1971). *Eur. J. Pharmac.* **16**, 380–384.

Halmi, K. A. and Noyes, R. (1972). *Biol. Psychiat.* **5**, 211–215.

Hanlon, L. W., Romaine, M., Gilroy, F. J. and Dietrick, J. E. (1949). *J. Amer. med. Assoc.* **139**, 688–692'

Harris, C. A. and Jenner, F. A. (1969a). *J. Physiol.* **200**, 59P.

Harris, C. A. and Jenner, F. A. (1969b). *J. Physiol.* **203**, 73P–74P.

Hullin, R. P. and Johnson, A. M. (1970). *Life Sci.* **9**, 9–20.

James, J. R. and Reilly, E. (1971). *Southern med. J.* **64**, 1322–1327.

Johnson, G., Macario, N., Gershon, S. and Korein, J. (1970). *J. nerv. ment. Dis.* **151**, 273–289.

Kerry, R. J., Liebling, L. I. and Owen, G. (1970). *Acta psychiat. scand.* **46**, 238–243.

Kusumi, Y. (1971). *Dis. nerv. Syst.* **32**, 853–854.

Larson, C., Kochar, M. S. and Wang, R. I. H. (1972). *J. clin. Pharmacol.* **12**, 459–464.

Lavender, S., Brown, J. N. and Berrill, W. T. (1973). *Postgrad. med. J.* **49**, 277–279.

Lazarus, J. H. and Bennie, E. H. (1972). *Acta Endocrinol.* **70**, 266–272.

Ljunggren, J. G., Sedvall, G., Levin, K. and Fyrö, B. (1971). *Acta endocrinol.* **67**, 784–792.

Mayfield, D. and Brown, R. G. (1966). *J. psychiat. Res.* **4**, 207–219.

Mellerup, E. T., Thomsen, H. G., Bjørum, N. and Rafaelsen, O. J. (1972). *Acta psychiat. scand.* **48**, 332–336.

McKusick, V. A. (1954). *J. clin. Invest.* **33**, 598–610.

Moracci, E. (1931). *Arch. Fisiol.* **29**, 487–492 and 493–511.

Murphy, D. L., Goodwin, F. K. and Bunney, W. E. (1971). *Amer. J. Psychiat.* **127**, 1559–1561.

Nelson, D. H., Sandberg, A. A. and Palmer, J. G. (1952). *J. clin. Invest.* **31**, 843–849.

O'Connell, R. A. (1970). *Int. Pharmacopsychiat.* **4**, 30–34.

O'Connell, R. A. (1971). *Compreh. psychiat.* **12**, 224–229.

Platman, S. R. and Fieve, R. S. (1968). *Archs gen. psychiat.* **18**, 591–594.

Plenge, P. K., Mellerup, E. T. and Rafaelsen, O. J. (1973). *Int. Pharmacopsychiat.* **8**, 234–238.

Prien, R. F., Caffey, E. M. and Klett, C. J. (1971). *Dis. nerv. Syst.* **32**, 521–531.

Radomski, J. L., Fuyat, H. N., Nelson, A. A. and Smith, P. K. (1950). *J. Pharmacol. exp. Ther.* **100**, 429–444.

Ramsey, T. A., Mendels, J., Stokes, J. W. and Fitzgerald, R. C. (1972). *J. Amer. med. Assoc.* **219**, 1446–1449.

Rask-Madsen, J., Baastrup, P. C. and Schwartz, M. (1972). *Brit. med. J.* **2**, 496–498.

Reilly, E., Halmi, K. A. and Noyes, R. Jr. (1973). *Int. Pharmacopsychiat.* **8**, 208–213.

Roberts, E. L. (1950). *Med. J. Aust.* **37**, 261–262.

Rogers, M. P. and Whybrow, P. C. (1971). *Amer. J. Psychiat.* **128**, 158–163.

Samuels, A. J. (1951). *J. clin. Invest.* **30**, 941.

Schou, M. (1957). *Pharmacol. Rev.* **9**, 17–58.

Schou, M. (1959). In "Neuropsychopharmacology" (P. B. Bradley, P. Deniker and C. Radouco-Thomas, eds), pp. 687–690. Elsevier, Amsterdam.

Schou, M. (1969). *Psychopharmacologia* **1**, 65–73.

Schou, M., Amdisen, A., Jensen, S. E. and Olsen, T. (1968a). *Brit. med. J.* **3**, 710–713.

Schou, M., Amdisen, A. and Trap-Jensen, J. (1968b). *Amer. J. Psychiat.* **125**, 520–527.

Sedvall, G., Jönsson, B., Pettersson, U. and Levin, K. (1968). *Life Sci.* **7**, 1257–1264.

Shopsin, B. and Gershon, S. (1971). *Archs gen. psychiat.* **24**, 320–327.

Shopsin, B., Johnson, G. and Gershon, S. (1970). *Int. Pharmacopsychiat.* **5**, 170–182.

Shopsin, B., Friedman, R. and Gershon, S. (1971). *Clin. Pharmacol. Ther.* **12**, 923–928.

Sivadon, P. and Chanoit, P. (1955). *Ann. méd. Psychol.* **113**, 790–796.

Smith, S. G. and Lasater, T. E. (1950). *Proc. Soc. exp. Biol. Med.* **74**, 427–431.

Stancer, H. C. and Kivi, R. (1971). *Lancet* **2**, 985.

Stern, R. L. (1949). *J. Amer. med. Assoc.* **139**, 710–711.

Surawicz, B. (1964). *Mod. Concepts. cardiovasc. Dis.* **33**, 875–880.

Talso, P. J. and Clarke, R. W. (1951). *Amer. J. Physiol.* **166**, 202–208.

Tangedahl, T. N. and Gau, G. T. (1972). *New Engl. J. Med.* **287**, 867–869.

Trautner, E. M., Morris, R., Noack, C. H. and Gershon, S. (1955). *Med. J. Aust.* **42**, 280–291.

Van der Velde, C. D. (1971). *Amer. J. Psychiat.* **127**, 1075–1077.

Villeneuve, A., Gautier, J., Jus, A. and Perron, D. (1972). *Lancet* **2**, 502.

Williams, J. A., Berens, S. C. and Wolff, J. (1971). *Endocrinol.* **88**, 1385–1388.

Wolff, H. P., Vessei, P., Kruck, F., Roscher, S., Brown, J. J., Dusterdieck, G., Lever, A. F. and Robertson, J. I. S. (1968). *Lancet* **1**, 257–261.

Wolff, J., Berens, S. C. and Jones, A. B. (1970). *Biochem. biophys. Res. Commun.* **39**, 77–82.

33

THE EFFECTS OF LITHIUM ON BASIC CELLULAR PROCESSES

SUSAN JOHNSON

I. Introduction

The lithium ion has multiple effects upon metabolism, as previous chapters have amply indicated. It is seldom possible to determine which effects are primary and which arise secondarily as a consequence of more fundamental actions of lithium, so interwoven is the fabric of biochemical reactions making up the body's metabolism. It may, however, be possible to account in part for the variety of the metabolic changes brought about by lithium, by considering those processes which appear to be common to all metabolic pathways. Enzymes are necessary components of biochemical processes and are also known to be particularly sensitive to the conditions of the milieu in which they operate: the efficiency with which they promote their associated reactions is modified by variations in such factors as temperature, pH, and the concentrations of various substances. Enzymes might well, therefore, be expected to respond to changes in tissue levels of lithium, and the consequences of such changes would undoubtedly extend beyond the immediate bounds of the

533

particular enzyme-dependent processes, showing up in all other associated processes to some extent. Thus, interference with the enzymatic basis of active transport mechanisms could lead to essential reactants of a wide range of metabolic pathways not being transported to appropriate sites. This chapter will examine some of the evidence of lithium involvement in enzyme action. As proteins, enzymes are dependent upon mechanisms of protein synthesis. There is some evidence that lithium may have effects upon the structure and metabolism of ribonucleic acid (RNA) and deoxyribonucleic acid (DNA), both of which are intimately concerned with the elaboration of protein molecules. This too will be considered in the present chapter.

The maintenance of cellular metabolism requires the expenditure of energy. Lithium has been shown to have some influence upon the provision of energy by the hydrolysis of ATP, and to act in various ways upon those organelles, the mitochondria, which seem to be most intimately involved with this aspect of energy metabolism. The evidence for this will also be reviewed.

Mellerup and Jørgensen, in Chapter 21, have made the point that, in the final analysis, the effects of lithium may be traceable to the replacement by lithium ions of some other cation or cations with which lithium shares one or more physico-chemical characteristic. In the following discussion the actions of lithium will be set in the context of effects produced by other cations, and in particular the ions of the Group I alkali metals.

II. Lithium and Enzymes

The mechanisms of enzyme action are extremely complex and still only partially understood. The roles of monovalent cations in general, and of lithium in particular, in determining enzyme activity have been vigorously studied in the last decade.

There have been many *in vitro* studies of the effects of lithium on enzyme activity at various biological levels (e.g., using purified enzyme extracts, tissue homogenates, tissue slices, and organ cultures) as well as many *in vivo* studies, but this work has so far failed to provide any general principles which might explain the therapeutic action of lithium in the treatment of recurrent endogenous affective disorders. Nevertheless, lithium-induced enzyme effects are so widely documented that there is no reason to suppose that a connection with therapeutic efficacy might not eventually be established.

A. *In vitro* studies

It is not possible to define precisely the mechanisms by which monovalent cations affect enzyme activity but several views have been put forward. Suelter (1970), in reviewing enzyme reactions activated by monovalent cations, has favoured the concept of a ternary complex being formed between the monovalent cation, enzyme and substrate, and thereby preventing, impairing, or possibly facilitating, the action of the enzyme upon the substrate. Lowenstein (1960) and Melchior (1965) have suggested that a complex may be formed consisting of monovalent cation and ATP, a concept based on studies of the role of monovalent cations in phosphoryl transfer reactions; as Suelter (1970) points out, however, not all enzymes activated by monovalent cations catalyse phosphoryl transfer reactions, and some more general mechanism must therefore be sought.

Evans and Sorger (1966), in a review of the effects of mineral elements on enzyme systems found in a whole variety of animals and plants, suggested that monovalent cations might act by changing the structural conformation of enzymes, particularly at points on the enzyme molecule which acted as reactive sites. They proposed that the conformation of univalent cation-activated enzymes may be flexible and dependent on the cationic environment. Thus many monovalent cation-activated enzymes function in environments containing K^+, NH_4^+ or Rb^+ whilst other ions, such as Li^+ and $Tris^+$ may produce conformations in the enzymes which make them unsuitable for taking part in catalysis or associated reactions.

There are many instances in the literature of cation-sensitive enzyme processes. For example, Black (1951) found yeast aldehyde dehydrogenase to be activated by K^+ and Rb^+ but not by Li^+, Na^+ or Cs^+. Li^+ was the most effective of the latter three ions in inhibiting the activating effect of K^+ and Rb^+. The inhibition was not competitive, the addition of Li^+ ions failing to lead to a significant increase in the amount of K^+ ions required to produce a maximum reaction rate. However, in a later study of univalent cation effects on the same enzyme, Sorger and Evans (1966) found Li^+ and Na^+ to be inhibitors of the activating properties of K^+ and Rb^+, Li^+ being more effective than Na^+ as a competitive inhibitor of K^+. Li^+ was less effective than Na^+ as a protector from heat inactivation. The order of effectiveness in reactivating the enzyme after prolonged dialysis against Tris buffer was $K^+ > Rb^+ > Na^+ > Li^+ > Tris^+$. In other studies, Inoue and Iwata (1971) demonstrated that Li^+ and Na^+ inhibited the stimulatory effect of Ca^{++} on the enzyme thiamine diphosphatase.

The hydrated atomic radii of the various cations has been cited as the critical factor in determining the effect of the ions on various enzymes (Evans and Sorger, 1966; Sorger and Evans, 1966). The advocates of this view point to the fact that enzymes activated by K^+, NH_4^+ and Rb^+ are activated little or not at all by Li^+ and Na^+, and relate this observation to the hydrated atomic radii of 5·32, 5·37 and 5·09 Å respectively for K^+, NH_4^+ and Rb^+, which are small compared with 7·9 and 10·0 Å respectively for Na^+ and Li^+ (Kachmar and Boyer, 1953). This point, however, will be taken up and discussed in further detail later in this chapter.

In contrast to the examples mentioned above of enzyme inhibition by alkali metal cations, conformations more suitable for catalysis are sometimes produced in the presence of the larger hydrated ions. For example, poly-β-hydroxybutyric depolymerase is activated by Li^+ and Na^+ but not by K^+, NH_4^+ or Rb^+ (Sierra and Gibbons, 1963). Setlow and Lowenstein (1968), in a study of the effects of the chlorides of lithium, sodium and potassium on the activity of calf brain adenylate deaminase, found lithium chloride to be the most effective activator of the enzyme in the absence of ATP (which activates the enzyme) and the most effective de-inhibitor of the enzyme in the presence of GTP (which inhibits the enzyme). The chlorides of lithium, sodium and magnesium all increase the activity of several oxidative enzymes (succinic dehydrogenase, DPN-diaphorase, and several others) in astrocytes grown from explants of rat cerebral cortex cultured in plasma clots (Friede, 1964). Kiseleva (1972) reported that lithium carbonate in concentrations of $1 \cdot 1 \times 10^{-4}$, $2 \cdot 2 \times 10^{-4}$ and $1 \cdot 1 \times 10^{-3}$ M, increased monoamine oxidase activity of rat brain homogenates by 44, 48 and 24·4% respectively. Electrical stimulation and the presence of various ions such as K^+, NH_4^+, Cs^+, Rb^+ and choline, increase respiratory rate, aerobic glycolysis, and the breakdown of creatine phosphate and ATP in brain slices, but only in the presence of Na^+ (Hertz and Schou, 1962): Li^+, unlike the other ions, was found to produce a stimulated respiration without the aid of Na^+ as a cofactor. The stimulating ions differed in the amount of each required to produce stimulation; for example, NH_4^+ was 10 times as active as Rb^+ and 25 times as active as Li^+. They fell into the following order of effectiveness in stimulating activity: $NH_4^+ > Cs^+ > Rb^+ = K^+ > Li^+ >$ choline. Hertz and Schou suggested that the stimulating activities expressed the relative affinities of the ions for particular stimulating sites in, or on, the brain cells.

If monovalent cations do in fact influence enzyme activity by changing structural conformation of enzyme molecules (which, as Suelter (1970) pointed out, is not incompatible with the idea of ternary complex formation) then detection of these changes by various physical means should correlate with observed changes in enzyme activity. A number of studies designed to demonstrate this have met with varying degrees of success. Warren et al. (1966) argued that the criteria for concluding that the effects of monovalent cations on enzyme activity are structural are firstly that the ions ordered by Von Hippel and Wong (1964) on the basis of physical methods should remain in the same order on the basis of their capacity to inhibit (or activate) a given enzyme, and secondly that the order of inhibitory (or activatory) effectiveness of the ions should be the same for radically different enzyme systems. Von Hippel and Wong (1964) found that various cations and anions could be ordered by their capacity to alter the organized structure of a variety of macromolecules such as DNA, collagen, gelatin and ribonuclease. The results of Tonomura et al. (1962) using myosin, and of Robinson and Jencks (1965) using a model polypeptide, were in general agreement with those of Von Hippel and Wong (1964), the effectiveness of the disrupting activity of the cations being $Li^+ > Na^+ > K^+ > Cs^+$. This is also the order of decreasing size of the hydrated ions. These studies were all carried out using high concentrations of ions. Warren *et al.* (1966) studied the effects of neutral salts in high concentrations (0·3 to 3·0M) on the activity of myosin nucleoside triphosphatase, trypsin, estradiol-17β dehydrogenase, lactate dehydrogenase, and fumarase, enzymes deliberately chosen for their wide differences. The effectiveness of ions in inhibiting the activity of each of these enzymes was again in the same order as that noted by Von Hippel and Wong (1964). Wilson *et al.* (1967), using non-physiological concentrations of salts (0·5 to 0·86M) found an inverse correlation between the known capacities of univalent cations to activate pyruvate kinase and their capacity to perturb tryptophan residues of the enzyme. In addition, the activating ability of an ion was found to be related to the protective effect which it could exert against the inactivating effects of incubation: thus, incubation of pyruvate kinase with non-activator cations $Tris^+$, $(CH_3)_4N^+$, and Li^+, resulted in a loss of 50% of the initial activity within 24h, whereas activity was maintained at normal levels after incubation with the activator cations K^+, Rb^+ and NH_4^+. In studies of the structural conformation of myosin, using a paramagnetic and a fluorescent label, Cheung and Cooke (1971) found that the alkali metal ions altered the molecular structure of the enzyme in the vicinity of the label. The results with the maleimide spin label, in which the maximum conformational change was seen in the presence of K^+ suggested, however, that the effects of alkali metal ions may not always be graded according to ionic size.

Not all studies have been able to show that changes in enzyme structure accompany changes in activity when the cationic environment is varied. Wildes *et al.* (1971), for example, found that although structural changes in the enzyme pyruvate kinase in the presence of different cations could be demonstrated by means of circular dichroism spectra, the changes did not correlate with the known activating abilities of the ions. The concentration of alkali cation used seems to be an important factor in determining the outcome of experiments in this area. Studies which have demonstrated correlations between effects on structure and effects on enzyme activity have tended to use ion concentrations which are, in physiological terms, high. Work with physiological levels of the cations has frequently failed to show this structure–activity correlation, even though enzyme activity continues to be affected. Thus the different effects noted by Wilson *et al.* (1967) on the structure of pyruvate kinase (see above) when cation concentrations between 0·5 and 0·86M were used, were not seen when concentrations of 0·1M were employed instead. In order to maintain the structural change hypothesis even for physiological concentrations of cations, Warren *et al.* (1966) have suggested that activity changes at low salt concentrations may result from subtle conformational changes which are undetectable with presently available methods. From this they argued that if a given enzyme exhibits two activity forms because it exists in two structural forms, the two activity forms should differ in sensitivity to the same ordered sequence of ions. This was found to be the case for native and *p*-chloromercuribenzoate (CMB)-modified myosin. CMB partially blocks sulphhydryl groups. ATPase activity of native and CMB-modified myosin are similar when assays are carried out in the absence of salts; in the presence of a 0·6M salt solution CMB-modified myosin is less sensitive to inhibition of activity by monovalent cations than is native myosin, having an activity two or three times greater than the latter in the same salt solution. The order of sensitivity to salt inhibition remains the same for the two forms of the enzyme, viz., $Li^+ > Na^+ > K^+ > Cs^+ > (CH_3)_4N^+$.

Betts and Evans (1968a) suggested that binding of activator ions to charged groups on the protein molecules may lead to conformations which expose active sites, these sites remaining buried in the molecule when non-activator ions are bound. In search of evidence to support this hypothesis they studied the effects of K^+ (an activator) and Li^+ (a non-activator), at a concentration of 0·1M, on the electrophoretic mobility and substrate binding of the enzyme pyruvate kinase. They were unable to demonstrate any ion-induced conformational change in the enzyme by the electrophoretic technique they used and each molecule of enzyme bound the same number of molecules of ADP or phosphoenolpyruvate regardless of whether activating K^+ or non-activating Li^+ was present in the medium. Thus, sites for substrate binding are apparently available whether activator ion is present or not. Betts and Evans concluded that, if either ion does indeed induce a conformational change in the enzyme, it must be important at some later stage in the process, and must also be very small so as not to be detected by the methods used. In a subsequent paper, Betts and Evans (1968b) pointed out the importance of considering the buffer system used in any assessment of the importance of monovalent cations in enzyme activation. When Tris was used as the buffer in studies of pyruvate kinase and acetaldehyde dehydrogenase a K_a for K^+ was obtained which varied as a result of varying buffer concentration.

B. *In vivo* studies

Just as there are apparent discrepancies between the results of studies using different concentrations of lithium in *in vitro* experiments, so also are there differences between *in vitro* and *in vivo* findings. Relatively long-term lithium administration under *in vivo* conditions simulates the therapeutic situation more closely than do *in vitro* studies, and has been employed in several investigations of the effects of lithium ions on specific enzyme activity.

Perkinson *et al.* (1969) used the *in vivo* technique to make a comparative study of the effects of lithium with those of various tricyclic antidepressant compounds, and showed that lithium, amitriptyline and desiprimine shared the property of being competitive, reversible inhibitors of butyrylcholinesterase. The various salts of sodium, potassium, calcium and magnesium showed no selective inhibition of this enzyme, a finding which is particularly interesting in view of data from *in vitro* studies indicating stimulatory or inhibitory properties of these substances on a variety of other enzymes. Abreu and Abreu (1972) noted a highly significant increase in brain succinate dehydrogenase activity in mice treated for 80 days with lithium carbonate in the drinking water in a dose range corresponding to therapeutic levels. *In vitro* addition of lithium carbonate to mouse brain homogenate before succinate dehydrogenase activity determination did not, however, change the enzyme activity. Similar dissociation between *in vitro* and *in vivo* findings was reported in later studies by the same investigators: long-term (108 days) administration of lithium carbonate to mice in the same concentrations as used in their previous studies, was found by Abreu and Abreu (1973) to result in a significant inhibition of aconitase activity in brain homogenates. Attempts to demonstrate a similar effect of lithium carbonate *in vitro* by adding the salt (up to 0·5 mg) to the incubation medium were, however, unsuccessful. There are no studies reported in the literature to indicate at what stage of lithium administration *in vivo* the changes in the activity of brain succinate dehydrogenase and aconitase become detectable. In hypothesising about the mechanisms involved it would be important to know whether the enzyme activity change occurred early in the period of lithium administration or whether it was an effect which was dependent upon chronic administration. The finding that long-term *in vivo* administration of lithium in therapeutic doses can lead to changes in specific enzyme activity which cannot be detected when lithium is added directly to the enzyme system *in vitro* raises the possibility that any structural change in the enzyme molecule which lithium brings about is produced indirectly. It may be that lithium alters the metabolic processes involved in enzyme synthesis, leading to the production of an enzyme molecule having subtle conformational changes and changed activity characteristics. Such effects on enzyme conformation could occur at any one of the many steps in protein synthesis, and perhaps even as far back in the chain as the DNA molecule.

The suggestion that there may be some degree of separation between lithium as a causal factor and changed enzyme activity as the ultimate consequence, has received support from some interesting studies by Vacquier (1971) on developing Sand Dollar larvae. In these larvae, β-1,3-glucanohydrolase (β-glucanase) activity is first noted at the time of differentiation of the digestive tract, some 24h after the first cleavage, and the enzyme activity increases during subsequent development. When lithium chloride was added to the sea water medium during the first 8h of development there subsequently appeared a marked increase (23%) in the maximum specific activity of β-glucanase some 16h later. Despite the fact that the enzyme activity was not established at the time of lithium administration, and also that the lithium was no longer present in the sea water medium when the enzyme activity increase became manifested, the causal

T

connection between lithium and changed enzyme activity is clear. It is difficult to see how lithium could produce a delayed effect of this kind except by modifying gene expression via an alteration in protein synthesis. Vacquier noted, in the same study, that the rate of synthesis of RNA and protein was decreased by 14 and 20% in the lithium chloride-treated larvae. Whilst Vacquier states that "these data remain quite uninterpretable because of a lack of knowledge of the effects of LiCl on macromolecular synthesis in developing systems" (p. 16) they do, nevertheless, provide some support for an indirect effect of lithium on enzyme synthesis *in vivo*.

III. Lithium and Protein Synthesis

The possibility that lithium may exert effects on protein synthesis mechanisms has also received support from a number of other studies. Turkington (1968), in an examination of the effects of cations on the initiation of DNA synthesis by mammary epithelial cells maintained in organ culture, showed that Li^+ and NH_4^+ ions acted in the G1 phase of the cell cycle to delay the onset of DNA synthesis and to produce a corresponding decrease in the mitotic index. No effects of a similar nature were noted when other cations (Na^+, K^+, Mg^{++} or Ca^{++}) were used. Lithium had no effect on DNA replication rate during the S phase once replication had been initiated. This inhibition by Li^+ of the induction of DNA synthesis in cells preparing for proliferation would be expected to retard the expression of new differentiated functions in progeny cells. A lithium-induced inhibition of DNA synthesis was also observed by Volm *et al.* (1970) who incubated *Tetrahymena pyriformis* (a ciliate) with lithium chloride and measured the uptake of tritiated thymidine, leucine and uridine. The authors concluded that Li^+ produced its effects during DNA replication and transcription. A similar conclusion had earlier been reached by Berg (1968) who found that whilst lithium chloride had no effect on protein synthesis during cleavage of the egg of the sea urchin *Lytechinus*, there did occur a sharp drop in protein synthesis at the end of cleavage in embryos treated with lithium. The low rate of protein synthesis was thereafter maintained in subsequent development. The drop in synthesis coincided in timing with that produced by actinomycin-D and this led Berg to conclude that the Li^+ effect was primarily upon protein synthesis at the transcription level, there being a decrease in DNA-dependent RNA.

Many of the studies of lithium effects on protein synthesis and associated mechanisms have involved the use of *in vitro* concentrations of Li^+ ions considerably larger than would be encountered *in vivo* during normal clinical usage. Even so, the findings of such investigations may not be without some significance. Thus, Kaji and Kaji (1964) found that lithium chloride in high concentrations inhibited the specific attachment of sRNA to ribosomes and split the 70S ribosomes into 30S and 50S particle subunits. Under the same conditions lithium chloride did not prevent the attachment of poly-uridylic acid to 30S ribosomes, nor the reaction of aminoacyl sRNA synthetase. Levine *et al.* (1966) examined the effects of various monovalent cations on the aminoacyl transfer reaction (i.e., the transfer of amino acids from aminoacyl sRNA to polypeptides on ribosomes) and showed that the effectiveness of the cations in stimulating the reaction was greatest with NH_4^+ and least with Li^+ and Cs^+, with K^+, Na^+ and Rb^+ occupying intermediate positions. The activity of the cations in polypeptide synthesis was correlated with crystal radius and entropy of formation at $25°C$, and negatively correlated with the radius of the hydrated ion. Similar findings were reported by Suzuka and Kaji (1968) who found that 0.1 to $0.5M$ concentrations of lithium chloride inhibited the binding of aminoacyl tRNA to ribosomes either in the presence or absence of messenger RNA, an effect which was partially reversed by NH_4^+ or K^+. The 70S ribosomes were completely dissociated into 50S and 30S subunits in $0.2M$ lithium chloride, an effect which was reversible on removal of the lithium salt. The ability of ribosomes to synthesis polyphenylalanine in the presence of polyuridylic acid was also recovered on removal of lithium chloride: this reversible effect was antagonized by the presence of a low concentration of NH_4^+. Igarashi *et al.* (1971) found that NH_4^+ and Li^+ were able to substitute for Mg^{++} in the role of stimulating aminoacyl tRNA formation.

Lithium may affect the binding of proteins to nucleic acids. Perry and Kelley (1968) noted that lithium chloride caused cleavage of ribosomal proteins from ribosomal RNA, and Bielka *et al.* (1970) subsequently demonstrated that ribosomes could be dissociated into RNA and protein fractions by high concentrations of a variety of monovalent cations. This property of lithium has been utilized by virologists in separating viral DNA from capsid and internal core proteins. Neurath *et al.* (1970), for example, employed lithium iodide for this purpose and referred to a suggestion made by Kurtz and Harrington (1966) that specific binding of lithium halides to peptide linkages leads to conformational changes in the polypeptides. According to Neurath and his colleagues, such binding might lead to disruption of the viral nucleoprotein core into its constituent proteins and nucleic acids.

Whilst *in vitro* studies have indicated quite clearly that Li^+ ions do produce alterations in nucleic acid metabolism, there is as yet little definitive information on the nature of Li^+-RNA or Li^+-DNA interactions. Several physico-chemical studies, which may have some bearing on this matter, have been reported in the literature, though it is seldom easy to relate the findings directly to events occurring in biological systems. Ross and Scruggs (1964a, b) studied the effects of adding small quantities of alkali metal ions on the electrophoretic mobility of DNA. Mobility was generally reduced, with Li^+ producing a greater effect than either Na^+ or K^+. The depression of mobility was considered to arise from a reduction of charge in the DNA, the viscosities of the solutions being nearly identical. The authors concluded that the alkali metal ions attach to single phosphate groups (an alkali ion bridge between two phosphate groups being unlikely in view of their wide separation). This view was based on comparisons of the electrophoretic data with earlier work on long-chain polyphosphates, but has received some more recent confirmation from studies reported by Rupprecht and Forslind (1970). These investigators examined the amount of alkali metal incorporated into a film of highly orientated DNA prepared by a wet spinning method, and they noted a linear increase with electrolyte concentration. Each phosphate group in DNA was found to have one alkali metal counter ion.

The relative binding of alkali metals with a variety of polynucleotides was further investigated by Barber and Noble (1966) who used the critical salt concentration of cetyltrimethylammonium precipitation of the polynucleotides as a criterion of counter ion binding. The strength of specific binding of alkali metal ions with calf thymus DNA, rRNA, sRNA and polyuridylic acid, was directly correlated with the crystal radii of the counter ions, i.e., $Li^+ > Na^+ > K^+ > Rb^+ > Cs^+$. Kuznetsov et al. (1967), observing that various studies of the thermal stability of DNA in the presence of alkali metal ions have not always resulted in the ions being ordered according to the lyotropic series, suggested that interactions between alkali metal ions and DNA macromolecules were of a more specific nature. They undertook studies involving the replacement of one alkali metal ion by another to observe the effects of changed ionic surroundings on DNA secondary structure as indexed by viscosity and fusion temperature. In general, fusion temperature was raised as the counter ions increased in degree of hydration, but the direct proportionality observed between fusion temperature and hydration energy for Cs^+, NH_4^+, K^+ and Na^+ broke down for Rb^+ and Li^+, the DNA salts of the latter two ions being much higher than expected. The strengths of affinity of DNA followed the order $Li^+ > Na^+ > Rb^+ > K^+ > NH_4^+ > Cs^+$. On the basis of previous work (Kuznetsov et al., 1963) in which cation absorbability on polystyrene sulphonic acid cationic exchange resin was shown to follow the reverse sequence, Kuznetsov et al. (1967) concluded that DNA could be viewed as a soluble ion exchanger, the affinities for Rb^+, and especially for Li^+, being anomalously high. The picture was complicated somewhat by the finding that the order of affinities varied slightly with changes in ionic strengths of the alkali metal solutions. Cation affinities for DNA were also studied by Shapiro et al. (1969) who examined the relative affinities of several small weakly bound cations for DNAs of varying base compositions. A dialysis competition technique, which is particularly sensitive to small differences in binding affinity, was used. The authors found that Na^+, Li^+, Cs^+ and K^+ as well as arginine, lysine and tetralysine, were bound equally strongly to DNAs of any base composition.

Whilst the greater part of the work on lithium and RNA has been conducted using *in vitro* systems and may, therefore, not be entirely representative of what actually happens in living systems, there is some evidence linking the therapeutic effectiveness of lithium in manic-depressive patients with changes in RNA metabolism. Anumonye *et al.* (1968) noted that uric acid excretion increased in the early phase of remission from hypomanic or depressive states, whether the remission was spontaneous or brought about by lithium treatment. Dewar and Reading (1971) pointed to these findings as indicating a possible involvement of RNA metabolism in the process of mood change since uric acid is an end product of purine catabolism, and they therefore set out to investigate the effects on brain RNA metabolism of prolonged administration of therapeutic dose levels of lithium (0·15 mg/g/day for 13 days) to rats. Intraventricular injections of 6-^{14}C orotic acid were given, and radioactive labelling of cerebral RNA fractions assessed at intervals between 2 and 24 h after the injection. At 2 h the lithium-treated rats showed elevated RNA synthesis: this was followed by a rapid and progressive decline in labelling over the next 8 to 24 h. By contrast, the control rats exhibited a progressive increase in labelling over the 24 h period, there being no initial burst of synthetic activity 2 h after the orotic acid injection. In the lithium-treated animals RNA synthesis was resumed after 48 h, but at a reduced rate. Dewar and Reading concluded that lithium apparently elevated RNA turnover rates, and this effect seemed to be specific to brain material since parallel investigations using liver RNA exhibited no effect of lithium. Several possible explanations are put forward by Dewar and Reading. Lithium may, for example, cause pool size changes in available nucleotide constituents of RNA. Alternatively, it may operate at the membrane level, changing the transport of labelled orotic acid so that more becomes available for RNA synthesis. A third possibility is that lithium produces a direct effect on brain RNA polymerase or ribonuclease.

Lithium effects on protein synthesis may eventually be found to result from several quite distinct mechanisms, effective at different levels in the progression from DNA to full elaboration of the protein molecule.

IV. Lithium and ATPase

A group of enzymes which have been found to be responsive to lithium ions and to other ions of the alkali metal series, consists of the various ATPases which are involved in membrane active transport processes. Whittam and Wheeler (1970) have commented that the nature of the ATPase reaction in cell membranes has become the central issue in investigations of active transport mechanisms. ATP is utilized in providing energy for two major aspects of cellular activity: on the one hand it supports general cellular metabolism, and on the other it powers the active transport mechanisms by which ions and other substances are transferred across cell membranes. The two components are presumably in dynamic balance and Whittam (1962b) has noted that a variation in the one will therefore be expected to result in a feedback control on the rate of supply of energy to the other. A change in membrane ATPase activity brought about by the administration of lithium would result in a concomitant alteration of energy availability for cellular metabolism as well as in changes in active transport across the cell membrane (Figure 1). A knowledge of the way in which lithium affects ATPase activity and of the relative differences between Li⁺ ions and the biologically important Na⁺ and K⁺ ions in this respect, may therefore prove to be of fundamental importance in understanding the metabolic correlates of clinical change during lithium therapy.

Enzyme actions have been studied using a variety of techniques and, as will become clear in the ensuing discussion, each technique poses its own special problems of interpretation. In particular, when enzymes are studied in cell-free systems the results may not be of direct relevance to cellular processes since differential ionic concentrations across cell membranes are known to have marked effects on enzyme activation or inhibition. This was pointed out by Whittam (1962b) who suggested that erythrocyte ghosts might appropriately be used to measure the effects on membrane ATPase activity of variations in external and internal cation concentrations. Whittam (1962a) and Glynn (1962) showed that Na⁺ ions stimulate ATPase activity from outside the erythrocyte ghost whilst K⁺ ions stimulate activity from the inside, the two ions acting synergistically. Whittam (1962b) prepared erythrocyte ghosts contain-

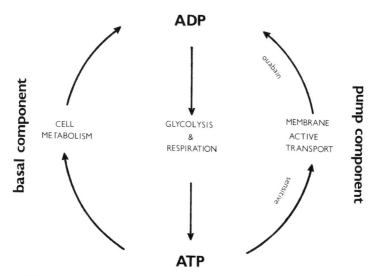

FIG. 1. ATP, derived from ADP by oxidative phosphorylation, is utilized in two main ways by the cell, i.e. to support ouabain-sensitive active transport mechanisms at the cell membrane, and to provide energy for cellular metabolism.

ing ATP and one of the cations Li^+, Na^+, K^+, Rb^+ or Cs^+ and showed that in a K^+-free external medium the rate of hydrolysis of ATP and its inhibition by ouabain were largely independent of the kind of internal alkali metal ion. In a K^+-containing medium, however, ATPase activity was increased by internal Li^+ or Na^+ but not by K^+, Rb^+ or Cs^+. The ouabain-sensitive component of enzyme activity was also greater with Li^+ and Na^+ than with the other ions. Internal Li^+ thus appeared to be similar to Na^+ in acting synergistically with external K^+ to stimulate ATP hydrolysis. In further experiments, Whittam (1962b) examined the effects of alkali metals in the external medium on ATP hydrolysis in ghosts loaded internally with Na^+ ions. The effectiveness of the ions in increasing ATPase activity above the level produced by external Na^+ was $K^+ > Li^+ > Cs^+ > Rb^+$; the increased enzyme activity was abolished by ouabain. Whittam pointed out that the similarity of the effects of external Cs^+ and Rb^+ to that of K^+ was not surprising in view of the fact that these ions are pumped like K^+ into human erythrocytes, but stimulation by external Li^+ was unexpected since Li^+ does not itself appear to be transported. Lithium ions thus appear to be able to replace both external K^+ and internal Na^+ ions and are unlike other alkali metals in possessing the ability to stimulate ATPase activity from both sides of the erythrocyte membrane.

Work such as that of Post et al. (1960) and Dunham and Glynn (1961) has emphasized the close correspondence existing between the ability of Na^+ and K^+ ions to stimulate membrane ATPase activity and to stimulate their own transport, a finding which has been interpreted as meaning that ion transport and ATPase activity are essentially coupled functions, and also that the ions stimulating the ATPase are the same as those being transported. Willis and Fang (1970) have produced data which do not support this conclusion in the case of lithium. These investigators worked with kidney slice preparations in preference to erythrocytes, noting that in kidney tissue the net ionic movement is rapid as compared with that occurring in erythrocytes, the kidney tissue also being rich in $Na^+ + K^+$-activated ATPase. Lithium ions were found to replace internal Na^+ and external K^+ in stimulating ouabain-sensitive respiration and also in stimulating $Na^+ + K^+$-dependent ATPase activity, confirming the findings of Whittam (1962a, b). This occurred only as a synergistic effect in the presence of either Na^+ or K^+. The uptake of K^+ was abolished when Li^+ was substituted for K^+ in a Na^+ medium. There was no net extrusion of Li^+ from Li^+-loaded slices in a Li^+ medium. These results raised the possibility that Li^+-stimulated transport-related ATPase activity may be uncoupled from the actual translocation of Li^+ ions.

ATPase activity in light microsomal preparations of rabbit skeletal muscle was studied by Askari and Fratantoni (1964) and Fratantoni and Askari (1965). They found ATPase activity in the absence of Na^+ and K^+, the activity being promoted further by monovalent cations in the order:

$K^+ > NH_4^+ = Rb^+ > Na^+ > Li^+ = Cs^+$. There are considerable difficulties in placing unequivocal interpretations upon this work, however. In the first place, both Li^+ and Cs^+ ions, though slightly stimulating on ATPase activity at low ionic concentrations, were inhibitory at concentrations in excess of 5mM, abolishing the stimulatory effects of K^+ and Na^+ and inhibiting the basic ATPase activity which occurred in the absence of these ions. Secondly, no synergism was reported between Na^+ and K^+, and ouabain was without effect on ATPase activity. The earlier work (Askari and Fratantoni, 1964) had shown that $Na^+ + K^+$-activated ATPase could be converted fairly readily into Na^+ *or* K^+-activated ATPase by sonification, thereby suggesting that orientation of the enzyme molecule within the membrane is an important factor in determining the nature of ion activation. The findings of Fratantoni and Askari (1965) may be rendered equivocal by a possible disturbance of the enzyme orientation during microsomal preparation; this would account for the failure of these investigators to note Na^+/K^+ synergism. Fratantoni and Askari draw attention to the importance of the preparative methods used in all studies of this kind, noting, for example, that ATPase prepared from liver mitochondria by treatment with deoxycholate is actually inhibited by Na^+ and K^+ and stimulated by Mg^{++} or Ca^{++}.

Dawson and Whittam (1970) approached the question of alkali metal effects on ATPase activity by considering the incorporation of $^{32}P_i$ into ATP by glycolytically inert erythrocyte ghosts. When the ghosts are rich in K^+ and low in Na^+ and the culture medium is high in Na^+ and free of K^+, the $^{32}P_i$ incorporation is partly inhibited by ouabain; this portion of ATP elaboration is thereby indicated as resulting from reversal of the membrane sodium pump mechanism and is referred to as the "pump" component to distinguish it from the "basal" component located within the cell (see Fig. 1). Stimulation of ATPase activity at the membrane will inhibit the pump component of $^{32}P_i$ incorporation; stimulation of intracellular ATPase will inhibit the basal component. Dawson and Whittam found that replacement of external Na^+ by other alkali metal ions resulted in inhibition of $^{32}P_i$ incorporation, the ions being effective in the following order: $K^+ = Rb^+ > Cs^+ > Li^+$. When internal K^+ ions were replaced by other cations it was found that K^+, Rb^+ and Cs^+ had no effect on $^{32}P_i$ incorporation, but that Li^+ and choline would support very little incorporation. All these effects were on the pump component of ATP synthesis. In contrast to the other alkali metal ions, Li^+ inhibited basal incorporation of $^{32}P_i$ by over 30%. The order of effectiveness of the alkali metal ions in inhibiting the pump component of $^{43}P_i$ incorporation was the same as that demonstrated by Whittam and Ager (1964) for the activation of $Na^+ + K^+$-dependent ATPase in erythrocytes, by Forte *et al.* (1967) for the activation of microsomal phosphatase derived from the gastric mucosa, and by Izatt *et al.* (1969) for the binding to various antibiotics and cyclic polyethers which increase biological membrane permeability (to alkali metal cations in particular).

Recent work by Gutman *et al.* (1973a) has served to emphasize the difficulties involved in extrapolating from the results of *in vitro* studies to conclusions about living systems, as far as lithium effects on ATPase are concerned. Gutman and his co-workers pointed to work by Ho *et al.* (1970) in which treatment with lithium had led to elevated Na^+ and decreased K^+ intracellular concentrations in various tissues, especially brain, in rats; such changes, they argued, indicated involvement of sodium-potassium pump mechanisms and accordingly they investigated the effects of Li^+ ions on microsomal $Na^+ + K^+$-dependent ATPase and Mg^{++}-dependent ATPase in a variety of mammalian tissues. Their results indicated wide differences in lithium effects according to the tissue used, a finding which could not have been predicted from *in vitro* studies. In brain tissue no change was noted in ATPase activity, despite the results reported by Ho *et al.* (1970) of marked changes in intracellular K^+ and Na^+ concentrations. Gutman *et al.* suggested that the brain changes in ion distrubition might in fact be secondary to some action produced by lithium on neural activity and not a direct result of changes in ion pump processes. In material from the mucosa of the colon there was a significant lithium-induced decrease in $Na^+ + K^+$-dependent ATPase activity, but a corresponding increase in Mg^{++}-dependent ATPase activity, resulting in a net ATPase activity change of non-significant proportions. Gutman and his colleagues suggested that the $Na^+ + K^+$-activated ATPase might become converted into the Mg^{++}-activated type, resulting in the total microsomal ATPase remaining the same, but the capacity of the sodium pump being reduced. Lithium elevated $Na^+ + K^+$-dependent ATPase activity in salivary gland preparations, particularly in parotid material, and this, it was suggested, might indicate increased conservation of sodium in the face of lithium-induced natriuresis. This work seems to indicate that lithium has a selective effect on microsomal ATPase activity, the effect being confined to those epithelial tissues which are able to develop considerable sodium gradients. Further studies by Gutman *et al.* (1973b) have served to confirm this general conclusion. In experiments on the effects of various concentrations of lithium chloride on microsomal ATPase activity in kidney cortex, medulla and papilla, it was found that enzyme activity was elevated to a marked degree in medullary tissue, there being no significant effect on the cortex and an inhibition of activity in the papilla.

Many of the *in vitro* investigations of ionic influences on ATPase activity have been set up to examine either monovalent or divalent cations but have tended to ignore the possibility that there may occur interactions between the two ionic species in the *in vivo* situation. There are, however, several reports in the literature of studies in which this possibility has been made explicit. In these cases the experimenters either added Ca^{++} or Mg^{++} to the *in vitro* system containing univalent ions, or added specific divalent ion chelating agents

(EDTA, EGTA, etc.) to ensure the absence of the divalent ions. The results of such studies, which presumably bear closely upon the situation obtaining in living systems where both univalent and divalent ions have interwoven functions, are interesting but frequently extremely difficult to interpret, at least in any simple manner. For example, the activation of myosin ATPase by EDTA was found by Bowen and Kerwin (1954) and by Kielley et $al.$ (1956) to be reduced by monovalent ions, the order of inhibitory effectiveness being: $Na^+ > Li^+ > Rb^+ > K^+ > NH_4^+$. The significance of such findings is, however, obscure in view of reports that different sequences of inhibitory effectiveness may be found when myosin ATPase is activated by other agents such as Ca^{++} (Warren et $al.$, 1966). The question received further attention from Kelemen and Mühlrad (1969) who examined the effects of various monovalent ions on the ATPase activity of native and covalently modified myosins in the presence of different effectors such as Ca^{++}, Mg^{++} and EDTA. With Ca^{++} and Mg^{++} ions sequences of inhibitory effectiveness of alkali metal ions were found which were similar to those reported by Warren et $al.$ (1966), though ionic concentration changes were important in determining the precise sequence. With EDTA, Kelemen and Mühlrad broadly confirmed the findings of Bowen and Kerwin (1954) and Kielley et $al.$ (1956). Covalent modification of myosin ATPase, which involved blocking the —SH and —NH_2 groups influencing enzymatic activity, resulted in no change in the orders of inhibitory effectiveness of monovalent ions, but generally reduced the sensitivity of myosin to the monovalent cations present. Of particular interest in the results reported by Kelemen and Mühlrad is the finding that, in the presence of EDTA, Na^+ ions are markedly more efficient than NH_4^+ ions in inhibiting ATPase activity (a ratio of $1:3,550$ was quoted for ATPase activity in the presence of the two types of ion). In view of findings by Seidel (1969) showing that, in the presence of EDTA, myosin catalyses ATP hydrolysis if K^+, NH_4^+ or Rb^+ are available, but not if Na^+ or Li^+ are substituted, Kelemen and Mühlrad (1969) concluded that there may exist a specific cation binding site which directly influences ATP splitting, and that when NH_4^+ or K^+ is bound to this site activity is high, but is reduced to near zero when the bound cation is Na^+ or Li^+. The higher affinity of divalent cations for this binding site would explain the loss of the extreme sensitivity of the system to the species of monovalent cation when Ca^{++} or Mg^{++} are added, and would also account for the recovery of this sensitivity on the addition of EDTA. The earlier work by Seidel (1969) had also drawn attention to the importance of divalent cations in determining monovalent ion effects on ATPase activity. He demonstrated that myosin ATPase activity was stimulated by NH_4^+, Rb^+ and K^+ (in that order) with Cs^+, Na^+ and Li^+ having little or no effect, and Na^+ and Li^+ actually being inhibitory when activity was stimulated by K^+. However, when EDTA was added to the system there was an intensification of the differences between the ionic effects: the stimulatory action of

NH_4^+ was markedly increased and elevations occurred in the stimulatory effects of K^+ and Rb^+ too. The low ATPase activity previously noted in the presence of Cs^+, Na^+ and Li^+ was depressed even further. Both Li^+ and Na^+ not only retained their inhibitory effects when K^+ was the ATPase activator, but showed them to a greater degree.

Katz (1968) reported that Mg^{++}-activated actomyosin ATPase activity was higher in the presence of Na^+ than the other alkali metal ions, the order being $Na^+ > K^+ > Rb^+ > Cs^+ > Li^+$. The differences between the ion effects were, however, concentration-dependent. Katz also pointed out that there was a lack of correlation between the effects of the ions on ATPase activity and their non-specific structure disrupting effects, i.e. $Li^+ > Na^+ > K^+ > Cs^+$.

In some more recent work on divalent-monovalent cation interactions, Costa et al. (1972) have examined the effects of alkali metal ions on the utilization of acetyl phosphate as a substrate for Ca^{++} uptake into the sarcoplasmic reticulum of skeletal muscle. This uptake had previously been shown to be inhibited by Li^+, Na^+ and K^+, but no inhibition had been found when ATP was used as the substrate instead of acetyl phosphate (De Meis, 1969; De Meis and Hassel-bach, 1971). Breakdown of acetyl phosphate by acetyl phosphatase is Mg^{++}-dependent and it is upon this enzyme that Li^+, Na^+ and K^+ presumably exert their inhibitory effects. Costa and his colleagues re-examined the alkali metal effects in the presence of EGTA to eliminate the additional enzyme stimulation provided by the presence of Ca^{++} ions. They found that the order of inhibition of Mg^{++}-dependent acetyl phosphatase activity by alkali metal cations was $Na^+ > Li^+ > K^+$. In the absence of EGTA and with Ca^{++} ions added to the preparation, the alkali metal ions increased the Ca^{++}-activated portion of acetyl phosphatase activity.

It is clear that, the closer the *in vitro* investigations approach the situation existing *in vivo*, the more complicated is the picture which emerges of the relationship between ATPase activity and the ionic environment. The investigations reviewed here are representative of the kinds of study being pursued in this area and future work may provide the generalizations which will unite the apparently disparate findings yielded so far.

V. Lithium and Mitochondria

Lithium may exert effects on ATP metabolism not only by modifying ATPase activity but also by operating at the level of the mitochondria where ATP is reconstituted from ADP as a result of oxidative phosphorylation. For example, the transfer of the adenine nucleotides ATP and ADP across mitochondrial membranes is under the control of the enzyme adenine nucleotide translocase. This transfer process has been found to be sensitive to the effects of various cations (Meisner, 1971). The ATP/ADP exchange in rat liver and heart mitochondria is stimulated by 10mM $Tris^+$, Na^+, Mg^{++}, Li^+ and K^+ to more or less equal extents, though Meisner points out that the effect may be dependent to some extent upon the concentrations of adenine nucleotides present. The relative lack of differential cation effects led Meisner to conclude that it was the positive charge on the ions, rather than their specific nature, which was important in determining the translocation process and he suggested that the positive charge facilitated the binding of adenine nucleotides to the mitochondrial membrane: subsequent translocation, he proposed, was cation-independent. Whatever the precise details of the mechanisms involved, it is clear that any variations in the ionic environment of mitochondria such as must inevitably occur during lithium administration, are bound to have an effect upon ATP/ADP translocation rate, and hence upon energetic metabolism in general.

Using Li^+ ion concentrations approximating serum levels established during lithium therapy, Krall (1967) showed that there were measurable effects of lithium on isolated rat brain mitochondria. ADP-deficient mitochondrial respiration was inhibited by Li^+ concentrations below 10mm, but enhanced with concentrations in excess of this figure. The stimulatory effect of lithium was greater than that usually observed with K^+, but less than that produced by Na^+. The effect was, in part, dependent upon the presence of EDTA. Simic and Gulidova (1970) reported concentration-dependent effects of Li^+ ions on oxidative phosphorylation in isolated cat brain mitochondria, concentrations between 10 and 15mm generally decreasing phosphorylative activity. This is in contrast to some earlier reports (e.g. Chappell and Crofts, 1965; Mitchell, 1966) that the addition of monovalent cations to freshly isolated mitochondria does not affect the efficiency of oxidative phosphorylation. It may be that as yet undetermined aspects of the techniques involved are critical in determining the outcome of experiments in this area.

There is still considerable doubt attached to the mechanisms whereby univalent cations enter mitochondria. Several writers (e.g., Chappell and Crofts, 1965; Mitchell, 1966) have noted that, under normal circumstances, the mitochondrial membrane is generally impermeable to cations and protons, though univalent ions may be transported into mitochondria against concentration gradients in the presence of appropriate membrane permeability-increasing agents and an oxidizable substrate or ATP (Moore and Pressman, 1964; Chappell and Crofts, 1965; Graven et al., 1966) and there is general agreement that the inner mitochondrial membrane is the site of the permeability barrier and cation transporting system. Divalent cations have been implicated in monovalent cation transport processes, though the evidence is indirect. For example, the addition of Mg^{++} chelating agents (such as EDTA or citrate) to liver mitochondria preparations has been observed to result in a cycle of mitochondrial swelling and shrinkage (Azzi et al., 1966). The rate of swelling was high in a medium rich in lithium chloride, decreased in sodium chloride, and negligible in the presence of potassium chloride. Noting that the swelling phase was associated with respiration- or ATP-dependent ejection of H^+ ions from the mitochondria with univalent cation uptake as a concomitant effect, whilst shrinkage was accompanied by the loss of univalent cations, Azzi and his associates presented a hypothetical model of mitochondrial membrane permeability to univalent cations. They suggested that OH^- and H^+ ions are separated by the mitochondrial membrane (the H^+ ions being on the outside) as a result of electron transport mechanisms in the respiratory chain. The resulting membrane potential of 210 mV leads to an influx of cations to restore electrochemical equilibrium. A cation concentration gradient is thereby established which, in its turn, creates an osmotic potential and causes water uptake and a consequent swelling of the mitochondria. Inhibition of respiratory chains in the mitochondria results in a loss of energy needed to maintain the cation gradient and the cations passively diffuse out of the mitochondria down the concentration gradient. The mitochondria thus shrink, respiratory mechanisms again commence functioning and the cycle of swelling begins once more. Addition of Mg^{++} to the medium inhibits swelling or causes the shrinkage of swollen mitochondria, leading Azzi et al. (1966) to propose that the membrane bound Mg^{++} controls mitochondrial permeability to univalent cations.

There is some evidence of an ability of mitochondrial membranes to discriminate between the different alkali metal cations. Moore and Pressman (1964), for example, demonstrated that in mitochondria treated with valinomycin (a permeability increasing agent) the respiratory-dependent production of acid was facilitated by K^+ ions but could also be supported by Rb^+ or Cs^+; Na^+ and Li^+ were, however, ineffective. A similar grouping was also reported by Chappell and Crofts (1965), who showed that cation-H^+ exchange was more effective with K^+, Rb^+ and Cs^+ than with Na^+ or Li^+ in gramicidin-treated mitochondria. The relatively greater efficiency of K^+/H^+ exchange over that of Na^+/H^+ exchange was also shown by Judah et al. (1965). The organization of alkali metal cations into two groups, one containing Li^+ and Na^+, and the other containing K^+, Rb^+ and Cs^+, as far as mitochondrial membrane permeability is concerned, seems to be a finding of some generality. Cereijo-Santalo (1968), for example, reported the same grouping when mitochondrial membrane permeabilities were progressively increased by the use of various agents such as alcohols, Triton-X-100, dinitrophenol, or certain antibiotics. However, when the membrane permeabilities were increased by a process of progressive acidification the ability of cations to enter the mitochondira increased in order of decreasing hydrated ionic radius: $Cs^+ > Rb^+ > K^+ > Na^+ > Li^+$. Cereijo-Santalo proposed that the permeability of the mitochondrial membrane was determined by the appearance of flaws or pores though which the hydrated ions could pass. This point will be taken up again in section VI.

Although the transport mechanisms still remain essentially unelucidated, there is evidence that mitochondria have some affinity for monovalent cations. Gear and Lehninger (1968) demonstrated that various monovalent cations would bind to rat liver mitochondria in exchange for released H^+ ions, the relative ease with which the exchange occurred being: $Li^+ > NH_4^+ > chol-ine > Na^+ > K^+ > Rb^+ > Tris^+$. It appears that the mitochondria behaved like particles in an ion exchange resin, the substitution of cations for H^+ ions occurring rapidly and not being dependent upon electron transport or related coupling mechanisms, or upon the presence of any agents increasing membrane permeability. Similar findings have been reported by Sanui and Pace (1959) in relation to cation binding to rat liver microsomes, and in this earlier work the data were also interpreted on the basis of a simple ion exchange process.

In the *in vivo* situation, the mitochondria may be subjected to many influences, both direct and indirect, as a result of lithium administration. The extensive effects of lithium on endocrine systems have already been reviewed (Chapter 27) and it may be significant that, as Cereijo-Santalo (1968) has pointed out, there have appeared occasional reports of hormonal influences on mitochondrial permeability (Rasmussen *et al.*, 1964) and swelling (Tapley and Cooper, 1965; Lehninger and Neubert, 1961; Neubert and Lehninger, 1962), any or all of which effects might have far-reaching implications for energy metabolism.

VI. Discrimination Between Alkali Metal Ions

In the study of lithium effects at a cellular or subcellular level, it is inevitable that a good deal of attention should be focused upon the manner in which alkali metal ions in general, and lithium ions in particular, cross various membranes. It has frequently been held that the hydrated ionic radius is a critical factor in determining differential membrane selectivity of ions, the implication being that the hydrated ions pass through pores of various radii in the membrane concerned. Similar size considerations have entered into discussions, reviewed earlier, of the ways in which alkali metal ions might modify enzyme structure and hence activity. These views have arisen as a result of the frequent finding that ion selectivity sequences happen to fall either in the order of hydrated ion sizes (the lyotropic series) or in the order of non-hydrated ion sizes. That this view may in fact be over-simplified has been suggested by several authors. Villalonga *et al.* (1969) comment that little use now attaches to the concept of cell membranes as simple sieves or diffusion systems, and they list various types of alternative models which have been proposed, including charged channel systems, mechanisms involving saltatory conveyance of materials from one specific binding site to another (Eisenman *et al.*, 1967; Ling, 1967), various carrier molecules, and membrane phase transitions. From their own studies of L-α-dipalmitoyl lecithin monolayers spread on alkali ion solutions, Villalonga and his colleagues suggest that the dimensions of pores in phospholipid bilayers may change according to the specific ions passing through them. The question was also considered by Diamond and Wright (1969) in a review of the general problem of discrimination between the alkali metal cations in non-living and biological systems. These authors noted that the five cation types, Li^+, Na^+, K^+, Rb^+ and Cs^+ may be permuted in 120 different ways, only 11 of which appear with any degree of regularity in biological systems. These sequences are:

1	Cs	Rb	K	Na	*Li*	: order of increasing hydrated size
2	Rb	Cs	K	Na	*Li*	
3	Rb	K	Cs	Na	*Li*	
4	K	Rb	Cs	Na	*Li*	
5	K	Rb	Na	Cs	*Li*	
6	K	Na	Rb	Cs	*Li*	
7	Na	K	Rb	Cs	*Li*	
8	Na	K	Rb	*Li*	Cs	
9	Na	K	*Li*	Rb	Cs	
10	Na	*Li*	K	Rb	Cs	
11	*Li*	Na	K	Rb	Cs	: order of increasing *non*-hydrated size

The first sequence (increasing hydrated ion size) is separated from the final sequence (increasing non-hydrated ion size) by an intermediate series of nine transitional steps, each of which involves inverting a single pair of ions in the previous sequence. It is the fact that the transitional sequences occur at all in living systems which led Diamond and Wright to emphasize the necessity for a more complicated model of ion selection mechanisms than one based simply on size. They pointed out that "the use of 'hydrated sizes' to explain data other than the data from which they were calculated has virtually disappeared from texts of physical chemistry" (p. 613) and that the only model to provide a consistent explanation of the 11 sequences is one proposed by Eisenman (1961, 1962) in which the main considerations are based upon coulombic forces exerted by water and membrane negative charges on the cations.

VII. Concluding Remarks

Between the psychological and social effects of lithium carbonate administered therapeutically to manic-depressive patients, and the metabolic actions of lithium at the cellular and subcellular levels, there is a large conceptual gap, and it seems unlikely that the two types of description will ever prove to be fully intertranslatable. Nevertheless, many of the biochemical and physiological changes which accompany the clinically valuable and the unwanted toxic effects of lithium treatment may eventually be better understood by examining fundamental cellular processes, and this approach may also lead to advances in our knowledge of the mechanisms underlying the origins and development of the affective disorders.

In the present chapter a necessarily selective review of the literature relating to lithium effects on basic cellular processes has indicated that processes such as enzyme activity, protein synthesis, nucleic acid metabolism, and the mechanisms associated with the provision of energy for a wide range of metabolic functions, are all sensitive to modifications in the ionic environment. Lithium administration, leading to extensive changes in ionic balance both intra- and extra-cellularly, inevitably affects all these important functions. The wide spectrum of biochemical and physiological correlates of lithium therapy, as indicated in previous chapters, may eventually be susceptible to a more unified explanation if the various individual effects may be related to a few changes within cells or at cell membranes.

Progress in this area has already been considerable. Because it represents a meeting point for many disciplines advances may occur on several different fronts, though it may frequently be difficult to interrelate the findings from different types of experiment.

One of the most hopeful trends has involved the use of *in vivo* studies in parallel with, or to complement, studies in *in vitro* systems, and the realization that, in biological systems, univalent cations exert their actions in a complex electrochemical environment in which divalent and other ionic species may produce extensive modifications in the observed effects. As these factors become more widely incorporated into the laboratory experiments we may expect to be provided with information relating more directly to the therapeutic use of lithium.

Lithium is only one of a group of univalent cations, the alkali metals, all of which have uniquely interesting properties. If the work on basic cellular mechanisms tells us anything, it is that we cannot afford to ignore questions such as the interrelationships between these ions and the mechanisms which govern their differential selectivity in biological systems.

References

Abreu, L. A. and Abreu, R. R. (1972). *Nature New Biology* **236**, 254–255.
Abreu, L. A. and Abreu, R. R. (1973). *Experientia* **29**, 446.
Anumonye, A., Reading, H. W., Knight, F. and Ashcroft, G. W. (1968). *Lancet* **1**, 1290–1293.
Askari, A. and Fratantoni, J. C. (1964). *Biochim. biophys. Acta* **92**, 132–137.
Azzi, A., Rossi, E., Azzone, G. F. (1966). *Enzym. biol. clin.* **7**, 25–37.
Barber, R. and Noble, M. (1966). *Biochim. biophys. Acta* **123**, 205–207.
Berg, W. W. (1968). *Expl cell Res.* **50**, 133–139.
Betts, G. F. and Evans, H. J. (1968a). *Biochim. biophys. Acta* **167**, 190–193.
Betts, G. F. and Evans, H. J. (1968b). *Biochim. biophys. Acta* **167**, 193–196.
Bielka, H., Grummt, F. and Schneiders, I. (1970). *Acta biol. med. germ.* **24**, 705–709.
Black, S. (1951). *Archs Biochem.* **34**, 86–97.
Bowen, W. J. and Kerwin, T. D. (1954). *J. biol. Chem.* **211**, 237–240.
Cereijo-Santaló, R. (1968). *Can. J. Biochem.* **46**, 55–61.
Chappell, J. and Crofts, A. (1965). *Biochem J.* **95**, 393–402.

Cheung, H. C. and Cooke, R. (1971). *Biopolymers* **10**, 523–529.
Costa, M. G. P., Peres, G. and De Meis, L. (1972). *Ann. Acad. Brasil. Ciênc.* **44**, 577–579.
Dawson, A. G. and Whittam, R. (1970). *Biochim. biophys. Acta.* **203**, 590–592.
De Meis, L. (1969). *J. biol. Chem.* **244**, 3733–3738.
De Meis, L. and Hasselbach, W. (1971). *J. biol. Chem.* **246**, 4759–4764.
Dewar, A. J. and Reading, H. W. (1971). *Psychol. Med.* **1**, 254–259.
Diamond, J. M. and Wright, E. M. (1969). *A. Rev. Physiol.* **31**, 581–646.
Dunham, E. T. and Glynn, I. M. (1961). *J. Physiol.* **156**, 274–281.
Eisenman, G. (1961). *In* "Symposium on Membrane Transport and Metabolism." (A. Kleinzeller and A. Kotyk, eds.) pp. 163–179. Academic Press, New York.
Eisenman, G. (1962). *Biophys. J.* **2**, 259–323.
Eisenman, G., Sandblom, J. P., and Walker, J. L. (1967). *Science* **155**, 965–966.
Evans, H. J. and Sorger, G. J. (1966). *A. Rev. plant Physiol.* **17**, 47–61.
Forte, J. G., Forte, G. M. and Saltman, P. (1967). *J. cell. Physiol.* **69**, 293–304.
Fratantoni, J. C. and Askari, A. (1965). *Biochim. biophys. Acta* **99**, 259–269.
Friede, R. L. (1964). *J. Cell Biol.* **20**, 5–15.
Gear, A. L. and Lehninger, A. L. (1968). *J. biol. Chem.* **243**, 3953–3962.
Glynn, I. M. (1962). *J. Physiol.* **160**, 18P–19P.
Graven, S. N., Lardy, H. A., Johnson, D. and Rutter, A. (1966). *Biochem.* **5**, 1729–1734.
Gutman, Y., Hochman, S. and Strachman, D. (1973a). *Int. J. Biochem.* **4**, 315–318.
Gutman, Y., Hochman, S. and Wald, H. (1973b). *Biochim. biophys. Acta*, **298**, 284–290.
Hertz, L. and Schou, M. (1962). *Biochem. J.* **85**, 93–104.
Ho, A. K. S., Gershon, S. and Pinckney, L. (1970). *Archs int. Pharmacodyn. Ther.* **186**, 54–65.
Igarashi, K., Yoh, M. and Takeda, Y. (1971). *Biochim. biophys. Acta* **238**, 314–323.
Inoue, A. and Iwata, R. (1971). *Biochim. biophys. Acta* **242**, 459–469.
Izatt, R. M., Rytting, J. H., Nelson, D. P., Haymore, B. L. and Christensen, J. J. (1969). *Science* **164**, 443–444.
Judah, J. D., Mclean, A. E., Ahmed, K. and Christie, G. S. (1965). *Biochim. biophys. Acta* **94**, 441–449.
Kachmar, J. F. and Boyer, P. D. (1953). *J. biol. Chem.* **200**, 669–682.
Kaji, A. and Kaji, H. (1964). *Biochim. biophys. Acta* **87**, 519–522.
Katz, A. M. (1968). *Biochim. biophys. Acta* **162**, 79–85.
Kelemen, G. Sz., and Mühlrad, A. (1969). *Acta biochim. biophys. Acad. Sci. Hung.* **4**, 349–356.
Kielley, W. W., Kalckar, H. M. and Bradley, L. B. (1956). *J. biol. Chem.* **218**, 653–659.
Kiseleva, I. P. (1972). *Vopr. med. Zhym.* **18**, 449–506.
Krall, A. R. (1967). *Life Sci.* **6**, 1339–1344.
Kurtz, J. and Harrington, W. F. (1966). *J. molec. Biol.* **17**, 440–455.
Kuznetsov, I. A., Kustova, L. V., Gorshkov, V. I. and Panchenkov, G. M. (1963). Vestnik Mosk. Gos. Univ. No. 2, 10. (Quoted by Kuznetsov *et al.*, 1967).
Kuznetsov, I. A., Mezentsev, A. N., Moshkovskii, Yu Sh. and Lukanin, A. S. (1967). *Biophysics* **12**, 425–430.
Lehninger, S. L. and Neubert, D. (1961). *Proc. natn. Acad. Sci. U.S.A.* **47**, 1929–1931.
Levine, H., Trindle, M. R. and Moldave, K. (1966). *Nature* **211**, 1302–1303.
Ling, G. (1967). *Science* **155**, 301–302.

Lowenstein, J. M. (1960). *Biochem. J.* **75**, 269–274.

Meisner, H. (1971). *Biochem.* **10**, 3485–3491.

Melchior, J. B. (1965). *Biochem.* **4**, 1518–1522.

Mitchell, P. (1966). *Biol. Rev.* **41**, 445–460.

Moore, C. and Pressman, C. (1964). *Biochem. biophys. Res. Commun.* **15**, 562–567.

Neubert, D. and Lenninger, A. L. (1962). *J. biol. Chem.* **237**, 952–958.

Neurath, A. R., Stasny, J. T. and Rubin, B. A. (1970). *J. Virol.* **5**, 173–178.

Perkinson, E., Ruckart, R. and Da Vanzo, J. P. (1969). *Proc. Soc. exp. Biol. Med.* **131**, 685–689.

Perry, R. P. and Kelley, D. E. (1968). *J. molec. Biol.* **35**, 37–59.

Post, R. L., Merrit, C. R., Kinsolving, C. R. and Albright, C. D. (1960). *J. Biol. Chem.* **235**, 1796–1803.

Rasmussen, H., Fischer, J. and Arnaud, C. (1964). *Proc. natn. Acad. Sci. U.S.A.* **52**, 1198–1201.

Robinson, D. R. and Jencks, W. P. (1965). *J. Amer. chem. Soc.* **87**, 2470–2479.

Ross, P. D. and Scruggs, R. L. (1964a). *Biopolymers* **2**, 79–89.

Ross, P. D. and Scruggs, R. L. (1964b). *Biopolymers* **2**, 231–236.

Rupprecht, A. and Forslind, B. (1970). *Biochim. biophys. Acta* **204**, 304–316.

Sanui, H. and pace, N. (1959). *J. gen. Physiol.* **43**, 1325–1331.

Seidel, J. C. (1969). *J. biol. Chem.* **244**, 1142–1148.

Setlow, B. and Lowenstein, J. M. (1968). *J. biol. chem.* **243**, 6216–6221.

Shapiro, J. T., Stannard, B. S. and Felsenfeld, G. (1969). *Biochem.* **8**, 3233–3241.

Sierra, G. and Gibbons, N. E. (1963). *Can. J. Microbiol* **9**, 491–497.

Simic, S. and Gulidova, G. P. (1970). Paper presented at CINP Congress, Prague.

Sorger, G. J. and Evans, H. J. (1966). *Biochim. biophys. Acta* **118**, 1–8.

Suelter, C. H. (1970). *Science* **168**, 789–795.

Suzuka, I. and Kaji, A. (1968). *J. biol. Chem.* **243**, 3136–3141.

Tapley, D. F. and Cooper, C. (1956). *J. biol. chem.* **242**, 341–348.

Tonomura, Y., Sekiya, K. and Imamura, K. (1962). *J. biol. Chem.* **237**, 3110–3115.

Turkington, R. W. (1968). *Experientia* **24**, 226–228.

Vacquier, V. D. (1971). *Devel. Biol.* **26**, 11–16.

Villalonga, F., Fernandez, M., Rotunno, C. and Cereijido, M. (1969). *Biochim. biophys. Acta* **183**, 98–109.

Volm, M., Schwartz, V. and Wayss, K. (1970). *Naturwiss.* **57**, 250.

Von Hippel, P. H. and Wong, K. Y. (1964). *Science* **145**, 577–583.

Warren, J. C., Stowring, L. and Morales, M. F. (1966). *J. biol. Chem.* **241**, 309–316.

Whittam, R. (1962a). *Biochem. J.* **84**, 110–120.

Whittam, R. (1962b). *Nature* **196**, 134–136.

Whittam, R. and Ager, M. E. (1964). *Biochem. J.* **93**, 337–348.

Whittam, R. and Wheeler, K. P. (1970). *A. Rev. Physiol.* **32**, 21–60.

Wildes, R. A., Evans, H. J. and Becker, R. R. (1971). *Biochim. biophys. Acta* **229**, 850–854.

Willis, J. S. and Fang, L. S. T. (1970). *Biochim. biophys. Acta* **219**, 486–489.

Wilson, R. H. Evans, H. J. and Becker, P. R. (1967). *J. biol. Chem.* **242**, 3825–3832.

INDEX

Motor functions—*continued*
  swimming to exhaustion, 343
  unsteadiness, 213, 342
  visual-motor performance, 334, 342, 346
  weakness, 342
Muscle, lithium in, 274
Mydriasis, 417
Myxoedema; see Thyroid

Organo-lithium compounds, 353
Orotic acid, 543
Osteoporosis, 371
Ouabain, 276, 435, 468, 487, 505, 544, 545
Overdose, 204
Ovulation, 248
2-Oxoglutarate, 499, 500, 501, 502, 504, 505

N

Negativism, 107
Neural tube, 242
Neurosecretion, 465
Neurotic states, 88
Neurotransmitters; see Transmitter substances
Non-episodic disorders, 93
Non-manic-depressive disorders, 85, 110, 146, 150
Noradrenaline, 327, 391, 411, 414, 415, 416, 417, 422, 430, 431, 438, 485, 486, 488, 489, 492, 494, 512
  brain concentrations, 416, 418
  retention, 420
  storage, 416
  synaptosome concentration, 416
  synthesis, 418
  turnover, 420
  uptake, 416, 420
Norepinephrine; see Noradrenaline
Normetanephrine, 415, 416, 420
Normalizing effect, 102
Normothymotic, 82
Nortriptyline, 47, 254, 255
Nucleic acid, 541

O

Observer bias, 72
Oedema; see Renal system
Obsessive-compulsive neurosis, 110
Old age disorders, 150
One-trial passive avoidance, 322
Organic acids, excretion, 499–506
  tissue levels, 502–504

P

Patient management, 143–163, 166
  anaesthetics, danger of, 149, 150, 161
  communicating with patient, 153
  dietary advice, 149, 150, 157, 162
  duration of treatment, 59, 79
  family support, 156, 158, 162
  fluid intake, 149, 162
  interviews, 147, 156, 158
  motivation, 154
  physical examination, 147
  pregnancy, q. v.
  preparations, choice of, q.v.
  rejection of treatment, q.v.
  salt tablets, 163
  surgical operations, 161
  urination frequency, 157
  weight gain, explanation of, 157
Palate, 248
Panic, 81
Paranoid traits, 81
Pargyline, 438
Parkinsonism, 94
Perchlorate test; see Thyroid
Periodic catatonia, 88, 89, 92
Periodicity, 348
Perphenazine, 111
Personality,
  abnormal, 88
  aggressive, 110
  deviations, 81
  sociopathic, 87
pH, intracellular, 500
Pheniprazine, 418
Phenylquinone, 341
Phobic reactions, 110
Phosphoenolpyruvate, 382, 538

T